THE ROYAL COLLEGE OF SURGEONS OF ENGLAND

Atlas of SURGICAL PATHOLOGY

Edited by

JOHN L. TURK

M.D., D.Sc., F.R.C.S., F.R.C.P., F.R.C.Path.,
Sir William Collins Professor of Pathology,
Royal College of Surgeons, London

CHRISTOPHER D. M. FLETCHER

M.B., B.S., M.R.C.Path.,
Senior Lecturer (Honorary Consultant),
and Director of Soft Tissue Tumour Unit,
Department of Histopathology
St Thomas's Hospital (U.M.D.S.), London

Gower Medical Publishing · London · New York

Distributed in USA and Canada by:
J B Lippincott Company
East Washington Square
Philadelphia, PA 19105
USA

Distributed in UK and Continental Europe by:
Gower Medical Publishing
Middlesex House
34–42 Cleveland Street
London W1P 5FB
UK

Distributed in Australia and New Zealand by:
Harper and Row (Australia) Pty Ltd
PO Box 226
Artarmon
NSW 2064
AUSTRALIA

Distributed in South East Asia, Hong Kong, India and Pakistan by:
Harper and Row (Asia) Pty Ltd
37 Jalan Pemimpin 02–01
Singapore 2057

Distributed in Japan by:
Nankodo Company Ltd
42–6 Hongo 3–chome
Bunkyo-Ku
Tokyo 113
JAPAN

Project editor: Lucy Hamilton
Design and page layout: Image
Index: Susan Ramsey
Publisher: Fiona Foley
Production: Susan Bishop

Library of Congress Cataloging-in-Publication Data
Royal College of Surgeons atlas of surgical pathology/edited by John L. Turk and Christopher D.M. Fletcher.
Includes index.
1. Pathology, Surgical – Atlases. I. Turk, J.L. II. Fletcher, Christopher D.M. III. Royal College of Surgeons of England. IV. Title: Atlas of surgical pathology.
(DNLM: 1. Pathology, Surgical – atlases. WO 517 T888)
RD57.R75 1991
617'.07'0222–dc20

British Library Cataloguing-in-Publication Data
Atlas of surgical pathology.
I. Fletcher, C.D.M. II. Turk, J.L.
617.0022

ISBN 0-397-44843-0

Typesetting by Image Communications
Text set in Bembo
Originated in Singapore by Chroma Graphics
Produced by Imago. Printed in Singapore 1991

CONTENTS

CONTRIBUTORS

Osteoarticular System — **Peter G. Bullough** M.B., Ch.B., Chief of Orthopaedic Pathology, The Hospital for Special Surgery, Professor of Pathology, Cornell University Medical College, New York

Nervous System — The late **William Blackwood** F.R.C.S.Ed., F.R.C.P.Ed., F.R.C.Path., formerly Emeritus Professor of Neuropathology, University of London, Institute of Neurology, London

Alimentary System — **Basil C. Morson** C.B.E., V.R.D., M.A., D.M.Oxf., F.R.C.P., F.R.C.S., F.R.C.Path., Consulting Pathologist, St. Mark's Hospital and Consultant Pathologist, The London Clinic, London

Ashley B. Price M.A., F.R.C.Path., Consultant Histopathologist, Northwick Park Hospital and Clinical Research Centre, Harrow

Peter J. Scheuer M.D.D.Sc.(Med.), F.R.C.Path., Professor of Histopathology, University of London, Honorary Consultant Histologist, Royal Free Hospital, London

Respiratory System — **Herbert Spencer** M.D., Ph.D., F.R.C.S., F.R.C.P., F.R.C.Path., Emeritus Professor of Morbid Anatomy, University of London, formerly Professor of Morbid Anatomy, St. Thomas's Hospital Medical School, London

Cardiovascular System — **Robert F.H. Anderson** M.D., F.R.C.Path., Joseph Levy Professor of Paediatric Cardiac Morphology, Cardiothoracic Institute of London, Honorary Consultant, Brompton Hospital, London

Urinary System — **Richard C.B. Pugh** M.D., F.R.C.S., F.R.C.Path., Consulting Pathologist, St. Peter's Hospital and The Institute of Urology, London

Reproductive System — **Harold Fox** M.D., F.R.C.Path., F.R.C.O.G., Professor of Reproductive Pathology, University of Manchester, Honorary Consultant Histopathologist, St. Mary's Hospital, Manchester

Richard C.B. Pugh M.D., F.R.C.S., F.R.C.Path., Consulting Pathologist, St. Peter's Hospital and The Institute of Urology, London

Phillip H. McKee F.R.C.Path., Senior Lecturer and Honorary Consultant in Histopathology, St. Thomas's Hospital Medical School, London

Endocrine System — **Sheldon C. Sommers** M.D., Scientific Director, Council for Tobacco Research, Consultant Pathologist, Lenox Hill Hospital, New York

Haemopoietic and Lymphoreticular Systems — **John E. Pettit** M.D. Otago, F.R.C.P.A., F.R.C.Path., Associate Professor of Haematology, University of Otago, Dunedin, New Zealand

Skin — **Phillip H. McKee** F.R.C.Path., Senior Lecturer and Honorary Consultant in Histopathology, St. Thomas's Hospital Medical School, London

Soft Tissues — **Phillip H. McKee** F.R.C.Path., Senior Lecturer and Honorary Consultant in Histopathology, St. Thomas's Medical School, London

FOREWORD

The Wellcome Museum of Pathology at the Royal College of Surgeons was founded in 1951 under a grant from the Wellcome Trust to set up Museums of Pathology and Anatomy to be separate from the Hunterian Museum which had been partially demolished by an incendiary bomb in 1941. It became operational as a teaching unit in 1954 and was officially opened by Sir Henry Dale in 1955.

The museum thus took over the role of the pathological collection of the Hunterian Museum based on John Hunter's original collection which had been purchased by Parliament in 1799 and entrusted to the care of the Company of Surgeons, later the Royal College of Surgeons of England. The number of pathological specimens in the original catalogue prepared by the first Conservator, John Hunter's assistant and amanuensis, William Clift, was 1,709. Between 1830 and 1846, 600 specimens had been added by donation and 1,208 had been purchased from the private museums of Sir Astley Cooper, Liston and other surgeons. The second catalogue was prepared by Edward Stanley and Sir James Paget separate from the catalogue of the physiological collection in 1846. The third catalogue was prepared between 1878 and 1882 again by Sir James Paget with the help of Dr. J.F. Goodhart and Mr. A.H.G. Doran. Paget, who had been President of the College in 1876, did the greater part of the work undertaking all the arrangement of headings, references, cross references and indices. The three would meet on Saturday afternoons and go over all the new specimens together. This was a considerable effort, as the pathological section had by now increased by a further 1,750 specimens. This catalogue was published in 1882 and there was a subsequent edition in 1909 prepared under the supervision of the then Pathological Curator, S.G. Shattock. When the museums of the College were destroyed in May 1941, there were approximately 15,000 pathological specimens of which only 3,000 survived. Half of these were Hunter's original specimens which had been stored underground. The rest, approximately 1,500, were re-assembled and formed the basis of the new Wellcome Museum of Pathology under the Conservatorship of Professor Geoffrey Hadfield with Dr. L.W. Proger as Pathology Curator. As well as starting the Wellcome Museum of Pathology, Dr. Proger re-arranged Hunter's pathological collection and wrote a new catalogue of Hunterian pathology specimens which was published in 1966.

At the present time, the Wellcome Museum of Pathology contains 2,169 specimens, representative of all the important branches of surgical pathology. Most of the pre-war specimens have been replaced. The only ones which remain are illustrative of conditions common in the pre-antibiotic era that are hardly seen now. The present breakdown of specimens is as follows:

444	Bones, Joints, Muscles
144	Nervous system and Special Sense Organs
425	Alimentary system
144	Respiratory system
186	Circulatory system
151	Urinary system
47	Female Genital system
22	Pathology of Gestation
78	Endocrine system
83	Skin and Connective Tissue
60	Haemopoietic system
31	Breast
168	Teratology
121	Histological specimens

The museum covers 3,108 square feet and is divided into ten bays. Its main function is to display a broad spectrum representing all aspects of surgical pathology. It is well lit by a diffuse illuminated ceiling. The specimens are mounted in perspex boxes and the mounting fluids are regularly changed to give maximum visual effect. All the specimens are accompanied by a description and there is a unique collection of individual histological slides. The museum is used at the present time by postgraduate students from all over the world, preparing for the final F.R.C.S., and College examinations are also held in the musum.

It is hoped that the availability of this atlas will open up the museum to much wider use by teachers of pathology and students from Universities and Colleges all over the world. In this way some of the traditions started by John Hunter and continued by his successors over two centuries can be carried to a worldwide forum. Moreover, this atlas might also be considered a modern descendant of Sir James Paget's catalogues, making the contents of the museum available to every classroom of surgery and pathology.

I should like to acknowledge the work of successive Curators of the museum, particularly Dr. L.W. Proger and Dr. M.S. Israel for preparing the working catalogue of the museum. The atlas is dedicated to the many surgeons and pathologists who have contributed new material to the museum. Finally, particular credit must go to Mr. L.F. Young who has skilfully prepared and mounted the specimens for a quarter of a century.

John L. Turk
Conservator

PREFACE

While a museum of pathological specimens of the size and extent of the Royal College of Surgeons is of immense historical value, its principal *raison d'être* is to provide teaching material at both the undergraduate and postgraduate level.

This atlas has been prepared as an aid to learning. It has been produced principally for the use of surgeons in training, particularly with the final Fellowship examination in mind. It should, additionally, be of value to pathologists, largely perhaps from the pictorial rather than textual point of view. It is also hoped that this atlas will be used by hospitals or medical schools who are unable to maintain their own collection of specimens – in other words to act as a 'portable' museum.

In terms of the material included, there is an undoubted bias towards surgical conditions. This is inevitable since the majority of specimens have been donated by surgeons rather than by pathologists; as such very many of the tissues have been obtained at operation and, less frequently, in the post-mortem room. However, despite the preponderance of 'surgical' specimens, the principal medical conditions are also covered in each volume. Some diseases are, by necessity, omitted since no single museum could ever be comprehensive; yet, on the few occasions where examples of important disease processes have been unavailable in the College collection, individual pathologists and other museums, have very generously filled the gaps and are gratefully acknowledged in the text. Conversely, where the museum has had a surfeit of material which would have added nothing here by repetition (there are 15 examples of Meckel's diverticulum and 9 of renal adenocarcinoma), we have had the unhappy task of rejecting the poorer examples for which we hope the contributors will forgive us.

Much of the teratological material, along with unique examples of bizarre congenital malformations, has been purposely omitted. The atlas is already quite extensive and it was felt that, other than in the case of clearly defined syndromes or disease entities, isolated cases showing idiopathic and inexplicable developmental abnormalities were of limited teaching value, particularly to the surgeon.

Undoubtedly it can be argued that formalin-fixed material in pots is inferior, from the aesthetic point of view, to fresh tissue. In compiling a collection of this size this is, again, inevitable: it would take a large number of individuals a very, very long time to obtain good, photogenic examples of all the conditions included in this atlas. Such material is usually compiled for a single volume atlas referring to only one of the anatomical systems.

Each of the legends has been substantially rewritten from the museum catalogue and, in isolated cases, the diagnosis has been amended in line with accepted current terminology: this has been aided by reference to original histological material which the museum retains in many cases.

The legends are divided into three sections, comprising a brief clinical history where available, a description of the salient macroscopical features and, finally, a concise and hopefully up-to-date resumé of the important clinicopathological information regarding the condition shown. This latter is, by virtue of available space, brief, being largely intended for the benefit of surgeons, and does not include any histological detail unless absolutely necessary.

Christopher D.M. Fletcher
St. Thomas's Hospital U.M.D.S.

1. CARDIOVASCULAR SYSTEM

HEART

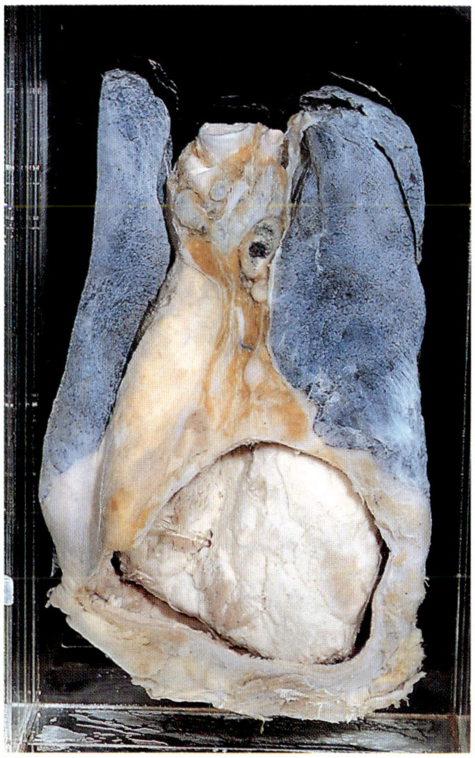

1.1 Atrial Septal Defect

This is a post-mortem specimen from a 55-year-old man with Down's syndrome who died of bronchopneumonia. He had been in congestive cardiac failure for some time prior to death.

The heart has been opened from behind to show dilatation of the right atrium (right) with a large defect in the fossa ovalis due to deficiency of its flap valve (septum primum). Note the marked right ventricular hypertrophy (bottom right), normally 3-5mm in thickness. There is also dilatation of the pulmonary trunk (top left).

Atrial septal defects are not uncommon and, if small, may remain entirely asymptomatic. When undetected in childhood, the majority of cases present in middle age with atrial fibrillation and progressive congestive cardiac failure due to the left-to-right shunt. The defects are conventionally divided into four major anatomical groups: defects within the fossa ovalis or so-called secundum defects (which account for 90 per cent); so-called primum defects, which are really atrioventricular septal defects (5 per cent); sinus venosus defects (5 per cent), and a very rare group that occurs at the site of the orifice of the coronary sinus. In the first group, failure of the septum primum to develop leaves a persistent ostium secundum or deficiency in the flap over the fossa ovalis. The so-called 'ostium primum' defect occurs when the bridging leaflets in an atrioventricular septal defect are fused to the crest of the ventricular septum, confining the shunt to atrial level. Because of the abnormal form of the atrioventricular junction and valve, there is usually a coexistent valvar abnormality ('cleft' mitral valve). In sinus venosus defects, in which either the caval or pulmonary veins are connected to both right and left atrial chambers, the interatrial communication is outside the confines of the true atrial septum. This is also the case with the coronary sinus defect, which exists because the sinus itself is 'unroofed' in its passage along the left atrioventricular junction.

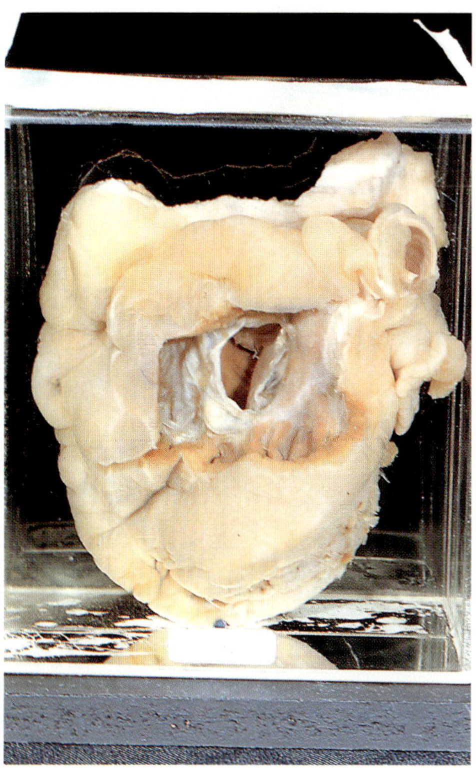

1.2 Ebstein's Anomaly

This is a post-mortem specimen from a 51-year-old man who died following a severe attack of anginal-type pain. In the past he had been discharged from the army on account of an uncertain cardiac abnormality and 5 months previously he had suffered a right-sided intracerebral haemorrhage.

The heart is hypertrophied and dilated, weighing 560g at autopsy. It has been opened through the right ventricle to view the tricuspid valve from below. The antero-superior leaflet of the tricuspid valve (left) is extremely large and extends downwards into the right ventricle where it was attached near the apex. The mural (inferior) and septal leaflets are deficient and adherent to the ventricular wall. As a consequence, the inlet portion of the right ventricle is continuous with the right atrium and is separated from the apical trabecular and outlet components, which function as a small right ventricle. The remaining functional tricuspid orifice measures about 2.5cm in diameter and there is atrial dilatation. There was also a patent foramen ovale (not shown in this view).

Ebstein's anomaly is characterised by an abnormally orientated tricuspid valve in which the annular attachments of the septal and mural valve leaflets are located more towards the apex of the right ventricle than usual. As a result, at least half of the ventricle becomes functionally a part of the atrium with associated dilatation. There is usually a coexistent atrial septal defect of some kind. The clinical consequences depend upon the degree of downward displacement and functional obstruction that ensues, which is largely related to the precise form and distal attachments of the antero-superior leaflet. In the presence of a large atrial septal defect, patients with this anomaly usually present in childhood with cardiac failure and cyanosis, while those that are less severely affected may remain asymptomatic well into adult life.

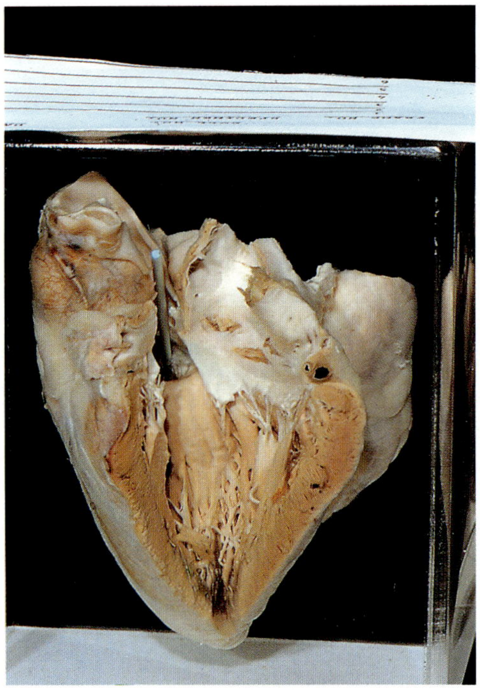

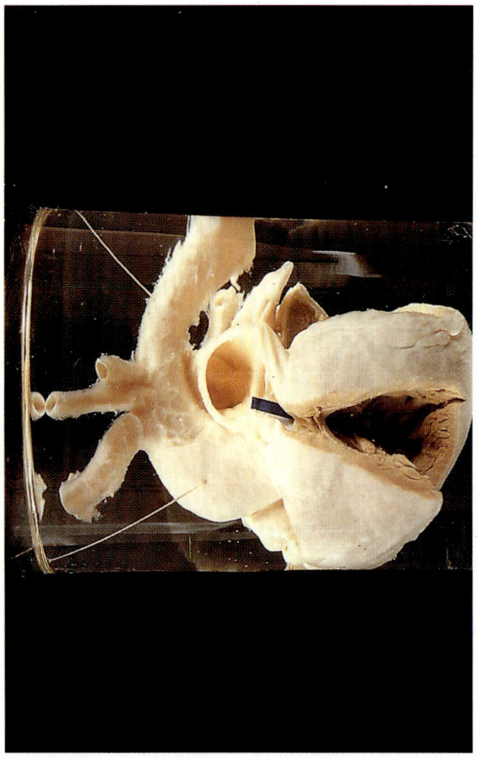

1.4 Pulmonary Atresia

No clinical details are available.

This infant's heart has been dissected to show persistence of the infundibular muscle between the pulmonary trunk (above) and the right ventricle (below). A blue rod marks the tiny ostium. The pulmonary valve leaflets are located above the obstruction and the pulmonary artery is dilated. Note also the marked right ventricular hypertrophy. Associated with this anomaly was a very large ventricular septal defect, not apparent in this view.

Congenital pulmonary atresia describes any malformation which renders the pulmonary circulation separate from the ventricles (i.e. allowing no blood flow from the heart to the lungs). The 3 commonest forms are an imperforate pulmonary valve, a persistent blind-ending myocardial infundibulum (as here) or absence of part or all of the pulmonary trunk. There may be an associated ventricular septal defect or, when the septum is intact, hypoplasia of the right ventricular cavity, produced by gross hypertrophy of the wall.

1.3 Ventricular Septal Defect

This is a post-mortem specimen from a 20-year-old man who suffered from the congenital rubella syndrome. He was mentally subnormal and was known to have a ventricular septal defect. While out for a walk, he collapsed and died suddenly; at autopsy there was also a patent ductus arteriosus.

The left side of the heart has been opened to show a large perimembranous ventricular septal defect, marked by a blue probe, just beneath the cusps of the aortic valve. The left circumflex coronary artery, seen in cross-section (upper right) is completely occluded by thrombus; this was probably the immediate cause of death. Note also the left ventricular hypertrophy.

Ventricular septal defects are more common than those in the atrium and their consequences are dependent upon their size and position. Small defects may remain asymptomatic (Maladie de Roger) and may only be detectable by the presence of a pansystolic murmur, while up to 50 per cent of lesions may close spontaneously or diminish in size. Large shunts typically present in infancy with heart failure or increased pulmonary vascular resistance, which may lead to reversal of the shunt (Eisenmenger's syndrome). Most often the defect occurs around the membranous part of the septum, just below the aortic valve, and results from deficient formation of the muscular components of the septum (perimembranous defect). Less frequently, the lesion is in the true muscular septum and, at this site, may be multiple. A third type of defect results from absence of the outlet component of the septum (doubly committed subarterial or 'supracristal' defect). It should not be forgotten that ventricular septal defects are occasionally acquired, following myocardial rupture due to infarction.

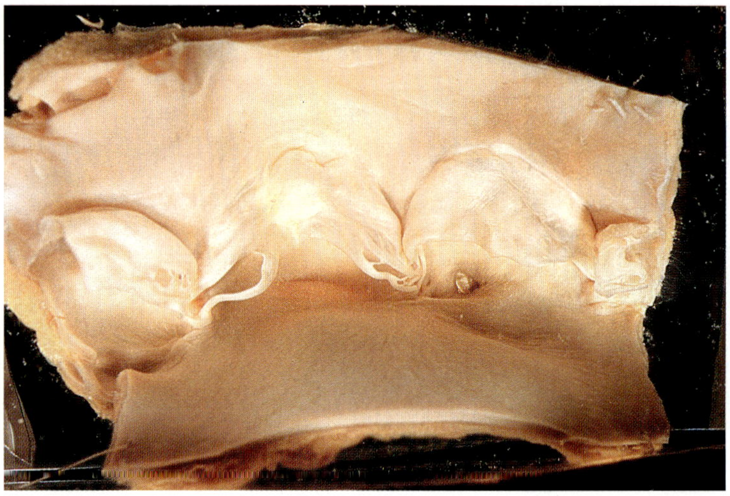

1.5 Aortic Valve: Fenestration of the Leaflets

This was an incidental finding at post-mortem in a soldier who died of gas poisoning during the First World War.

This aortic valve, seen in a close-up view, shows several small gaps beneath the surface of two of the cusps.

Fenestration of arterial valve leaflets is a very common finding at post-mortem and is probably of no functional significance. Whether it represents a congenital anomaly or an acquired lesion is uncertain but the incidence is higher in patients with hypertension or a dilated valve orifice.

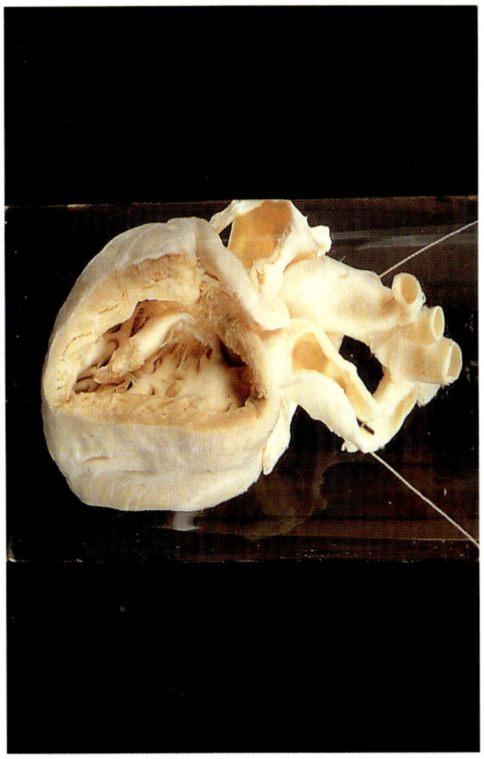

1.6 Patent Ductus Arteriosus

This is a post-mortem specimen from a 7-month-old girl who had been noted to have a loud systolic murmur from birth but had not developed cyanosis or clubbing.

The heart has been dissected to show a large, widely patent ductus arteriosus (top right) which joins the pulmonary trunk to the aortic arch. The right ventricle is hypertrophied and the foramen ovale was patent (not seen in this view).

Persistent patency of the ductus arteriosis for more than a short time after birth (other than in premature infants) may represent either a primary congenital anomaly of the ductal wall or may be secondary to intra-uterine rubella infection. The majority of such cases are amenable to prompt surgical correction or pharmacological manipulation with prostaglandin inhibitors. Complications in untreated cases (now almost unknown) included left ventricular failure (due to constant volume overload as blood in the aorta is returned to the pulmonary circulation) and infective endocarditis.

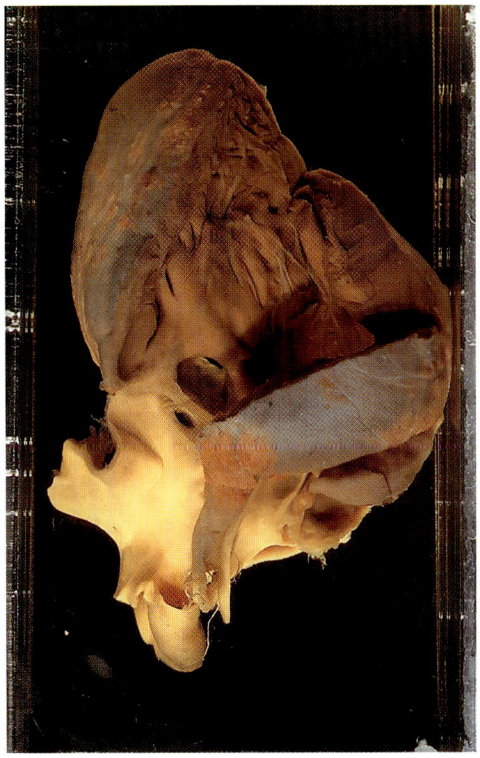

1.7 Complete Transposition

This is a post-mortem specimen from a 4½-year-old boy, who had been noticed to be cyanosed from birth. He was found to have a loud pansystolic murmur and the pulmonary arteries were unusually prominent on a chest X-ray. He remained chronically unfit and failed to thrive, dying eventually with a right temporal lobe abscess which complicated an attack of otitis media.

The right ventricle has been opened to show that the aorta (top right) arises from it and slightly overrides the interventricular septum. A large ventricular septal defect is visible posteriorly. The pulmonary trunk arose posteriorly from the left ventricle (discordant ventriculo-atrial connection). The foramen ovale was also patent (not apparent in this view).

Complete transposition is a relatively common congenital malformation which is characterised by concordant atrioventricular but discordant ventriculo-arterial connections. The clinical consequences depend entirely on the presence of other anomalies since, without either a ventricular or atrial septal defect or patency of the ductus arteriosus, complete transposition is incompatible with life. Nowadays most cases are amenable to surgical intervention. (Courtesy of the Gordon Museum, Guy's Hospital Medical School)

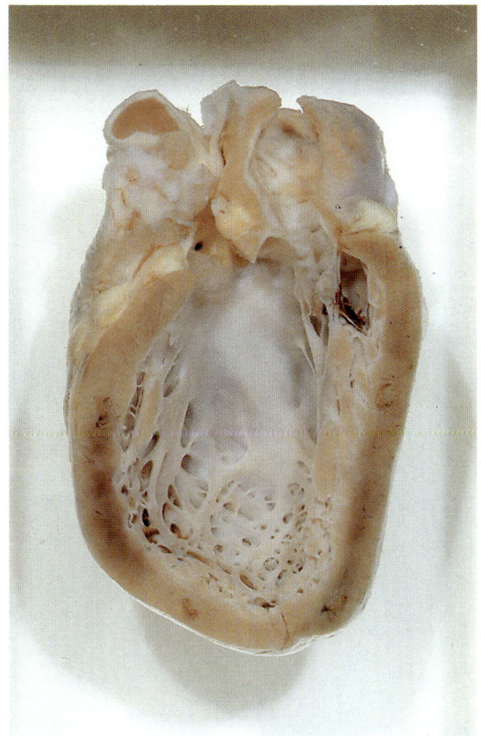

1.8 Primary Endocardial Fibro-elastosis

This is a post-mortem specimen from an infant who died in cardiac failure.

The left side of this infant's heart has been opened to show dilatation and hypertrophy of the left ventricle, associated with a thickened, pale, opaque endocardium. This distinctive endocardial appearance has been likened to porcelain.

Endocardial fibro-elastosis is a rare congenital abnormality characterised by the development of a thick layer of collagen and elastin on the surface of the myocardium. Usually it is a secondary event, as seen in the hypoplastic left heart syndrome. When it is a primary phenomenon, the left ventricle is predominantly affected and the consequent decrease in compliance leads to ventricular dilatation and mitral incompetence. There may be other associated congenital heart defects. This condition should not be confused with endomyocardial fibrosis, a cardiomyopathy seen most often in Africans (see Figure and Legend 1.48).

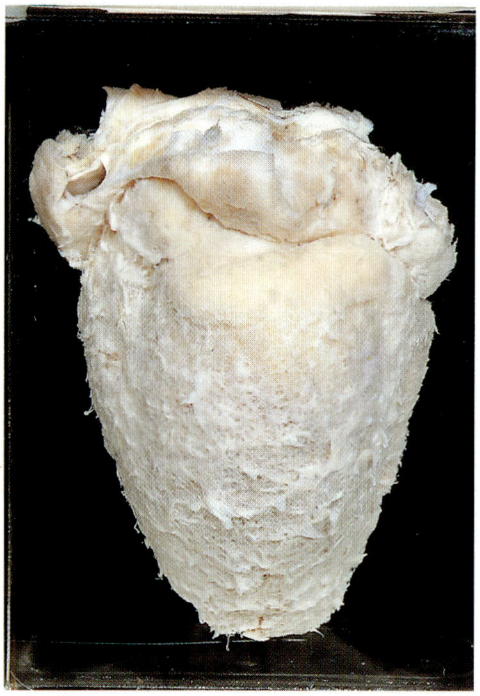

1.9 Fibrinous Pericarditis

This is a post-mortem specimen from a 17-year-old boy with Down's syndrome who presented with a one month history of vomiting and diarrhoea. On admission there was marked oedema and ascites with evidence of pericarditis. He was found to have acute glomerulonephritis (which was confirmed at autopsy) and he died one month later.

The parietal pericardium has been dissected off to show that the visceral pericardium is covered by a pale, shaggy fibrinous exudate, an appearance known as 'bread and butter' pericarditis.

Acute pericarditis may occur as a primary disease, usually due to viral infection (e.g. Coxsackie B), but is most often a secondary phenomenon related to a preceding adjacent or systemic pathological process. Common local causes include pulmonary or pleural infection (e.g. bacterial pneumonia or tuberculosis), metastatic tumour, and acute myocardial infarction. Less frequently, relapsing pericarditis may complicate myocardial infarction several weeks after the acute event (Dressler's syndrome) and this is thought to be an autoimmune process due to the formation of antibodies to damaged cardiac muscle proteins. Other systemic causes include uraemia (due to acute or chronic renal failure, the probable cause in this case), rheumatic fever, systemic lupus erythematosus, and polyserositis.

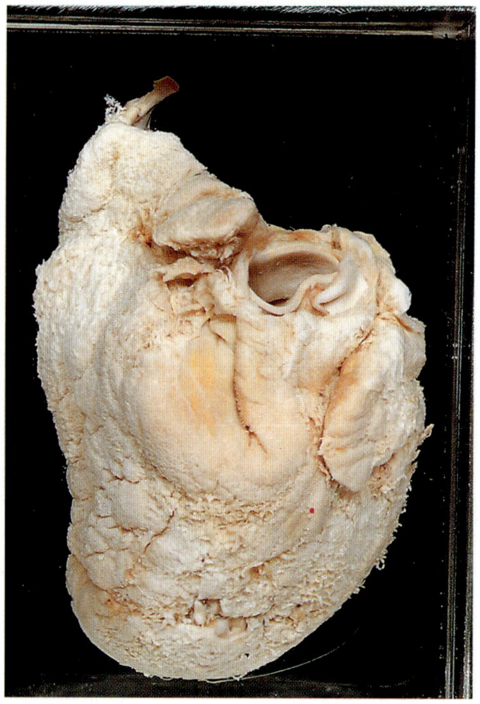

1.10 Fibrinopurulent Pericarditis

This is a post-mortem specimen from a 50-year-old woman who had been unwell for one week, but with no specific symptoms. She seemed to be recovering but was found dead on the bedroom floor. At autopsy there was a large right-sided pleural empyema and a pericarditis.

The visceral pericardium is covered in a florid, shaggy exudate which has a yellowish appearance.

This is another example of classical 'bread and butter' fibrinous pericarditis; however in this case there is a purulent component. The culinary term is derived from the fact that this appearance resembles that of a buttered sandwich, in which one of the slices of bread has been abruptly removed from the other.

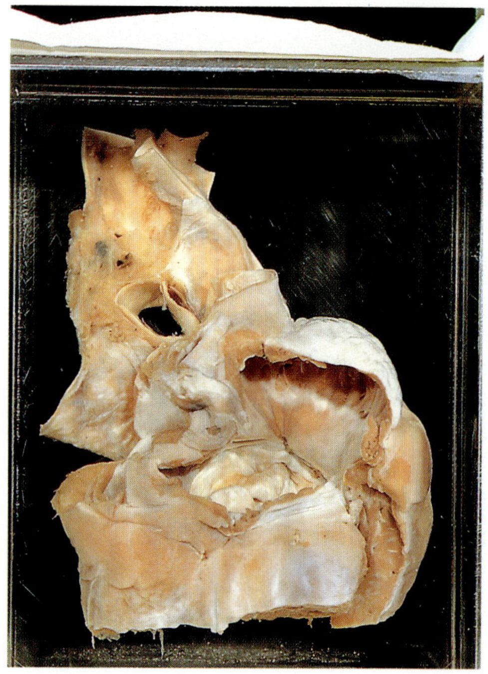

1.11 Tuberculous Pericarditis

No clinical details are available.

The heart with part of the lungs and mediastinum are shown, all of which are mutually adherent to one another. The heart is dilated and the visceral pericardium is covered in pale, opaque caseous material. A number of enlarged caseous lymph nodes are visible in the mediastinum. At autopsy the lungs, when complete, showed the typical features of tuberculosis.

Tuberculous pericarditis is almost always associated with pulmonary infection and is said to result from the lymphatic spread of bacilli from mediastinal nodes. The consequent effusion is often blood-stained. There is often dense fibrosis and scarring of the pericardial layers in cases which eventually heal. The appearances may then closely resemble Pick's disease (idiopathic constrictive pericarditis). Another cause of granulomatous pericarditis, which may have a similar macroscopic appearance, is fungal infection (e.g. blastomycosis).

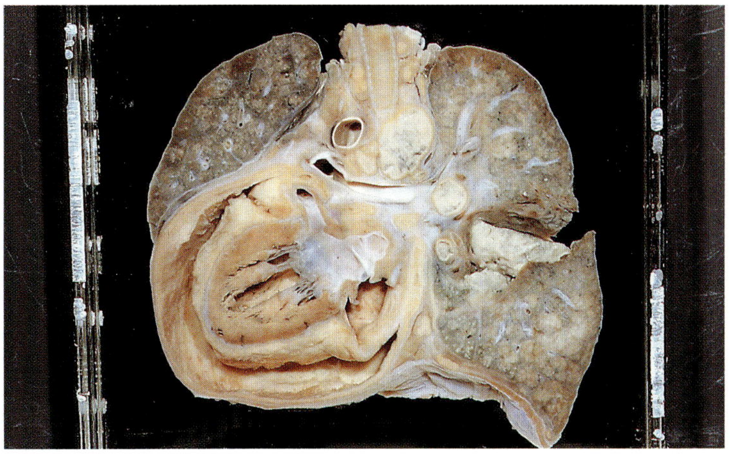

1.12 Tuberculous Pericarditis

This is a post-mortem specimen from a 3-year-old girl who had always been in poor health. Six months previously she had had measles followed by bronchopneumonia, since which time she had suffered from a persistent cough and dyspnoea. Later she developed cervical lymphadenopathy but the Mantoux text was repeatedly negative. She eventually presented with pericarditis and died.

A coronal section through the heart and lungs, viewed posteriorly, shows florid tuberculous bronchopneumonia. There are obvious enlarged, caseous lymph nodes in the mediastinum. The pericardium is grossly thickened and is covered in caseous material. Macroscopically-evident tubercles are present in the parietal pericardium (upper left).

This is another good example of tuberculous pericarditis.

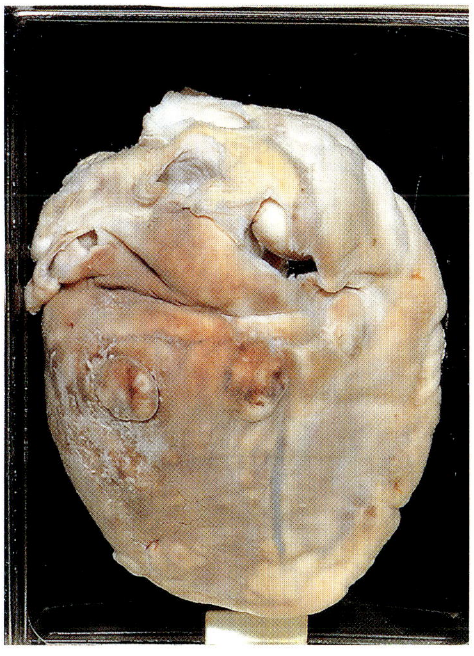

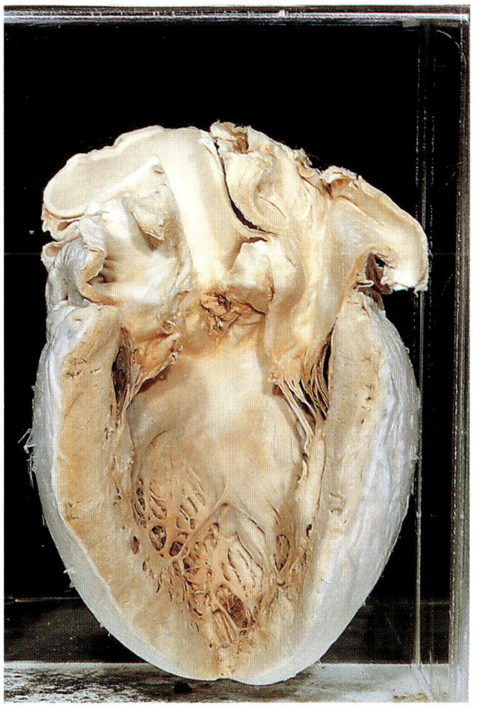

1.13 Pericarditis due to Metastases

This is a post-mortem specimen from a 59-year-old woman who presented with a mass in the region of the right shoulder. She rapidly developed enlarged lymph nodes in the neck and groin and, at autopsy, there was carcinomatosis with tumour masses in the cerebellum, adrenals, skeleton, heart and many lymph nodes. The primary site of the neoplasm remained undetermined.

Two flattened nodules of metastatic tumour, measuring approximately 2cm in diameter, are visible in the epicardium. There is a surrounding serosanguinous exudate.

Pericardial metastases are not uncommon in any case of disseminated malignant disease but are particularly seen in cases of carcinoma of the bronchus, breast or stomach. Occasionally direct local invasion of the pericardium by a primary tumour may occur, most often a bronchial or oesophageal carcinoma, a pleural mesothelioma or a thymoma.

1.14 Aortic Valve: Infective Endocarditis

This is a post-mortem specimen from a 39-year-old man who was severely mentally subnormal. He was admitted to hospital, following prolonged self-neglect, and was found to have pneumonia with septicaemia and gangrenous feet. He died 4 days later and autopsy revealed, in addition to the cardiac lesion, multiple systemic emboli with a cerebellar infarct.

The left side of the heart has been opened through the mitral valve to reveal marked ventricular hypertrophy and dilatation, associated with a stenotic aortic valve. The leaflets are thickened and contracted: one of the commissures (upper centre) is covered by friable, large, reddish vegetations with consequent partial destruction of the valve substance.

Infective endocarditis usually occurs on a previously abnormal valve (traditionally known as subacute endocarditis). This accounts for about 80 per cent of cases. The remaining 20 per cent affect a normal valve, in which circumstance the infection tends to be acute and fulminant. In cases with a pre-existent valvar abnormality, which is most often rheumatic or congenital in nature, local alterations in blood flow lead to turbulence and the formation of microthrombi. Organisms, particularly *Streptococcus viridans* and other Gram-positive cocci, may accumulate either at the site of low-pressure 'eddies' or colonise the microthrombi. The most frequent means by which these organisms enter the bloodstream are: minor dental procedures; catheterisation or instrumentation of the urinary tract; during childbirth, or in the course of a systemic infection. Any of these may give rise to an asymptomatic bacteraemia. Patients with normal valves tend to have some other predisposition, very often being intravenous drug abusers or immunocompromised individuals. More virulent organisms, particularly *Staphylococcus aureus*, are usually isolated in this group. The mitral valve is most often affected in either group, followed by the aortic valve (with or without coexistent mitral involvement). It should be remembered, however, that in drug addicts the right-sided heart valves are more likely to be infected. Other organisms, including viruses, fungi, mycobacteria, spirochaetes or *Rickettsiae*, may occasionally be responsible, particularly in immunocompromised individuals.

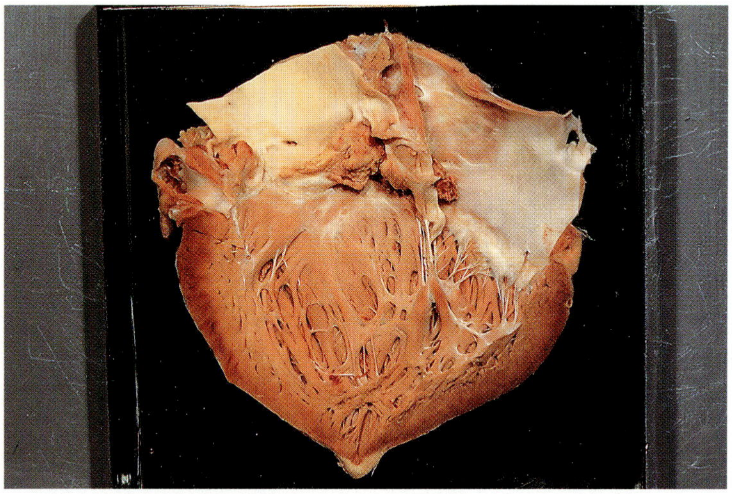

1.15 Aortic Valve: Infective Endocarditis

This is a post-mortem specimen from a 35-year-old man, who had felt generally unwell for a few weeks and who suddenly became seriously ill and died.

The left side of the heart has been opened through the mitral valve to show large, haemorrhagic vegetations attached to the congenitally bifoliate aortic valve. These have virtually destroyed the valve leaflet and the infective process has ulcerated through the ventricular wall into the left atrium just above the mitral valve (upper right).

Destruction or perforation of an affected valve leaflet and necrosis of the adjacent myocardium are well-recognised complications of infective endocarditis. Other complications include the development of cardiac failure (due to impaired valve function), systemic arterial embolisation by fragmented vegetations (as in the previous case), septic infarction or mycotic aneurysm formation at the site of embolisation, cutaneous petechial haemorrhages and glomerulonephritis due to immune complex deposition.

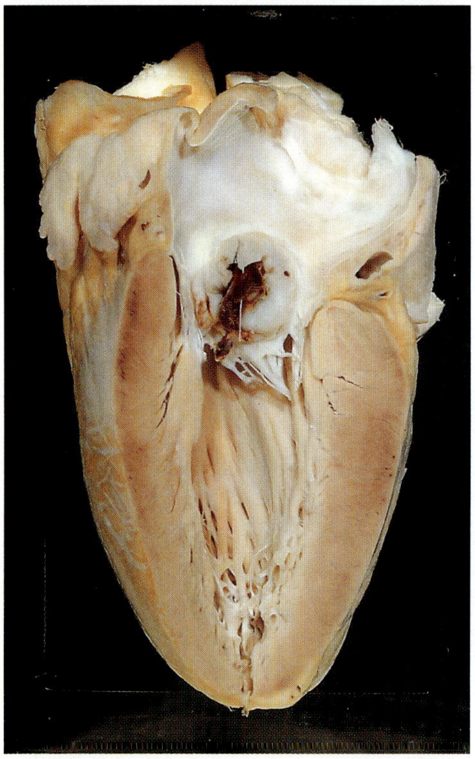

1.16 Mitral Valve: Infective Endocarditis

This is a post-mortem specimen from a 41-year-old man, with known long-standing mitral stenosis and aortic incompetence due to rheumatic heart disease, who developed severe left ventricular failure and died.

The heart has been dissected to show the left ventricle, atrium and mitral valve. There is marked left ventricular hypertrophy. Projecting from the atrial surface of the mural leaflet of the mitral valve is a massive thrombotic vegetation, which has ulcerated, and from which streptococci were cultured.

This case serves to demonstrate the severe valvar damage that infective endocarditis may induce.

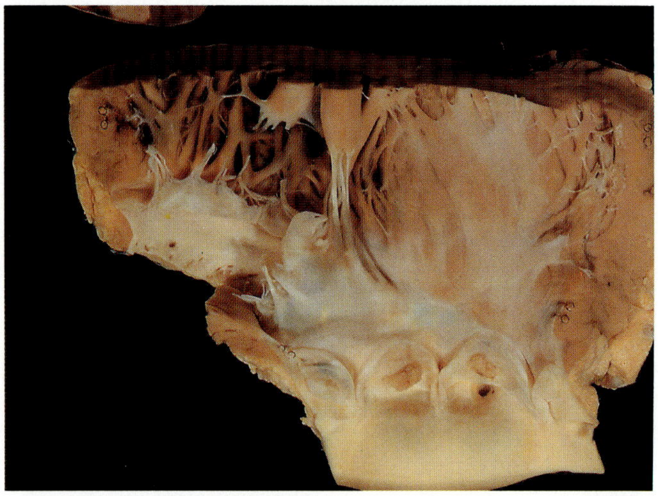

1.17 Aortic Valve: Non-Infective Thrombotic Endocarditis

This was an incidental finding at post-mortem in a 38-year-old woman who died of disseminated squamous carcinoma of unknown primary origin.

Attached to the leaflets of the aortic valve (above) are large, greyish vegetations. There is no evidence of any pre-existent rheumatic or congenital valvular disease.

Non-infective thrombotic endocarditis is an unusual, but not uncommon, condition which predominantly occurs in patients with a malignant neoplasm. It is thought to be a consequence of idiopathic hypercoaguability and may be associated with embolic or other thrombotic phenomena. (Courtesy of the Gordon Museum, Guy's Hospital Medical School)

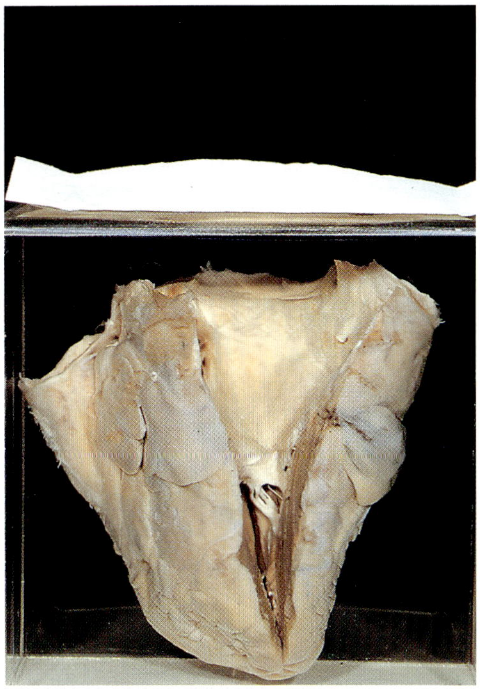

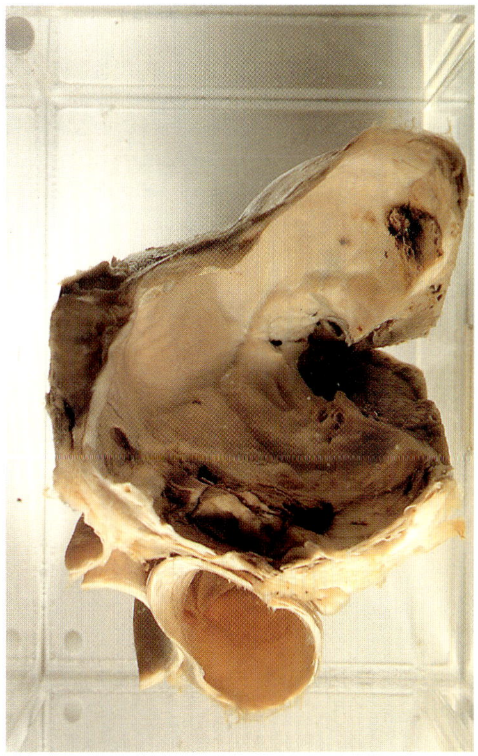

Mitral stenosis is the single commonest valvar defect and is almost always due to an episode of rheumatic fever in the past, although very rarely the lesion is congenital. Rheumatic fever is a multisystem disease, now fairly uncommon in the Western world. It results from the development of cross-reacting antibodies to ß-haemolytic *Streptococcus pyogenes*. It therefore most often occurs a few weeks after a minor streptococcal infection, usually of the upper respiratory tract, and typically affects young children. While the principal early feature is a non-suppurative polyarthritis, a pancarditis also develops. The latter is characterised by a fibrinous pericarditis, a granulomatous myocarditis and a diffuse endocarditis which predominantly affects the heart valves (particularly the mitral and aortic). This valvar inflammation with ulceration induces the deposition of platelet thrombi (producing characteristic small vegetations, see Legend 1.22). Healing by fibrosis leads to thickening, shortening and adherence of the leaflets and chordae tendinae, hence the rigid 'fish-mouth' mitral orifice which is both stenotic and incompetent. Myocardial involvement is characteristically most marked in the posterior wall of the left atrium. This also heals by fibrosis, leaving a pale area known as MacCullum's patch (as in this case). Other features of rheumatic fever may include skin rashes or nodules, a polyarthritis, pneumonitis and encephalitis, leading to Sydenham's chorea. Complications of mitral stenosis include atrial fibrillation (with or without the development of mural thrombus and systemic emboli), pulmonary hypertension and, later, infective endocarditis (see Legend 1.14 et seq.).

1.18 Mitral Stenosis

This is a post-mortem specimen from a 91-year-old woman who had suffered an attack of rheumatic fever at the age of 13. She eventually died with signs of ischaemic heart disease following insertion of a hip prosthesis for a fracture. At autopsy a large aneurysm of the aortic arch was also found.

The left side of the heart has been opened to show marked atrial dilatation, ventricular hypertrophy and a very small ventricular cavity (1.18a). The leaflets of the mitral valve are thickened and opaque and the posterior wall of the left atrium is pale and scarred, with adherent thrombus (1.18b).

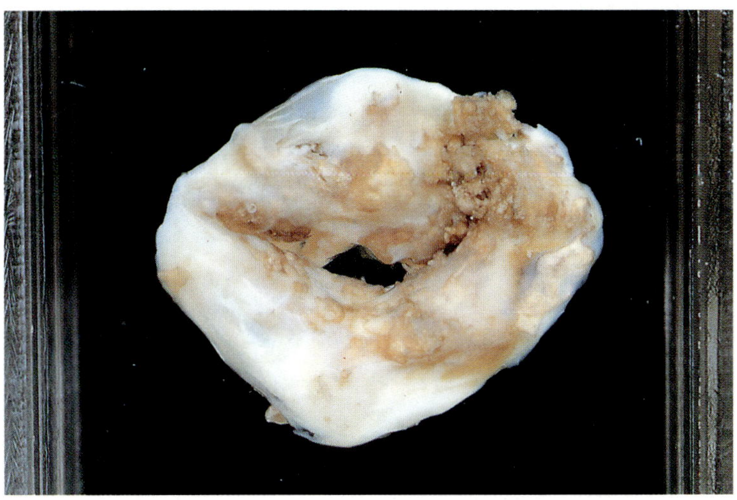

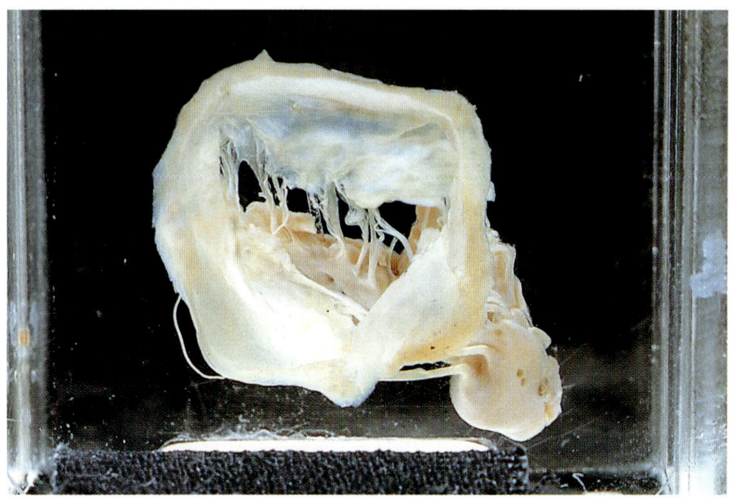

1.19 Mitral Stenosis

This specimen was excised from a 40-year-old man who had intractable cardiac failure due to rheumatic mitral stenosis and who had required two closed mitral valvotomies in the past. His condition did not improve so the diseased mitral valve was excised and replaced by a Starr-Edwards valve.

The diseased valve, viewed from above (1.19a) shows severe stenosis with a narrow, slit-like orifice which has been extended to the right by previous valvotomy. The valve leaflets are thickened and calcified and show adherent thrombus. The chordae are barely visible, at the lower margin on the orifice as very thick, short fibrous bands. A normal mitral valve is shown (1.19b) for comparison.

This case demonstrates well the classical rigid, small mitral orifice that is seen in rheumatic heart disease and which both impedes flow from the left atrium in diastole and allows flow back into the atrium during systole. Note that while 50 per cent of patients with rheumatic heart disease have mitral involvement alone, up to a further 35 per cent manifest both mitral and aortic dysfunction.

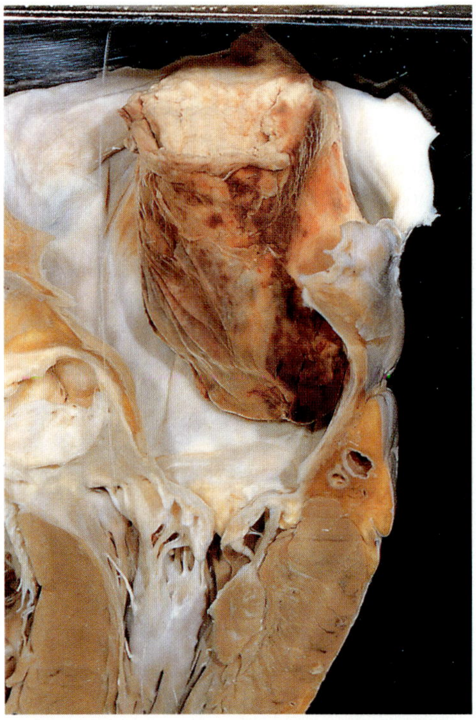

1.20 Mitral Stenosis with Left Atrial Thrombosis

This is a post-mortem specimen from an 80-year-old woman, who was known to have had rheumatic heart disease and chronic bronchitis. A year prior to her death she underwent amputation of her right leg for arterial thrombosis. She died following an operation to remove further thrombus from the left femoral artery.

The left side of the heart has been opened to show marked dilatation of the left atrium. The mitral valve is severely stenosed with fibrosis and contracture of the valve leaflets and chordae tendinae. Adherent to the posterior atrial wall is a large, cylindrical mass of thrombus, measuring 5.5×3.5×2.5cm.

As previously stated, rheumatic mitral stenosis is frequently complicated by thrombosis in the left atrium, particularly if there is coexistent atrial fibrillation, which is common. This is a serious complication because the risk of systemic embolisation by fragments of the thrombus is high, as seen in this case. Clearly the clinical consequences of such emboli will depend upon the arterial site at which they lodge. Very occasionally, they are large enough to occlude the aorta itself. Atrial thrombi may also act as a kind of ball valve which sits on top of the mitral valve during diastole, thus impeding atrial emptying and exaggerating the stenosis.

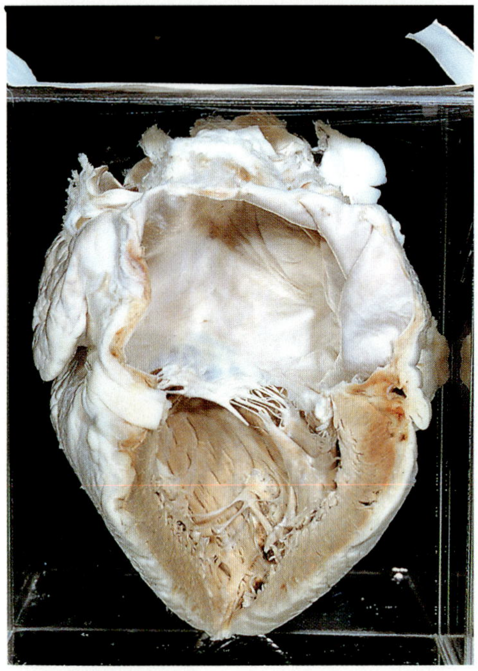

1.21 Mitral Incompetence with Massive Hypertrophy

This is a post-mortem specimen from a 75-year-old woman, known to have rheumatic mitral valve disease, who died having developed senile dementia.

The left side of the heart has been opened to show an enormously dilated left atrium and a greatly hypertrophied left ventricle. In the fresh state, the heart weighed 1020g. The mitral valve is markedly dilated, being more than twice the normal circumference, and its leaflets are thickened and opaque. The chordae tendinae are shortened and fibrotic. The aortic valve (not apparent in this view) was also thickened and incompetent.

This is an example of 'cor bovinum', the type of massive cardiac enlargement which is only seen in cases with both mitral and aortic incompetence resulting in gross volume overload. It is almost invariably rheumatic in origin.

Rheumatic endocarditis is the commonest cause of mitral incompetence and is a consequence of shortening and distortion of the valve leaflets and chordae which then prevent valve closure. Other causes of mitral incompetence include ischaemic heart disease (either by papillary muscle fibrosis or rupture due to infarction), functional stretching of the mitral valve ring in left ventricular dilatation, or myxoid degeneration of the valve leaflets (seen in the elderly or Marfan's syndrome) which results in mitral leaflet prolapse.

The principal complication is left ventricular failure (due to volume overload) but atrial fibrillation, pulmonary hypertension and infective endocarditis may occur (although less commonly than in mitral stenosis).

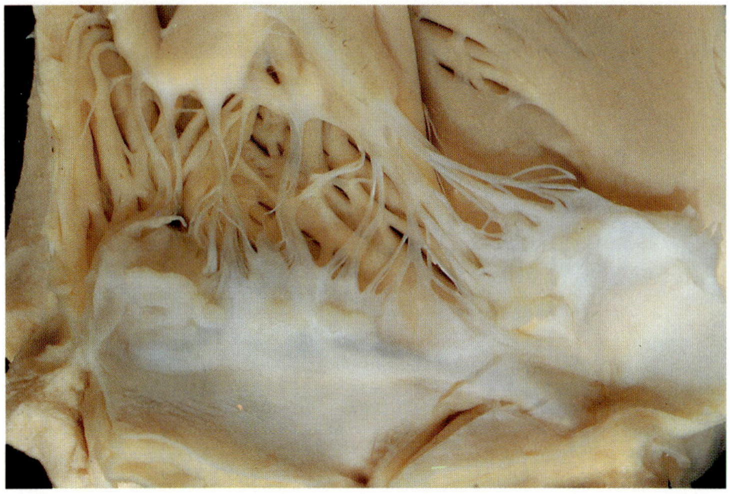

1.22 Mitral Incompetence with Recurrent Acute Rheumatic Endocarditis

This is a post-mortem specimen from a 35-year-old man who had developed mitral incompetence following an attack of rheumatic fever at the age of 13. Five weeks before his death he had suffered from an acute sore throat which was complicated by increasing dyspnoea. He collapsed suddenly and died.

A close-up view of this mitral valve shows a row of small, pale vegetations lying along the line of valve closure.

These vegetations represent fibrin and platelet deposition at the site of the acute valvitic process. They are noticeably smaller and paler than those of infective endocarditis. Recurrence of acute rheumatic fever is a well recognised feature of rheumatic heart disease but is typically only seen in children and young adults. (Courtesy of the Gordon Museum, Guy's Hospital Medical School)

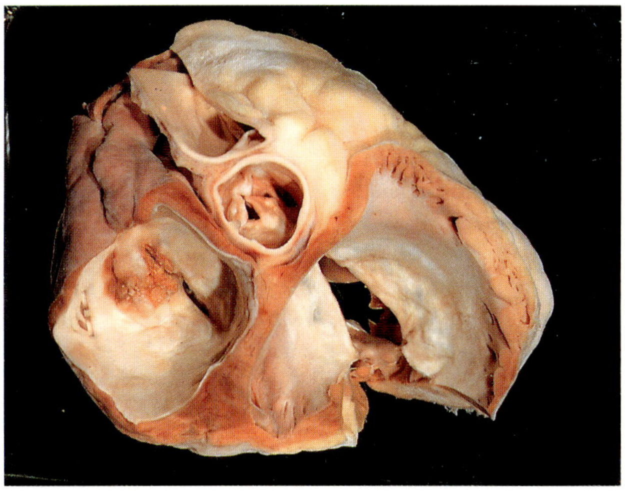

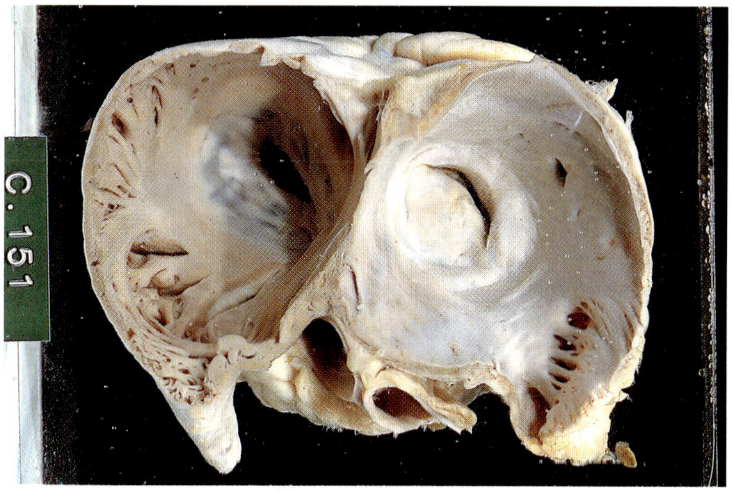

1.23 Mitral and Aortic Stenosis

This is a post-mortem specimen from a 20-year-old woman who had had an attack of Sydenham's chorea at the age of 12 followed by two further attacks of rheumatic fever in her teens. She developed increasing dyspnoea and cardiac failure and had signs of aortic stenosis with left ventricular hypertrophy. Despite all treatment, she died.

A transverse section through the heart at the level of the atria, viewed from above, shows a pale, dilated left atrium (bottom left), with mural thrombus, at the back of which the mitral valve is reduced to a narrow slit-like orifice. The aortic valve (middle) is also tightly stenosed and shows nodular calcification of the fibrotic cusps.

As previously stated, damage to both the mitral and aortic valves occurs in up to 35 per cent of cases of rheumatic heart disease. The valves on the right side of the heart are uncommonly affected, but this case does show some pallor and fibrosis of the tricuspid valve (bottom right) suggestive of rheumatic involvement.

1.24 Combined Mitral and Tricuspid Stenosis

This is a post-mortem specimen from a 40-year-old woman, known to have suffered from rheumatic fever as a child, who suddenly collapsed and died.

A transverse section through the atria, viewed from above, shows marked dilatation of both cavities. The mitral valve (left) shows severe stenosis with marked fibrosis of the valve leaflets: note also the endocardial fibrosis of the anterior left atrial wall. The tricuspid valve (right) is similarly stenotic, due to fusion of the valve leaflets, but the fibrotic process is less marked.

Up to 5 per cent of patients with rheumatic heart disease have coexistent damage to the mitral and tricuspid valves and this is the commonest cause of tricuspid stenosis. Rarer causes of the latter include the carcinoid syndrome or a congenital malformation. (Courtesy of the Gordon Museum, Guy's Hospital Medical School)

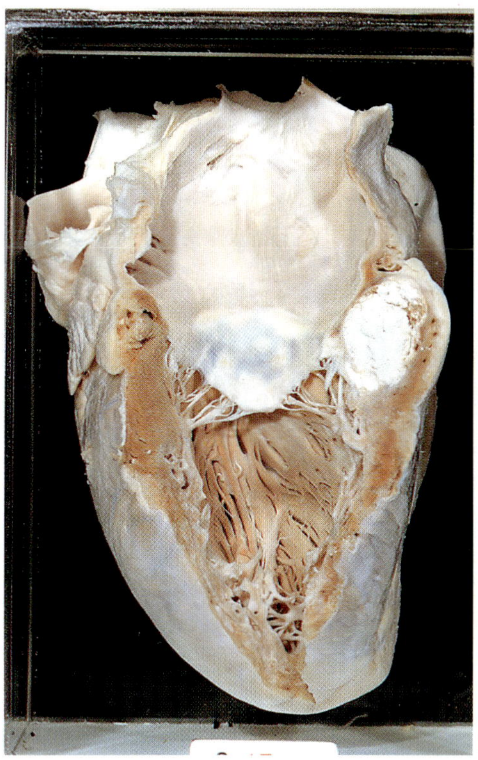

1.25 Calcification of the Mitral Valve Ring

This is a post-mortem specimen from an elderly woman, with known long-standing hypertension who suddenly collapsed and died.

The left side of the heart has been opened to show atrial dilatation and mild ventricular hypertrophy. The mitral annulus shows massive calcification which extends deeply into the myocardium (best seen on the right). The valve leaflets and chordae are healthy.

Calcification of the mitral valve ring (annulus fibrosus) is a common degenerative process which is thought to be an ageing phenomenon. Females are predominantly affected for reasons which are not apparent. The calcium deposition commences in the angle between the valve leaflets and the ventricular wall and may extend to involve either the adjacent leaflets or the myocardium. This results in marked rigidity of the valve and hence often functional incompetence. The development of overlying thrombosis or infective endocarditis are the commonest complications.

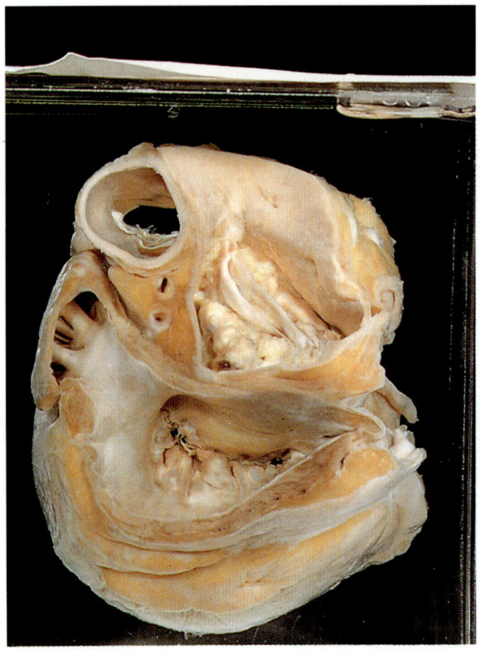

1.26 Calcific Aortic Stenosis

This is a post-mortem specimen from an elderly man, known to have had symptoms of heart disease, who suddenly collapsed and died.

A transverse section through the heart, near the base of the left atrium, shows the aortic valve (bottom right) to have only two leaflets. The valve leaflets are massively calcified and nodular and the orifice is reduced to a very narrow slit. The left atrium and mitral valve (bottom left) and the pulmonary valve (top right) appear normal.

In the majority of cases, stenotic aortic valves are heavily calcified and are of the congenitally bifoliate type. The aetiology of this relatively common developmental anomaly is unknown. Less often, calcific aortic stenosis may be seen simply as a manifestation of the ageing process. Other causes of aortic stenosis, not necessarily associated with calcification, are rheumatic heart disease and various congenital malformations. Complications of aortic stenosis include coronary ischaemia, left ventricular failure, sudden death and infective endocarditis.

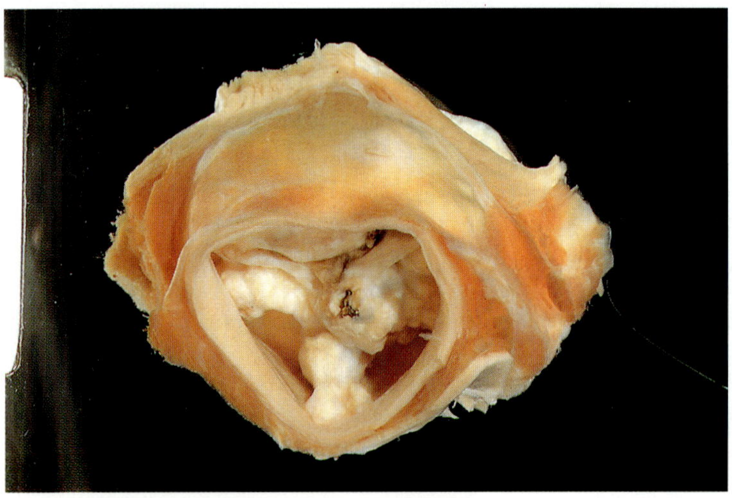

1.27 Calcific Aortic Stenosis with Infective Endocarditis

No clinical details are available.

The aortic valve, which has a normal trifoliate configuration in this case, shows prominent nodular calcification. The margins of the leaflets are fused, however, reducing the valve orifice to a narrow slit, one leaflet being covered with small haemorrhagic vegetations.

While this example of aortic stenosis most probably represents the effects of rheumatic heart disease with superadded terminal infective endocarditis, fusion of the valve cusps may sometimes be seen as a congenital phenomenon which is frequently followed by calcification.

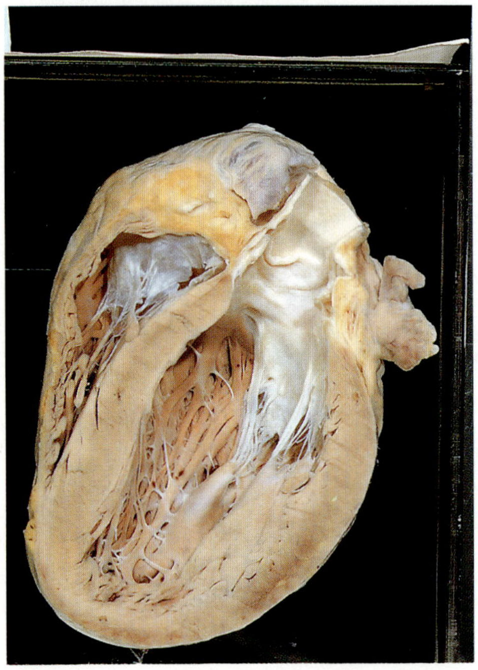

1.28 Aortic Incompetence

This is a post-mortem specimen from a 49-year-old man who was found dead in bed. He was known to have had rheumatic fever while in his early twenties.

The left side of the heart has been opened to show very marked ventricular dilatation and hypertrophy. The aortic valve (top left) shows thickened, contracted leaflets, leaving an enormously expanded valve orifice.

Aortic incompetence is most often a consequence of rheumatic heart disease (see Legend 1.18) but may also be due to dilatation of the aortic root as seen in syphilitic aortitis or Marfan's syndrome. It may also be a feature of ankylosing spondylitis or Reiter's disease in which widening of the attachments of the valve leaflets occurs. Congenitally bifoliate valves are also occasionally incompetent.

Complications of aortic incompetence are often only a late feature of the disease (because of ventricular compensation) but include left ventricular failure and the development of bacterial endocarditis.

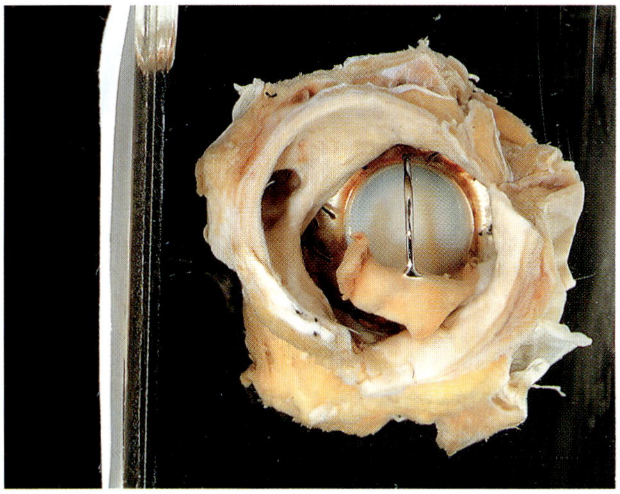

1.29 Starr-Edwards Prosthesis in the Aortic position

This is a post-mortem specimen from a 67-year-old man, who had originally presented with aortic incompetence due to rheumatic heart disease. He had undergone valve replacement 7 years previously but represented with severe acute left ventricular failure and died. At autopsy there was thrombus adherent to the prosthesis and embolic infarcts in the small intestine, kidney and spleen.

The aortic root, viewed from above, shows a Starr-Edwards ball-valve prosthesis. The aortic rim of the metal cage has become endothelialised, at which site the ante-mortem thrombosis had occurred.

The Starr-Edwards prosthesis, a very popular mechanical valve that has been used for many years, works by the ball being forced onto the metal cage during systole and falling back on the metal ring during diastole. Tissue overgrowth, thrombosis and mechanical dysfunction are the commoner causes of failure in mechanical prostheses.

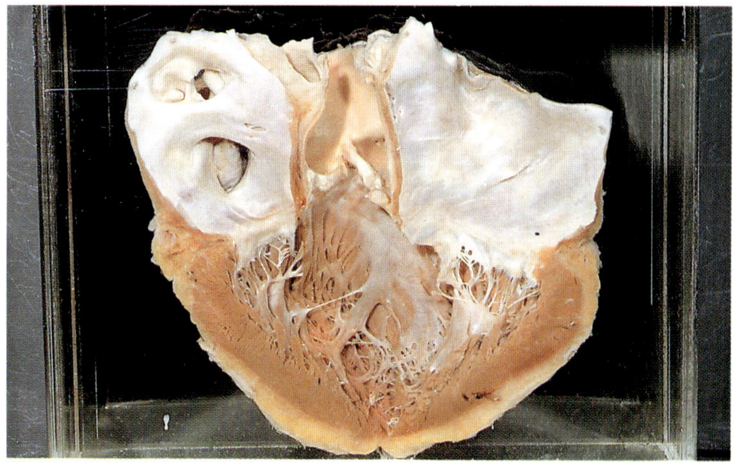

1.30 Calcified Aortic Valve Homograft

This is a post-mortem specimen from a 65-year-old woman, who had presented with rheumatic aortic valve disease and had undergone homograft valve replacement 8 years previously. She died of a cerebral embolism.

The left side of the heart has been widely opened to show ventricular dilatation and hypertrophy. The aortic valve graft (centre top) shows heavy calcification of the cusps; in the unopened state, the valve orifice was severely stenosed. In contrast the bisected mitral valve appears normal.

Bioprostheses (i.e. homografts or xenografts which are usually porcine), when they fail, tend to do so as a consequence of degenerative changes, such as calcification, fibrosis, and tearing or perforation of the cusps. They are less prone to undergo tissue overgrowth or thrombosis than mechanical prostheses.

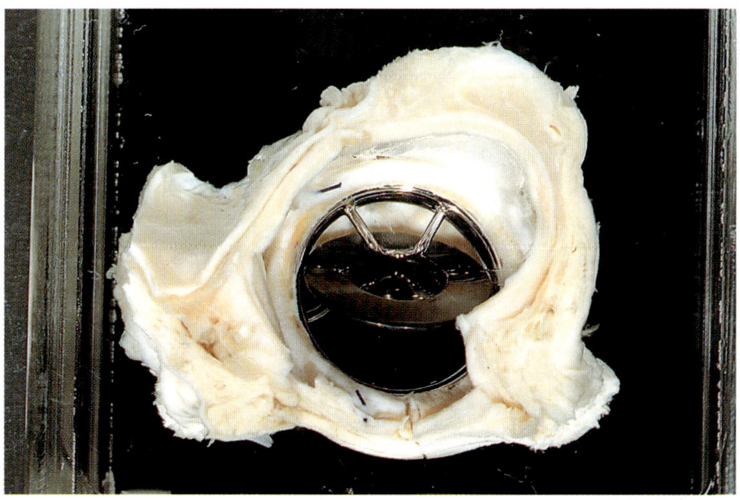

1.31 Aortic Valve with Björk-Shiley Prosthesis

This is a post-mortem specimen from a 76-year-old man who had undergone valve replacement for calcific aortic stenosis almost 2 years previously. He died of widespread metastases from a rectal carcinoma.

The aortic valve, viewed from above, has been replaced by a metallic Björk-Shiley tilting-disc prosthesis which is completely healthy.

The Björk-Shiley prosthesis is another very popular mechanical prosthesis and works by the disc tilting away from the metal ring (at the base) during systole and then falling back to occlude the ring during diastole.

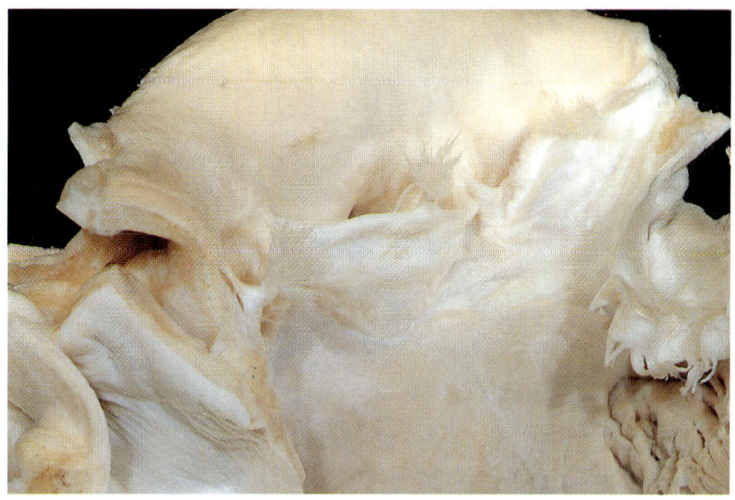

1.32 Lambl's Excrescences

These were an incidental finding at post-mortem. No further clinical details are available.

This close-up view of the aortic valve shows small, tuft-like papillary excrescences projecting from the centre of each cusp.

Lambl's excrescences, while previously regarded by some as organised vegetations, are now thought to represent an ageing phenomenon and are characterised by small fibro-elastic 'polyps' which develop at the site of valve closure; the mitral or aortic valves are most often affected. They are of no clinical significance *per se* but may possibly act as the originating site for infective endocarditis.

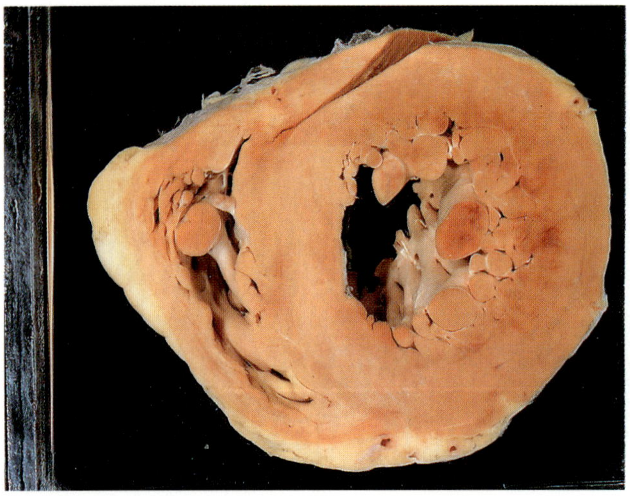

1.33 Left Ventricular Hypertrophy due to Hypertension

This is a post-mortem specimen from a 60-year-old man who died of a cerebral haemorrhage. He had presented with a 3 year history of transient cerebral ischaemic attacks and was found to have a blood pressure of 240/140mmHg.

A transverse section through the ventricles, viewed from below, shows marked hypertrophy of the left ventricular myocardium, measuring almost 25mm (normally 13-15mm) in cross-section. The heart weighed 480g at autopsy.

Systemic hypertension is the commonest cause of left ventricular hypertrophy. Up to 90 per cent of cases of hypertension are 'essential' or idiopathic in type. Aetiologically it is thought that genetic and environmental factors (such as cigarette smoking, obesity, stress and salt intake), perhaps in association with an endogenous failure of the renin-angiotensin system or of cellular sodium transport, may be responsible. Essential hypertension is commonest from the 4th decade onwards, affects females more than males, and coloured peoples more than Caucasians. The overall incidence in the British adult population is about 20 per cent. Ten per cent of cases of hypertension occur secondarily to an identifiable cause, such as chronic renal disease (e.g. glomerulonephritis, interstitial nephritis, polycystic disease or diabetic nephropathy), renal artery stenosis, Conn's syndrome, Cushing's syndrome, phaeochromocytoma, or pregnancy. Coarctation of the aorta leads to localised hypertension in the head, neck and upper limbs. At least 90 per cent of hypertensives follow a so-called 'benign' course but have a reduced life expectancy, largely as a consequence of myocardial infarction or cerebral haemorrhage. A small proportion will develop so-called 'malignant' or 'accelerated' hypertension, an acute phenomenon characterised by renal failure, papilloedema and an even greater risk of cardiac or cerebral injury. This group have a much poorer prognosis.

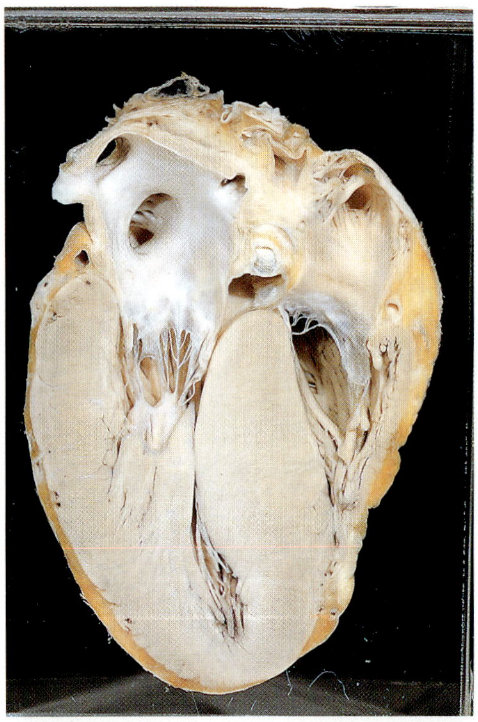

1.34 Left Ventricular Hypertrophy with Malignant Hypertension

This is a post-mortem specimen from a 53-year-old woman who presented with a 2 year history of increasing ankle oedema and dyspnoea. More acutely she had developed anorexia and repeated vomiting. Examination revealed a blood pressure of 300/155mmHg, associated with marked left ventricular hypertrophy and retinal haemorrhages. Biochemical tests showed the patient to be in severe renal failure and despite all treatment, she died with increasing uraemia 3 weeks later.

A four-chamber section of the heart is viewed from behind to show massive left ventricular hypertrophy, the septum measuring over 25mm in cross-section at the outflow tract. In the fresh state, the heart weighed 866g and there was a fibrinous pericarditis (not apparent in this view).

This is another particularly good example of left ventricular hypertrophy due to hypertension. Other causes of left ventricular hypertrophy include aortic stenosis or incompetence, aortic coarctation, various congenital cardiac anomalies, hypertrophic cardiomyopathy, severe anaemia, thyrotoxicosis or Paget's disease.

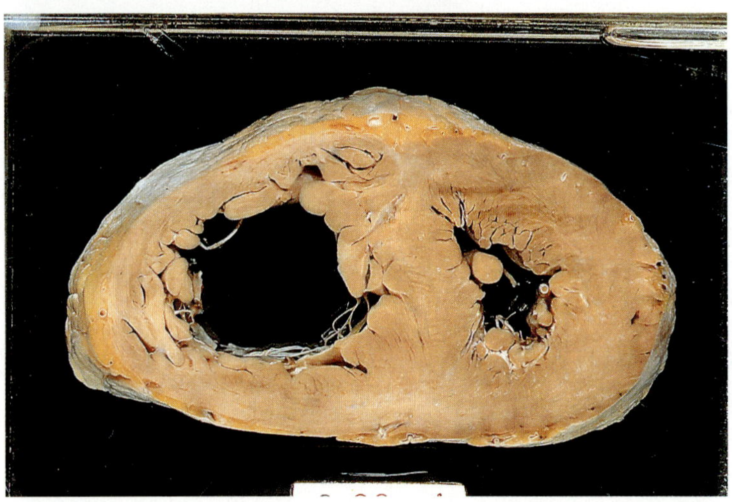

1.35 Right Ventricular Hypertrophy

This is a post-mortem specimen from a 62-year-old man who suddenly collapsed and died. He had suffered from long-standing chronic bronchitis and had developed cor pulmonale.

A short axis section of the ventricles is viewed from beneath. The left ventricle (on the right of the picture) is moderately hypertrophic measuring up to 20mm in cross-section but there is no dilatation. In contrast, the right ventricle shows marked myocardial hypertrophy (measuring 10mm in cross-section, normally 3-5mm) and dilatation of its cavity. Note also the patchy, pale foci of ischaemic scarring in the left ventricular wall.

Right ventricular hypertrophy is almost always a consequence of pulmonary hypertension (i.e. increased pulmonary vascular resistance), the commonest causes of which are mitral stenosis, long-standing left ventricular failure, repeated pulmonary emboli or interstitial lung damage (usually inflammatory in nature). Other rare predisposing factors include stenosis of the pulmonary valve or an atrial or ventricular septal defect. When pulmonary hypertension (of whatever cause) eventually leads to right ventricular hypertrophy, the combination is known as cor pulmonale. Thereafter congestive cardiac failure, with all its sequelae, commonly ensues.

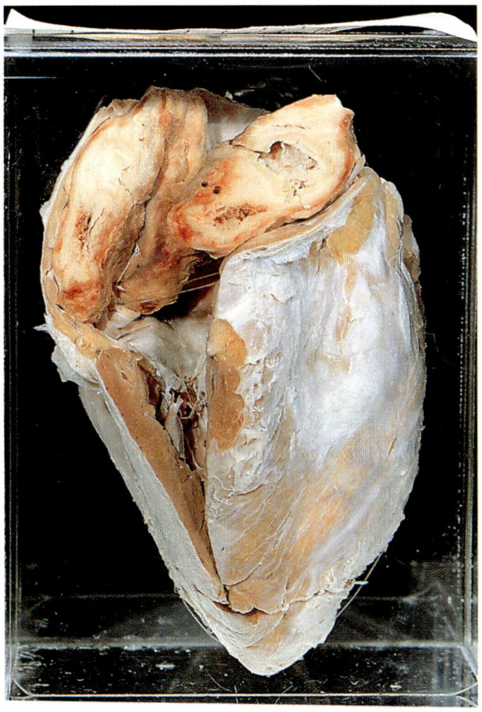

1.36 Cor Pulmonale with Right Atrial Thrombosis

This is a post-mortem specimen from a 64-year-old woman who was found dead in bed. She was a long-standing chronic bronchitic and was said to be in heart failure.

The right atrium has been opened to show dilatation. Adherent to the atrial wall is a mass of laminated thrombus, which measures 4.5cm in maximum diameter. The tricuspid valve appears normal. At autopsy there was also marked mitral stenosis, of probable rheumatic origin (not seen in this view).

The combination of chronic bronchitis and mitral stenosis has probably led to considerable pulmonary hypertension in this patient, thus leading to dilatation and hypertrophy of the right-sided heart chambers. In these circumstances, right atrial thrombosis is an occasional finding and may lead to pulmonary embolism.

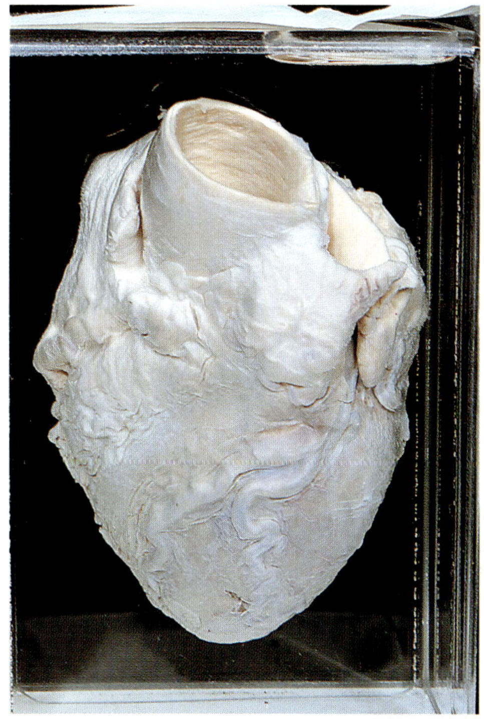

1.37 Senile Atrophy

This is a post-mortem specimen from an 84-year-old woman, known to suffer from Parkinson's disease, who died of bronchopneumonia following an operation to pin and plate a fracture of her left femur.

The heart is very small, weighing approximately 135g, and almost completely lacks epicardial fat. The coronary arteries appear very tortuous as a consequence of myocardial shrinkage.

Myocardial atrophy, while a feature of almost any wasting disease, is commonest with advancing age. It is characterised by a diminution in size and number of cardiac muscle fibres with a corresponding relative increase in brown lipofuscin pigment (representing the lipid remnants of effete organelles). The aetiology of cardiac atrophy with advancing age is probably multifactorial, being related to a comparatively poor or reduced dietary intake, a decreased functional demand and an almost invariable reduction in coronary arterial blood flow.

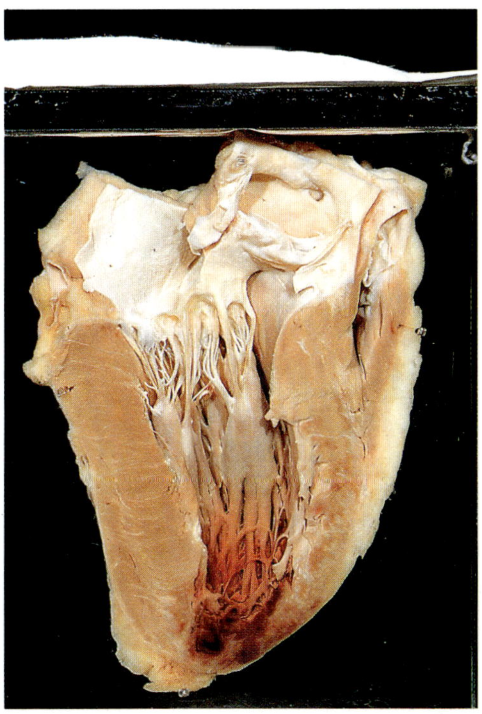

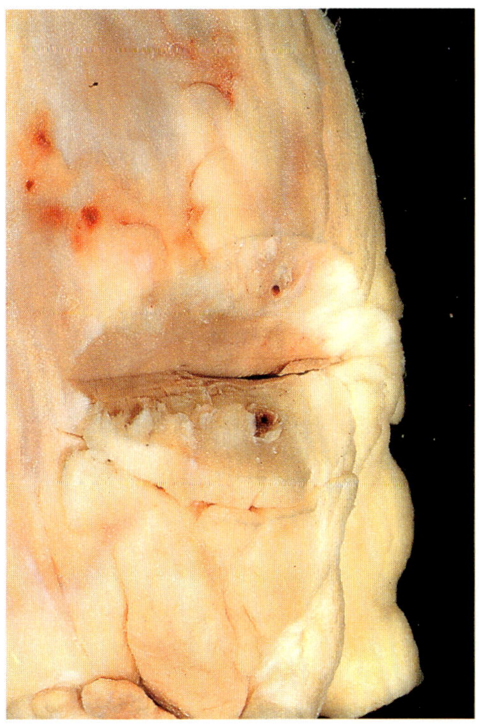

1.38 Acute Myocardial Infarct

This is a post-mortem specimen from a 56-year-old man who had suffered from anginal chest pain on exertion for 4 years. He presented acutely with similar pain which persisted despite rest and his usual medication. An electrocardiogram (ECG) showed evidence of acute myocardial infarction and left bundle branch block. He died 5 days later.

The parietal part of a long axis section through the left ventricle (1.38a) shows an ill-defined area of haemorrhagic infarction in the apical and anterior myocardium and the adjacent papillary muscles. The remainder of the anterior wall shows patchy pale fibrosis and some atrophy, compatible with long-standing ischaemic damage. A cross-section through the left anterior descending coronary artery of the same patient (1.38b) shows marked atheromatous stenosis and total occlusion by overlying thrombus.

Myocardial infarction is the single commonest cause of death in Britain and the United States and, in the vast majority of cases, is a consequence of atheroma (see Legend 1.60 et seq.) of the major epicardial coronary arteries. Atheroma (usually with overlying thrombosis) leads to narrowing (or occlusion) of the coronary arterial lumen which, in turn, reduces the myocardial blood supply and hence the oxygen supply. Then, when myocardial oxygen demand exceeds the diminished supply, ischaemic necrosis of the heart muscle occurs. Myocardial infarcts are more common in men than in women and more frequent in white than coloured peoples, although the latter are often affected at an earlier age. Males are most usually affected in the 6th and 7th decades, females tending to be 10-15 years older. Recognised risk factors are largely the same as for the development of atheroma and include hypertension, cigarette smoking, hyperlipidaemia (particularly low density lipoprotein) and diabetes mellitus. In females, the contraceptive pill (particularly if high in oestrogens) is also an important contributory element. Complications of myocardial infarction include sudden death (usually due to ventricular arrhythmias) which occurs in up to 30 per cent of patients, ventricular mural thrombosis with systemic embolism, ventricular rupture, cardiac aneurysm formation and the development of acute (or delayed) pericarditis (see Legend 1.9).

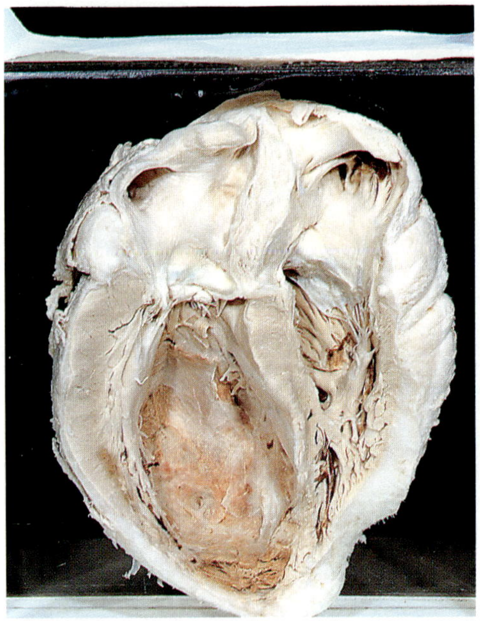

1.39 Acute Myocardial Infarct with Mural Thrombosis

This is a post-mortem specimen from a 72-year-old woman, who died suddenly having suffered a myocardial infarct 3 weeks previously.

This is a four chamber section through the heart in the plane of the mitral and tricuspid valves, viewed from behind. Note the area of fairly recent transmural myocardial infarction in the anterior and apical walls of the left ventricle. In the apical region there is massive destruction of muscle, such that the wall is thinned and dilated. At this site, there is a thick layer of adherent endocardial thrombus.

The vast majority of myocardial infarcts are localised transmural lesions as shown here. A proportion are distributed subendocardially and may extend as a broad band around most of the ventricle (see Legend 1.40). The thinned ventricular apical component, seen in this case, which is at least partly replaced by fibrous scar tissue (suggestive of infarction at an earlier date than the stated clinical history), is beginning to show early aneurysmal dilatation (see Legend 1.43).

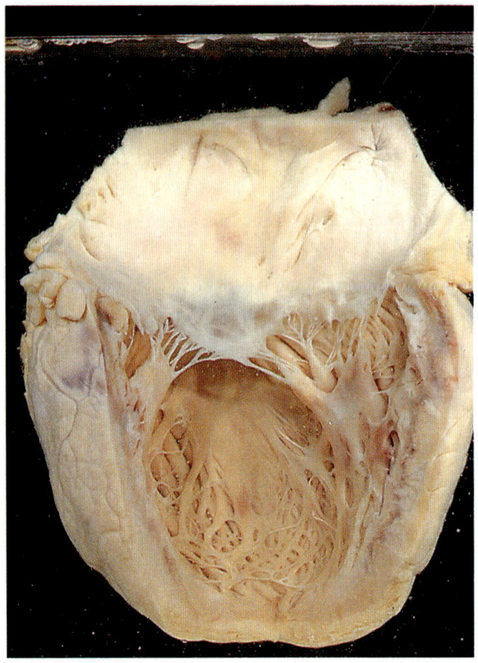

1.40 Acute Subendocardial Myocardial Infarct

This is a post-mortem specimen from a 67-year-old diabetic woman, who developed pains in her chest and neck and collapsed. She died in hospital following repeated cardiac arrests.

The left side of the heart has been opened to show a zone of reddish infarction extending beneath the endocardium along almost the whole parietal ventricular wall. Note also involvement of the papillary muscles. In addition there are foci of pale myocardial fibrosis (right) indicative of previous ischaemia.

Subendocardial myocardial infarcts are outnumbered by the transmural type by at least 20 to 1. They are thought to be due to extreme coronary hypoperfusion as a result of hypotension (of whatever cause), in the presence of a compromised ventricular blood supply. In other words, they are not typically associated with acute occlusion of a coronary artery. In this case, the left circumflex coronary artery showed organised, previous thrombus only. (Courtesy of the Gordon Museum, Guy's Hospital Medical School)

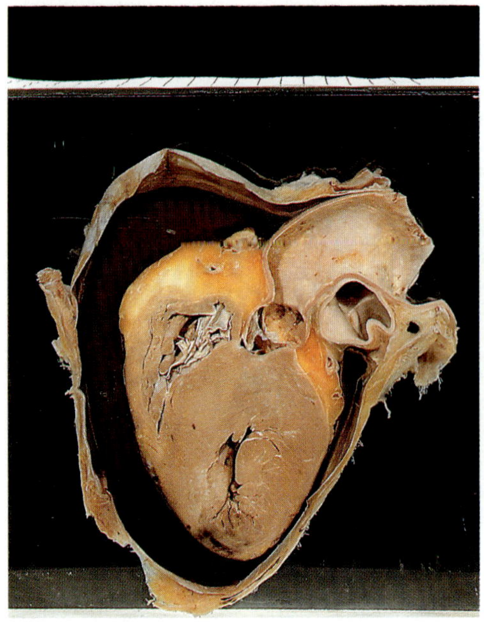

1.41 Haemopericardium due to a Ruptured Myocardial Infarct

This is a post-mortem specimen from an 84-year-old woman who died suddenly.

A section through the heart and pericardium shows that the pericardial sac is filled and distended by blood clot which envelopes the entire heart. At the apex of the hypertrophied left ventricle is an area of brownish discolouration indicating the presence of a recent myocardial infarct which has ruptured.

Haemopericardium is most often due to a ruptured myocardial infarct and is responsible for up to 10 per cent of the fatalities resulting from coronary thrombosis. This complication usually occurs within one week of the primary event, before scar tissue begins to form, and is commonest in elderly females or patients with full-thickness transmural infarction. Other causes of a haemopericardium include a dissecting aortic aneurysm (see Legend 1.75) or trauma.

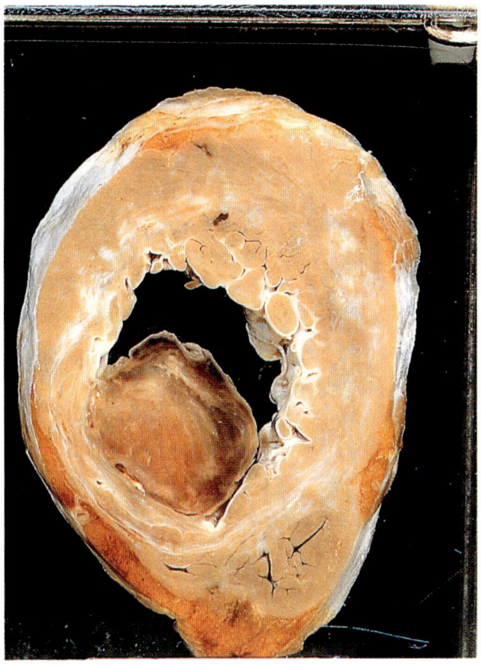

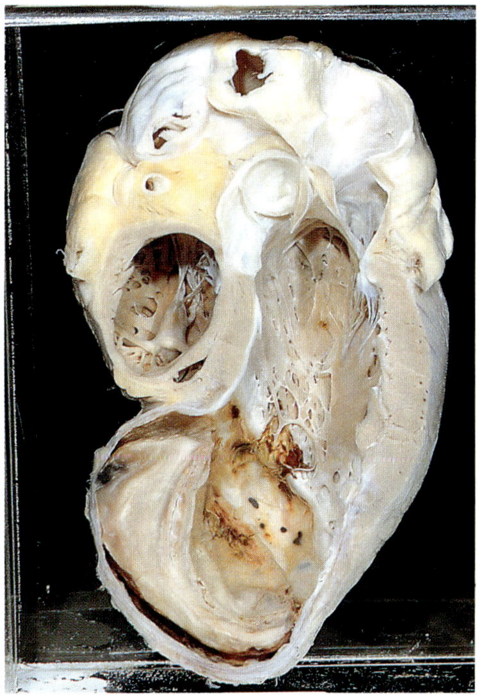

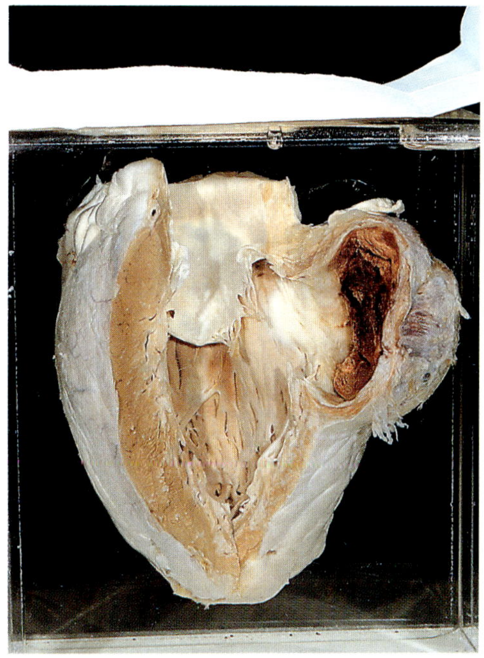

1.42 Healed Myocardial Infarct with Mural Thrombosis

This is a post-mortem specimen from a 61-year-old woman who died suddenly. She was a known hypertensive who had suffered a myocardial infarct 7 years previously since which time she had experienced occasional attacks of chest pain and dyspnoea.

This is a transverse section through the left ventricle near the apex, viewed from beneath. Note the extensive fibrous scarring of the myocardium, manifest as irregular pale foci, which indicates long-standing ischaemia. At the lower left, there is a dense band of fibrosis with myocardial thinning indicative of healed infarction. Adherent to the endocardium at this site is a mass of old laminated thrombus on the surface of which is a layer of more recent blood clot.

Following myocardial infarction, granulation tissue is apparent at the site of necrosis about one week after the primary event. After 3 weeks the first collagen fibres are laid down and eventual healing by fibrous scar tissue is complete after 2-3 months, depending upon the size of the infarct. Mural thrombi, as here, are often complicated by systemic emboli.

1.43 Ventricular Aneurysm following Myocardial Infarction

This is a post-mortem specimen from a 55-year-old man who suddenly collapsed and died. He had suffered a myocardial infarct 4 years previously.

A coronal section through both ventricles shows massive aneurysmal dilatation of the left ventricular cavity, which extends anteriorly as a thin-walled sac measuring 8cm in diameter. Note that the wall of the aneurysm (i.e. the anterior myocardium) consists solely of a thin layer of fibrous tissue. The sac contains a large, laminated thrombus.

True ventricular aneurysms usually develop gradually over a period of months following transmural myocardial infarction. The inelastic fibrous scar tissue is repeatedly stretched during systole and the wall becomes progressively thinner. Complications include the development of intraluminal thrombus (with possible consequent systemic embolism) and, less commonly, rupture. False aneurysms are occasionally encountered at the site of myocardial rupture when the resultant haematoma becomes walled-off by the epicardium.

1.44 Ventricular Aneurysm following Myocardial Infarction

This is a post-mortem specimen from a 64-year-old man who was found dead in bed. At autopsy the cause of death was shown to be a coronary thrombosis. No further clinical details are available.

The left ventricle has been opened to show marked mural hypertrophy. An aneurysmal sac, measuring 5cm in maximum diameter, projects from the upper part of the postero-lateral wall. At this site, the myocardium consists of pale fibrous tissue and the saccular lumen contains organised thrombus.

This is another typical example of a left ventricular aneurysm.

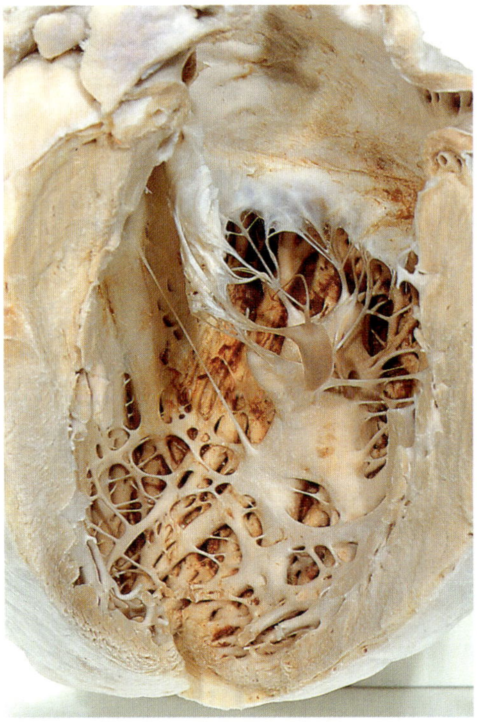

1.45 Congestive Cardiomyopathy

This is a post-mortem specimen from a 19-year-old man, who was incidentally found to have an enlarged heart while being examined following an epileptic fit. He developed severe congestive cardiac failure and collapsed and died soon afterwards.

The left ventricle, which has been opened, is greatly dilated and also shows a degree of mural hypertrophy. The mitral valve, although structurally normal, is incompetent as a consequence of the ventricular dilatation with resultant atrial hypertrophy and dilatation. Note the marked pallor of both the endocardium and myocardium.

A cardiomyopathy is by definition any myocardial disorder *for which no cause can be found*, in particular in the proven absence of ischaemia, hypertension, valvar or inflammatory disease. Idiopathic cardiomyopathies are currently classified into four main types; congestive, hypertrophic, constrictive (restrictive) and obliterative. The WHO recently proposed a three type classification (dilated, hypertrophic and restrictive) which is not yet widely accepted. Idiopathic congestive cardiomyopathy typically presents with severe progressive, congestive cardiac failure at any age and is thought to be due to an as yet unidentified cardiotoxic agent (or agents), although some cases are familial. The heart in these patients is typically large, dilated and flabby and there may be endocardial thrombosis. It should be noted that an identical appearance may be seen in chronic alcohol abuse, beri-beri, acromegaly, Freidreich's ataxia, various muscular dystrophies, or following childbirth. While the mechanism in a given case may not be precisely clear, these examples, which are not truly idiopathic, should not strictly be labelled as cardiomyopathies.

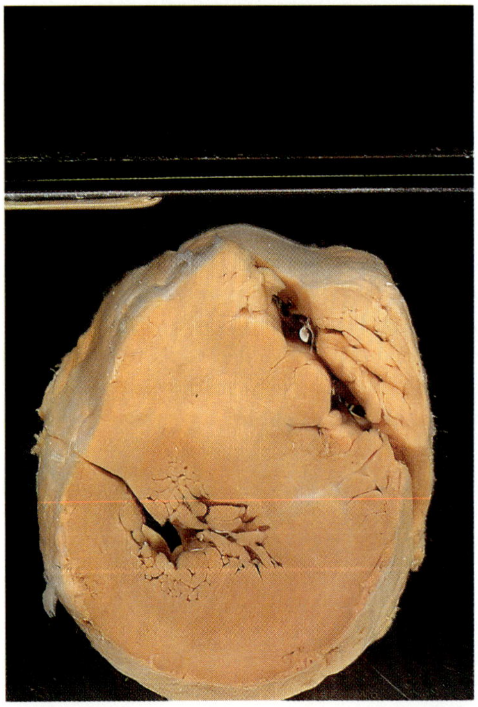

1.46 Hypertrophic Cardiomyopathy

This is a post-mortem specimen from a 14-year-old schoolboy, who appeared completely fit and healthy but suddenly collapsed and died.

A transverse section through the ventricles, viewed from beneath, shows massive left-sided myocardial hypertrophy, particularly of the interventricular septum, associated with pallor of the heart muscle. The heart weighed 400g in the fresh state.

Hypertrophic cardiomyopathy may be seen at any age but is commonest in adolescents and young adults. It is characterised by asymmetrical cardiac hypertrophy, affecting predominantly the left ventricle. The principal haemodynamic consequences are impaired left ventricular compliance and obstruction of the outflow tract leading to subvalvar aortic stenosis. Many cases appear to be familial, being inherited by an autosomal dominant trait. While the majority present with cardiac failure, this condition is a well-recognised cause of sudden death. (Courtesy of the Gordon Museum, Guy's Hospital Medical School)

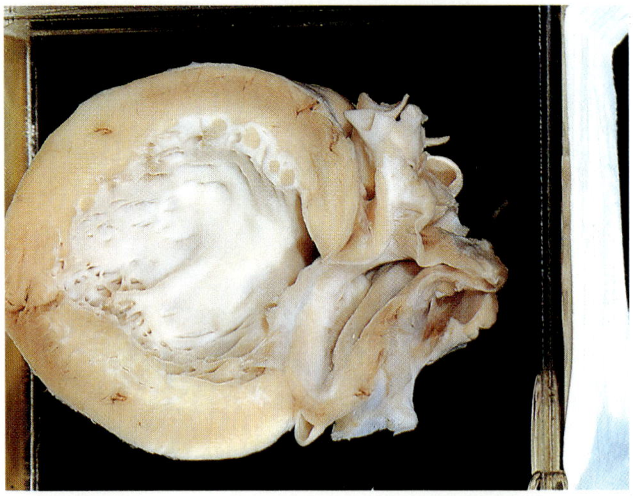

1.47 Constrictive Cardiomyopathy (Endocardial Fibro-elastosis)

This is a post-mortem specimen from a 5-month-old boy who died in cardiac failure.

The left side of the heart has been opened to show ventricular dilatation with marked pallor and thickening of the endocardium. Note also that the subendocardial portion of the myocardium is unusually pale.

Primary endocardial fibro-elastosis is a congenital abnormality, which typically presents in infancy and is characterised by deposition of collagen and elastic tissue between the endocardium and myocardium of the left ventricle. Some prefer to classify this lesion as a developmental anomaly rather than a true cardiomyopathy (see Legend 1.8). The accumulation of this fibro-elastic tissue leads to relative rigidity and reduced compliance of the ventricular wall, hence the term constrictive or restrictive. It should be noted that this lesion is sometimes associated with other cardiovascular or systemic malformations. In adulthood, a very similar appearance may be seen in amyloidosis, although this is not a true cardiomyopathy.

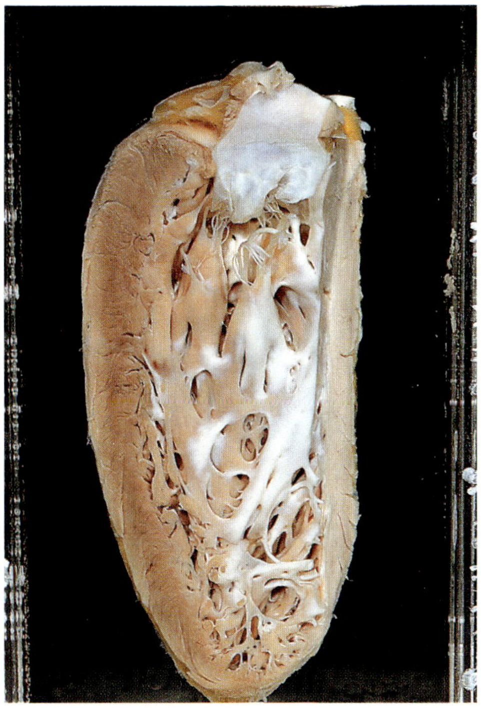

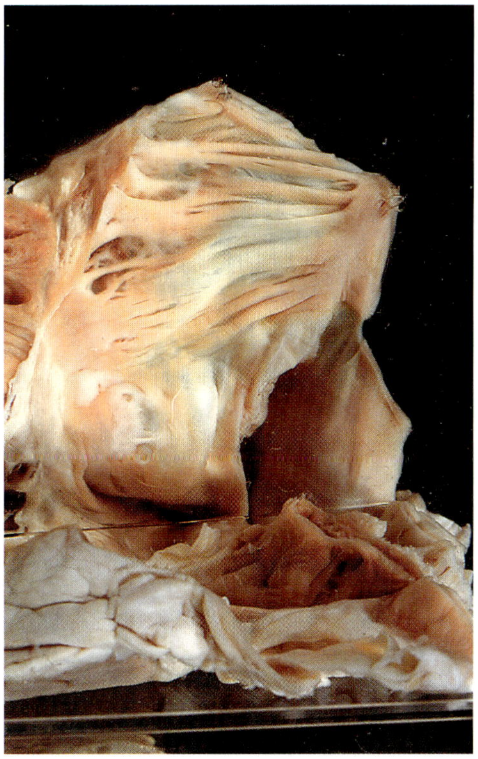

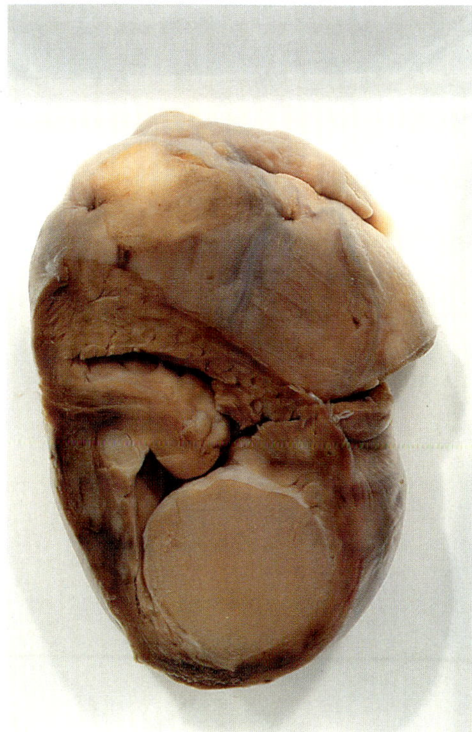

1.48 Obliterative Cardiomyopathy

This is a post-mortem specimen from a 67-year-old man who, for the past 3 years, had developed increasingly severe left ventricular failure with cardiomegaly in the absence of hypertension or any evidence of ischaemic heart disease. Latterly, severe congestive cardiac failure with atrial fibrillation supervened and he died.

Part of the left ventricle has been opened to show marked endocardial fibrosis, particularly over the papillary muscles. The myocardium appears relatively normal.

Obliterative cardiomyopathy may be theoretically divided into two principal subtypes: endomyocardial fibrosis (largely a disease of tropical Africans in whom it is common), which tends to produce massive endocardial thickening with a resultant marked reduction in size of the ventricular cavity (often with overlying thrombosis), and Löeffler's endocarditis (more often seen in Caucasians), which produces less severe fibrotic thickening and is often associated with an eosinophilic pneumonia. This case does not seem to fall into either category.

1.49 Right Atrium and Tricuspid Valve: Carcinoid Syndrome

This is a post-mortem specimen from a 62-year-old man, who presented with a one year history of intermittent diarrhoea and reddish-blue discolouration of the face. Examination revealed irregular hepatomegaly and a variable cardiac murmur. The finding of a grossly elevated urinary 5-hydroxyindole acetic acid excretion, presumed to be due to a small intestinal primary tumour with liver metastases, confirmed the diagnosis of the carcinoid syndrome. The patient died 15 months later.

The right atrium has been opened to show patchy pale endocardial thickening. The tricuspid valve (bottom right) shows similar changes, which are not so well seen.

Up to 50 per cent of patients with the carcinoid syndrome (see Chapter 3) develop cardiac complications, most often characterised by fibrosis of the right-sided heart valves and endocardium. Typically, tricuspid incompetence and/or pulmonary stenosis result from thickening and shortening of the valve leaflets thus leading to congestive cardiac failure. Toxic metabolites of kallikrein, a peptide secreted by carcinoid tumours, are thought to be pathogenetically responsible. (Courtesy of the Gordon Museum, Guy's Hospital Medical School)

1.50 Congenital 'Rhabdomyoma'

This is a post-mortem specimen from a 1-day-old baby girl who died from an intracranial haemorrhage.

Two well-circumscribed masses are apparent in this section of the left ventricular myocardium, the larger (above) projecting into the ventricular cavity.

Cardiac 'rhabdomyomas' are hamartomatous malformations characterised by the accumulation of large amounts of glycogen within myocardial cells. They are typically seen in infancy and are very frequently multiple. The clinical consequences are extremely variable but up to 50 per cent of affected infants have coexistent tuberose sclerosis (epiloia). (Courtesy of the Gordon Museum, Guy's Hospital Medical School)

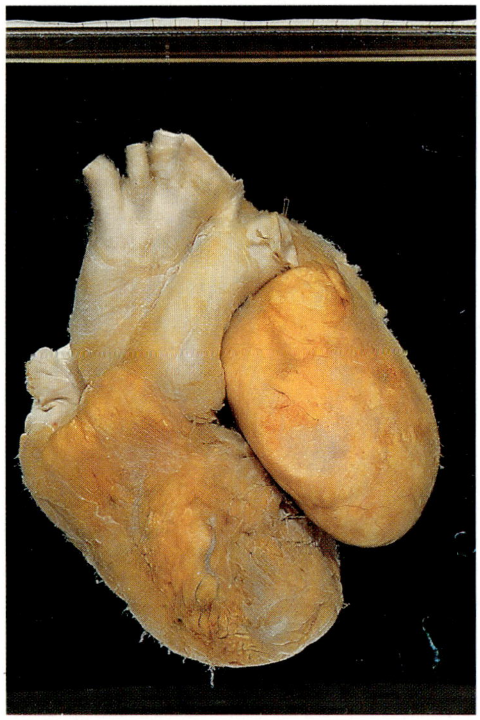

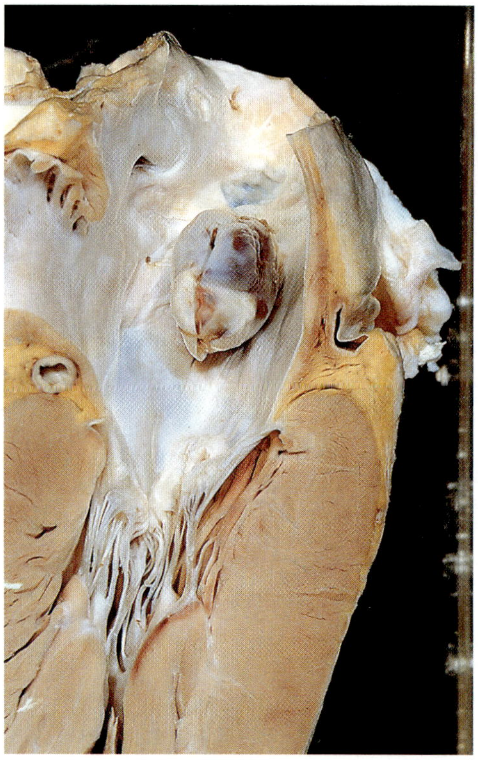

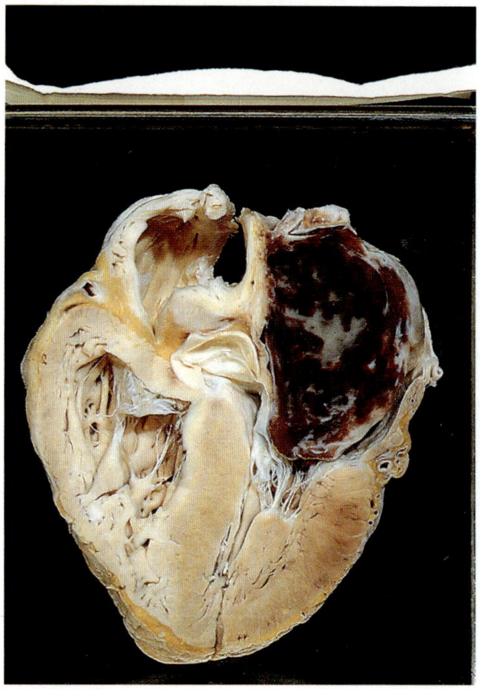

1.51 Pericardial Lipoma

This was an incidental finding at post-mortem in an 80-year-old man who died of a myocardial infarct.

Arising from the visceral pericardium at the root of the great vessels, just beneath the pulmonary trunk, is a large, well-circumscribed fatty mass. The tumour, which is ovoid in shape, is almost as large as the heart and, in the fresh state, projected into the pericardial cavity.

Tumours of adipose tissue in the heart are extremely uncommon but most often take the form of lipomatous hypertrophy of the interatrial septum, a condition seen in the elderly which may give rise to arrhythmias. True lipomas are even more rare; they may be intramyocardial (often associated with tuberose sclerosis in young adults) or pericardial, as in this case, in which circumstance the patients are usually older and asymptomatic.

1.52 Left Atrial Myxoma

This was an incidental finding at post-mortem in a 66-year-old hypertensive woman who died of a cerebral haemorrhage.

The left side of the heart has been opened to show a rounded, polypoid and gelatinous tumour, measuring 1.5cm in diameter, arising from the interatrial septum just below the fossa ovalis. Note the marked left ventricular hypertrophy, a probable consequence of this patient's hypertension.

Cardiac myxomas are by far the commonest primary tumours of the heart. They arise most often in adulthood, in either sex, and typically present either with the features of mitral valve disease or with systemic emboli; they often remain asymptomatic (as in this case). The vast majority develop as pedunculated lesions in the left atrium, the right atrium being the second most common site. The ventricles are only rarely affected. The precise nature of these benign lesions has been a source of controversy. Many have held the view that they simply represent organised, rather myxoid thrombi. The current consensus is that these myxomas are true neoplasms, derived from subendocardial tissues, which show only primitive mesenchymal differentiation.

1.53 Left Atrial Myxoma

This is a post-mortem specimen from a 46-year-old woman, who died having been admitted in a confused state with severe congestive cardiac failure and atrial fibrillation.

A section through the heart shows the left atrium to be distended and filled by a large, haemorrhagic mass, measuring 7cm in diameter, which arises in the region of the fossa ovalis. The tumour is occluding, and projecting through, the mitral valve orifice. Note the hypertrophy of both the right and left ventricular myocardium.

Clearly there has been extensive haemorrhage into this myxoma, which has probably contributed to its considerable size. It is apparent that such lesions, in obstructing the mitral valve may present clinically with the features of mitral stenosis. In this case, the tumour had given rise to pulmonary hypertension and right ventricular hypertrophy.

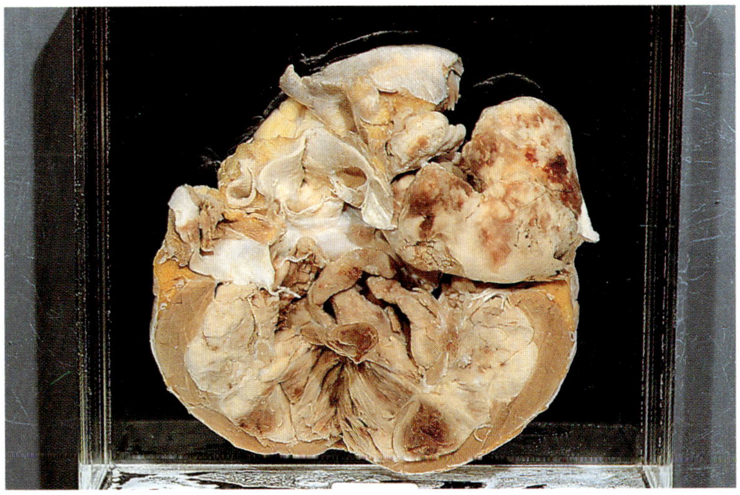

1.54 Pleomorphic Rhabdomyosarcoma

This is a post-mortem specimen from a 57-year-old man, who presented with a 4 year history of anginal chest pain on exertion and two suspected myocardial infarcts. He was admitted with unremitting chest pain and dyspnoea. Further infarction was suspected and there was evidence of mitral regurgitation. His course in hospital was punctuated by an intermittent pyrexia (for which no cause could be found) and repeated exacerbations of his chest pain, after one of which he collapsed and died. At autopsy, there was no evidence of myocardial infarction or of coronary arterial disease but a large tumour was found in the left side of the heart, with metastases in the small bowel.

The left side of the heart has been opened to show a large, focally haemorrhagic mass virtually obliterating both the ventricular and atrial cavities, which are extremely dilated. The precise myocardial site of origin is no longer identifiable. In the fresh state, the heart weighed 800g.

Primary sarcomas of the heart, of whatever histological type, are exceedingly rare. While angiosarcomas are most often encountered, rhabdomyosarcomas are the second commonest type. Cardiac rhabdomyosarcoma is typically a lesion of adulthood and may arise in any of the four chambers. Symptoms are often non-specific although cardiac murmurs are frequently detected. The prognosis is generally very poor.

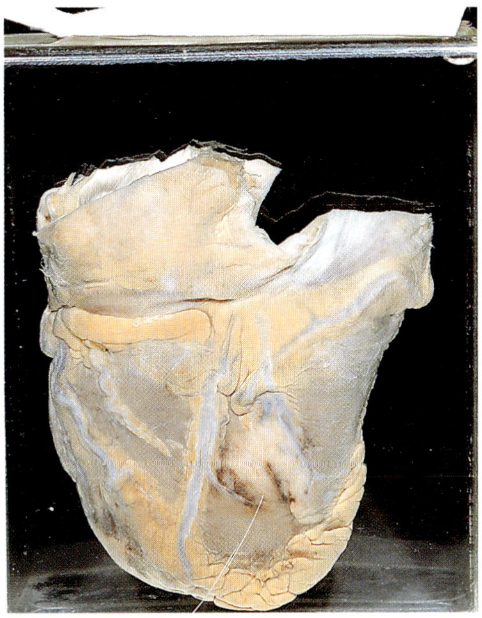

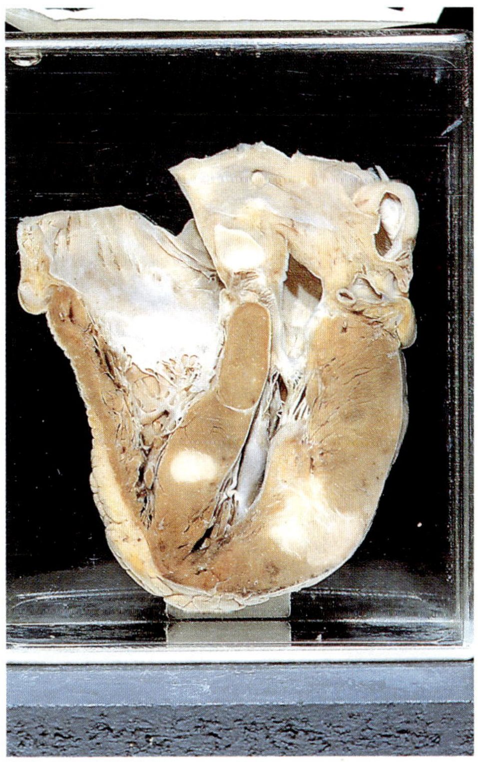

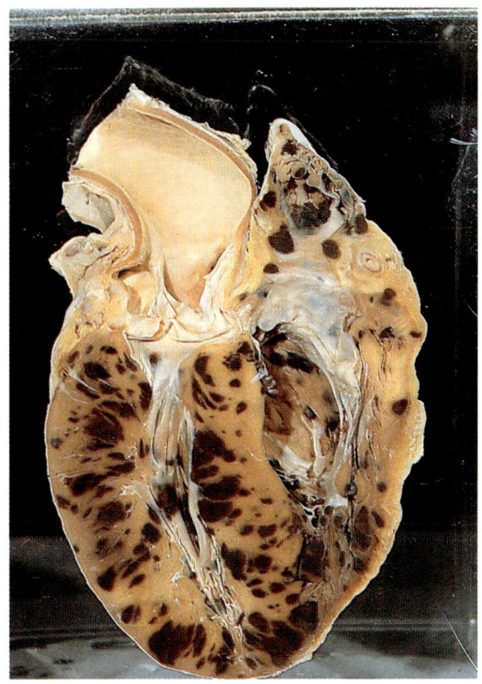

1.55 Metastatic Bronchial Carcinoma

This is a post-mortem specimen from an 89-year-old woman, who died following a short history of non-specific pulmonary symptoms. Autopsy revealed a squamous cell carcinoma of the right upper lobe bronchus with metastases in the mediastinum, pleura, vertebral column and heart.

The external surface of the heart (1.55a) shows a large, pale tumour nodule, with a haemorrhagic margin, situated beneath the visceral pericardium. A section through the heart (1.55b) shows two similar intramyocardial deposits.

Secondary deposits from malignant neoplasms elsewhere in the body are the commonest tumours seen in the heart, outnumbering primary benign or malignant cardiac lesions by at least 30-fold. Of all patients with disseminated malignant disease, up to 15 per cent have cardiac metastases. The commonest primary sites of origin are carcinomas of the lung, breast, large bowel and stomach, closely followed by malignant lymphoma. While the majority of such metastases are asymptomatic, patients may present with features of cardiac failure, arrhythmias or a pericarditis.

1.56 Metastatic Malignant Melanoma

This is a post-mortem specimen from an adult male who had undergone excision of a cutaneous malignant melanoma over the right iliac crest 18 months previously. He rapidly developed lymph node and hepatic metastases, followed by bony and cutaneous deposits with melaninuria and he died.

A section through the heart shows numerous pigmented deposits of metastatic melanoma throughout the myocardium.

The incidence of metastatic malignant melanoma in the heart is comparatively low, largely because this tumour is substantially less common than the carcinomas mentioned in Legend 1.55. Of those patients dying of disseminated melanoma, a very high proportion have cardiac deposits.

BLOOD VESSELS

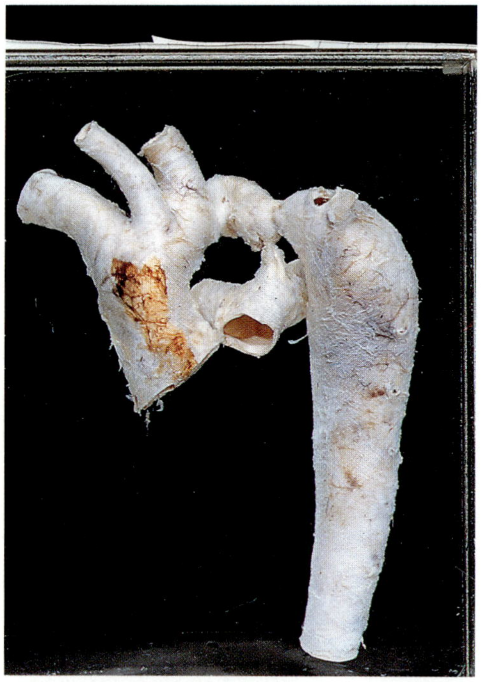

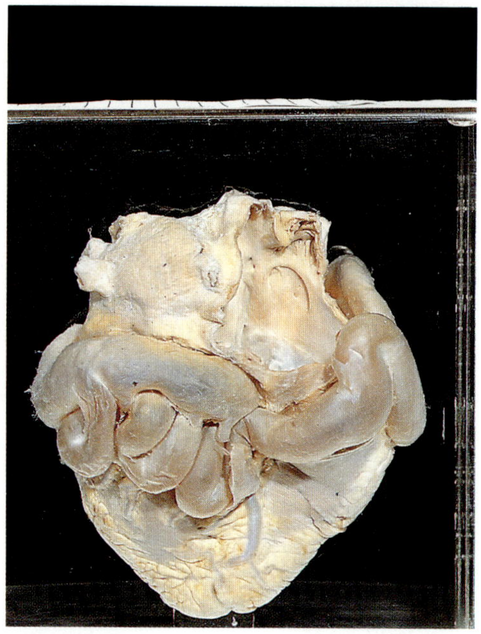

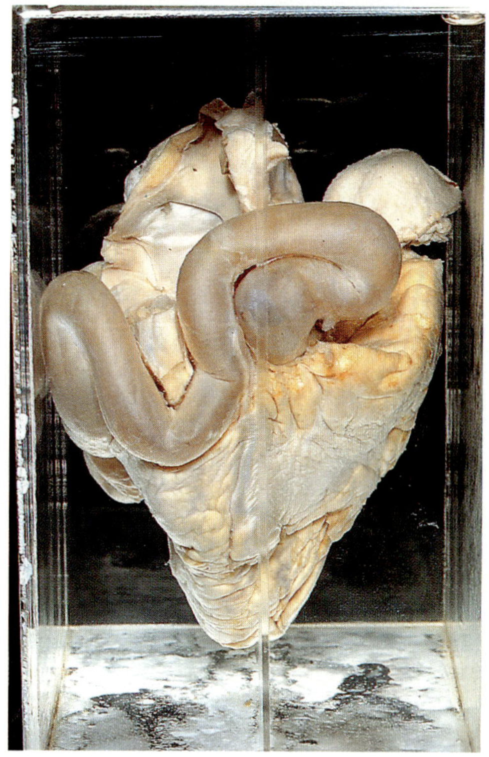

1.57 Thoracic Aorta: Coarctation

This is a post-mortem specimen from a 53-year-old man who collapsed and died suddenly. He had a history of rheumatic heart disease.

The thoracic aorta is mounted to show moderate luminal narrowing distal to the origin of the left subclavian artery and severe stenosis beyond the level of the ligamentum arteriosum, which is the rudimentary remnant of the ductus arteriosus and is included in the specimen with the pulmonary arteries. Note the proximal dilatation of the innominate, left common carotid and subclavian arteries and the post-stenotic dilatation of the descending aorta.

Coarctation is a congenital anomaly of the thoracic aorta, which is more common in males and may be associated with Turner's syndrome. In infancy, the stenosis, which is most commonly situated just proximal to a patent ductus arteriosus, is often associated with other cardiac malformations and the prognosis is therefore variable. In adulthood, the ductus is nearly always closed (as in this case) and there are no other malformations. An extensive collateral circulation commonly develops in this group between the pre- and post-stenotic portions. Complications in reasonably long-standing cases include marked left ventricular hypertrophy and hypertension in the upper part of the body.

1.58 Coronary Artery: Cirsoid Aneurysm

This is a post-mortem specimen from an adult male who died suddenly. No further clinical details are available.

The unopened heart, which is enlarged, is viewed anteriorly (1.58a). There is massive dilatation of the right coronary artery, which travels as a thin-walled trunk, measuring 2cm in diameter, along the atrioventricular groove taking an extremely tortuous course. It passes to the posterior surface of the heart (1.58b) where it anomalously enters the coronary sinus, which is also markedly dilated.

Cirsoid aneurysms are uncommon arteriovenous malformations, which are most often seen in the meninges or brain. They represent the result of an abnormal communication between the arterial and venous systems and, as such, are usually characterised by marked venous dilatation. They are particularly prone to be complicated by haemorrhage.

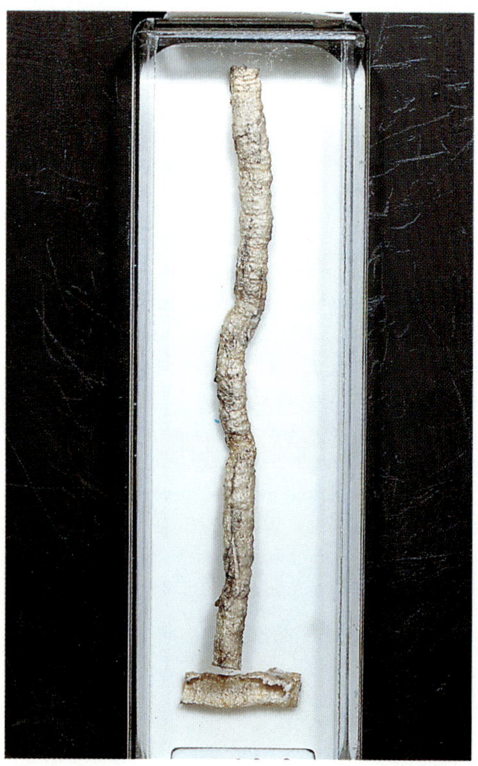

1.59 Femoral Artery: Medial Calcification (Mönckeberg's Sclerosis)

No clinical details are available.

Apparent from both the adventitial (above) and intimal (below) surfaces of this artery are numerous concentric, pale rings, which are composed of calcium. Note that the vessel is held rigid in an almost pipe-like form.

Mönckeberg's sclerosis is characterised by the accumulation of large amounts of calcium in the media of arteries (particularly those in the pelvis and lower limb) and in the aorta. It probably represents part of the ageing process, being more common from the 5th decade onwards, and also develops more fequently in patients with chronic renal failure and diabetes mellitus. In general it is of no clinical significance, typically being detected only radiologically in the living patient, but it may occasionally interfere with vascular access or surgery in patients with renal failure.

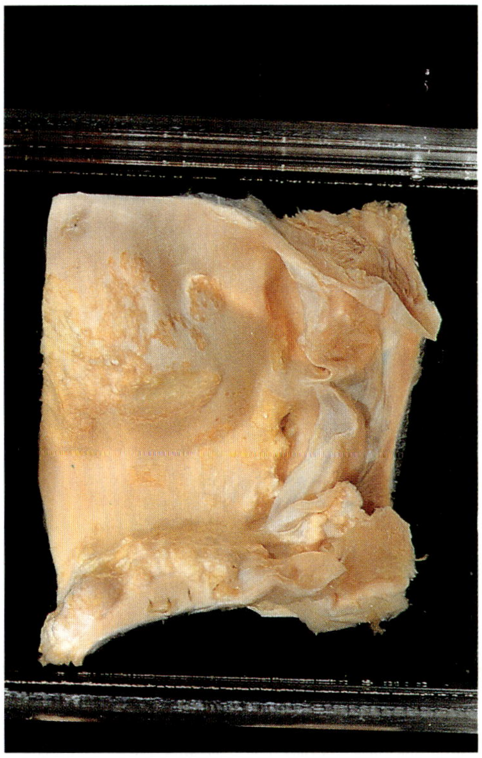

1.60 Ascending Aorta: Atheroma

This was an incidental finding at post-mortem in an 87-year-old woman who died of ischaemic heart disease.

The root of the ascending thoracic aorta, with the aortic valve cusps, is shown. The intimal surface of the aorta is elevated and roughened by irregular plaques of focally calcified, pale atheroma.

Atheroma (Greek – αθεϱε – porridge) is the single commonest *root* cause of death in the Western world, being responsible for the vast proportion of ischaemic heart disease, cerebrovascular, and peripheral vascular disease. It is defined as a lesion consisting of intimal, arterial thickened plaques, composed mainly of lipid and fibrous tissue.

Atheroma is ubiquitous in all parts of the world in which society has become 'Westernised', particularly with regard to dietary and smoking habits. While the earliest lesions may be apparent from adolescence, increasing age correlates very significantly with a marked increase in the prevalence of the condition; males are more severely affected, at least until the 6th decade, when post-menopausal females start to 'catch up'.

Pathogenetically there remains much uncertainty about this important condition. The two longest standing theories are those of incorporation of repeated microthrombi (Rokitansky) and of the 'imbibing' of circulating lipids (Virchow). More recently, it has been demonstrated that the myofibroblasts within plaques are monoclonal in origin within each plaque, suggesting an unexplained 'neoplastic' phenomenon.

Aetiologicallly, known risk factors (other than increasing age or male sex) include high circulating levels of cholesterol or low-density lipoprotein, tobacco smoking, systemic hypertension, physical inactivity, diabetes mellitus and indefinable psychological 'stress' elements. Interestingly, circulating levels of high-density lipoprotein are *inversely* correlated with the development of atheroma.

Topographically, the aorta (most especially the abdominal portion) is worst affected, followed by coronary, limb, cerebral and mesenteric arteries. All arteries down to a diameter of only 2mm may be involved. The clinical consequences are dependent upon the site of the lesions.

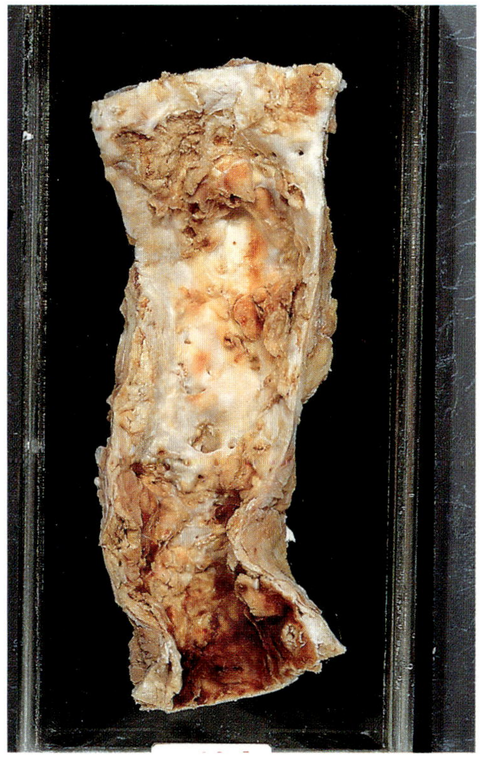

1.61 Descending Aorta: Atheroma

This was an incidental finding at post-mortem in an 85-year-old man, who died following a head injury.

A length of the descending thoracic aorta has been opened to show extensive atheromatous involvement. Many of the plaques show ulceration, haemorrhage and calcification.

The principal local complications that may occur within atheromatous plaques are haemorrhage (from small fragile vessels which grow into the plaque from the media), surface ulceration or fragmentation and overlying thrombosis (which may or may not be occlusive). In addition, underlying medial thinning commonly coexists and is associated with weakening of the vessel wall.

The principal effects, therefore, of complicated atheroma include vascular narrowing or occlusion (often with thrombosis), leading to ischaemia or gangrene. Emboli (composed either of atheromatous material or thrombus) may be shed from the surface and medial thinning predisposes to aneurysm formation.

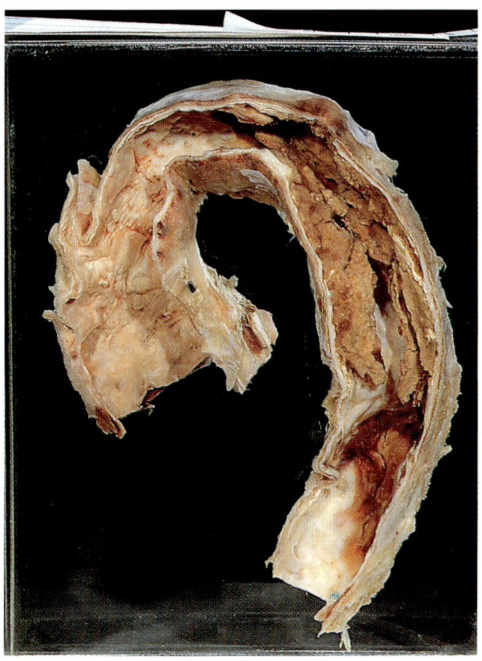

1.62 Thoracic Aorta: Atheroma with Massive Thrombosis

This is a post-mortem specimen from a 75-year-old woman who died of a ruptured saccular aneurysm of the proximal ascending aorta.

The aortic arch (distal to the fatal aneurysm) and descending aorta are shown. Proximally the terminal portion of the dilated aneurysmal lesion is apparent. The descending aorta shows intimal atheromatous thickening, over which lies an extensive layer of largely organised thrombus measuring 7cm in length. The lumen at this site is severely narrowed. The pale puckering of the intimal surface of the proximal aortic arch is highly suggestive of syphilitic aortitis (see Legends 1.69 et seq.).

This case shows both the effect of syphilis (the probable cause of the aneurysm) and of superimposed atheroma. The extent to which either pathological process led to this massive thrombosis cannot be determined accurately but, histologically, atheroma was the most probable cause.

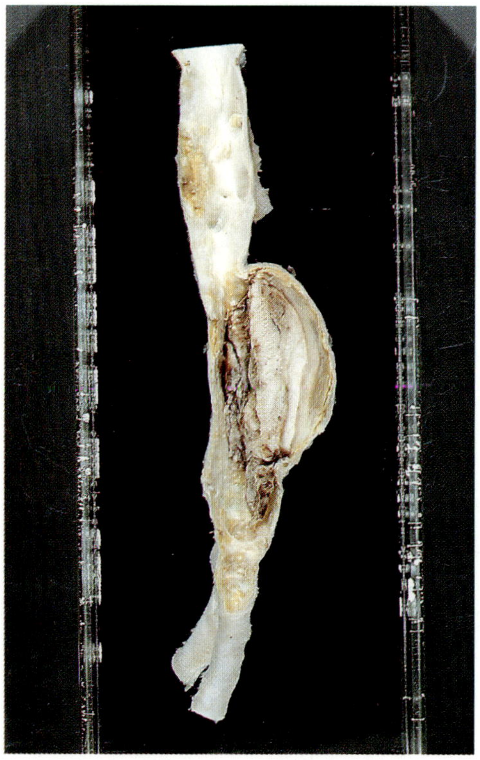

1.63 Abdominal Aorta: Atheromatous Saccular Aneurysm

This was an incidental finding at post-mortem in a 75-year-old woman, who died of a pulmonary embolism following a partial gastrectomy.

The abdominal aorta has been opened anteroposteriorly and is viewed from the right side. Projecting from the anterior surface, below the origin of the renal arteries, is a saccular aneurysm which measures 7cm in maximum diameter. The attenuated wall of the aneurysm shows calcific atheroma, as does the adjacent aorta and common iliac artery. The sac is filled with organised thrombus, which extends as a finger-like process towards the bifurcation.

Aneurysms, which are defined as localised dilatations of an arterial lumen, are a consequence of atheroma in the majority of cases (largely as a result of medial weakening). Atheromatous aneurysms, which are seen most often in elderly males, tend to affect predominantly the abdominal aorta or common iliac arteries. They typically adopt a fusiform or saccular configuration, as a consequence of the distending effects of an often elevated blood pressure.

Thrombosis within the aneurysmal sac almost invariably occurs and, to some extent, may delay or prevent rupture of the lesion which is the commonest and most dangerous complication. Rupture leads to massive haemorrhage, usually into the retroperitoneum or peritoneal cavity, and is very often fatal despite emergency surgical measures. Intrasaccular thrombus may, of itself, lead to gradual occlusion of the vascular lumen at the site of the aneurysm or may fragment, giving rise to systemic emboli (the consequences of which will depend on the vessel affected).

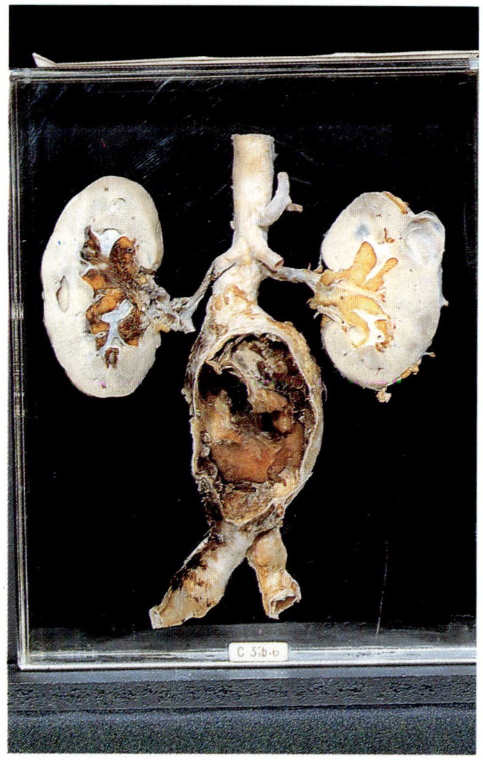

1.64 Abdominal Aorta: Ruptured Atheromatous Fusiform Aneurysm

This is a post-mortem specimen from a 57-year-old man who presented with acute severe pain in the right iliac fossa and collapsed. On admission to hospital, he was in severe hypotensive shock and there was a palpable abdominal mass. He died soon afterwards.

The abdominal aorta, with the kidneys and common iliac arteries, is viewed anteriorly. Distal to the origin of the renal arteries there is a fusiform aortic aneurysm, which measures 11cm in length and 7cm in maximum diameter. The aneurysmal sac has been opened to show extensive calcific atheroma of its walls and massive intraluminal organised and fresh thrombus. There had been extensive right-sided retroperitoneal haemorrhage in the fresh state, traces of which are apparent at the hilum of the right kidney and along the right common iliac artery.

This is a classical example of the commonest form of aneurysm in the Western world.

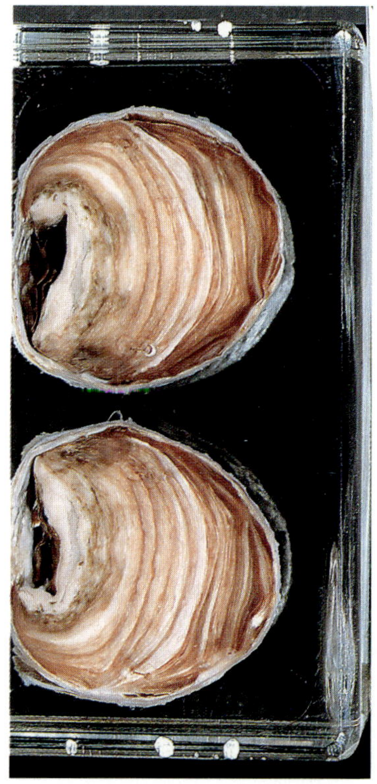

1.65 Abdominal Aorta: Atheromatous Aneurysm with Intraluminal Thrombosis

This was an incidental finding at post-mortem in a 77-year-old man who died of pneumonia.

This is a transverse section through a saccular aneurysm which was found just above the aortic bifurcation. The aortic wall is markedly attenuated and the lumen is virtually occluded by a mass of laminated, organised thrombus.

This case shows particularly well the appearances of progressive intra-aneurysmal thrombosis with luminal stenosis.

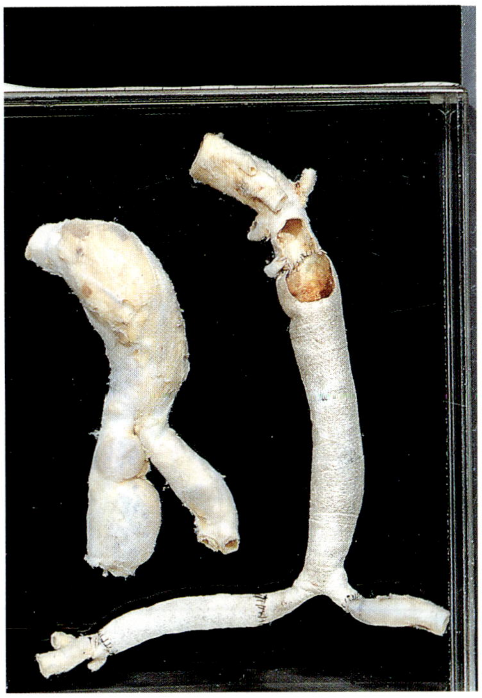

1.66 Abdominal Aorta: Aorto-bi-Iliac Synthetic Graft with Aneurysmectomy

These are surgical and post-mortem specimens from a 67-year-old man who presented with a pulsating abdominal mass. Laparotomy was performed at which a fusiform aortic aneurysm was found extending from just below the renal arteries to the bifurcation. There were further separate aneurysms of the common and internal iliac arteries. The aortic aneurysm was resected and replaced with a graft and the internal iliac arteries were ligated. Eight hours post-operatively, the patient developed an occlusion of the right external iliac artery which was treated by a further graft from the synthetic aorta to the right femoral artery. However, he died suddenly 15 hours after the second operation.

On the left is mounted the resected aortic aneurysm, which measures up to 4cm in diameter. Note also the fusiform dilatation of the left common iliac artery and the two saccular aneurysms of the right. On the right, the post-mortem specimen shows the synthetic grafts (that used to be made of Invalon) which were inserted.

The introduction of synthetic vascular grafts revolutionised the treatment of abdominal aortic aneurysms which, if left untreated, carry a high mortality. The results of surgery vary according to whether the aneurysmectomy is performed electively or as an emergency when the aneurysm has begun to leak. Under optimal conditions, the 5-year-survival and patency of the graft is approximately 90 per cent.

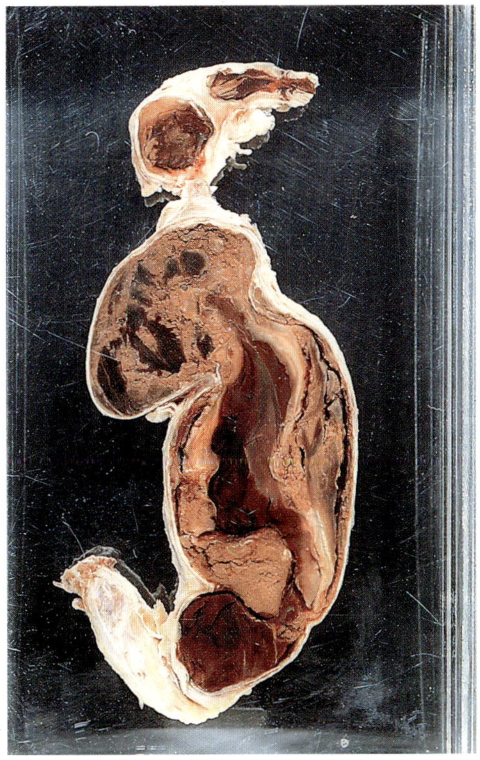

1.67 Popliteal Artery: Atheromatous Aneurysm

This specimen was resected from a 62-year-old man, who presented with a 2 week history of a painful right great toe associated more recently with progressive bluish discolouration of the rest of the right foot. There were palpable, pulsatile swellings in both popliteal fossae but no signs of ischaemia in the left leg. By-pass grafting of the aneurysm was not technically feasible and, shortly thereafter, a right above-knee amputation was performed.

This segment of the popliteal artery, which has been dissected from the amputation specimen, shows a large, fusiform aneurysmal sac, measuring 12.5cm in length and 5cm in maximum diameter. The wall of the aneurysm and adjacent artery are atheromatous and the lumen is focally occluded by laminated and fresh thrombus.

The major lower limb arteries are the most frequent site of atheromatous aneurysms after the abdominal aorta. In the leg, where such aneurysms are often multiple, ischaemic complications (due to occlusion or embolism) are much more common than rupture.

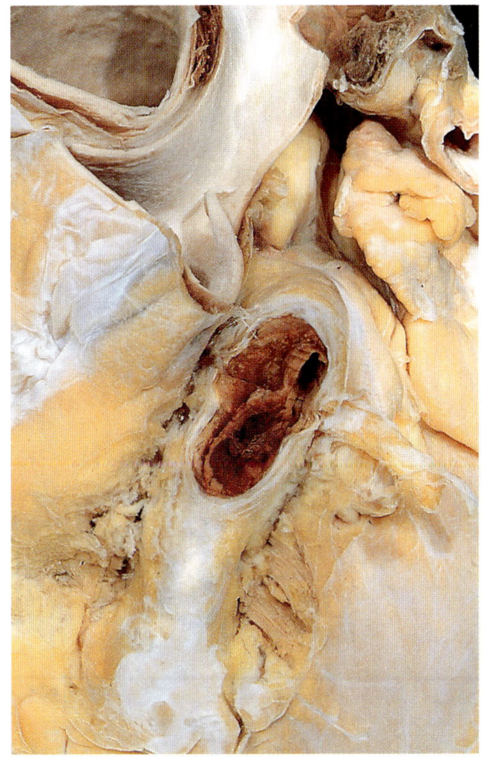

1.68 Coronary Artery: Atheromatous Aneurysm with Thrombosis

This is a post-mortem specimen from a 77-year-old woman, who died suddenly of a dissecting thoracic aortic aneurysm.

On the anterior surface of the heart, the left anterior descending coronary artery shows a fusiform aneurysmal dilatation which measures 1cm in diameter. The aneurysm has been opened to show that the vessel wall is atheromatous and the lumen is totally occluded by thrombus. It should be stressed that this lesion was anatomically quite separate from the dissecting aortic aneurysm.

As already stated, atheromatous fusiform aneurysms are most common in the abdominal aorta or the major arteries of the lower limb. They may occasionally be seen in smaller arteries, as in this case. Other rare causes of coronary artery aneurysms include polyarteritis nodosa and a congenital malformation connecting the artery to the coronary sinus (cirsoid aneurysm, see Figure and Legend 1.58).

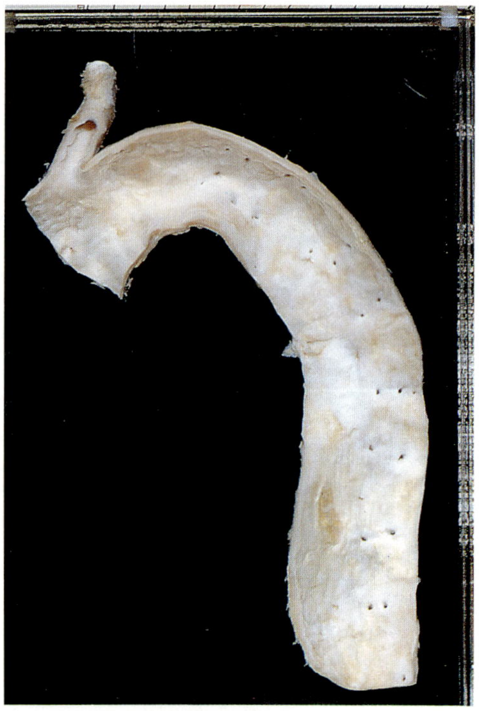

1.69 Thoracic Aorta: Syphilitic Aortitis

This is a post-mortem specimen from a 67-year-old woman, who died following a skull fracture. At autopsy the aortic valve was incompetent and there was left ventricular hypertrophy.

The distal aortic arch and descending thoracic aorta have been opened to show numerous small white plaques, separated by irregular thin grooved scars; this appearance is sometimes likened to tree-bark. In addition there are a few, uncomplicated yellowish plaques of atheroma.

Syphilitic aortitis is the commonest complication of tertiary infection but is only of clinical significance in a small proportion of cases. Pathogenetically a florid arteritis of the vasa vasorum leads to medial necrosis with scarring and intimal fibrosis. As a consequence the aortic wall is weakened and thereby dilatation often ensues, sometimes with aneurysm formation. In addition, the ostia of the coronary arteries may be narrowed by adjacent intimal fibrosis and the aortic valve often becomes incompetent due to dilatation of the valve ring and fibrosis of the valve cusps.

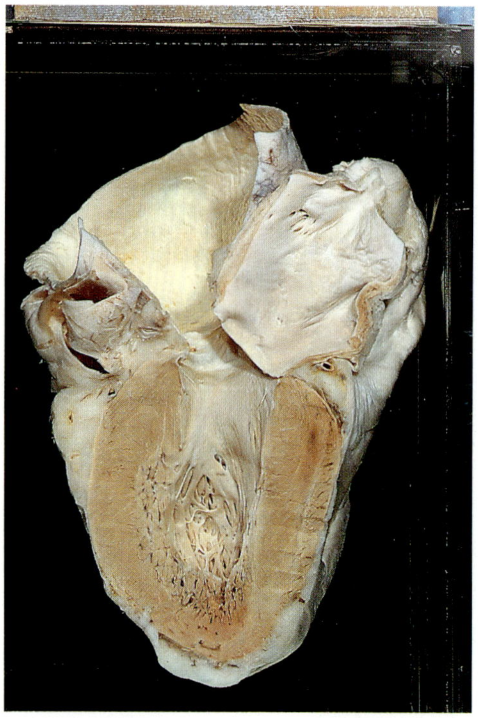

1.70 Ascending Aorta and Aortic Valve: Syphilis

This is a post-mortem specimen from a 71-year-old woman who collapsed and died suddenly of a coronary thrombosis. At autopsy, there was an aneurysm of the aortic arch.

The heart and proximal aorta have been opened; the aortic intima is pale and puckered and there is marked dilatation. The leaflets of the aortic valve are fibrotic and shortened, leading to incompetence which, in turn, has given rise to left ventricular hypertrophy. The posterior wall of the ventricle shows ischaemic scarring but the terminal infarct is not evident in this view.

These are the typical appearances of syphilitic aortitis, which is usually most severe in the proximal aorta and tends to tail off towards the diaphragm.

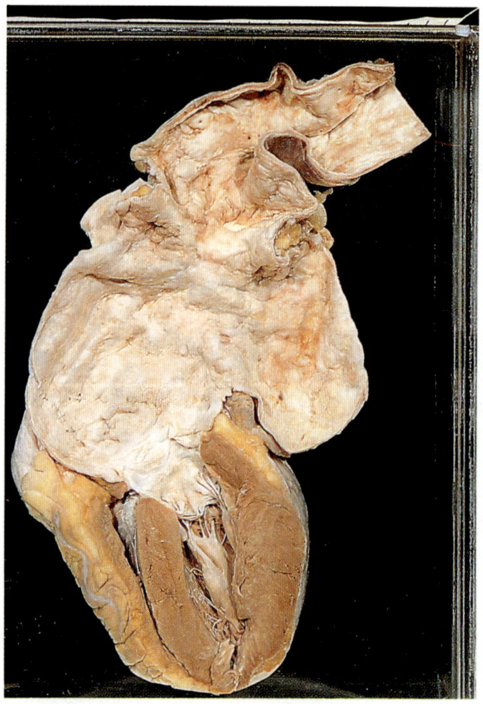

1.71 Ascending Aorta: Syphilitic Saccular Aneurysm

This was an incidental finding at post-mortem in a 75-year-old woman, who died suddenly of a coronary thrombosis.

The heart, ascending aorta and aortic arch are viewed anteriorly. There is a large saccular aneurysm of the ascending aorta, which measures 16cm in length and 10cm in maximum diameter. The intimal surface shows the typical fibrosis and scarring of the syphilitic aortitis with superimposed atheromatous plaques. Note also the left ventricular hypertrophy.

As already stated, aneurysmal dilatation of the proximal aorta, which may be fusiform or saccular, is a common complication of syphilitic aortitis (see Legends 1.69 and 1.70). Erosion or compression of adjacent structures, such as trachea or oesophagus, commonly ensues and rupture is almost invariably fatal. Syphilis is by far the commonest cause of aneurysms in the thoracic aorta but, surprisingly, only infrequently gives rise to similar lesions elsewhere.

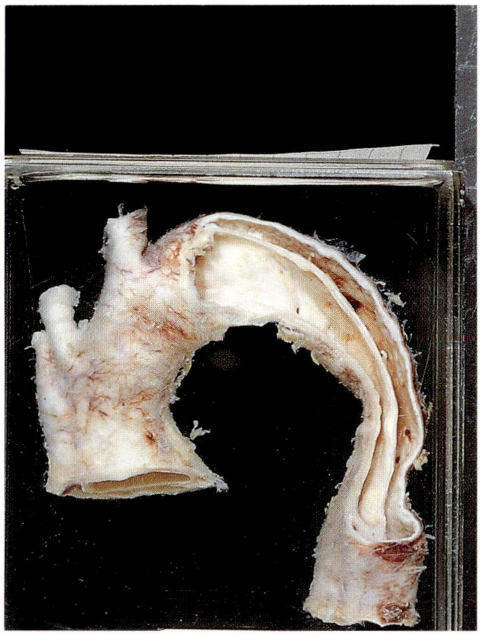

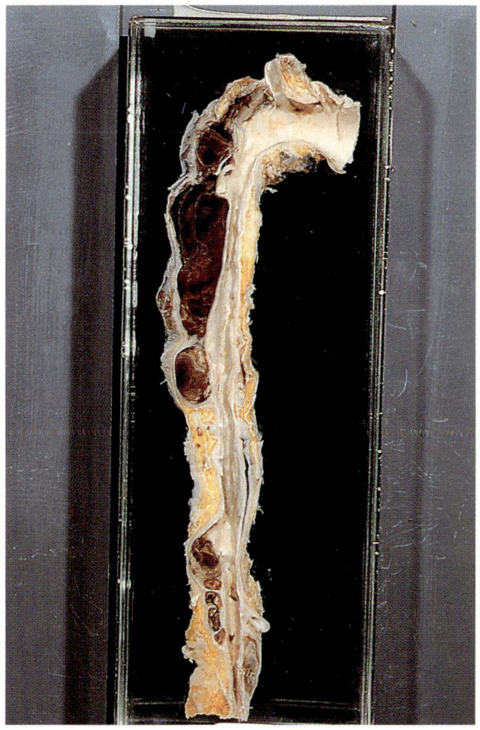

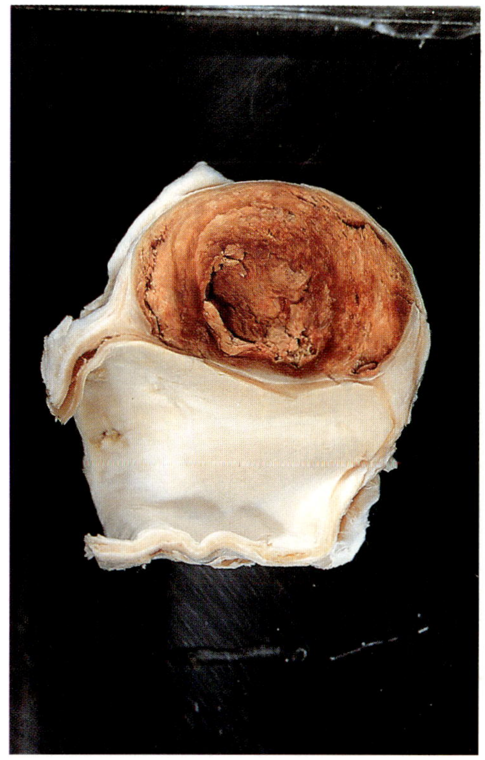

1.72 Thoracic Aorta: Dissecting Aneurysm

This is a post-mortem specimen from a 68-year-old man, known to have chronic bronchitis and cardiac failure who, following an acute episode of non-specific abdominal pain, collapsed and died. At autopsy there was a haemopericardium, due to a ruptured dissecting aneurysm.

The aortic arch has been partially opened to show a portion of this patient's dissecting aneurysm which, in the fresh state, extended from the aortic valve to the lower thorax. Note the double-barrelled lumen distal to the origin of the left subclavian artery; the wall of the 'false' lumen (above) is formed of the aortic adventitia and media (Erdheim's necrosis).

Dissecting aneurysms, which occur predominantly in the aorta, are characterised by the passage of blood into the vessel wall (through an intimal tear) where an intramural false lumen develops. This condition is commonest in the elderly, particularly males, and is most often the result of idiopathic mucoid degeneration of the media (Erdheim), frequently with coexistent hypertension. It is occasionally familial and is a well-recognised complication of Marfan's syndrome. The distance over which the false intramural lumen extends is extremely variable, but may reach as far as the lower limbs. Possible consequences include external rupture (which is usually fatal), internal rupture back into the true lumen (which may allow prolonged survival), and stenosis of arteries arising from the aorta, the lumen of which may be severely compressed by the intramural dissection.

1.73 Aorta: Dissecting and Saccular Aneurysms

This is a post-mortem specimen from a 58-year-old woman. No further clinical details are available.

The distal aortic arch, descending and abdominal aorta have been opened to show two separate lesions. Just distal to the origin of the left subclavian artery, there is an irregular intimal tear which communicates with a dissecting aneurysm, measuring 15cm in length. This lesion is filled with fresh thrombus. Distal to the origin of the renal arteries is a saccular atheromatous aneurysm, measuring 1cm in diameter. This lesion has ruptured into adjacent soft tissues, leaving a false aneurysm, 4cm in length, filled with organised thrombus.

The coexistence of these two lesions is probably fortuitous. The proximal aneurysm is entirely typical, while the lower one demonstrates well the difference between true and false aneurysms, the former being lined by a vessel wall and the latter simply being a localised haemorrhage, walled off by fibrous tissue.

1.74 Ascending Aorta: Localised Dissecting Aneurysm

This was an incidental finding at post-mortem in a 76-year-old woman, who died of cerebral infarction.

This short segment of the ascending aorta, measuring 3cm in length, has been opened to show a localised cavity containing organised blood clot in the aortic wall. At the lower left of the specimen, the proximal part of the mural dissection is visible although the actual intimal tear, which (in the fresh state) had healed, is not apparent in this view.

Dissecting aneurysms do, occasionally, remain very localised (as here) and may be entirely asymptomatic. In this circumstance, the intimal tear usually heals and the intramural blood clot is gradually organised into fibrous scar tissue.

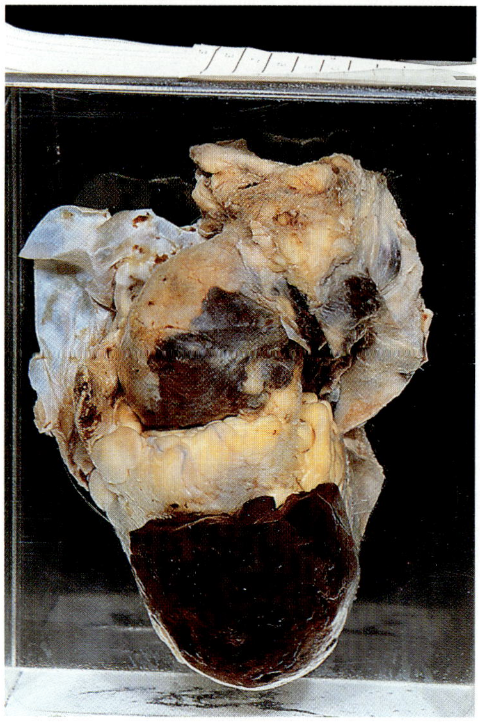

1.75 Haemopericardium due to a Dissecting Aortic Aneurysm

This is a post-mortem specimen from a 66-year-old woman who was known to be hypertensive and who had complained of pain in the chest and neck for 3 days prior to dying suddenly. At autopsy there was also a large cerebral haemorrhage.

The pericardium has been dissected off the heart to show a large mass of blood clot which filled the pericardial sac in the fresh state. This haemopericardium has resulted from bleeding through a tear in the wall of the intrapericardial segment of the ascending aorta (upper right) which, in turn, had resulted from a dissecting aneurysm in the aortic arch. The aneurysm has been left intact but the blood within it is visible through the attenuated aortic adventitia (top right).

The commonest complication of dissecting aneurysm is rupture through the outer vessel wall and, in the aorta, this most often results in massive intrapericardial or intrapleural haemorrhage which is almost always rapidly fatal. Retrograde dissection of such a lesion in the thoracic aorta may also occasionally give rise to myocardial infarction by disrupting and occluding the ostia of the coronary arteries.

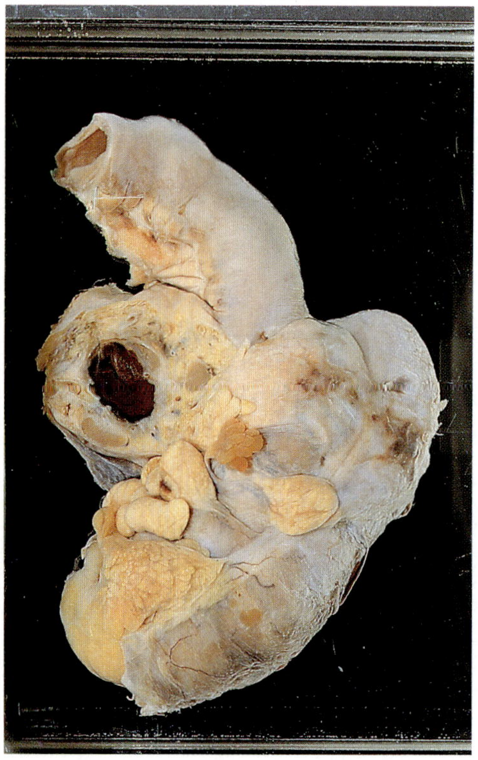

1.76 Ileocolic Artery: Mycotic Aneurysm

This specimen was excised from a 31-year-old man, who presented with severe abdominal pain and, at laparotomy, was found to have a leaking aneurysm of the ileocolic artery. One month previously he had been discharged from hospital following a 2 month episode of bacterial endocarditis due to *Streptococcus viridans*, which had responded to penicillin.

The distal ileum, caecum and proximal ascending colon with attached mesentery are shown. In the mesenteric fat is a rounded sac, measuring 2cm in diameter which is filled with fresh thrombus. The ileocolic artery is just visible entering the aneurysm at its superior aspect.

Mycotic aneurysms result from damage and weakening of an arterial wall due to colonisation by micro-organisms. These organisms (usually bacteria) infect the vessel by being deposited within a septic embolus, most often from vegetations in bacterial endocarditis. Such aneurysms are usually small but show a marked tendency to early leakage or rupture.

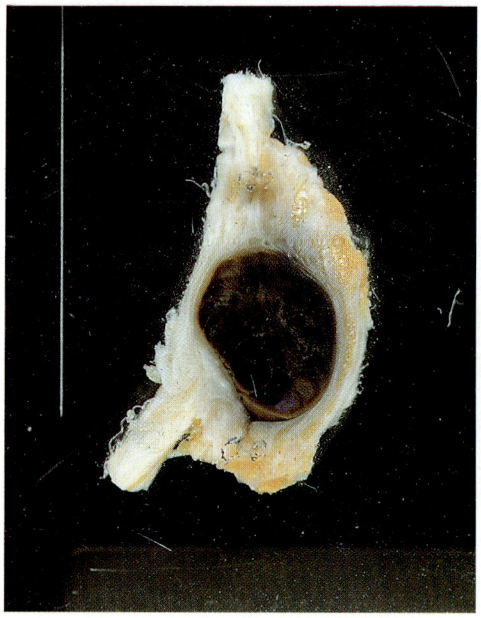

1.77 Radial Artery: Traumatic Aneurysm

This specimen was excised from a 55-year-old woman. One month previously she had been bitten on the wrist by a dog. Bleeding was controlled by local sutures but a fortnight later a swelling, which grew rapidly in the next week, developed under the scar.

Projecting from this portion of the radial artery is a saccular aneurysm, measuring 1.5cm in diameter, which contains fresh thrombus. The aneurysm is surrounded by a thin layer of fibrous tissue.

Traumatic aneurysms, which are a direct result of penetrating injury to an arterial wall, are usually 'false' in nature, in other words, they represent a localised, walled-off haemorrhage.

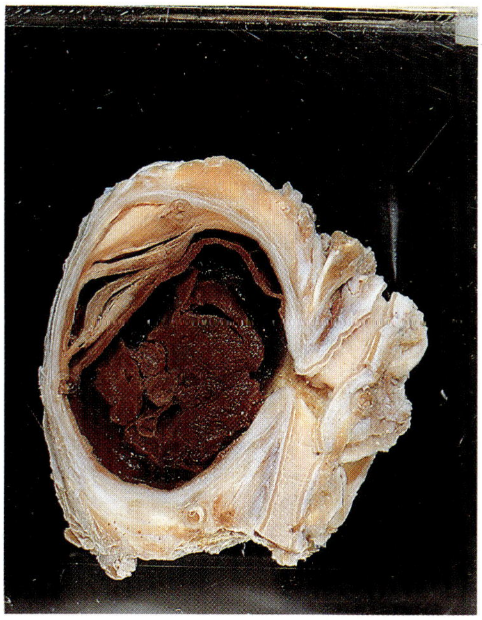

1.78 Femoral Artery: Traumatic Aneurysm

This specimen was excised from a 29-year-old soldier who had sustained a bullet wound in the thigh 5 months previously. Following the injury, he had developed cardiomegaly and a tachycardia indicative of an arteriovenous fistula.

Segments of the femoral artery and vein have been opened to show rounded openings in the walls of both vessels, which communicate with an aneurysmal sac, measuring 4cm in diameter. The sac contains laminated and fresh thrombus.

Penetrating arterial injuries are frequently associated with similar damage to the adjacent vein and a communication often develops between the two. In this circumstance the vein may become markedly dilated and the lesion may be referred to as a varicose aneurysm.

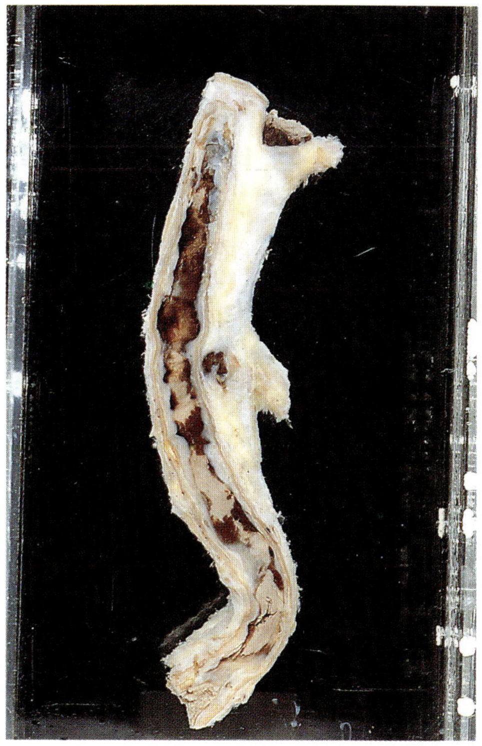

1.79 Femoral Artery: Thrombosis

This specimen was excised from a 76-year-old man, who developed ischaemic gangrene of the left lower leg and underwent mid-thigh amputation.

The distal portion of the femoral artery has been opened to show complete luminal occlusion over a considerable length by pale laminated thrombus; the wall is atheromatous. The femoral vein (right) is also thrombosed (visible at the superior aspect).

Thrombosis of this extent in a major artery is usually a consequence of embolisation, most often from the heart in which mural thrombosis may complicate a myocardial infarct or atrial fibrillation. Thrombus may also become dislodged from an aortic aneurysmal sac. Other local causes of arterial thrombosis include complicated atheroma and trauma. Pain and pallor develop rapidly in the affected limb and, unless surgical intervention is prompt, dry gangrene supervenes.

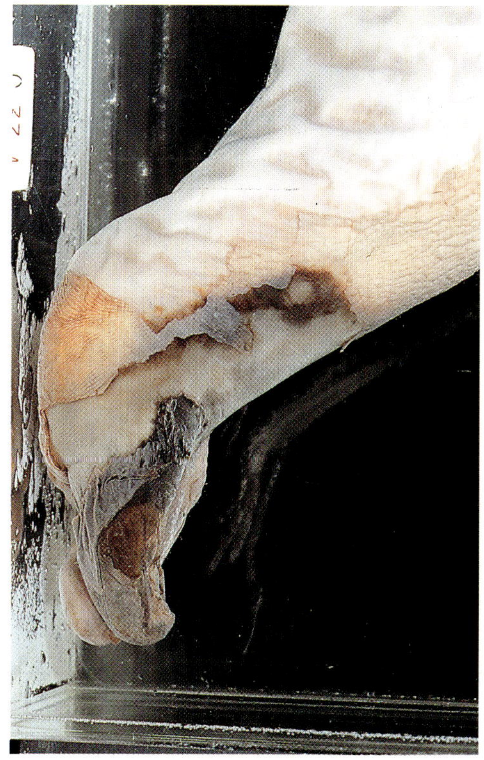

1.80 Foot: Ischaemic Gangrene

This is an amputation specimen from an 85-year-old man who presented with severe pain and paraesthesia in the left calf and foot. Examination revealed dark discolouration of the left great toe and one week later an above-knee amputation was performed.

There is marked blackish discolouration of the great toe and some adjacent skin. In addition much of the skin of the dorsum and sole of the foot is greyish, translucent and obviously necrotic.

Ischaemic ('dry') gangrene of a limb, which is predominantly seen in the leg, nearly always results from arterial occlusion proximally. This may be due to extensive atheroma with superadded thrombosis, an embolus (usually from the heart or a fragmented atheromatous plaque), thrombo-angiitis obliterans (Buerger's disease), or Raynaud's disease. Other causes include trauma and physical damage such as burning, freezing, trench foot or irradiation. Very rarely, venous gangrene may occur in which circumstance very extensive deep venous thrombosis leads to peripheral circulatory impairment (see Figure and Legend 1.84).

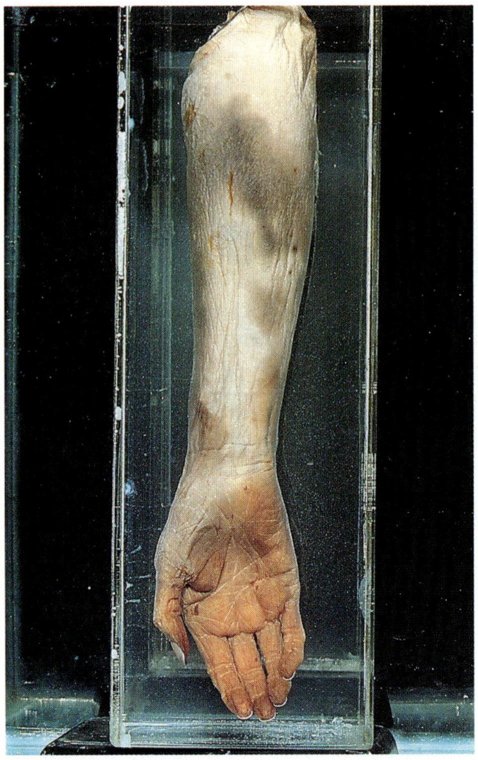

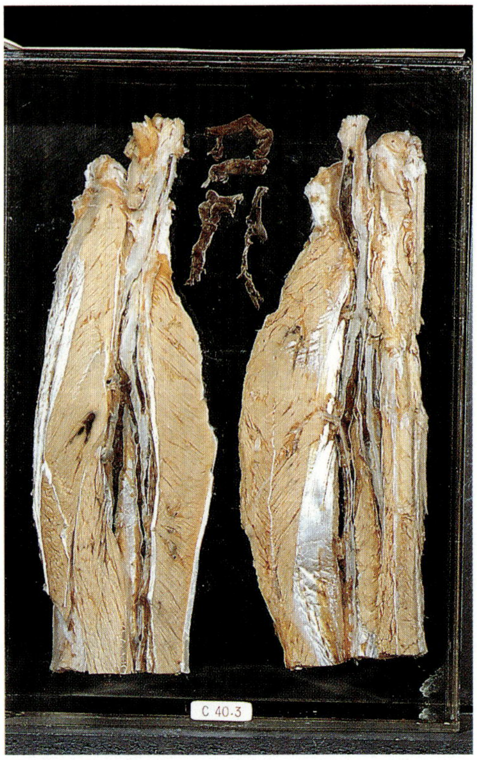

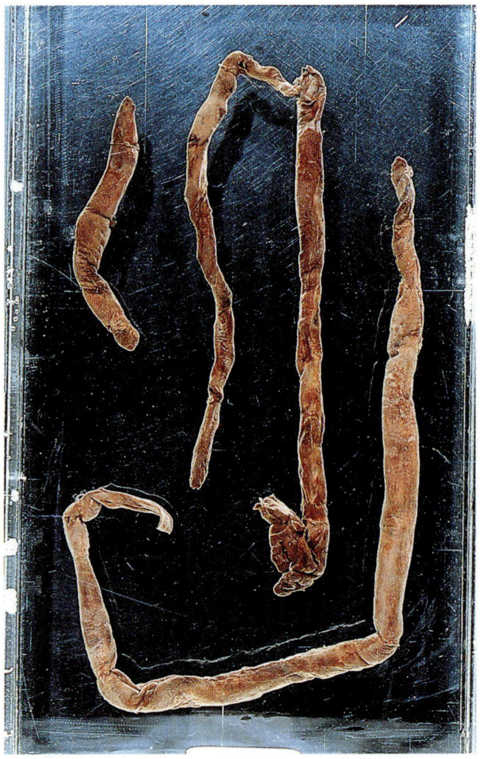

1.81 Arm: Ischaemic Gangrene

This is an amputation specimen from a 74-year-old woman, who presented with severe pain with anaesthesia and paralysis of the right arm. An embolus was removed from the axillary artery and the circulation to the limb was restored. The symptoms recurred 4 days post-operatively and gangrene rapidly developed, so the limb was amputated. The source of the emboli was thought to be endocardial thrombus due to atrial fibrillation.

The right lower arm, which has been amputated just above the elbow, shows extensive, multifocal gangrene with reddish-brown and black discolouration. Note the well-marked line of demarcation at the wrist.

Ischaemic gangrene of the arm is much less common than in the leg.

1.82 Calf Muscles: Deep Venous Thromboses

These are post-mortem specimens from a 62-year-old woman who collapsed and died 8 days after an exploratory laparotomy for ovarian carcinoma. Autopsy revealed multiple pulmonary emboli.

The calf musculature of both this patient's legs has been dissected to display the deep veins. The veins have been opened to demonstrate extensive thromboses. Between these two specimens are mounted several of the emboli removed from the patient's pulmonary arteries.

Deep venous thrombosis, which occurs principally in the lower limb musculature, is a very common condition. However, the true incidence is uncertain since many such thromboses, and sometimes pulmonary emboli, may remain clinically inapparent. In general terms, the principal pathogenetic factors which predispose to venous thrombosis are encompassed in Virchow's triad:

1) an alteration in the vessel wall;
2) an alteration in the blood flow, or
3) an alteration in the blood constituents (particularly with regard to coagulability).

The commonest causes are prolonged immobility (particularly after surgical operation), parturition, myocardial infarction, any debilitating illness (such as cancer), oral contraceptives, varicose veins or phlebitis, and any abnormality of coagulability (such as thrombocythaemia or polycythaemia). Much the most important complication is, of couse, pulmonary embolism (see Chapter 2).

1.83 Pulmonary Artery: Unfolded Embolus

This is a post-mortem specimen from a 64-year-old man, who suddenly collapsed and died 7 days after undergoing transvesical prostatectomy. At autopsy, one of the pulmonary arteries and its main branches were tightly plugged with thrombus and thrombi were detected in the deep veins of both calves.

The main portion of the pulmonary embolus has been unfolded to show its considerable length (over 60cm in total) and its calibre, which corresponds well with that of the major limb veins.

Large propagated thrombi such as this often give rise to massive pulmonary embolism (see Chapter 3) and sudden death.

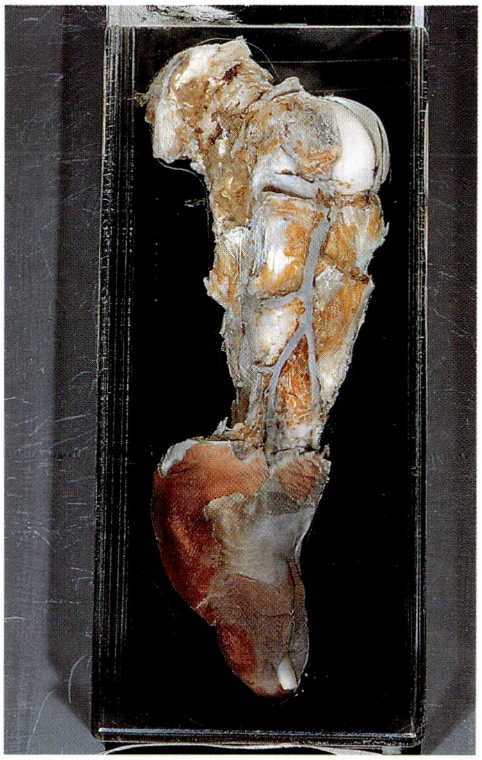

1.84 Foot: Venous Thrombosis with Gangrene

This is an amputation specimen from a 62-year-old woman who was admitted to hospital with a pulmonary embolism. Despite treatment with anticoagulants the left leg became cold, swollen and adopted a livid appearance. Circulation gradually returned except to the toes, which became gangrenous, and a Syme's amputation was performed. Venography had revealed extensive thrombosis of the femoral and great saphenous veins.

The left foot has been dissected to show established gangrene of the great toe (the other toes not seen in this view had a similar appearance). All the veins displayed are completely occluded by thrombus.

Venous gangrene, known as phlegmasia caerulea dolens, is extremely uncommon. It occurs when there is such massive and extensive deep venous thrombosis in the limb that blood flow becomes completely obstructed and the arterial supply is consequently impaired.

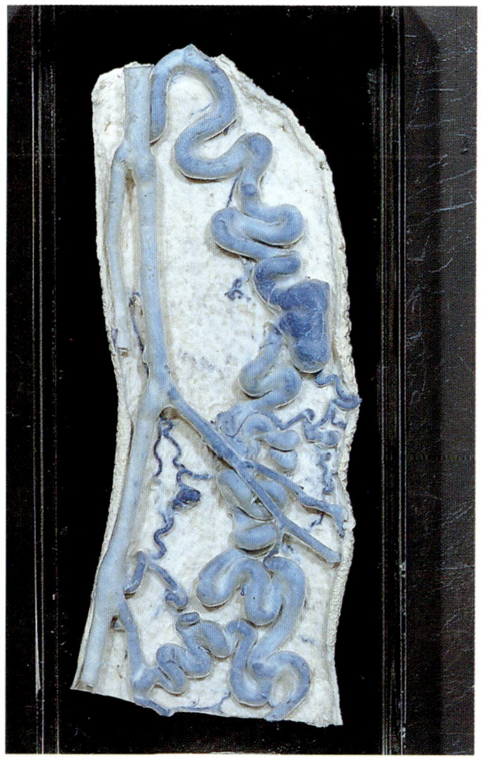

1.85 Leg: Varicose Veins

No clinical details are available.

The superficial veins of the inner side of the leg have been injected with dye to show a normal great saphenous vein (left) and a markedly dilated and tortuous, varicose vein running alongside and entering it above.

Varicose veins are defined as veins that have become irreversibly dilated and tortuous. Those of the lower limb are affected in the vast majority of cases of this very common condition, which is seen most often in young or middle-aged adults, particularly females. The majority of such lesions are thought to be due to an inherited or idiopathic abnormality of the venous walls or valves which, combined with the erect human posture, cannot accommodate the high venous pressure. Aggravating factors include prolonged standing or upright physical activity, pregnancy and congestive cardiac failure. A small proportion of cases occur secondarily to previous deep venous thrombosis.

Complications include phlebitis, oedema, epidermal atrophy, cutaneous ulceration and, very occasionally, haemorrhage.

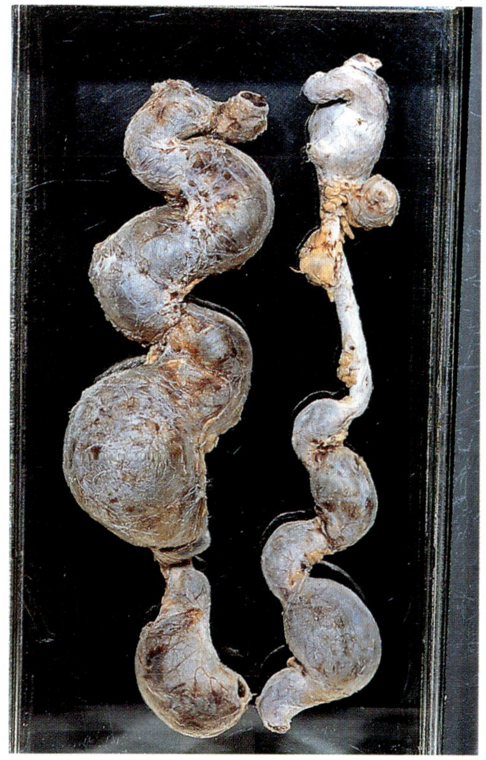

1.86 Leg: Varicose Veins

No clinical details are available.

Two segments of excised saphenous vein show marked tortuosity and dilatation, particularly that on the right.

These are the typical appearances of varicose veins.

2. RESPIRATORY SYSTEM

UPPER RESPIRATORY TRACT

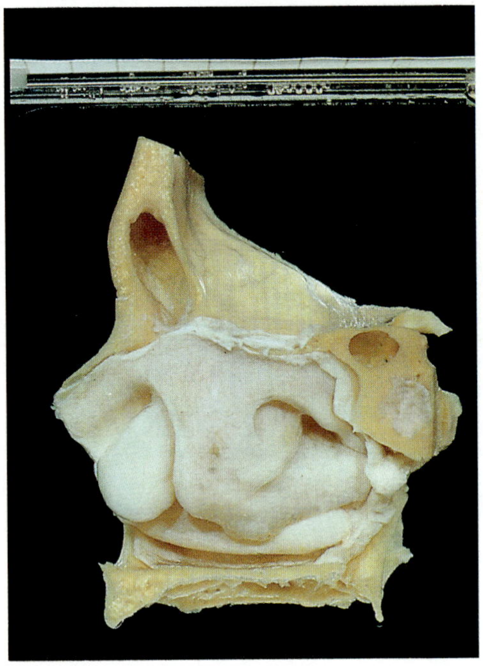

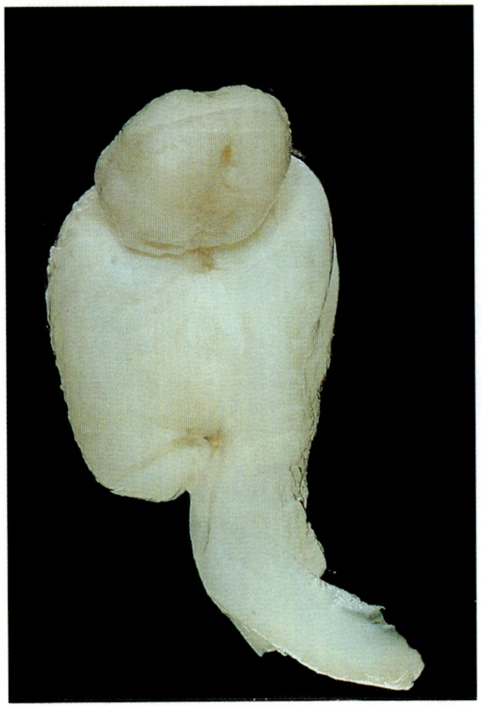

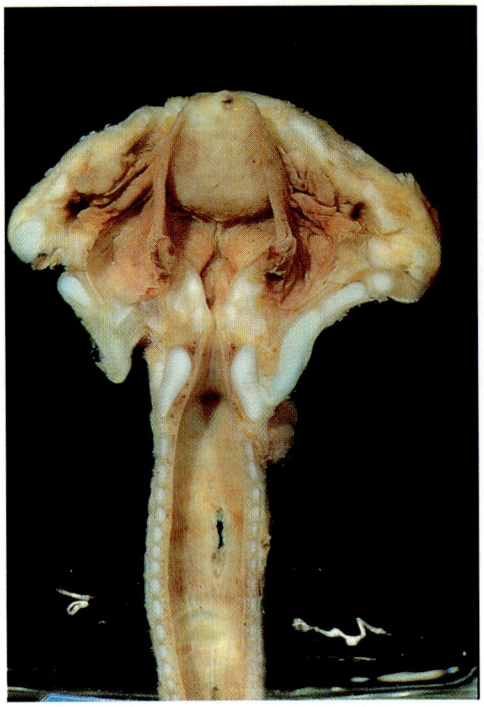

2.1 Nasal Fossa: Nasal Polyp

No clinical details are available.

This is a dissection of the right nasal fossa, showing a polypoid mass of oedematous tissue projecting from the lateral wall just anterior to the middle concha.

Nasal polyps are very common and represent protuberant oedematous epithelium of the nasal air passages. They arise most often in adulthood, particularly in men, and may be allergic or nonallergic in type. In obstructing the air passages, the nostrils become dilated and the external appearance of the nose may be altered, the polyps giving rise to broadening and obvious enlargement of the nose. Aetiologically, these polyps are thought to result from long-standing rhinitis or sinusitis in most cases.

2.2 Nose: Allergic Nasal Poylp

This specimen was excised from a 6-year-old boy who had had asthma since infancy and had developed progressive nasal obstruction over the previous 3 years.

The lesion is rounded, lobulated and gelatinous, measuring 3 × 1 × 1cm. Note the narrow smooth pedicle to which it is attached, being a further 2cm in length.

The allergic variant of nasal polyps are classically very oedematous, owing to the persistent local increase in vascular permeability due to recurrent Type I hypersensitivity reactions. They are classically seen in allergic rhinitis and hay fever.

2.3 Larynx: Congenital Stricture

This is a post-mortem specimen from a 2-year-old female infant who had suffered from frequent attacks of stridor and dyspnoea since birth. Latterly a tracheostomy was required but she died of pneumonia.

The larynx and trachea of the infant have been opened from behind to show a tight stricture at the level of the vocal cords, the glottic orifice being reduced to less than 1mm in diameter. The arytenoid cartilages are closely approximated and their vocal processes appear reduced in size. The laryngeal epithelium appears normal with no evidence of inflammation or scarring.

The aetiology of this laryngeal stenosis is not apparent. Recognised causes of a congenital laryngeal stricture include external compression of whatever source, a laryngeal web, a dermoid cyst, or congenital syphilis, of which the case here may be an example. Acquired stenoses, more often seen in adults, usually follow severe local inflammation, whether infective, chemical or traumatic in origin.

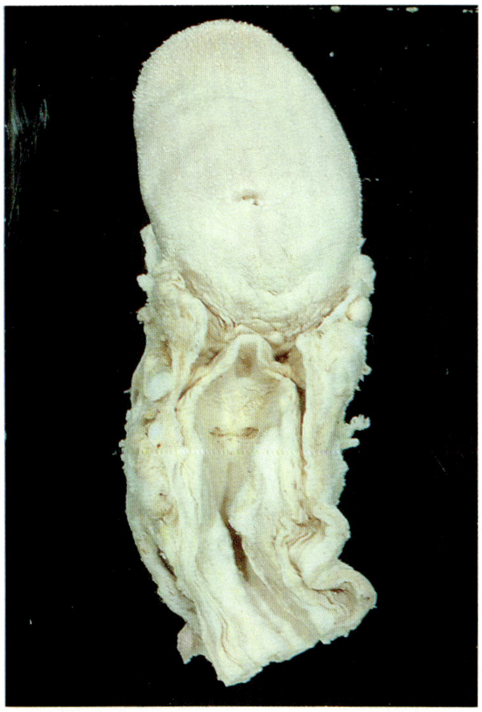

2.4 Larynx: Laryngomalacia

This is a post-mortem specimen from a 4-month-old boy who was found dead in his cot. He had suffered from intermittent stridor since birth and had also been noted to have multiple congenital skeletal malformations.

The tongue with the larynx and trachea, opened posteriorly, are shown. There is dilatation of the laryngeal lumen. The epiglottis is mildly enlarged and has a tubular contour.

Laryngomalacia is an extremely rare congenital anomaly, normally seen in association with similar changes in the trachea. The underlying abnormality at both sites is excessive flacidity or softening of their cartilaginous component. This leads to collapse of the laryngeal or tracheal walls with consequent stridor. A very few cases have been reported due to either polychondritis or congenitally absent cartilage. Most often, in otherwise fit children, the condition remits spontaneously in the 2nd or 3rd year of life.

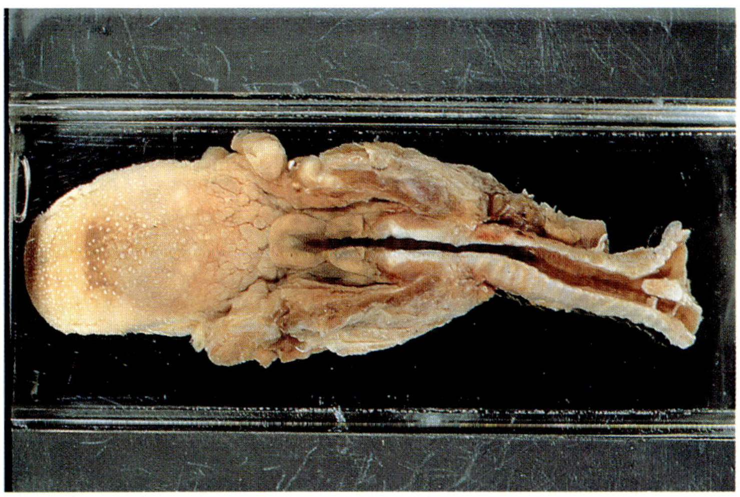

2.5 Larynx: Acute Epiglottitis

This is a post-mortem specimen from a 4-year-old girl who initially complained of a sore throat. She rapidly became very ill with severe dyspnoea and, despite all resuscitative measures, died approximately 20 hours after the onset of her illness. Culture of a laryngeal swab yielded a heavy growth of *Haemophilus influenzae* Type B.

The tongue with the larynx and trachea, opened posteriorly, are shown. There is intense swelling, with congestion, of the epiglottis and aryepiglottic folds. Note also the site of the tracheostomy, which was performed shortly before death, at the lower pole of the thyroid.

Acute epiglottitis is commonest in children between the ages of 2 and 7 years but is occasionally seen in adults. It is a rare illness of very rapid onset and the vast majority of cases are due to *Haemophilus influenzae.* While an associated septicaemia is common, in fatal cases death usually results from asphyxia due to severe epiglottic oedema.

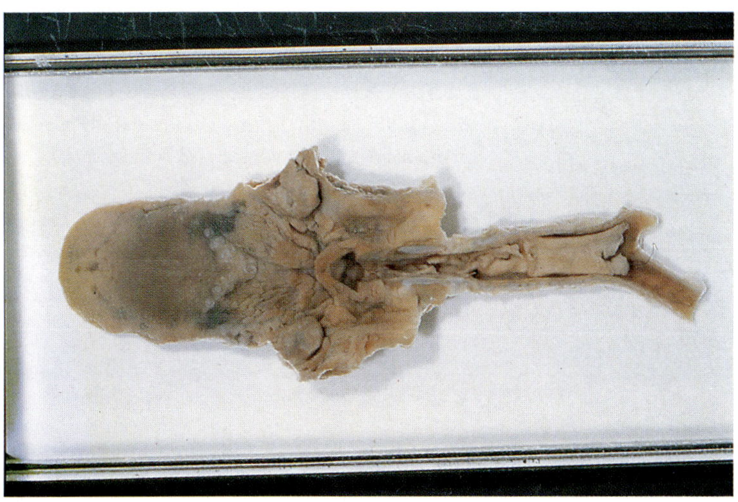

2.6 Larynx and Trachea: Diphtheria

This is a post-mortem specimen from an 8-year-old girl who, having apparently had a coryzal illness with a sore throat for one week, rapidly became dyspnoeic and died.

The tongue with the larynx, trachea and main bronchi, opened from behind, are shown. There is very marked laryngeal oedema and the characteristic false 'membrane', composed of ulcerated and sloughed respiratory mucosa, is clearly visible and extends as far as the main bronchi.

Diphtheria is due to infection by the Gram-positive bacillus *Corynebacterium diphtheriae.* This disease has become very rare in the Western world, largely as a result of improved living standards and immunisation, but remains an important cause of death in developing, dusty countries. The infection is most often respiratory, due to airborne droplet spread, but very occasionally diphtheritic wound infections occur. Small children are most often affected and, in addition to respiratory symptoms, systemic effects due to the elaboration of a potent exotoxin are usually seen; these include cardiac failure and polyneuritis.

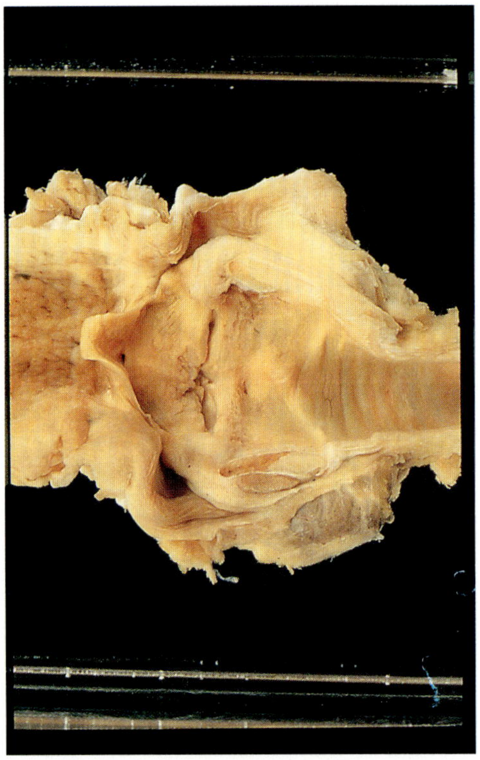

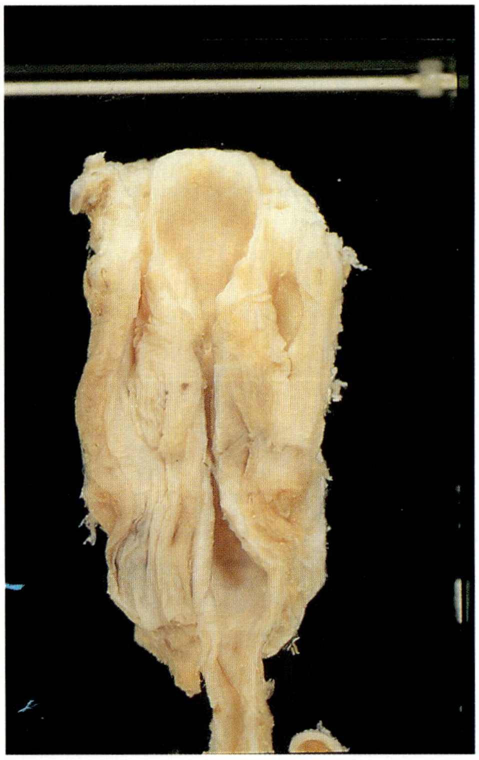

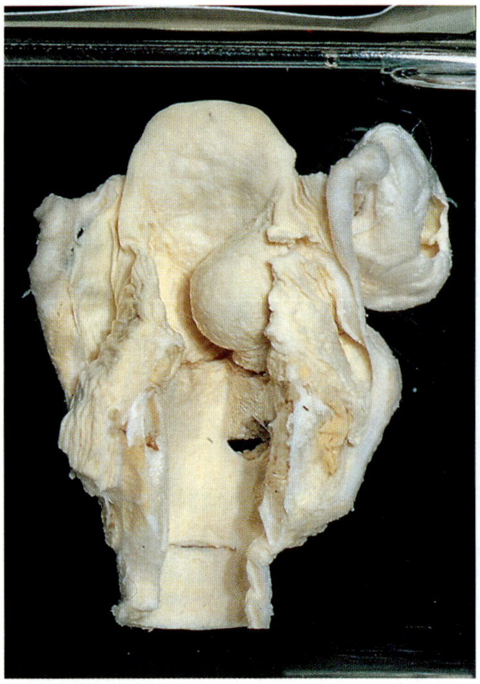

2.7 Larynx: Tuberculosis

This was an incidental finding at post-mortem in a 62-year-old diabetic woman who died of carcinomatosis. At autopsy, extensive pulmonary tuberculosis was also found.

The tongue and larynx, opened from behind, are shown. There is irregular, superficial mucosal ulceration in the region of the vocal cords.

Tuberculous laryngitis is comparatively uncommon but most often occurs in association with florid pulmonary infection. Extensive ulceration, as seen here, is characteristic and may extend to involve underlying cartilage. Prolonged infection frequently leads to extensive fibrosis with laryngeal stenosis and, clinically, such cases may be confused with a carcinoma. It should be noted that, occasionally, tuberculous laryngitis may predispose to the development of squamous carcinoma of the larynx.

2.8 Trachea: Syphilitic Stricture

This is a post-mortem specimen from a 73-year-old woman who had suffered from chronic laryngitis for several years. She had recently developed fainting attacks and died suddenly. At autopsy there was marked aortic incompetence and a fusiform aneurysm of the aortic arch.

The larynx and trachea have been opened posteriorly to show a tight tracheal stricture and irregular mucosal scarring.

Syphilitic laryngitis may be congenital or acquired and may take any of 3 forms: a primary chancre, which is extremely rare; secondary infection, which is manifest as mucosal congestion, or perichondritis; and tertiary infection, which may give rise to gummatous inflammation or ulceration. Scarring associated with either congenital infection or perichondritis occasionally results in stricture formation, as seen in this case.

2.9 Larynx: Mucous Cyst

This is a post-mortem specimen from a 50-year-old woman who presented with a 3 year history of hoarseness and dyspnoea. Laryngoscopy revealed a sessile cyst adjacent to the right aryepiglottic fold from which mucoid fluid was aspirated. The cyst, however, refilled over the next week and surgical excision was proposed. At operation, the patient's neck was extended for the purpose of intubation and respiratory arrest occurred from which she could not be resuscitated.

The larynx has been opened posteriorly to show a rounded cyst, measuring 1.5cm in diameter, just above the right aryepiglottic fold. This cyst is connected by a thin channel with a larger cyst situated in front of the hyoid bone, outside the larynx. Note the laryngotomy incision, beneath the cyst, which was performed during the attempted resuscitation.

Such laryngeal cysts most often arise as a consequence of obstruction of mucous glands, either due to inflammation or scarring. Lateral extension, as seen here, is unusual, but may indicate that this particular cyst arose as a consequence of degenerative mucoid change in the adjacent cartilage, as occasionally happens. Laryngeal cysts may be complicated by secondary infections or may attain a size sufficient to produce respiratory obstruction. In the case here, it was thought that extension of the neck led to the contents of the outer cyst being forced into the intralaryngeal moiety, thus producing complete laryngeal occlusion.

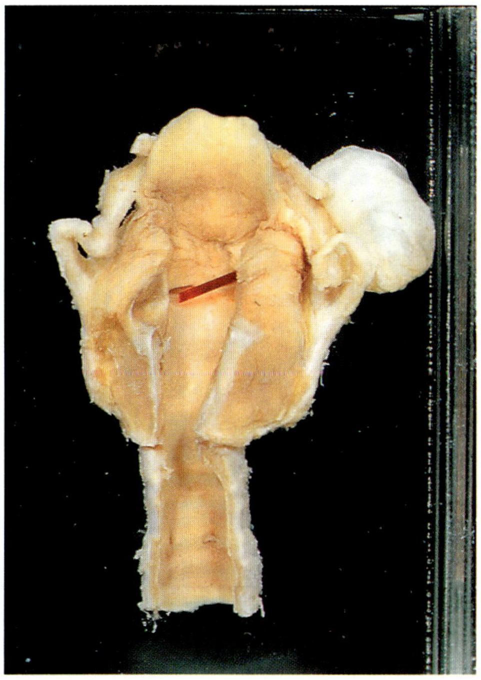

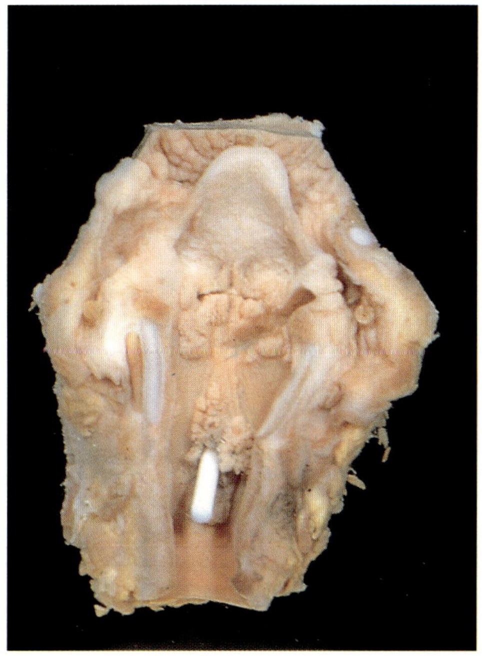

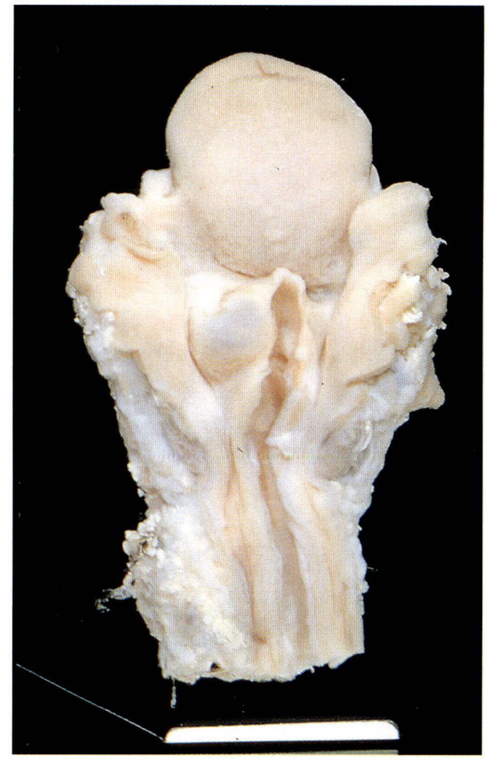

2.10 Larynx: Ventricular Laryngocele

This specimen was excised from a 40-year-old woman who had noticed a swelling in the neck since childhood. The lesion varied in size and could be enlarged by forced expiration. There were no laryngeal symptoms.

The larynx and upper trachea have been opened posteriorly to show a thin-walled, air-filled sac, situated outside the larynx anteriorly. The narrow aperture by which it communicates with the larynx is indicated by a small, red probe.

A laryngocele represents an air-filled cystic lesion of the laryngeal ventricle or saccule which is effectively a herniation or diverticulum of the laryngeal mucosa. It is comparable to the naturally-occurring cervical air pouches found in some species of monkey. It is probable, however, that this lesion is not purely atavistic since it is more common in patients with a chronic cough, glass-blowers and players of brass musical instruments. Occasional cases are complicated by infection or abscess formation.

2.11 Larynx: Paralaryngeal Dermoid Cyst

This is a post-mortem specimen from a 3-day-old infant who had intermittent, but severe, stridor from birth and died.

The tongue with the larynx and proximal trachea, opened posteriorly, are shown. Adjacent to the left lateral wall of the larynx is a smooth, thin-walled cyst, which projects into the pyriform fossa and displaces the larynx to the right.

Dermoid cysts at this site represent developmental anomalies derived from midline rests of embryonal cells. Similar lesions are not uncommonly found in the floor of the mouth or just beneath the mandible.

2.12 Larynx: Multiple Juvenile Squamous Papillomata

This is a post-mortem specimen from a 2-year-old boy who had been noticed to have a husky cry since birth. He had recently become cyanosed and a tracheostomy was performed. Bulky, wart-like lesions, diagnosed as squamous papillomata, were excised but 3 months later he collapsed and died during an attempt to reinsert the tracheostomy tube.

The larynx has been opened from behind to show numerous small, warty lesions along both the true and false vocal cords and surrounding the tracheostomy site, which is marked by a white probe.

Juvenile laryngeal papillomata are uncommon but are found in very young children of either sex. They are usually multiple and new lesions or local recurrences may necessitate repeated local excision over many years. While a viral aetiology has been postulated, the fact that these papillomata remit spontaneously at puberty is suggestive of a contributory endocrine factor. Very rarely, malignant change may occur, particularly in severe or long-standing cases. Squamous papillomata in adulthood are more common and usually solitary. They are thought to be related to chronic irritation and it is extremely unusual for adult lesions to either recur or progress to malignancy.

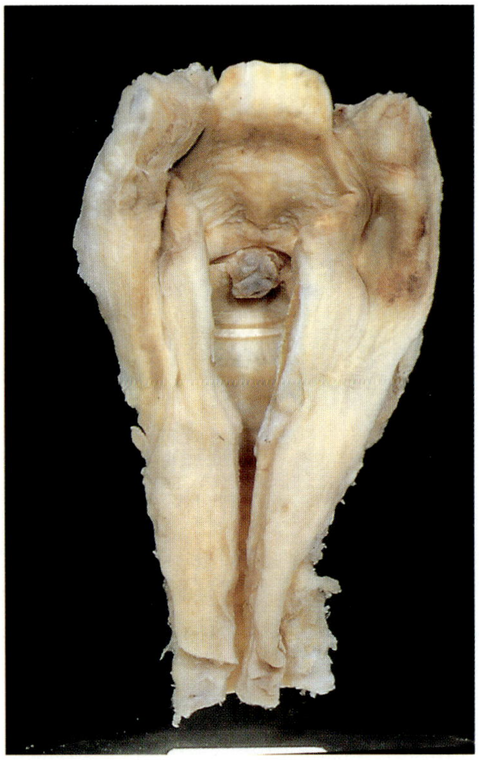

2.13 Larynx: Vocal Cord Polyp

This was an incidental finding at post-mortem in a 75-year-old man who had suffered from chronic bronchitis for many years.

The larynx and trachea have been opened posteriorly to show a pedunculated, 'mulberry-like' tumour arising from the right vocal cord adjacent to the midline. It measures approximately 1cm in diameter.

Polyps of the vocal cord (synonym: Singer's nodule, vocal abuse nodule) may occur in either sex at any age, although usually in adulthood, and are thought to arise as a direct result of either prolonged or strenuous use of the voice. Such abuse probably causes congestion, haemorrhage and stromal proliferation in the vocal cord, leading to polyp formation. Extensive neo-vascularisation often leads to a mistaken diagnosis of haemangioma and, macroscopically, the resemblance is clearly seen in the case here. True haemangiomas of the larynx are very rare and are usually found in children. Laryngeal polyps, due to abuse, have no malignant potential.

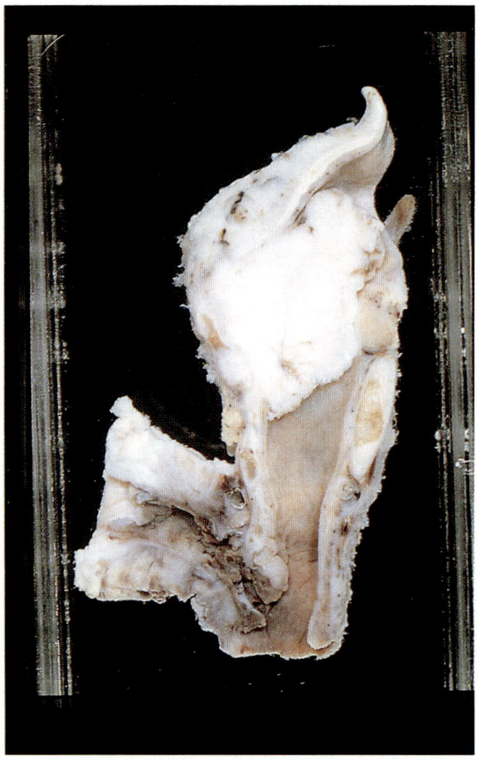

2.14 Larynx: Squamous Carcinoma

This specimen was excised from an 84-year-old man who first complained of hoarseness 2½ years previously. A small tumour was found arising from the right vocal cord and was treated by radiotherapy. Local recurrence and subglottic extension one year later necessitated reduction by diathermy and a tracheostomy. However, increasing dyspnoea and the development of dysphagia made total laryngectomy unavoidable.

This sagittal section through the larynx and upper trachea shows a large, pale mass of tumour occupying most of the right side of the laryngeal cavity, almost occluding the laryngeal inlet. The vestibular and vocal folds have been obliterated by the tumour, which has also invaded the anterior laryngeal wall. Note the fibrosis and haemorrhage around the tracheostomy site distally.

Squamous carcinoma of the larynx is not uncommon and occurs predominantly in the 6th and 7th decades, with a preponderance of males. Well-recognised aetiological factors include cigarette smoking and chronic laryngeal irritation. The glottic region is the commonest primary site and carries the best prognosis, while subglottic tumours are relatively unusual and are associated with a poor outlook. Supraglottic lesions fall between these two groups both in incidence and clinical behaviour. All these subgroups tend to an exophytic rather than ulcerative growth pattern, with a predilection for extensive local invasion prior to lymphatic dissemination. Five-year-survival is closely related to staging and the figure for fairly localised tumours is of the order of 80 per cent.

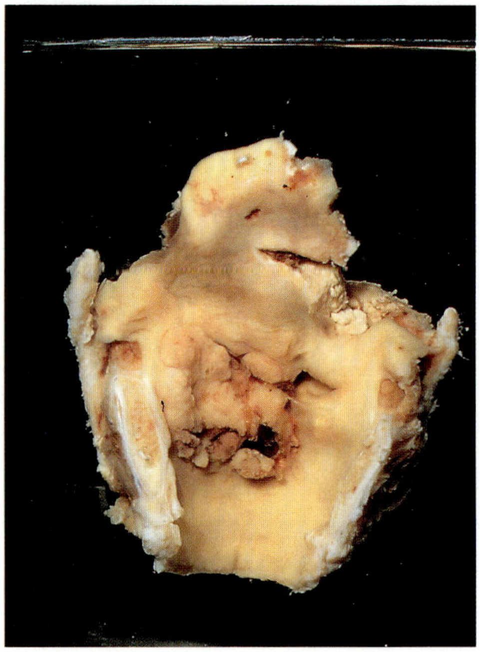

2.15 Larynx: Recurrent Carcinoma

This specimen was excised from a 64-year-old man who presented with a 6 month history of hoarseness. A large papillomatous neoplasm was excised with the left vocal cord and post-operative radiotherapy was given. Nine months later the tumour recurred, necessitating laryngectomy.

The larynx has been opened posteriorly to show an exophytic, focally ulcerated tumour arising in the region of the left vocal cord and extending both across the mid-line and superiorly.

Local recurrence following either local or radical excision for squamous carcinoma of the larynx is very common. This may be attributed either to implantation of malignant cells at operation or to undetected microscopic extension of the tumour beyond the original resection margins.

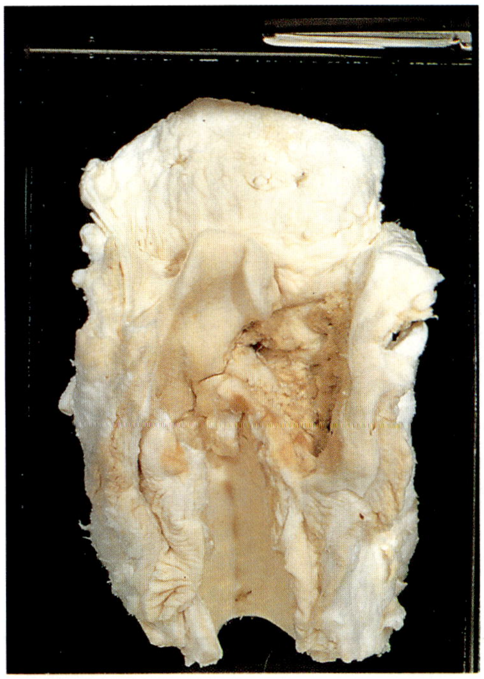

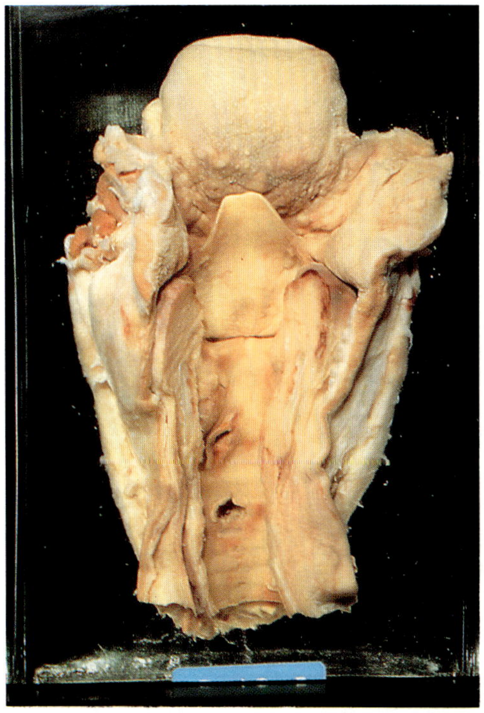

2.17 Larynx: Non-Hodgkin's Lymphoma

This is a post-mortem specimen from a 41-year-old man who presented with a sore throat and dyspnoea. The arytenoid region was swollen and the appearances suggested a post-cricoid carcinoma. The patient's dyspnoea became rapidly worse and, despite tracheostomy, he died.

The tongue with the larynx, opened from behind, are swollen. There is an ill-defined mass of pale tumour distending the aryepiglottic folds and spreading beneath the mucosa in the posterior and lateral laryngeal walls. There is evidence of recent haemorrhage into the upper part of the tumour which may have been responsible for the rapid deterioration in respiratory function.

While any laryngeal involvement in lymphoma is most often secondary to disseminated disease, both lymphocytic non-Hodgkin's lymphoma and Hodgkin's disease may occasionally arise primarily in the wall of the larynx. If mucosal ulceration supervenes, the macroscopical appearances may be indistinguishable from a laryngeal carcinoma.

2.16 Larynx: Carcinoma of Pyriform Fossa

This is a post-mortem specimen from a 56-year-old man who was known to have had an inoperable tumour in the neck for 6 months, the primary site being unclear. He developed extreme dyspnoea and died.

The larynx has been opened posteriorly to show an ulcerated neoplasm, which has arisen in the right pyriform fossa. There is extensive invasion and destruction of the base of the epiglottis and the right vocal cord.

Carcinoma of the pyriform fossa was previously classified as an 'extrinsic' laryngeal tumour. It is now better regarded as a laryngohypopharyngeal carcinoma and should be separated from post-cricoid tumours. This tumour principally affects the elderly, with a predilection for males. It is associated with smoking and carries a poor prognosis.

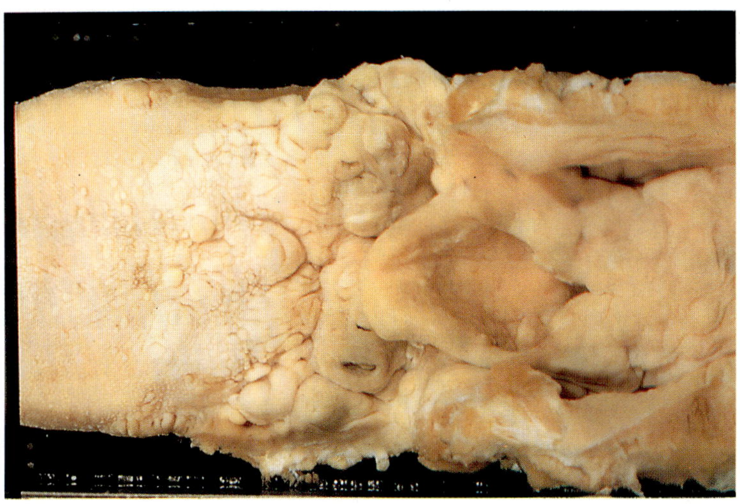

2.18 Larynx: Leukaemic Infiltration

This is a post-mortem specimen from a male who died with acute lymphoblastic leukaemia.

The tongue and larynx, opened posteriorly, show very prominent nodularity and enlargement of the lymphoid tissue, both at the base of the tongue and on the posterior laryngeal wall. Some of the nodules are clearly ulcerated.

Widespread expansive infiltration of lymphoid tissue and other organs is more commonly a feature of chronic leukaemias than acute cases.

LUNG

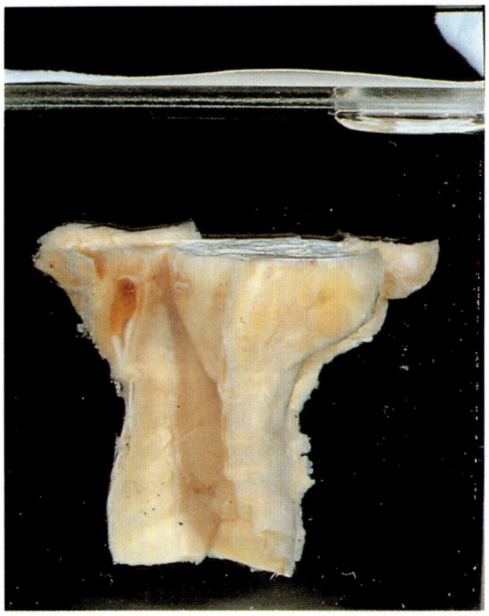

2.19 Larynx: Chondroma

This is a post-mortem specimen from an 84-year-old woman who suffered from progressive hoarseness, stridor and dysphagia. Terminally, she developed severe dyspnoea and died.

Part of the larynx and upper trachea have been opened from behind to show a rounded, cartilaginous tumour, measuring 2cm in diameter, which arises from the right ala of the thyroid cartilage. There is virtual obliteration of the right vocal cord and superior laryngeal opening. Note that the laryngeal mucosa remains intact but attenuated over the surface of the neoplasm.

Chondromas may arise in any of the laryngeal cartilages but are very uncommon; the cricoid cartilage appears to be the most frequent primary site. They are very slow-growing tumours, usually occurring in adulthood and may attain a size sufficient to interfere with respiration, as in the case here.

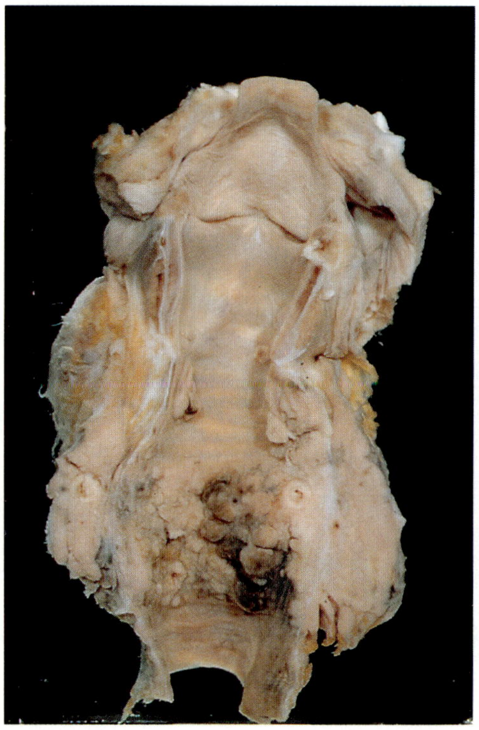

2.20 Trachea: Anaplastic Carcinoma

This is post-mortem specimen from a 71-year-old woman who complained of dyspnoea and haemoptysis for some months. She died before any treatment could be undertaken and, at autopsy, there were multiple hepatic metastases.

The larynx and upper trachea have been opened posteriorly to show an ulcerated, fungating tumour encircling the tracheal lumen. There is invasion of the tracheal wall, and adjacent lymph nodes are totally replaced by metastatic tumour. The thyroid gland is uninvolved.

Carcinoma of the trachea is rare but usually squamous in type. As is the case in most primary malignant tumours of the lower respiratory tract, cigarette smoking is the best recognised aetiological factor. The elderly are most often affected and almost invariable inoperability, largely owing to the tumour site, confers a very poor prognosis.

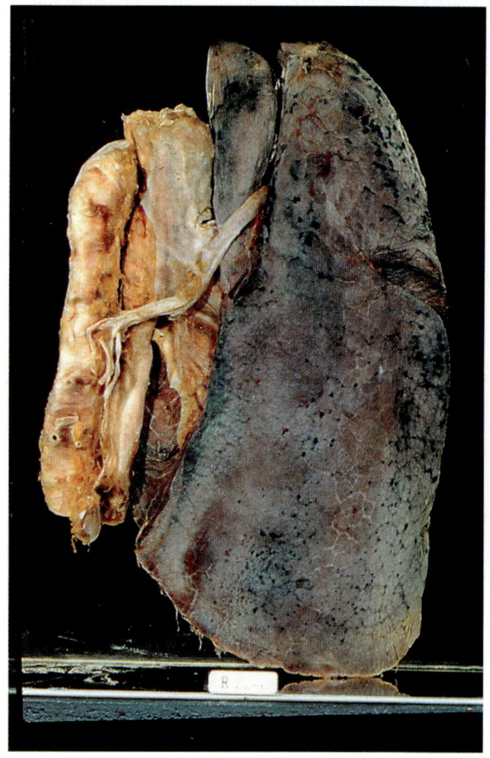

2.21 Azygos Lobe

This was an incidental finding at post-mortem in a 72-year-old man who died of intercurrent disease.

This is the posterior surface of the right lung which shows an abnormally located lobe, measuring 6.5 × 4 × 4cm, arising from the medial border of the upper lobe near its apex. The prominent azygos vein winds anteriorly around the base of the abnormal lobe.

The azygos lobe is a common congenital anomaly in which it is thought that a portion of the upper lobe, usually of the right lung, grows medially to the right posterior and common cardinal veins while the azygos vein travels laterally. A double fold of visceral pleura usually separates this portion from the remainder of the upper lobe. This malformation has no clinical significance.

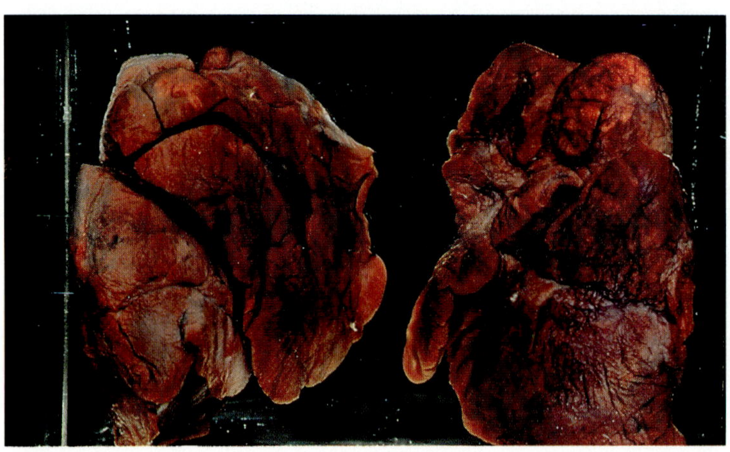

2.22 Congenital Abnormal Lobulation

These are post-mortem specimens from a 15-month-old boy with Down's syndrome (Trisomy 21) who died of a chest infection. At autopsy there were also cardiac and urinary developmental malformations.

Both lungs show multiple, irregular sub-lobulation of the main lobes such that there are 15 lobes altogether.

Such a degree of congenitally abnormal lobulation is unusual but has no especial relationship to Down's syndrome, other than to suggest a genetic basis for its development in the case here.

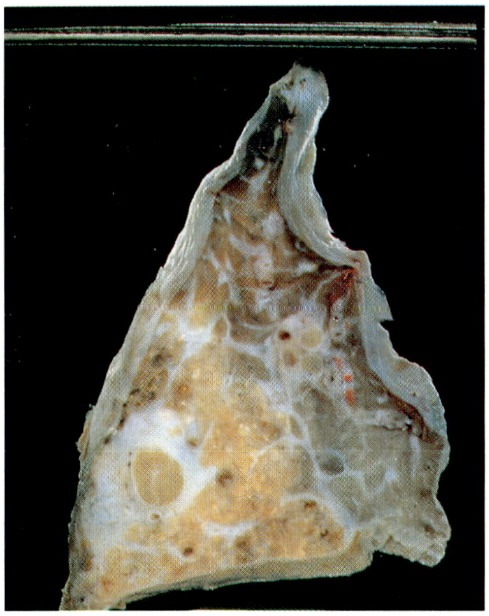

2.23 Intralobar Sequestration

This is a lobectomy specimen from an 8-year-old boy who had complained of a recurrent dry cough associated with intermittent pyrexia. A chest X-ray showed a fairly well-defined opacity in the postero-medial portion of the left lower lobe and bronchograms showed the normal basal bronchi to be displaced anteriorly by the lesion.

The left lower lobe has been sectioned to show a fairly well-demarcated, wedge-shaped lesion in the posterolateral region. The normal pulmonary arteries have been injected with red gelatin while the aberrant vessels, which had arisen from the aorta, have been delineated with tan-coloured gelatin. The abnormal area receives its vascular supply from the aberrant arteries and the bronchi do not communicate with the normal bronchial tree. There is marked consolidation with fibrosis and bronchiectasis in the sequestrated segment.

Pulmonary sequestration is defined as a portion of lung tissue having no connection with the normal bronchial tree. It may be extralobar, appearing as a non-functioning mass of accessory lung tissue, either intra- or extrathoracically, or intralobar in which the tissue is confined within one of the normal lung lobes. The origin of intralobar sequestrations remains unclear, being either an embryological anomaly or possibly the result of inflammation or scarring in early life. The presence of an anomalous arterial supply, in the case here, is very suggestive of a developmental malformation. Such lesions may remain clinically undetected or present with recurrent infection or haemoptysis, most often in childhood.

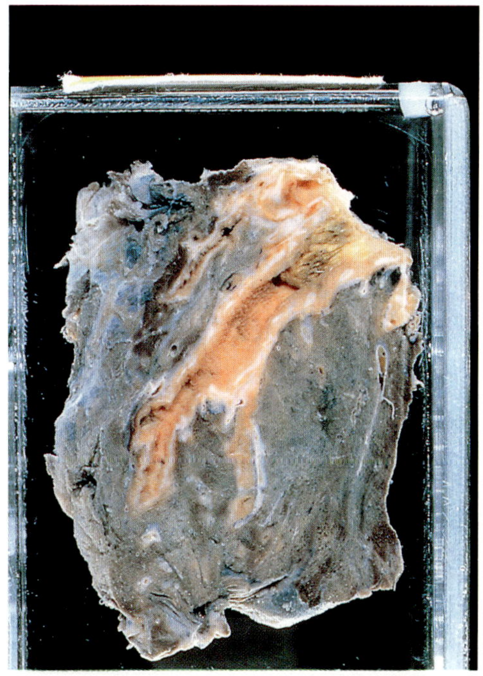

2.24 Impacted Foreign Body

This is a lobectomy specimen from a 29-year-old man who presented with a 10 month history of persistent coughing with occasional haemoptysis. He developed repeated pyrexial illnesses with gradual clubbing of the fingers and bronchoscopy revealed a haemorrhagic mass in the right lower lobe bronchus.

The right lower lobe has been sectioned to show obstruction of the principal bronchus by a flat piece of bone measuring 1cm in length. Distally there is marked bronchiectasis with associated collapse and inflammation.

Inhalation of foreign bodies is not unusual but is commonest in young children or the mentally ill. The consequences are dependent upon the irritant nature of the foreign body, its size and the degree or duration of obstruction. In a long-standing case, such as the one here, the development of bronchiectasis and scarring distally is to be expected. It is interesting to note that many patients, at all ages, fail to recognise the inhalation because any choking may be very short-lived.

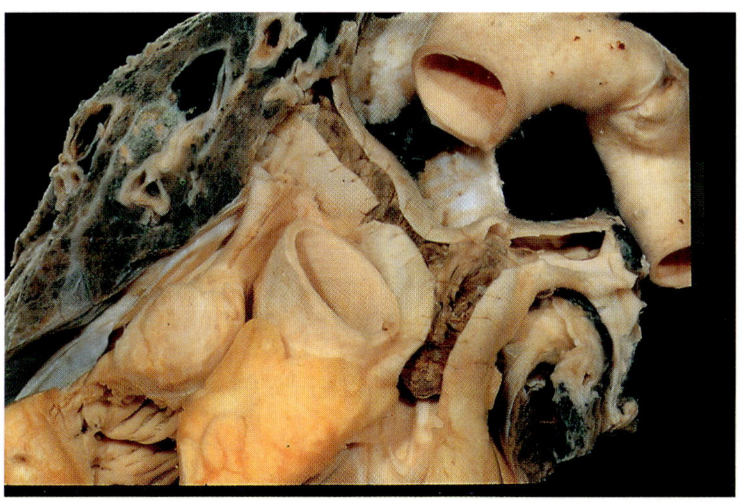

2.25 Pulmonary Embolism

This is a post-mortem specimen from a 50-year-old woman who suddenly developed severe dyspnoea and cyanosis 6 days after undergoing cholecystectomy. She collapsed and died rapidly.

This is a dissection of the great vessels and trachea adjacent to the heart. A massive thrombosis has occluded the main pulmonary artery, just proximal to its bifurcation (bottom right).

Pulmonary embolism is defined as occlusive impaction of any material in the pulmonary arterial system. In the vast majority of cases this is due to the passage of thrombus from the systemic venous system, most often the deep veins of the lower limbs. However, fat, amniotic fluid, tumour and air emboli should not be forgotten although none of these are intravascular in origin. The incidence of pulmonary embolism following deep venous thrombosis is uncertain since many thromboses and small emboli probably go undetected. Common predisposing causes include prolonged bed rest, particularly post-operatively, childbirth, post-myocardial infarction use of oestrogen-containing medication (including the contraceptive pill), congestive cardiac failure and hypercoagulability. Massive pulmonary embolism, as in the case here, is invariably fatal but smaller emboli, which are often multiple, are more common, resulting in variable impairment of both respiratory and right ventricular function.

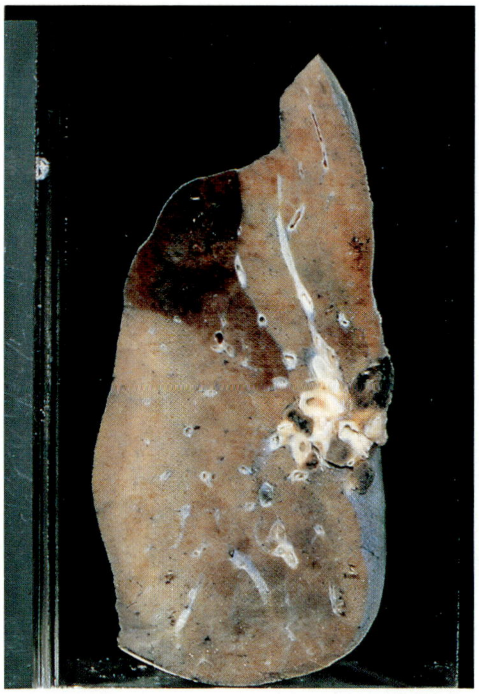

2.26 Red Infarct

This is a post-mortem specimen from a 43-year-old man who had suffered with post-rheumatic aortic stenosis since the age of 13. Latterly he developed congestive cardiac failure and died following an episode of haemoptysis associated with apparent pulmonary consolidation. At autopsy, several other pulmonary infarcts were present in the other lung.

A coronal section through the right lung shows a typical, dark-red, wedge-shaped area of infarction in the upper lobe. The branch of the pulmonary artery supplying this is visibly occluded by a small embolus. The remaining lung parenchyma shows patchy, rusty discolouration, indicative of long-standing venous congestion ('brown induration').

'Red' infarction of the lung, as seen here, reflects the fact that, while the affected tissue undergoes extreme congestion, true ischaemic necrosis only rarely occurs owing to the dual blood supply and anastomatic system provided by the bronchial arteries. Pulmonary infarction is seen most often in late adulthood and the overwhelming majority of cases are due to pulmonary embolism (see Legend 2.25).

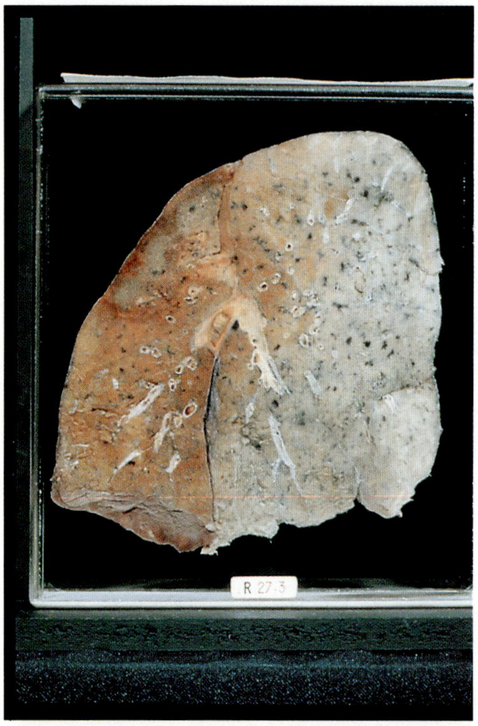

2.27 Red Infarct

This is a post-mortem specimen from an 80-year-old woman who died shortly after fracturing her left femur.

A coronal section through the right lung shows red infarction of the entire lower lobe. The corresponding branch of the pulmonary artery is occluded by thrombus, which was embolic in origin. The adjacent areas of the middle and upper lobes are mildly congested. Note that the apical segment of the lower lobe appears in isolation to have progressed to a true pale infarct.

Deep venous thrombosis, and therefore pulmonary embolism, is a common complication of fractures of the long bones of the leg. The development of an area of true ischaemic necrosis in this infarct probably reflects a degree of low-output cardiac failure in this patient.

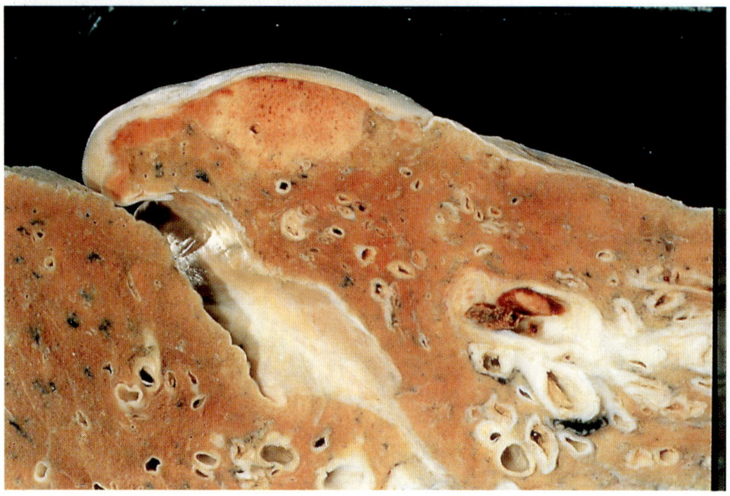

2.28 Pale Infarct

This is a post-mortem specimen from a 69-year-old woman who had suffered from multiple sclerosis for 30 years and latterly developed atrial fibrillation and congestive cardiac failure.

A section through the upper part of the left lower lobe shows a circumscribed area of pale necrosis, while the adjacent lung parenchyma is rather congested. Several branches of the pulmonary artery are occluded by thrombus.

Pale pulmonary infarction is very uncommon and occurs only when alveolar walls undergo ischaemic necrosis. This necessitates some impairment of the bronchial arterial supply, additional to the pulmonary arterial occlusion. The most frequent predisposing cause is left ventricular failure, particularly if associated with a low cardiac output and passive pulmonary venous congestion. Pale infarcts are often subpleural in location and may heal to leave a small, linear scar much smaller than the original bulk of lung tissue affected.

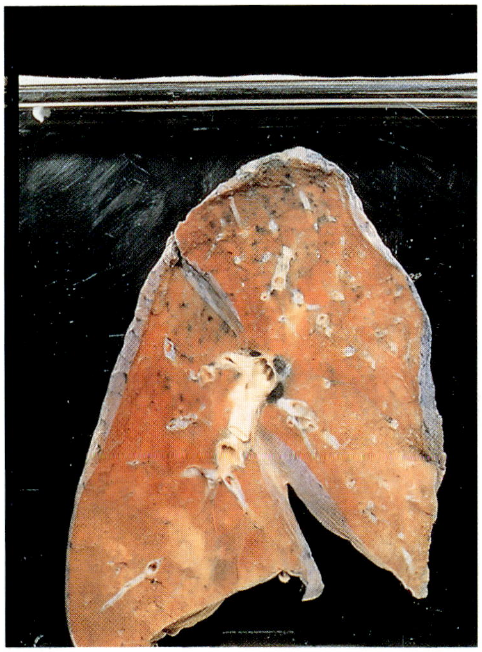

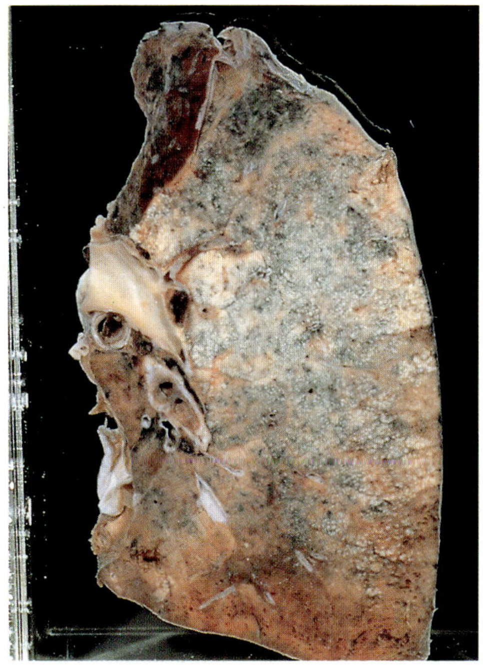

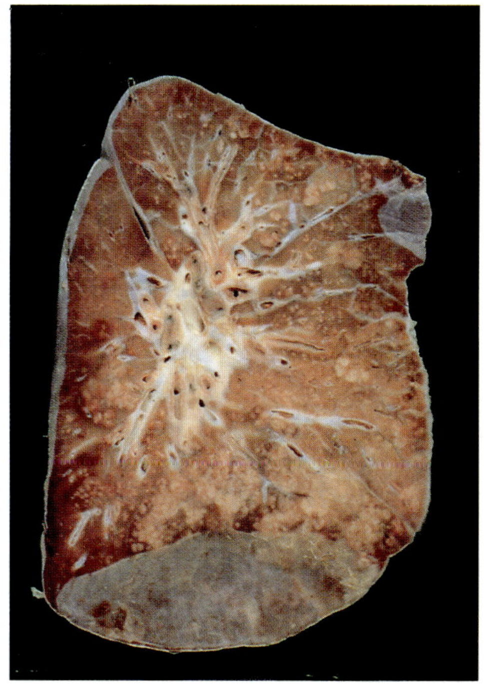

2.29 Bronchopneumonia

This is a post-mortem specimen from a 79-year-old diabetic woman, who died after being found collapsed at home with hypothermia and a chest infection.

A coronal section through the right lung shows confluent consolidation of the basal portion of the lower lobe and patchy consolidation of the middle lobe. The affected areas have a greyish-white appearance and are poorly demarcated from the remaining lung parenchyma, which is moderately congested.

Bronchopneumonia occurs most often in the elderly, the very young and immunosuppressed or debilitated patients. It is a multifocal disease which is largely centrilobular in distribution, being centred on the terminal and respiratory bronchioles, and which spreads largely by the air passages. Common predisposing factors include chronic obstructive airways disease and preceding viral respiratory infection. A very wide variety of organisms may be responsible, the commonest of which are *Streptococcus pneumoniae*, *S. pyogenes*, *Haemophilus influenzae* and *Staphylococcus aureus*. Infection acquired in hospital, particularly in patients already receiving antibiotics, is often due to the *Enterobacteriaceae*. Possible complications include the development of bacteraemia or septicaemia, a lung abscess or pleural empyema and adjacent suppurative pericarditis.

2.30 Confluent Bronchopneumonia

This is a post-mortem specimen from a 63-year-old man. No clinical details are available.

A coronal section through the lung shows very extensive pale consolidation which has largely become confluent, but is still visibly centrilobular in distribution in the lower portion of the lung. The main bronchus is very congested and inflamed.

Confluent consolidation, as seen here, simply represents progression of the infective process but may easily be confused with lobar pneumonia in appearance.

2.31 Suppurative Bronchopneumonia

This is a post-mortem specimen from a 13-year-old girl who, following a brief influenzal illness, was admitted with bronchopneumonia. A penicillin-resistant strain of *Staphylococcus aureus* was repeatedly isolated from her sputum and, despite intensive antibiotic therapy, she died.

A coronal section through this lung shows numerous small foci of pale consolidation throughout the parenchyma. In some areas, particularly the lower lobe, there are many small abscesses. The remaining lung tissue is markedly congested.

Suppurative bronchopneumonia, which is associated with the development of lung abscesses of varying size, is a particular feature of infection with either *S. aureus*, *Pseudomonas aeruginosa* or *Klebsiella pneumoniae* (Friedlander's bacillus). Occasionally, non-sporing anaerobes are responsible. Reasons given for the tendency of these organisms to cause suppuration include increased tissue destruction and lesional ischaemia due to the action of bacterial toxins on the adjacent blood vessels. Both staphylococcal and pseudomonas infections are commonly hospital-acquired and may run a fulminating course.

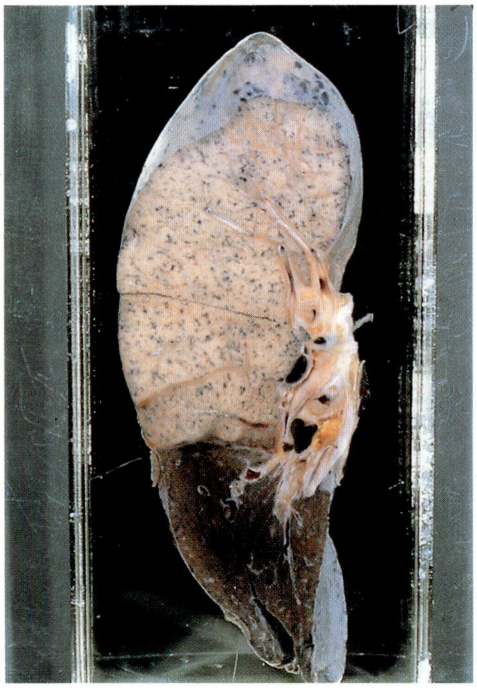

2.32 Lobar Pneumonia

This is a post-mortem specimen from a young soldier who was admitted to hospital during the First World War with signs of right upper lobe consolidation and very marked pyrexia. He became cyanotic and comatose and died 9 hours later.

A coronal section through the lung shows total consolidation of the upper lobe, which is uniformly greyish in colour. The lower lobe is intensely congested and shows a small area of red hepatisation at its apex.

Lobar pneumonia, in its classical form, has become uncommon since the advent of antibiotics, which have dramatically altered the course of the disease. Typically, previously fit young adults, with a preponderance of males, are most often affected. Up to 95 per cent of cases are caused by *Streptococcus pneumoniae*, especially Types 1, 2, 3 and 7. In the remaining 5 per cent, any of the organisms mentioned in Legend 2.30 may be isolated. The classical untreated case goes through 4 stages: acute congestion, which covers the 1st day of developing infection; red hepatisation, from the 2nd to 4th days, which is characterised by a brick-red, firm lung in which there is intense acute inflammation and extravasation of red cells; grey hepatisation (seen in the case here), from the 4th to 8th days, in which there is a massive accumulation of fibrin; and, finally, at around the 8th to 10th day, resolution, in which digestion and organisation of the inflammatory process occurs. In fatal cases, death usually occurs at the stage of grey hepatisation. Possible complications include septicaemia, abscess formation and pulmonary fibrosis, due to extensive organisation of the inflammatory exudate. The reasons given for the quite different appearance to bronchopneumonia include the dose and virulence of the infective organism and the tendency of the infection to spread along the air passages without causing any significant damage to the bronchial or bronchiolar epithelium.

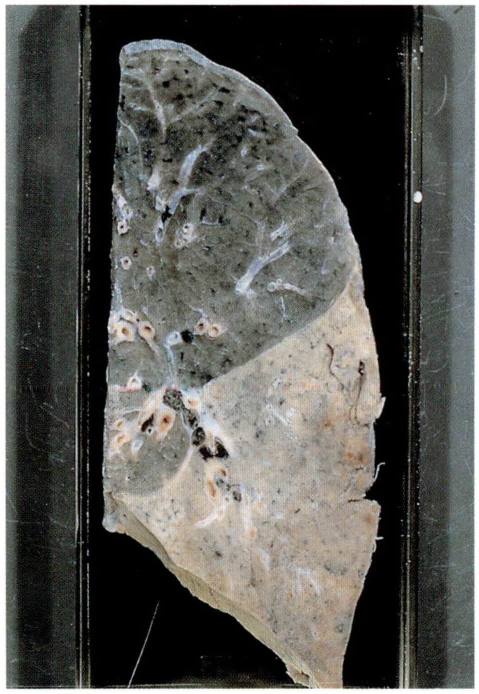

2.33 Lobar Pneumonia

No clinical details are available.

This coronal section through the left lung shows uniform, grey consolidation confined to the lower lobe. Note also the formation of an irregular abscess cavity in the apical segment of the affected lobe.

This is another classical example of grey hepatisation in lobar pneumonia, in this case complicated by a lung abscess. Possible causative organisms include Type 3 pneumococcus, *Klebsiella* and *Staphylococcus aureus*.

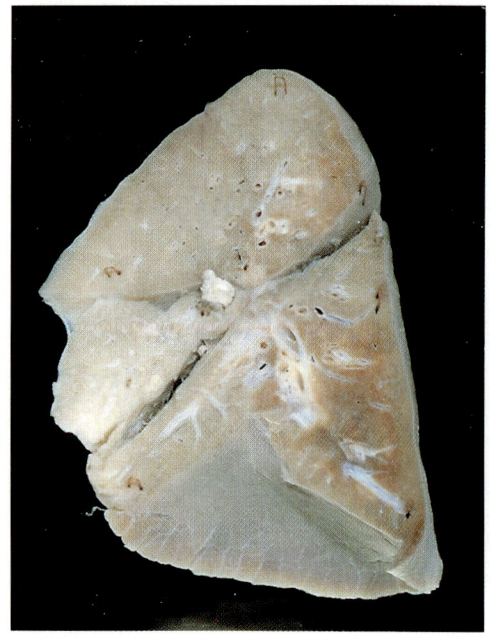

2.34 Primary Tuberculosis

This is a post-mortem specimen from a 3-year-old boy who died of pneumococcal bronchopneumonia.

A coronal section through the right lung shows fibrosis and shrinkage of the middle lobe. There is a small, clearly defined focus of caseous necrosis at the apex of the middle lobe and an enlarged caseous lymph node was found at the lung hilum. The lower lobe shows congestion and consolidation compatible with the terminal illness.

Primary pulmonary tuberculosis is now much less common in the indigenous population of the Western world than it was 40 years ago, but it remains an important source of morbidity and mortality in underdeveloped countries. The vast majority of cases are due to infection by *Mycobacterium tuberculosis* acquired by droplet spread; occasional cases may be attributed to atypical mycobacteriae. Children, adolescents and young adults are most often affected and develop the classical Ghon focus, a small subpleural caseous nodule which may be found in any lobe (cf. post-primary infection). The carriage of acid-fast bacilli to the hilar lymph nodes sets up infection there, which in combination with the Ghon focus is referred to as the primary complex. The majority of cases undergo spontaneous healing by fibrosis, with or without dystrophic calcification and ossification but may later re-present with reactivated infection. A proportion of patients, however, develop progressive infection which may be complicated by cavitation, miliary spread or bronchopneumonia.

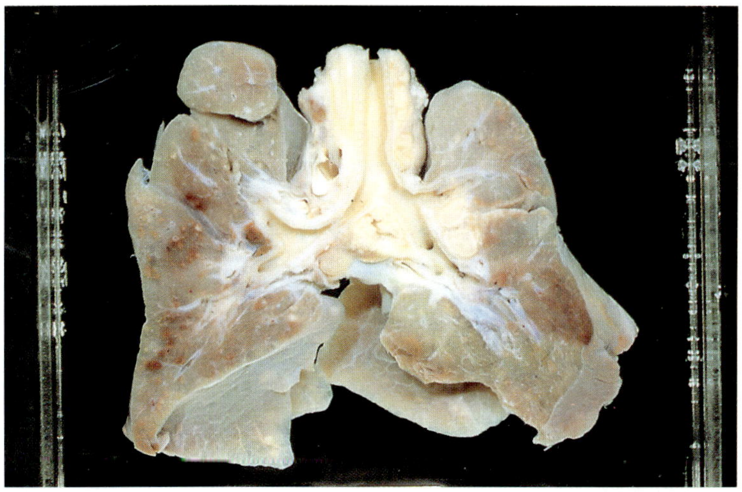

2.35 Primary Tuberculosis

No clinical details are available regarding this small child.

The trachea and lungs have been sectioned coronally to show prominent caseous enlargement of the lymph nodes at the right hilum, carina and along the right side of the trachea. In this particular example, the Ghon focus is not visible, but note that terminal haematogenous spread has given rise to numerous miliary tubercles, particularly in the left lung, many of which are surrounded by a small zone of congestion.

This case shows the typical features of lymph node involvement in primary tuberculosis and should be viewed in conjunction with Figure 2.34. As already stated, miliary spread is a comparatively uncommon, although not unusual, terminal event.

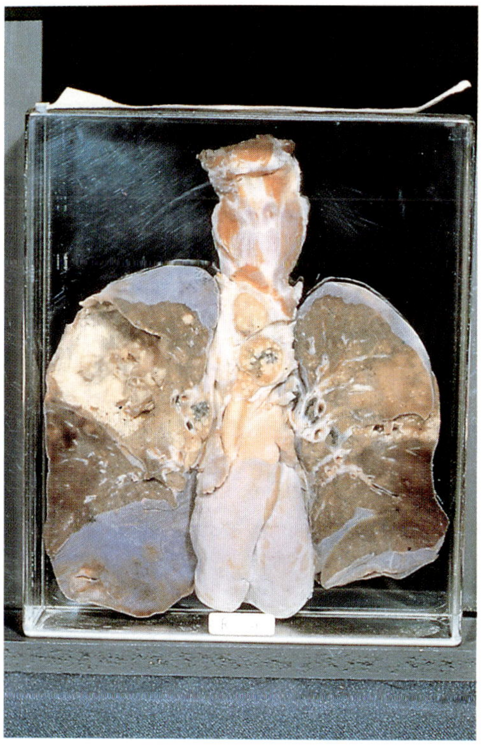

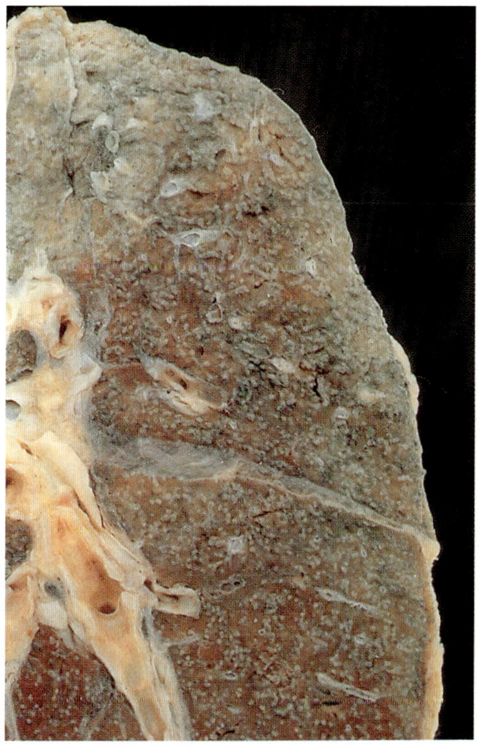

2.36 Primary Cavitating Tuberculosis complicated by Bronchopneumonia

This is a post-mortem specimen from a young adult male who died in Belsen concentration camp.

The lungs, heart, trachea and adjacent structures are shown. There is a large tuberculous cavity in the right upper lobe, which contains copious caseous material. The hilar and mediastinal lymph nodes show extensive caseous necrosis. In addition, there is widespread bilateral consolidation indicative of tuberculous bronchopneumonia. The heart is atrophic.

This is an example of primary infection which has failed to heal and has progressed to terminal bronchopneumonia. Such an event only occurs in a small number of cases and, in this patient, was probably a consequence of malnourishment and general debilitation.

2.37 Miliary Tuberculosis

This is a post-mortem specimen from a 35-year-old man who presented with a 2 month history of dyspnoea and intermittent pyrexia. After a brief period of improvement, he developed a swelling in the left testicle, meningitis and acid-fast bacilli were cultured from the urine. At autopsy, generalised miliary tuberculosis was found with caseous lesions in the right kidney and left epididymis.

A close-up view of the lung shows intense parenchymal congestion and innumerable, small, pale tubercles scattered throughout the lung substance. There are dense, fibrous pleural adhesions.

Miliary tuberculosis is almost solely a complication of primary infection, although very occasional cases may be seen in debilitated patients with post-primary disease. It is a result of haematogenous spread of bacilli, following rupture of either a caseous focus or lymph node into a blood vessel wall. This results in widespread dissemination of organisms throughout the body, which form smaller tubercles, resembling millet seed (hence the name), particularly in the spleen, liver, bone marrow, meninges and lungs. While, in the past, such an event was uniformly fatal, the availability of modern antibiotics is now often curative.

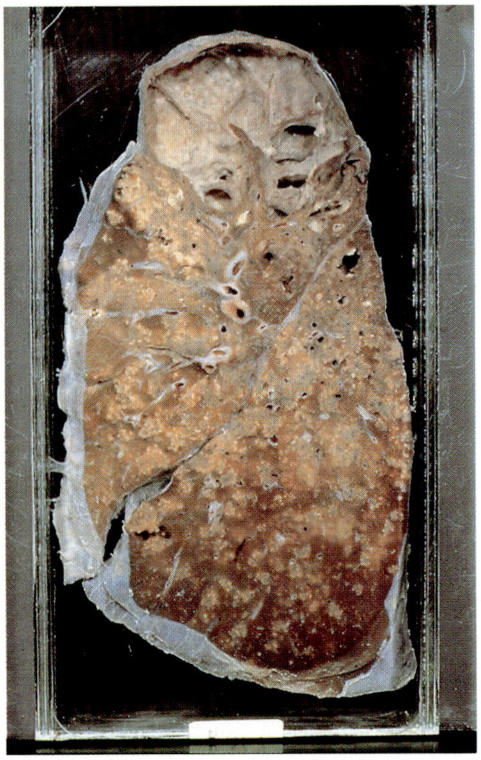

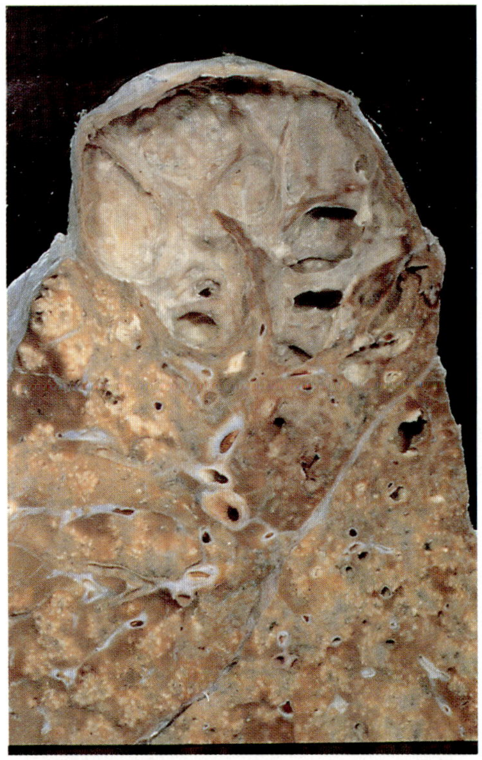

2.38 Post-Primary Tuberculosis

No clinical details are available.

A coronal section through one of the lungs shows extensive apical cavitation (2.38a and 2.38b). The cavities have thick fibrous walls and, adjacent to them, are numerous foci of caseous consolidation extending throughout the upper lobe and into the middle lobe. This therefore suggests that tuberculous bronchopneumonia has supervened.

Post-primary tuberculosis is most often due to exogenous reinfection with either the same or a different mycobacteria and seems only rarely to be a result of endogenous reactivation of pre-existent infection. Post-primary lesions classically are found in the lung apices, in the absence of a Ghon focus. Thereafter, they may cavitate and be complicated by bronchopneumonia, laryngotracheal or alimentary involvement. This cavitation is largely responsible for the droplet spread of infection to other individuals. In long-standing infection, secondary amyloidosis not uncommonly develops.

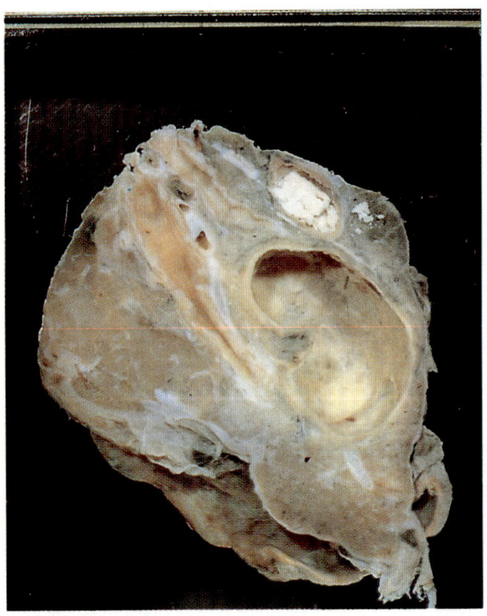

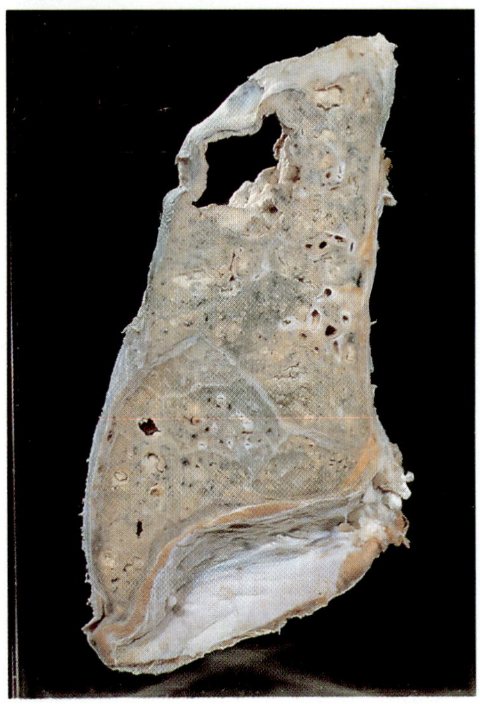

2.40 Post-Primary Tuberculosis complicated by Bronchopneumonia

This is a post-mortem specimen from a 27-year-old woman who had been ill with tuberculosis for 4 years prior to death.

A coronal section through the lung shows a large, irregular cavity in the upper lobe, measuring 5cm in maximum diameter. The cavity is lined by caseous material and fibrous tissue. In addition both upper and lower lobes show multiple foci of caseous bronchopneumonia, some of which are cavitating in the lower lobe.

These are the typical features of a fatal case of post-primary pulmonary tuberculosis. Rupture of an apical cavity into the bronchial tree leads to rapid dissemination of infection within the lung, thereby giving rise to the serious complication of bronchopneumonia.

2.39 Lung: Post-Primary Tuberculosis

This is a lobectomy specimen from a 21-year-old woman who had a 3 year history of pulmonary tuberculosis. Two members of her close family had recently died of tuberculosis.

The right lower lobe has been sectioned in the plane of the main bronchus to show a thick-walled cavity, measuring 3cm in maximum diameter. Just above this, at the apex of the lower lobe, is a small cavity, the lumen of which is completely filled with pale caseous material. The pleural surface shows ragged fibrous adhesions.

This is a good example of uncomplicated post-primary tuberculosis.

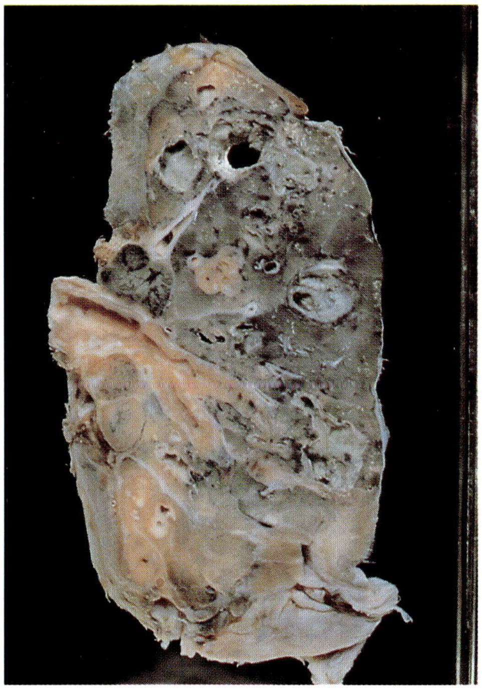

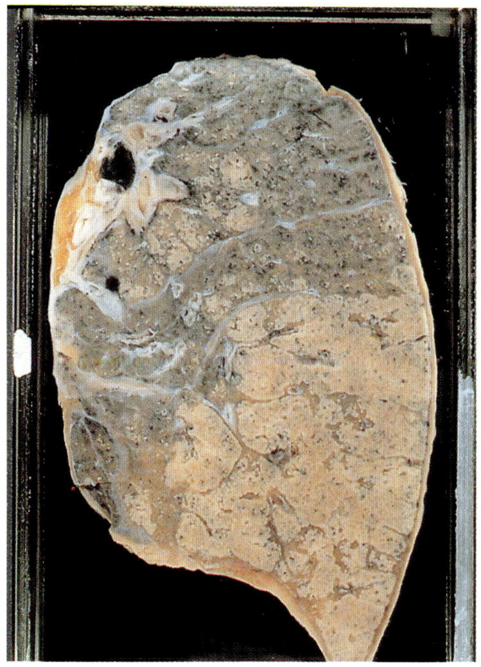

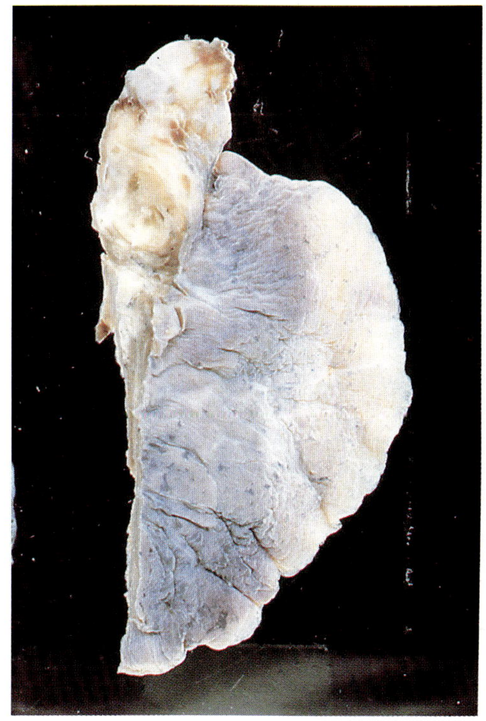

2.41 Post-Primary Tuberculosis with Secondary Bronchiectasis

This is a pneumonectomy specimen from a 33-year-old woman who complained of a productive cough for many years. Chest X-rays were interpreted as showing cystic change, fibrosis and bronchiectasis and the diagnosis of tuberculosis was only made histologically.

A coronal section through the left lung shows several, irregular cavities in the upper lobe which are lined by fibrous tissue. There are foci of caseous consolidation around the lower lobe bronchi, which, along with several smaller intermediate bronchi, show small saccular dilatations.

Fibrosis associated with tuberculous damage not infrequently leads to localised distortion and dilatation of parts of the bronchial tree, resulting in saccular bronchiectasis.

2.42 Tuberculous Bronchopneumonia

This is a post-mortem specimen from a 26-year-old woman who presented with a 2 week history of a cough and pyrexia. Despite all measures available at the time (1935), the disease progressed rapidly and she died 3 months later.

A coronal section through the left lung shows almost total consolidation of the lower lobe, the parenchyma being replaced by a mass of confluent caseous necrosis. The upper lobe is diffusely, but less severely, involved and there is marked pleural thickening.

Tuberculous bronchopneumonia may occur in primary infection, if the caseous cavity enters the bronchial tree, or more commonly, by the same mechanism in post-primary reinfection. In either case, this is usually an acute and very serious complication, which typically affects the lower lobes and is often fatal.

2.43 Cryptococcoma

This is a lobectomy specimen from a 41-year-old man who presented with a 4 month history of headaches. A routine chest X-ray revealed a mass in the right lung which was thought to be a bronchial carcinoma. A right middle lobectomy was performed but, post-operatively, the patient developed frank meningitis and died. At autopsy, there was a gelatinous basal meningitis from which cryptococci were cultured.

A portion of the right middle lobe shows a pale, gelatinous mass at its apex, foci of which have undergone cystic degeneration.

Cryptococcosis (synonym: torulosis) is due to infection by the fungus *Cryptococcus neoformans* and appears to be derived most often from birds' faeces. The disease occurs at any age and inhalation of the organism may result in small subpleural nodules, a large, granulomatous mass (as in the case here) or disseminated miliary nodules. Meningitis is a not uncommon complication and is almost always associated with an underlying, possibly undetected, pulmonary lesion.

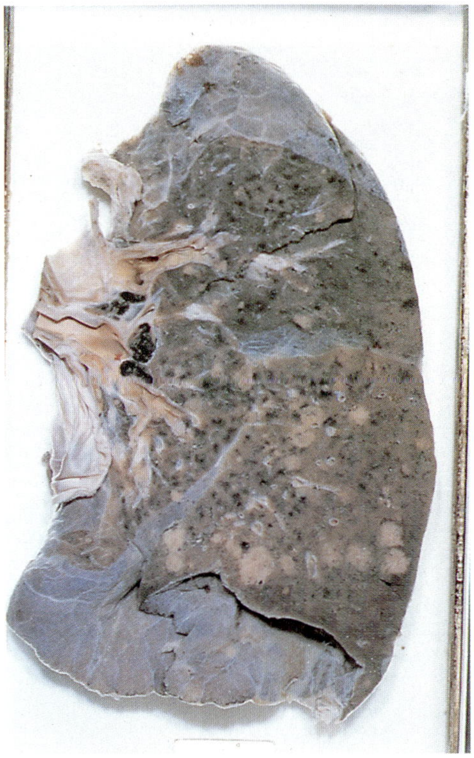

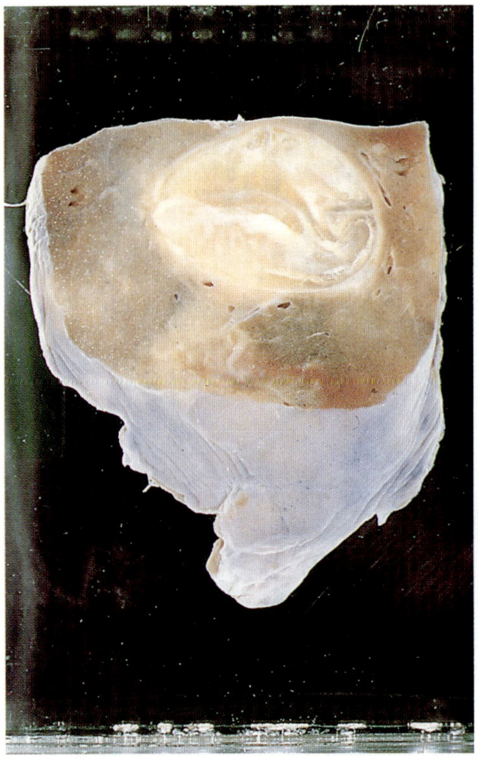

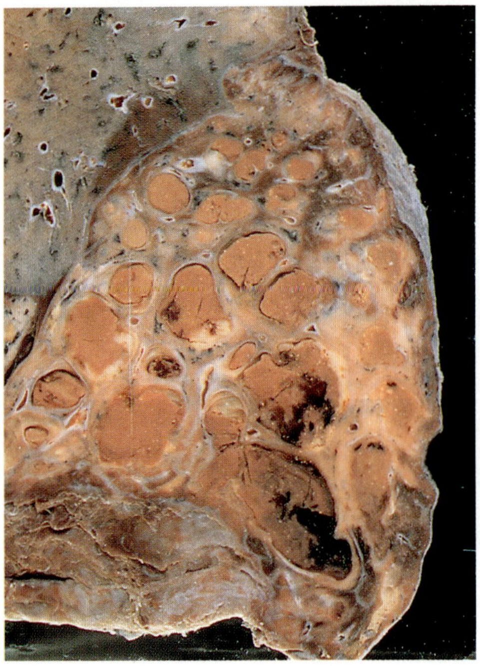

2.44 Melioidosis

This is a post-mortem specimen from a soldier who had served for many years in the Far East. He had suffered from the disease for the previous 5 years, with recurrent bacteraemia and fever and the culpable organism had been isolated from a subcutaneous abscess. Because this case preceded the development of suitable antibiotics, the patient's condition deteriorated and, at autopsy, foci of infection were also found in the liver, kidneys and spinal column.

This coronal section through the left lung shows numerous, rounded pale nodules, particularly in the lower lobe. These nodules represent the typical small abscesses of melioidosis.

Melioidosis is very uncommon in the Western world but is endemic in the Far East and South-East Asia. It is caused by the bacterium *Pseudomonas pseudomallei*, which may be cultured from the soil or stagnant water in endemic areas and is thought to be transmitted in rodent faeces. Infection may be acquired either by contamination of skin wounds, ingestion or inhalation and may follow either an acute, usually fatal, or chronic indolent course. Systemic dissemination is a common feature.

2.45 Hydatid Cyst

This specimen was excised from a 19-year-old Cypriot man, who was found to have a rounded mass in the left lung on routine chest radiography. He had recently developed a productive cough and haemoptysis and, at operation, the apical bronchus was found to communicate with the cyst.

The excised apical segment of the left lower lobe has been sectioned to show a well-circumscribed, laminated hydatid cyst. Much of the cyst's fluid content appears to have been lost via the bronchus.

Hydatid disease follows ingestion of the eggs of the tapeworm *Echinococcus granulosus*, and is most often seen in sheep-farming communities. The cysts are typically multilocular, containing numerous daughter cysts within which the brood capsules are formed. The organism is usually carried in the bloodstream to the lung from the small intestine, having first been ingested. Up to 30 per cent of cases may show pulmonary involvement and rupture of a cyst into the bronchial tree or pleural cavity is not uncommon. The diagnosis may be made by demonstration of cutaneous hypersensitivity to hydatid antigen, the Casoni test.

2.46 Bronchiectasis

This specimen was excised from a 42-year-old man who presented with a persistent chest infection. Bronchoscopy was performed at which a carcinoma, obstructing the right lower lobe bronchus, was found. Pneumonectomy was performed.

A coronal section through part of the right lower lobe shows numerous large bronchiectatic cavities, each of which contains coagulated serosanguineous material. The intervening lung parenchyma shows dense scarring. While there are adhesions in the oblique interlobar fissure, the middle lobe parenchyma is relatively normal.

This case falls into the category of atelectatic bronchiectasis, since it has resulted from chronic collapse distal to obstruction of a major bronchus. This form of bronchiectasis occurs most often in adulthood and the commonest cause is bronchial carcinoma. Bronchial dilatation is an inevitable consequence but the degree of epithelial and interstitial damage is dependent upon the duration of obstruction and the presence and persistence of infection. This case shows very advanced destructive changes.

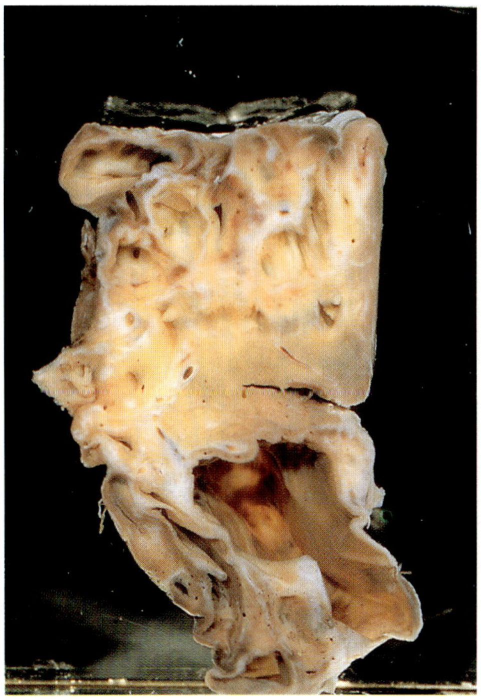

2.47 Bronchiectasis

This is a lobectomy specimen from a 6-year-old girl who had developed a persistent cough with foul-smelling sputum ever since an attack of whooping-cough and pneumonia in infancy. Bronchograms showed saccular bronchiectasis in the left lower lobe with similar, but less marked, changes in the right middle lobe.

This portion of the left lower lobe shows a number of smooth-walled, cyst-like spaces, measuring up to 3cm in diameter. The intervening lung parenchyma shows dense fibrosis and consolidation.

This is an example of saccular post-pneumonic infective bronchiectasis, which classically develops after an episode of bronchopneumonia in infancy, sometimes after whooping-cough or measles. The left lower lobe is typically affected and there is focal but extensive damage and destruction of smaller bronchi with peribronchial fibrosis. The cystic spaces represent gross saccular dilatations of the obliterated bronchi and are lined solely by interstitial tissue.

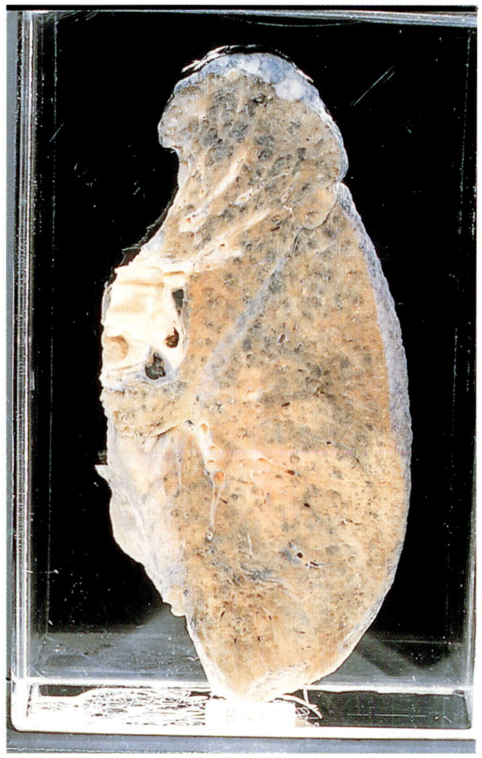

2.48 Panacinar Emphysema

This is a post-mortem specimen from an 88-year-old woman who was a heavy smoker and was known to suffer from chronic bronchitis. She died of bronchopneumonia and an additional finding at autopsy was an oat cell carcinoma arising in the right upper lobe bronchus.

A coronal section of the left lung shows large, almost confluent, dilated air spaces replacing entire lung acini. There is moderate anthracotic pigmentation and foci of pale bronchopneumonic consolidation are apparent in the lower lobe.

The definition of emphysema varies internationally: in the USA, irreversible enlargement or dilatation of the air spaces distal to the terminal bronchiole must be accompanied by destruction of adjacent lung tissue, while, in the United Kingdom, destruction is an 'optional' component. As a consequence, the American and WHO classification of emphysema includes 4 types: panacinar, centrilobular, paraseptal and irregular. In Britain, such entities as senile, compensatory and obstructive emphysema may also be included under the less strict definition. The pathogenesis remains unclear but seems to involve inflammatory destruction of the walls of air spaces, associated with a variable degree of air-trapping and a genetic predisposition. Panacinar emphysema implies dilatation and destruction of the alveoli and alveolar walls as well as the respiratory bronchioles and is classically seen in α_1-antitrypsin deficiency or following long-standing obstruction. It is not uncommonly associated with centrilobular emphysema and affects predominantly the lower lobes. A degree of panacinar or centrilobular emphysema may be found in up to 50 per cent of autopsies in the Western world but is the principal cause of death in only about 5 per cent. Panacinar emphysema, because of the increased lung damage as compared to centrilobular, tends to produce significant respiratory impairment and common causes of death include superadded infection, cor pulmonale and respiratory acidosis.

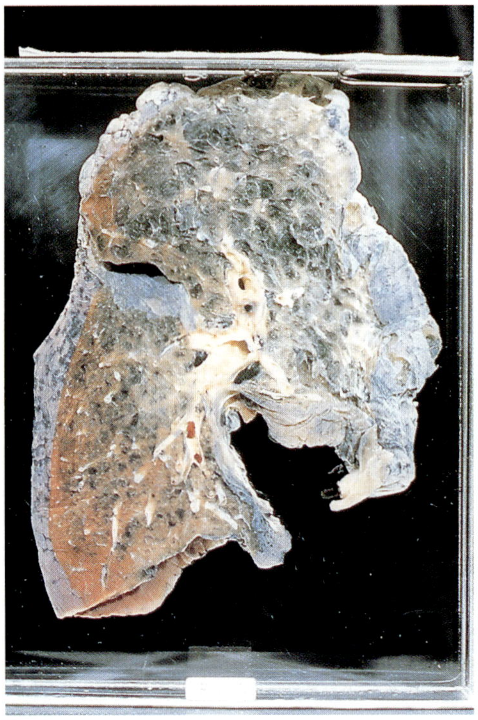

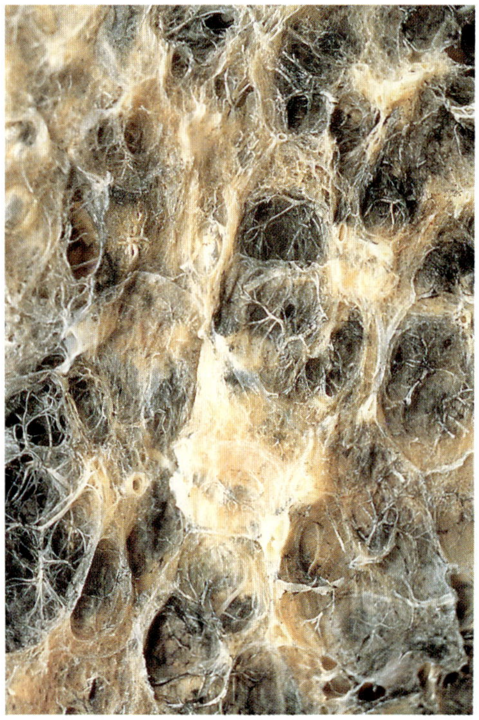

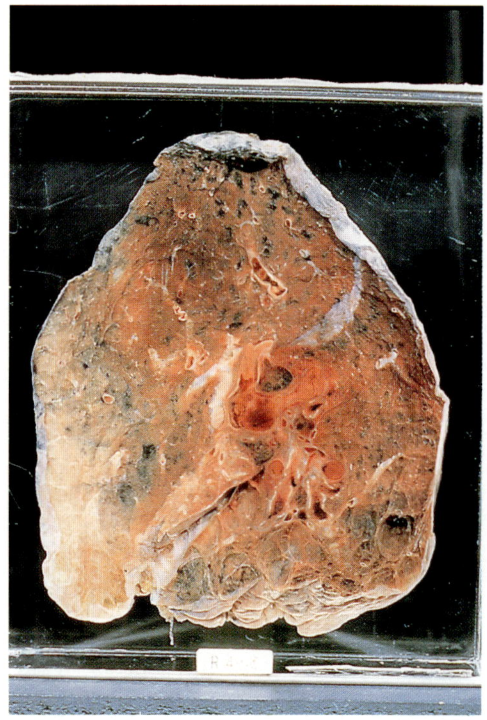

2.49 Centrilobular Emphysema

This is a post-mortem specimen from a 76-year-old man with known long-standing chronic obstructive airways disease, who died after massive bleeding from a gastric peptic ulcer.

A coronal section through the right lung shows multiple, small dilated air spaces, surrounded by anthracotic pigment, giving an almost nodular appearance to the upper lobe, which is predominantly affected (2.49a and 2.49b). Similar changes are, however, apparent in the lower lobe. At the lung apex there are several small bullae, not clearly seen in this view.

Centrilobular emphysema is probably the commonest, clinically significant, single form of emphysema and is characterised by dilatation and destruction of the respiratory bronchioles with sparing of the distal air spaces. It is classically seen in cigarette smokers, especially males and affects especially the upper lobes, in particular the lung apices. The contribution of chronic bronchitis or bronchiolitis in such individuals to pathogenetic lung damage is hard to determine, since both disease processes are usually advanced before presenting clinically. A very similar, though usually less extensive, change may be seen in coal workers' pneumoconiosis and is known as focal dust emphysema: destruction in this group is thought to be due to the inflammatory response initiated by dust-laden macrophages adjacent to the respiratory bronchiolar walls.

2.50 Irregular Emphysema

This is a post-mortem specimen from an 82-year-old man who had suffered from chronic bronchitis for many years.

A coronal section through the right lung shows a variety of changes. The lower lobe shows irregular dilated air spaces with several subpleural bullae and there is adjacent scarring with puckering of the overlying pleura. The middle lobe shows bronchiectasis with extensive fibrosis and consolidation. In addition, the main pulmonary artery, and several of its branches are occluded by fresh thrombus.

Irregular emphysema is characterised by inconsistent dilatation and destruction of the air spaces and shows no uniformity of distribution in the lung acini. It is typically associated with areas of parenchymal scarring, most often due to chronic bronchitis or tuberculosis. It is extremely common but usually asymptomatic, rarely causing any functional impairment.

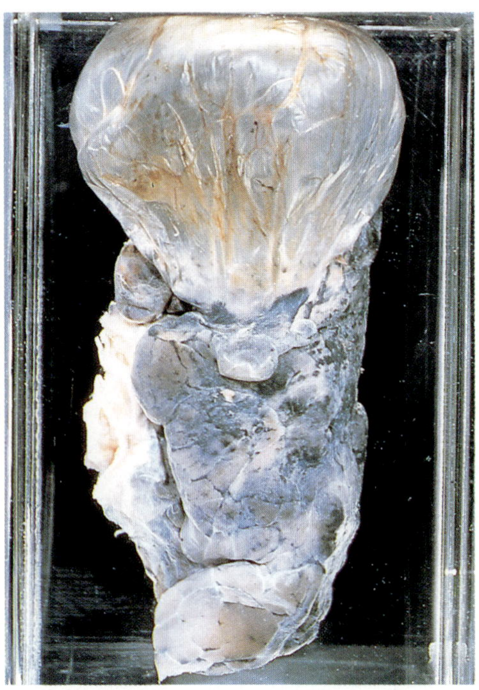

2.51 Paraseptal (Bullous) Emphysema

This is a post-mortem specimen from a 44-year-old schizophrenic man who had been in a mental hospital for the past 22 years. He died while undergoing surgery for carcinoma of the stomach.

Part of the right lung shows a large, thin-walled, air-filled sac, measuring 6cm in maximum diameter, projecting from the apical pleural surface. A similar, though smaller, bulla is visible subpleurally in the middle lobe (bottom).

Paraseptal or bullous emphysema is typified by dilatation and destruction of the alveolar ducts and alveoli with sparing of the proximal portion of the lung acinus. The definition of a bulla is a dilated air space greater than 1cm in diameter. It usually affects lung tissue adjacent to interlobular connective tissue septa or the pleura. The upper lobes are most often involved and the condition is commonly associated with pre-existent scarring or atelectasis. Bullae such as the one here may occasionally rupture, resulting in a pneumothorax.

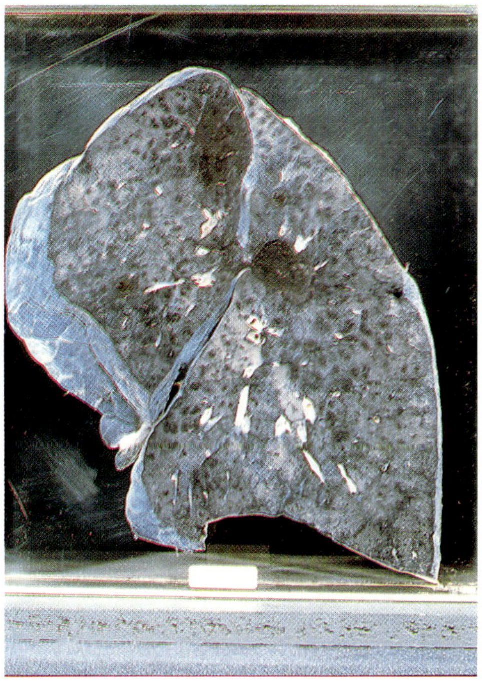

2.52 Coal-Workers' Pneumoconiosis

This is a post-mortem specimen from a 71-year-old man, who had worked all his life in a coal-mine.

A section through the left lung shows very intense, diffuse deposition of black coal dust throughout the lung parenchyma and in the hilar lymph nodes. The lung is over-expanded, due to centrilobular 'focal dust' emphysema, and there are several small fibrotic nodules, particularly in the lower lobe.

Coal-workers' pneumoconiosis may be divided into three types: simple, nodular and progressive massive fibrosis. The pattern seen in any particular case is dependent upon the silica content of the inhaled dust and the susceptibility of the affected individual.

The simple pattern, also known as dust reticulation, is due largely to the deposition of coal-dust alone in alveolar and respiratory bronchiolar walls, which gives rise to carbon pigmentation, and focal dust emphysema. The nodular variant is a consequence of focal fibrosis around areas of damage associated with silica and quartz particles. Progressive massive fibrosis, the most severe form, typically affects the upper lobes and may be induced by coexistent tuberculosis. Characteristically large, black, fibrotic masses are found, sometimes with central cavitation. Particular complications of coal-workers' pneumoconiosis include extensive vascular damage, leading to cor pulmonale, and tuberculosis, but there is no significantly increased risk of developing lung cancer.

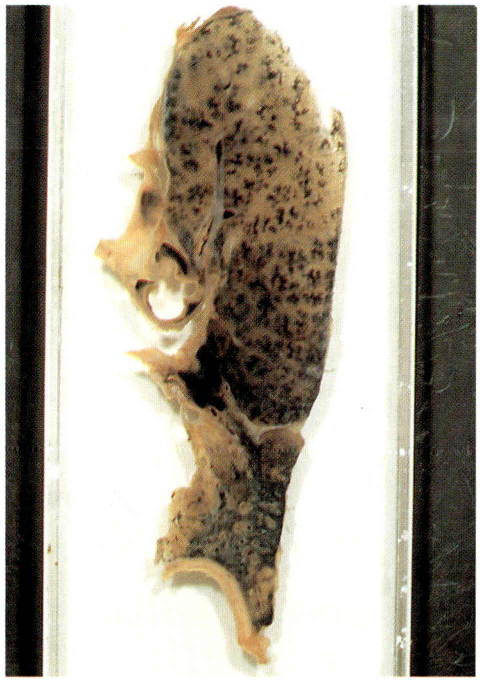

2.53 Asbestosis

This is a post-mortem specimen from a 48-year-old woman who, from the age of 17, had worked for 4 years in an asbestos factory. She first became dyspnoeic at the age of 27 and thereafter her condition deteriorated with an unremitting cough and, latterly, cor pulmonale.

A section through the left lung, in addition to diffuse anthrocotic pigmentation, shows collapse and dense fibrosis in the lower lobe, associated with bronchiectasis. The visceral pleura at the base of the lower lobe is grossly thickened and fibrotic. The upper lobe, particularly the apex, shows a degree of compensatory overaeration.

Asbestosis is not uncommon and affects particularly those who process asbestos and those who use it in the construction industries. The most frequent pathogenic types of asbestos fibre encountered are, crocidolite (blue) and amosite (brown), of which crocidolite is the most dangerous. The duration of exposure required to cause pulmonary changes may only be a matter of months and it is sometimes 25 years or more before symptoms develop. The consequent interstitial inflammation is followed by extensive fibrosis, the lower lobes being predominantly affected. Prolonged exposure to asbestos also confers a greatly increased risk of developing bronchial carcinoma, particularly in smokers, and asbestos workers are up to 1000 times more likely to develop a mesothelioma than other members of the population (see Legend 2.84).

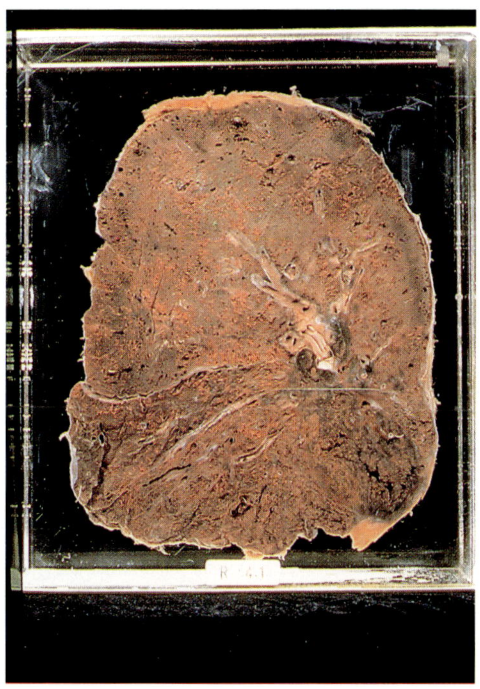

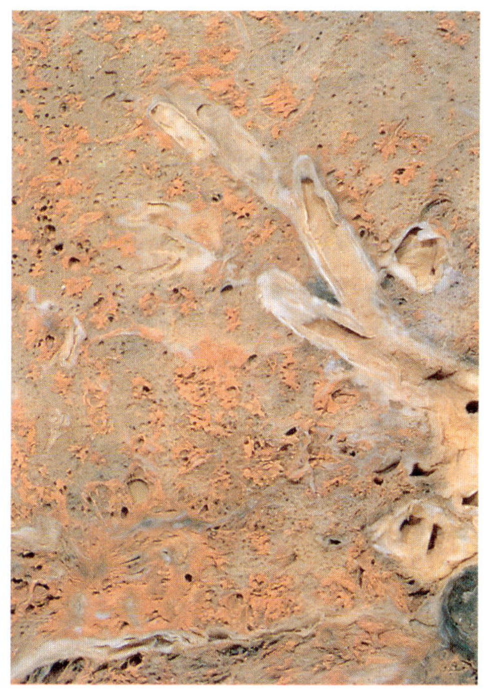

2.54 Haematite Pneumoconiosis

This is a post-mortem specimen from a 61-year-old man who had worked in haematite mines for 30 years. Ten years previously he had developed dyspnoea which had progressively worsened and he eventually died with cor pulmonale.

A coronal section through the lung shows parenchymal oedema and marked brick-red pigmentation (2.54a and 2.54b). Note the nodular and diffuse fibrosis with associated emphysematous changes. There are also dense, fibrous pleural adhesions, best seen at the top of this specimen.

Haematite pneumoconiosis is a form of siderotic lung disease, associated with the inhalation of iron oxide. While this condition is most often seen in iron ore miners, silver polishers and workers in steel or iron foundries may also be occasionally affected. Each of these groups may also develop silicosis. Pathogenetically, haematite pneumoconiosis may be divided into diffuse, nodular and massive fibrotic forms in exactly the same way as coal workers' pneumoconiosis (see Legend 2.52) and, as in that condition, is dependent upon the co-existence of silica and iron particles in the inhaled dust. Tuberculosis is a very common complication and there is also a predisposition to bronchial carcinoma, which may be attributed either to inhaled radioactive gases or it may arise in foci of parenchymal scarring in the lung.

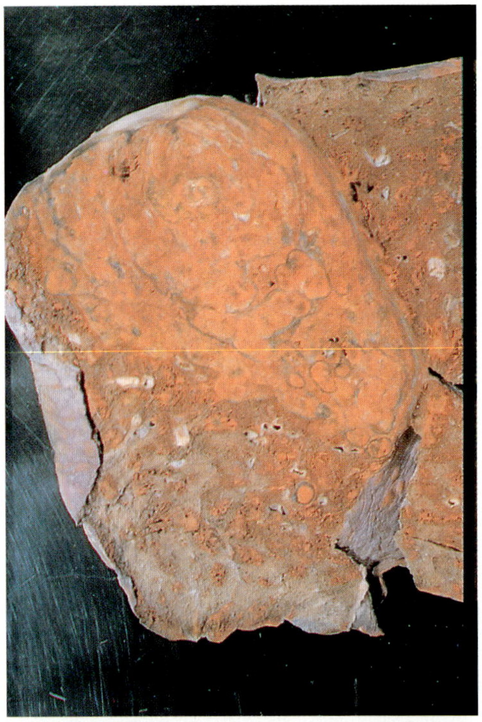

2.55 Haematite Pneumoconiosis

This is a post-mortem specimen from an elderly man who had worked in an iron-ore mine for 28 years. Latterly he was found to have extensive spinal tuberculosis with a psoas abscess and he died.

A section through the right upper lobe shows, in addition to brick-red pigmentation, a confluent, multinodular mass, measuring up to 7cm in diameter.

This is an example of massive fibrosis in a haematite lung, analogous in nature to that seen in coal workers' pneumoconiosis. The upper lobes are typically affected, with associated pleural fibrosis, and their appearance seems directly related to the silica content of the inhaled dust. This case also demonstrates, clinically, the frequency with which tuberculosis may complicate many of the pneumoconioses.

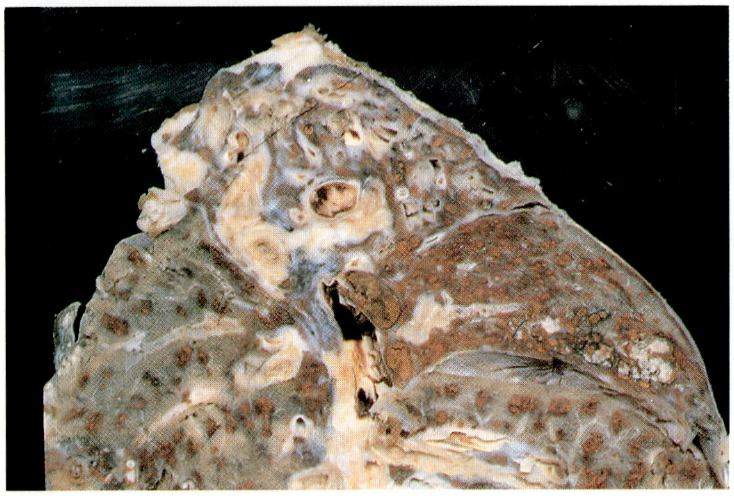

2.56 Haematite Pneumoconiosis with Squamous Carcinoma and Tuberculosis

This is a post-mortem specimen from a 61-year-old man who had been an iron-ore miner for 20 years and, latterly, had required numerous hospital admissions for deteriorating respiratory function.

A section through the upper lobe and apex of the middle lobe shows a variety of features. There is brick-red parenchymal pigmentation with focal fibrosis, a pale mass arising in the upper lobe bronchus which has infiltrated the upper lobe, small foci of caseous necrosis at the base of the upper lobe and an organised thrombus in the upper lobe branch of the pulmonary artery.

As already stated, tuberculosis is a not uncommon complication of haematite lung, as is bronchial carcinoma. The carcinoma may frequently develop away from the bronchial wall in an area of scarring. It is thought by some that the increased radioactivity in haematite mines may be responsible for this neoplastic change.

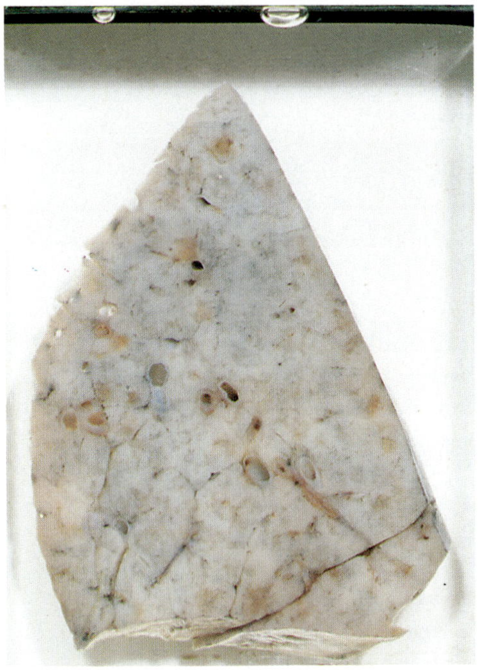

2.57 Alveolar Lipoproteinosis

This is a post-mortem specimen from a 25-year-old male metal worker. He first presented 4 years previously with dyspnoea and chest pain and was found on chest X-ray to have multiple pulmonary opacities. He recovered but returned 2 years later with bronchopneumonia. He gradually developed increasing dyspnoea, cyanosis and finger clubbing and eventually died in respiratory failure.

This section of lung shows uniform pale consolidation with some small foci of haemorrhage. The areas of consolidation have a typical uniform greyish appearance.

Alveolar lipoproteinosis is an idiopathic condition, first described in 1958, which appears to be a non-specific pulmonary response to an array of noxious substances, including various inorganic dusts and cytotoxic drugs. Males are more often affected, probably due to occupational factors. The disease is characterised by massive deposition of mucopolysaccharide and lipid within alveoli, probably as a result of hyperplasia and excessive, but abnormal, secretory activity of Type 2 pneumocytes. The clinical course is extremely variable, ranging from minimal to extreme impairment of respiratory function.

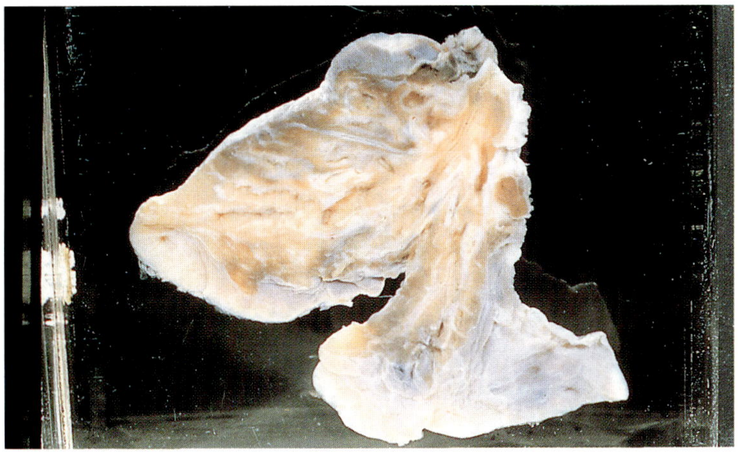

2.58 Atelectasis (Collapse)

This specimen was excised from an 8-year-old girl who had contracted pneumonia as a baby. She had remained well but was found to have substantial and irreversible collapse of the right middle and lower lobes, which were therefore removed. There was no evidence of obstruction or external compression.

The right middle and lower lobes have been sectioned coronally to show total collapse of the air spaces, leaving only solid pale lung parenchyma around the bronchial tree which shows some mild irregular dilatation.

Atelectasis, or collapse of lung tissue, may be subdivided into congenital and acquired types, the latter group being further classified as pressure, absorption or massive in type. Congenital collapse may be due to prematurity, hyaline membrane disease, proximal obstruction or congenital pulmonary anomalies. Pressure collapse, due to pleural compression, may be a result of a pneumothorax, haemothorax or pleural effusion. Absorption collapse is caused by total proximal (usually bronchial) obstruction of rapid onset. Massive collapse is seen most often in severe chest injuries. In the case here, the previous episode of pneumonia was probably a complication rather than the cause of this girl's collapsed lobes. More likely causes are congenital hypoplasia, incomplete expansion at birth or hyaline membrane disease, either probably being a consequence of prematurity.

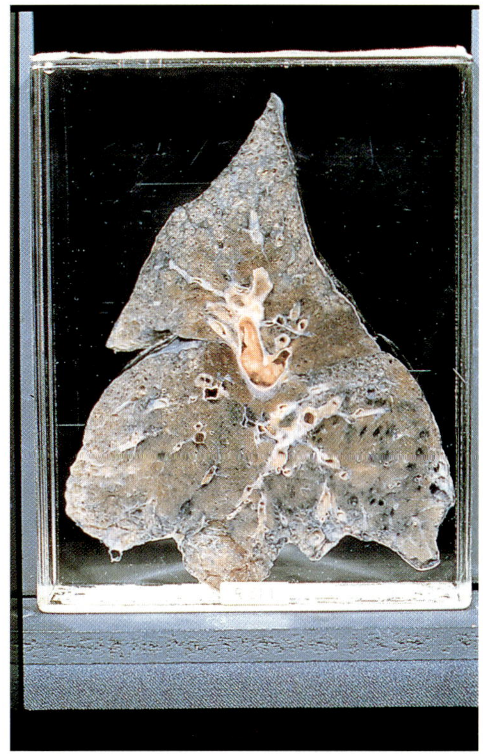

2.59 Idiopathic Fibrosing Alveolitis

This is a post-mortem specimen from a 63-year-old man who had suffered from bouts of dyspnoea for 14 years, more recently becoming continuous in nature. He was found to have diffuse pulmonary fibrosis for which no cause could be identified and he died.

The middle and lower lobes of the right lung have been sectioned coronally to show marked, diffuse, interstitial fibrosis, as a consequence of which there is compensatory dilatation of subpleural air spaces, giving some areas a honeycomb appearance. In addition, organising thrombus is apparent in a large pulmonary artery and there is adjacent red infarction.

Idiopathic fibrosing alveolitis (synonym: Hamman-Rich syndrome) is an uncommon condition, affecting males predominantly, which is thought to result from immunological damage to alveolar walls. It is a diagnosis of exclusion since very similar diffuse interstitial fibrosis may be seen in many other conditions, for example some of the pneumoconioses, extrinsic allergic alveolitis (e.g. farmer's lung) and connective tissue diseases (e.g. systemic lupus erythematosus or rheumatoid arthritis).

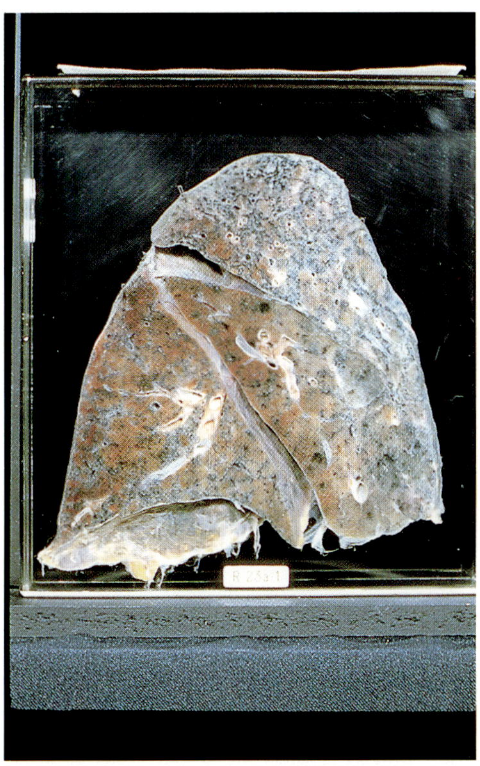

2.60 Radiation Fibrosis

This is a post-mortem specimen from a 61-year-old woman who had been treated for breast carcinoma by mastectomy and radiotherapy 5 years previously. She developed a cough and progressive dyspnoea and was assumed to have pulmonary lymphangitis carcinomatosa on chest X-ray. She died eventually with cor pulmonale, but at autopsy there was no evidence of metastatic carcinoma.

This lung, which was inflated prior to fixation, has been sectioned sagittaly to show dense, diffuse fibrosis in the apical and posterior segments. Anteriorly, there is pulmonary congestion and the pleural fibrous adhesions should be noted (bottom left).

Pulmonary fibrosis due to irradiation (synonym: radiation pneumonitis) is not uncommon and may follow therapeutic irradiation, or industrial or accidental exposure to radioactive materials. The degree of damage is dependent upon the duration of exposure, dose, and individual susceptibility. Interstitial fibrosis results from the exuberant reparative process that follows acute alveolar and bronchial damage. Note also that prolonged exposure to inhaled radioactive material may lead to the development of bronchial carcinoma without preceding interstitial fibrosis.

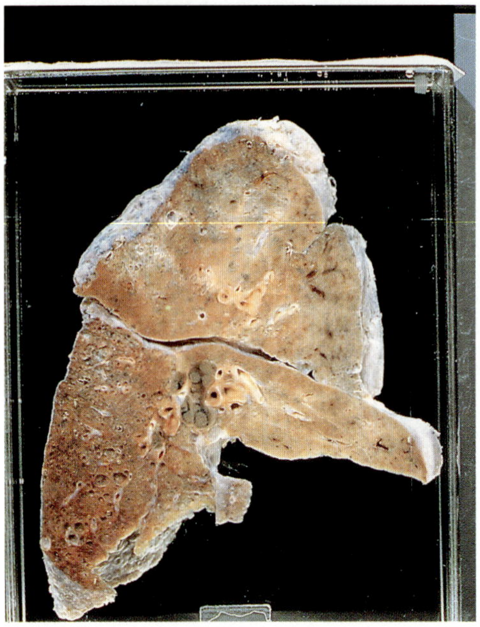

2.61 Systemic Sclerosis

This is a post-mortem specimen from a 35-year-old man who had been treated for progressive systemic sclerosis for several years.

In coronal section the left lung has a honeycomb appearance in the posterior segment of the lower lobe. In the upper lobe there are smaller foci of similar change. There is marked hilar lymphadenopathy, the nodes being greyish in colour.

Pulmonary involvement in progressive systemic sclerosis is well recognised and is characterised by diffuse interstitial fibrosis, honeycomb changes (particularly in the subpleural portions of the lower lobe) and pleural fibrous adhesions. Typically, females, usually in the 5th and 6th decades, are most often affected, as in scleroderma. Complications include the development of pulmonary hypertension and primary pulmonary adenocarcinoma, which may be bronchioalveolar in type.

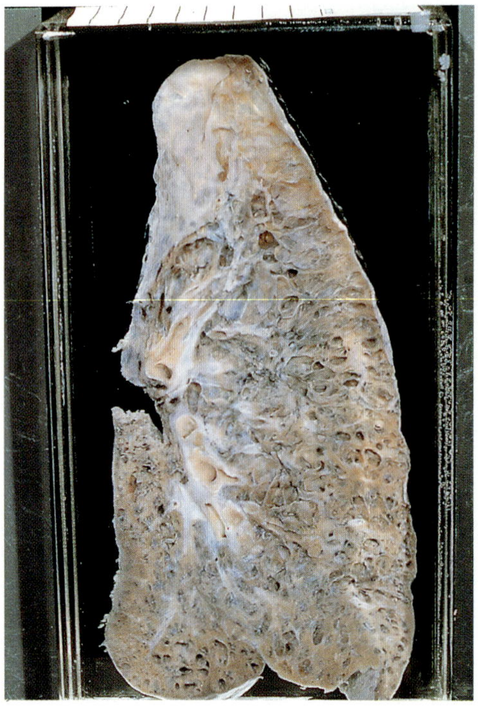

2.62 Honeycomb Lung

This is a post-mortem specimen from a 28-year-old man who was known to have multiple bony 'cysts', probably polyostotic fibrous dysplasia. Latterly, he developed chest pains with evidence of pulmonary consolidation, and he eventually died of pneumonia.

A coronal section through this lung shows innumerable thin-walled, cystic spaces, which measure up to 1cm in diameter. The entire lung parenchyma is uniformly affected.

Honeycomb lung represents the end-stage of a wide variety of pulmonary diseases. It is, therefore, a non-specific appearance, representing obliterative damage of some bronchioles and alveoli, with compensatory dilatation of the adjacent unaffected air passages. It is a common cause of cor pulmonale and pulmonary hypertension. Common preceding conditions include many of the pneumoconioses, particularly asbestosis, extrinsic allergic alveolitis, idiopathic fibrosing alveolitis, sarcoidosis, systemic sclerosis, rheumatoid arthritis and very extensive pneumonia or tuberculosis. In this case, the cause was not identified.

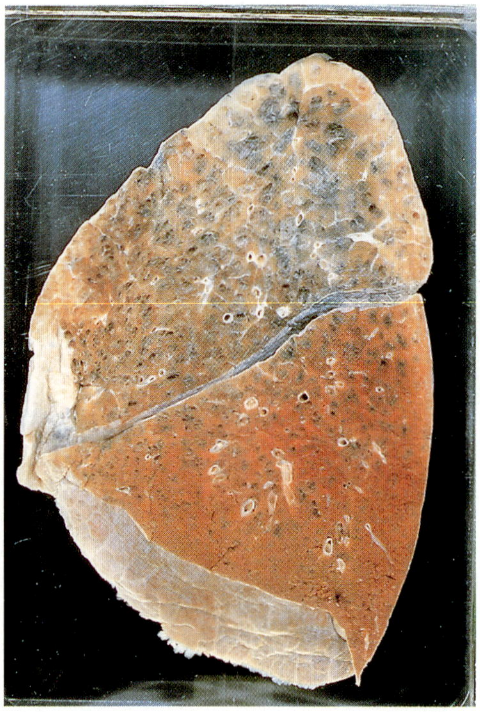

2.63 Idiopathic Pulmonary Haemosiderosis

This is a post-mortem specimen from a 43-year-old woman who was also known to have multiple sclerosis.

A coronal section through the lung shows marked, diffuse, reddish-brown parenchymal pigmentation, particularly of the lower lobe. The upper lobe also shows mild, centrilobular emphysema (see Legend 2.49).

Idiopathic pulmonary haemosiderosis (synonym: Ceelen's disease) is a rare condition which predominantly affects children and young adults, with an equal sex distribution. It is characterised by repeated focal intra-alveolar and intrabronchiolar haemorrhages, with no apparent cause, accompanied by the deposition of haemosiderin, hyperplasia of the alveolar epithelium and destruction of the elastic tissue in both alveolar and pulmonary vascular walls. Consequent fibrosis leads to pulmonary hypertension and cor pulmonale. The clinical course is unpredictable but in fatal cases, death usually results from intrapulmonary haemorrhage. Pathogenetically, it may be related to Goodpasture's syndrome, being autoimmune in origin but showing no renal involvement.

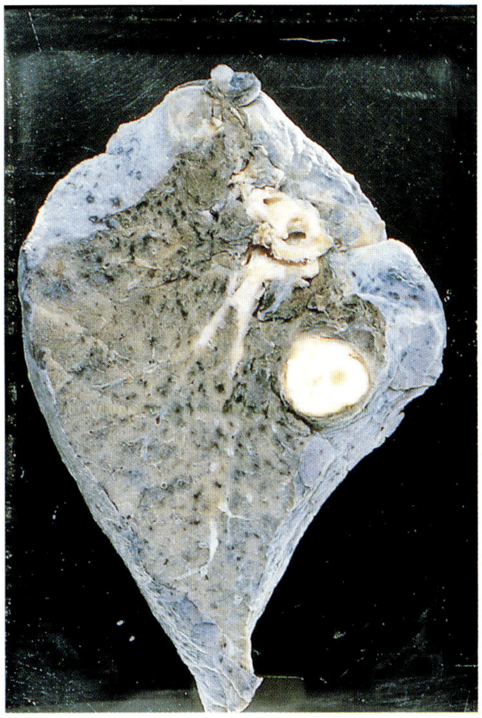

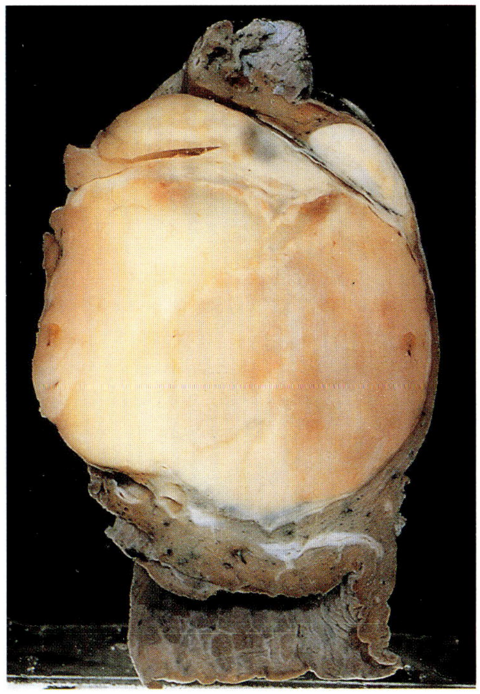

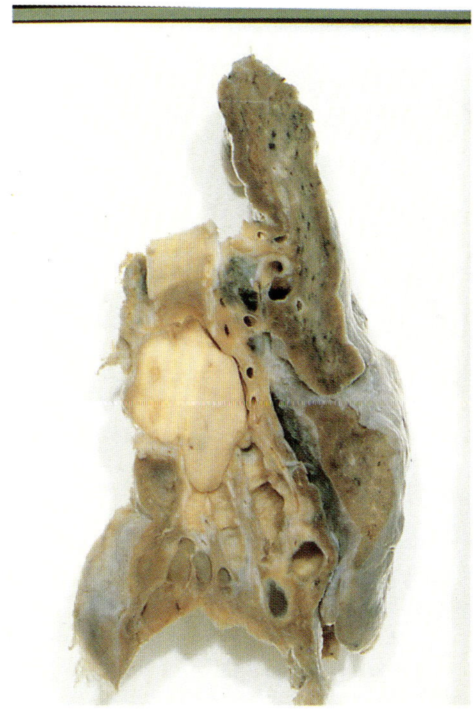

2.64 Hamartoma

This is a lobectomy specimen from a 60-year-old male smoker who complained of recurrent chest infections. A chest X-ray revealed a rounded opacity in the right lower lobe and operation was advised.

A section through the right lower lobe shows a well-circumscribed, pale mass, measuring 2cm in diameter, adjacent to the diaphragmatic surface.

Pulmonary hamartomas (synonym: adenochondroma) are not uncommon but are usually asymptomatic. Males are affected more frequently than females and these lesions may be solitary or, rarely, multiple. Classically, they are composed largely of cartilage, well-circumscribed and lobulated giving rise to a 'coin' lesion on chest X-ray. They have no potential for malignant change. Such hamartomas are most often subpleural in location. Not infrequently lobectomy is performed in the mistaken belief that the patient has a peripheral primary carcinoma.

2.65 Hamartoma

This specimen was excised from a 48-year-old woman who presented with non-specific discomfort in the right lower chest. A chest X-ray showed a well-defined tumour in the right lower lobe and lobectomy was performed.

A coronal section through the right lower lobe shows a well-circumscribed, nodular, yellowish tumour, measuring 5cm in maximum diameter. The pleura is attenuated over the lesion.

This is an unusually large example of a pulmonary hamartoma and, microscopically, could be classified as an adenofibromatous variant, being devoid of cartilage on this occasion.

2.66 Bronchial 'Adenoma'

This is a pneumonectomy specimen from a 36-year-old woman who presented with a 2 year history of intermittent haemoptysis. Chest X-ray showed a mass in the right lower lobe and bronchoscopy revealed an ulcerated endobronchial tumour. The right lung was excised.

A coronal section through the right lower lobe shows a rounded, lobulated neoplasm, arising from the wall of the main bronchus and projecting into the lumen. The tumour measures 3cm in maximum diameter and, in obstructing the bronchus, has caused marked distal bronchiectasis with collapse.

The term bronchial 'adenoma' is a misnomer for two reasons: firstly, it represents several distinct entities and, secondly, many cases should be regarded as low-grade malignant tumours. The commonest variety of this uncommon lesion is the bronchial carcinoid tumour, of which the case here is an example. Bronchial carcinoids are slow-growing tumours, typically occurring in middle age, and may grow into the bronchial lumen or submucosally. They may be responsible for ectopic hormone secretion, in particular 5-hydroxytryptamine, ACTH, ADH and insulin. Up to 5 per cent of cases metastasise. The other, much rarer, entities included under the heading bronchial 'adenoma' are the truly benign cystadenoma and mucoepidermoid adenoma, and the low grade malignant adenoid cystic carcinoma (synonym: bronchial cylindroma).

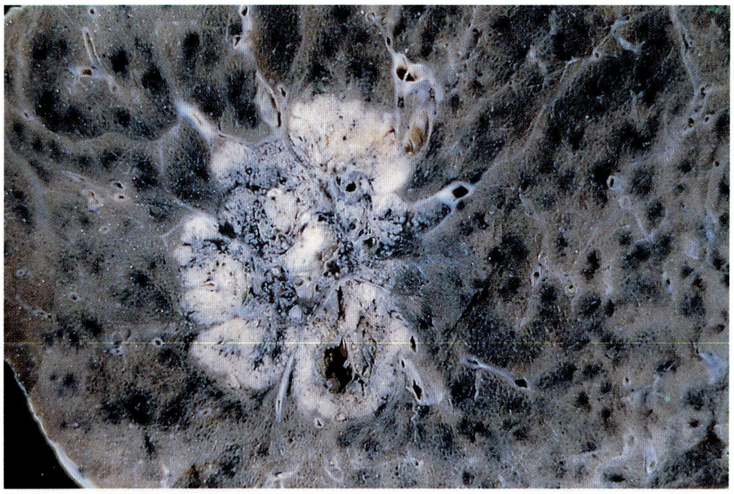

2.67 Squamous Cell Carcinoma

This is a lobectomy specimen from a 63-year-old man who had been a heavy smoker for many years. He was admitted to hospital with a 2 week history of pleuritic chest pain and haemoptysis and a chest X-ray revealed a mass in the right upper lobe.

A coronal section through part of the right upper lobe shows an irregular, pale neoplasm, which measures 4cm in maximum diameter, arising from one of the segmental bronchi. The lesion is fairly well circumscribed and shows central necrosis.

Carcinoma of the lung is, numerically, the single most common cause of death from malignant disease in the United Kingdom. The incidence is increasing, middle-aged and elderly adults predominating, and while in the past males were most often affected, the growing number of female smokers is leading to a more equal sex incidence. The most important aetiological agent by far is cigarette smoking; tumour incidence being directly proportional to the number of cigarettes smoked, the duration of the habit, and the tendency to inhale. There are over 200 proven carcinogens or co-carcinogens in cigarette smoke. Other important aetiological factors are occupational (workers exposed to radiation, uranium, asbestos, nickel, chromates and many others), urban pollution and previous scarring of the lung parenchyma. Fifty per cent of bronchial carcinomas are squamous in type, the remainder being divided between oat cell, adeno- and large cell anaplastic tumours. With the exception of adenocarcinoma, the majority arise in large bronchi adjacent to the lung hilum. Lymphatic spread occurs in the vast majority of cases and is often rapidly followed by haematogenous dissemination; metastases show a predilection for the adrenal, liver, bone and brain. Many other features will be covered in the subsequent legends; however, with reference to squamous carcinoma in particular, these tumours tend to a slightly less aggressive course than the anaplastic group with later metastasis. Even so, the overall 5-year-survival for all types of lung cancer is only of the order of 10 per cent. Squamous carcinoma may occasionally be responsible for the ectopic production of a parathormone-like substance, but inappropriate endocrine activity is much more a feature of oat cell carcinoma (see Legend 2.69).

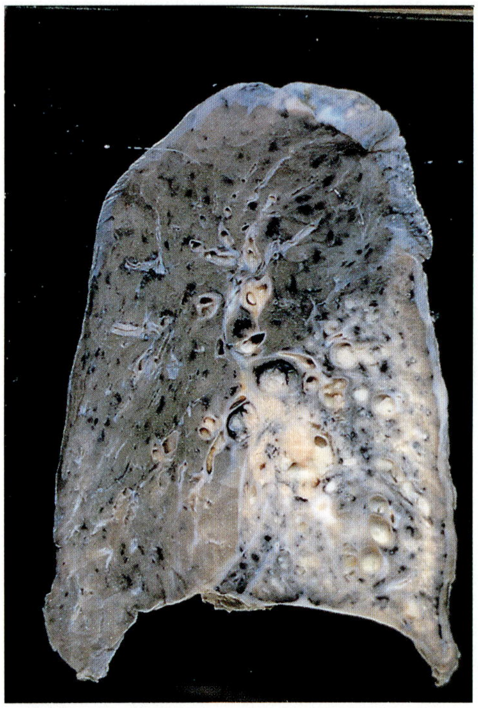

2.68 Squamous Cell Carcinoma

This is a pneumonectomy specimen from a 55-year-old man who developed a persistent cough and a lower lobe pneumonia. Bronchoscopy revealed a mass obstructing the right lower lobe bronchus which was deemed operable.

A coronal section through the right lung shows a pale neoplasm obstructing the main lower lobe bronchus and invading the adjacent parenchyma. Two anthracotic hilar lymph nodes are also clearly involved. Distal to the obstruction, the lower lobe is collapsed and shows marked bronchiectasis with pneumonic consolidation.

Proximity to the lung hilum makes very many cases inoperable; only 20 per cent of lung carcinomas are considered for surgery. A careful pre-operative search for metastases, utilising modern imaging techniques, usually means that only about 5 per cent of cases are treated surgically. The case here demonstrates three of the common local complications of intraluminal growth of bronchial carcinomas: distal atelectasis, bronchopneumonia or bronchiectasis are frequent presenting features.

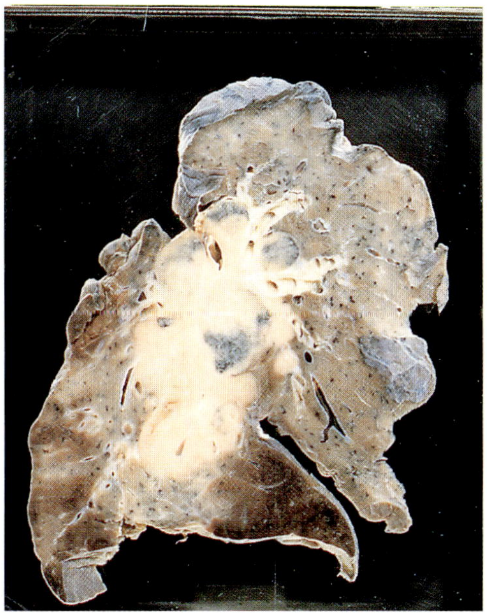

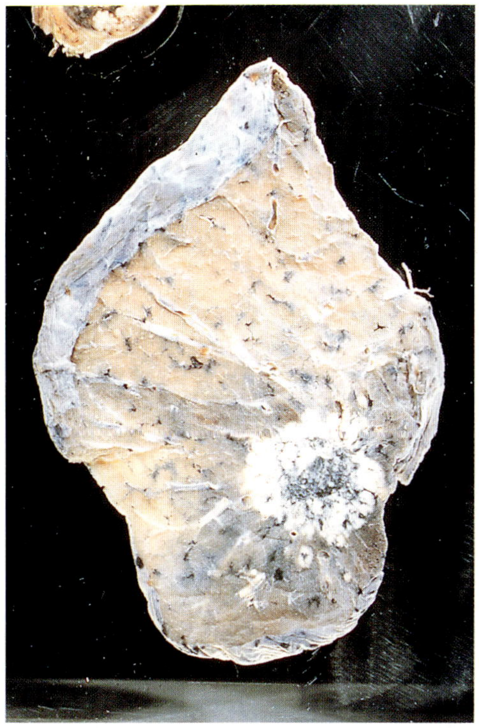

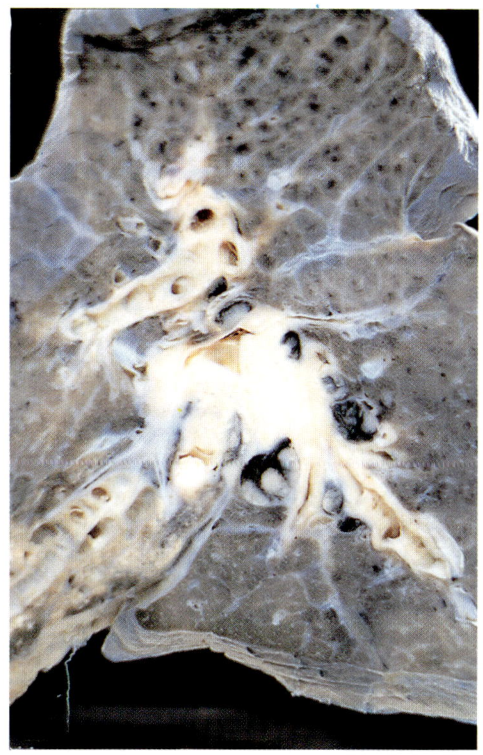

2.69 Oat Cell (Small Cell Anaplastic) Carcinoma

This specimen was excised from a 40-year-old man who presented with a 6 week history of a dry cough and pleuritic chest pain. X-rays showed collapse and consolidation of the left lower lobe and bronchoscopy showed rigid infiltration of the left lower lobe bronchus. A left pneumonectomy was performed, at which operation mediastinal lymph node involvement was noted.

A coronal section through the left lung shows a large, irregularly infiltrative pale neoplasm arising at the lung hilum. The lower lobe bronchus is virtually obliterated and the hilar lymph nodes are invaded in continuity with the main tumour mass. There is extensive infarction of the remainder of the lower lobe, suggestive of vascular occlusion or disruption by the tumour.

Oat cell (small cell anaplastic) carcinoma comprises about 20 per cent of all bronchial malignancies. While a proportion of cases may originate in bronchial neuroendocrine (APUD) cells (known as Kulchitsky cells), the majority probably represent totally undifferentiated tumours of bronchial respiratory epithelium. These tumours are the most prone to ectopic hormone production, in particular ACTH, ADH and 5-hydroxytryptamine, with the expected clinical results. Oat cell carcinomas, as a group, carry the worst prognosis of the common bronchial malignancies, being almost universally fatal within a year from the time of diagnosis, usually with very extensive and widespread metastases.

2.70 Adenocarcinoma

This is a lobectomy specimen from a 60-year-old woman who had a 2 year history of recurrent chest infections, more recently associated with haemoptysis and pleuritic pain. Bronchoscopy was normal but a chest X-ray revealed a rounded opacity in the posterior segment of the left upper lobe.

A section through the left upper lobe shows a rounded, pale neoplasm, measuring 2cm in diameter, just beneath the pleural surface posteriorly. The tumour has a well-defined, crenated margin and there are several smaller, adjacent tumour nodules.

Primary adenocarcinoma of the lung comprises about 15 per cent of all lung cancers when the bronchioalveolar group (see Legend 2.72) are included. Adenocarcinomas show an equal sex incidence and are typically peripherally located. They are often small tumours which have a particular tendency to arise in foci of scarring, associated with a previous healed infarct or tuberculosis, for example. These tumours tend to be slow growing and this, in combination with their frequent operability, confers a better prognosis than other lung carcinomas.

2.71 Large Cell Anaplastic Carcinoma

This specimen was excised from a 49-year-old man who presented with weight loss, a cough and chest pain. Chest X-ray revealed collapse and consolidation of the right middle lobe and at bronchoscopy there was an exophytic tumour obstructing the middle lobe bronchus. A right pneumonectomy was performed.

A coronal section through the right lung shows a pale neoplasm obstructing the major bronchi to the middle and lower lobes. The adjacent hilar lymph nodes contain obvious metastatic tumour. There is marked distal bronchiectasis and the middle lobe shows areas of pale consolidation.

Large cell anaplastic carcinoma comprises about 10 per cent of bronchial malignancies and is thought to represent totally undifferentiated examples of either squamous or adenocarcinoma. It carries a very poor prognosis, although not quite as dismal as oat cell carcinoma. Occasional examples may secrete human chorionic gonadotrophin, which can lead to gynaecomastia in males.

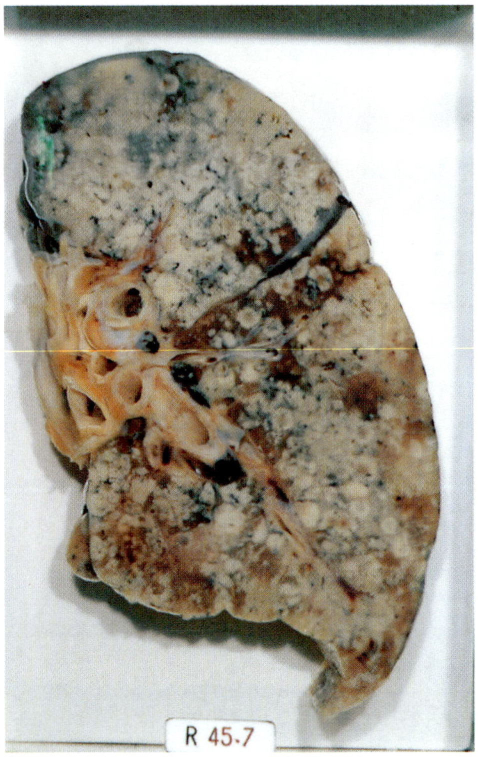

2.72 Bronchioalveolar Carcinoma

This is a post-mortem specimen from a 45-year-old man who presented with a 2 year history of cough and malaise. Chest radiography was suggestive of tuberculosis. However, despite empirical treatment, his condition deteriorated with increasing dyspnoea and haemoptysis and he died. At autopsy, other than a single involved lymph node at the carina, there was no evidence of metastasis elsewhere.

A coronal section through the right lung shows widespread, diffuse infiltration by pale tumour, having a nodular appearance in places. There is very little remaining normal parenchyma.

Bronchioalveolar carcinoma (synonym: malignant pulmonary adenomatosis) represents a specific variant of adenocarcinoma and comprises about 2 per cent of all primary lung malignancies. It is usually a well-differentiated tumour which is thought to arise either from alveolar or terminal bronchiolar epithelium and tends to spread throughout the air passages while preserving the septal and lobular architecture. The sex incidence is about equal and the age of presentation is very variable. While this tumour is slow-growing and usually metastasises late in the course of the disease, the 5-year-survival is only about 5 per cent. This is thought to reflect the fact that these neoplasms often present late or may be initially mistaken for an infective or diffuse interstitial disorder.

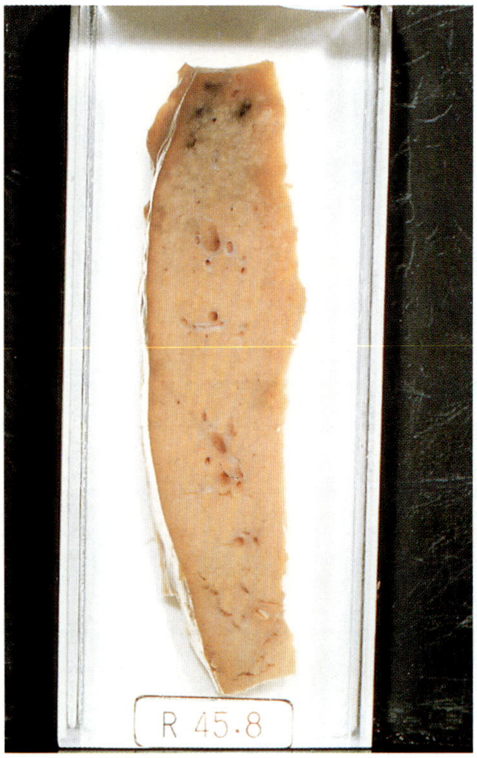

2.73 Bronchioalveolar Carcinoma

This specimen was excised from a 64-year-old woman who had a 2 month history of a productive cough. There were signs of right lower lobe consolidation both clinically and radiologically and adenocarcinoma cells were identified on sputum cytology. A lobectomy was performed.

A portion of the right lower lobe has been sectioned to show diffuse, pale consolidation which is only recognisable as tumour at the top of the specimen, where invasion is more focal.

This sample demonstrates well that diffuse involvement by bronchioalveolar carcinoma may give rise to an unusual appearance, not immediately identifiable as a neoplasm. It is hardly surprising that a chest X-ray in a case such as this might be misinterpreted, thus delaying an accurate diagnosis. Occasionally this tumour presents with a more multinodular pattern, mimicking multiple metastases. Such a finding should provoke a careful search for a primary adenocarcinoma elsewhere.

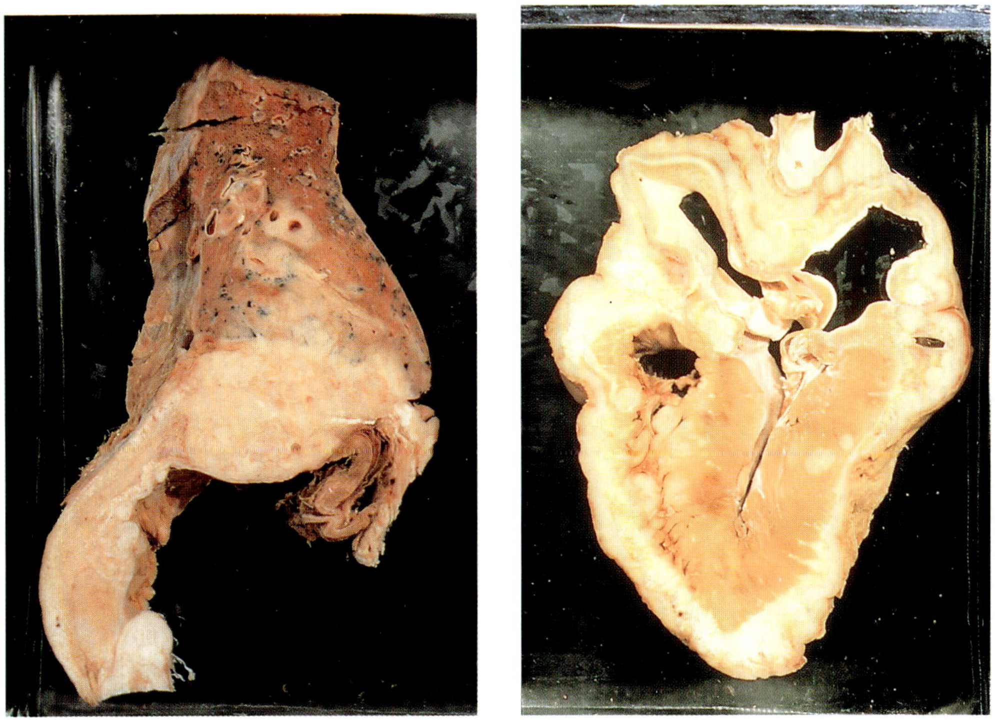

2.74 Anaplastic Carcinoma showing extensive Local Invasion

These are post-mortem specimens from a 70-year-old woman who died in congestive cardiac failure. At autopsy, in association with the primary lung tumour, metastases were found in lymph nodes, the pancreas, liver, right adrenal and thyroid.

The right lower lobe (2.74a) shows an ill-defined pale neoplasm which has diffusely and extensively infiltrated the densely adherent parietal pleura and diaphragm. A sagittal section through the heart (2.74b) shows similar diffuse extension throughout the parietal and visceral layers of the pericardium. The great vessels are likewise encased in tumour and there are discrete nodules in the myocardium.

This case demonstrates well some of the possible consequences of local invasion by any bronchial carcinoma. The patient effectively died of tumour-induced cardiac tamponade.

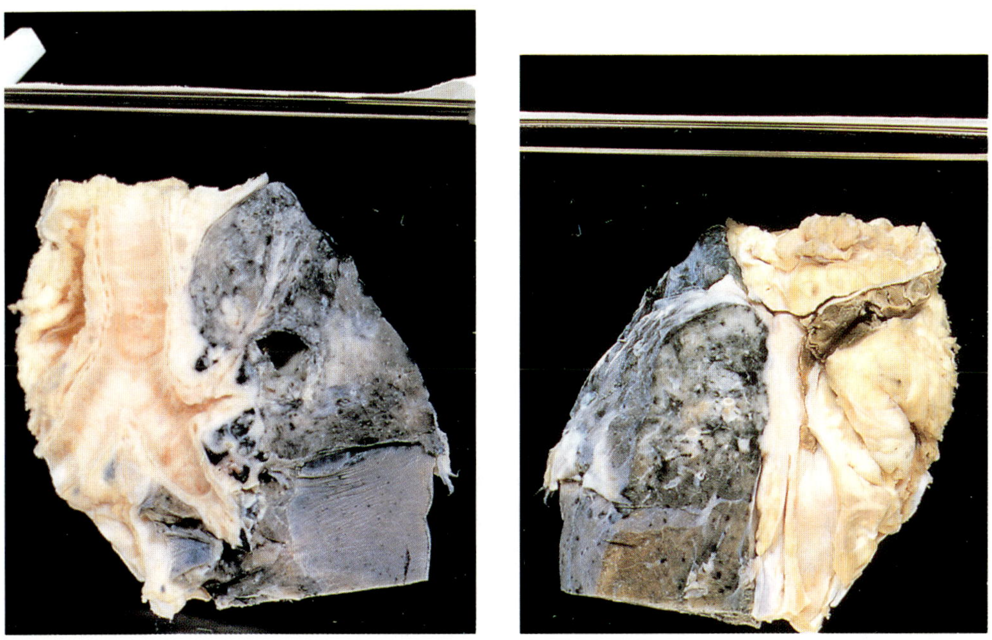

2.75 Bronchial Carcinoma with obstruction of the Superior Vena Cava

This is a post-mortem specimen from a 69-year-old man who presented with a persistent cough and weight loss. Bronchoscopy revealed obstruction of the right upper lobe bronchus and a biopsy showed squamous cell carcinoma. He rapidly developed features of superior vena caval obstruction, with intense oedema and congestion of the face and arms. Despite palliative radiotherapy, he died 4 months later.

A section through the right upper lobe and tracheal bifurcation, opened posteriorly, shows a pale neoplasm obstructing the upper lobe bronchus and extending to the lateral tracheal wall (2.75a). Distal to the tumour is an irregular abscess cavity, measuring 2cm in diameter. The superior vena cava (2.75b) can be seen to pass through a mass of enlarged, adherent hilar lymph nodes. Just above these, the wall of the vena cava is infiltrated by tumour and the narrowed lumen has eventually become occluded by overlying thrombus.

Local invasion of mediastinal structures is a common occurrence in bronchial carcinoma and obstruction of the superior vena cava with or without consequent thrombosis, is very well recognised. Palliation of the resultant distressing symptoms is usually achieved with radiotherapy, but does not prolong survival.

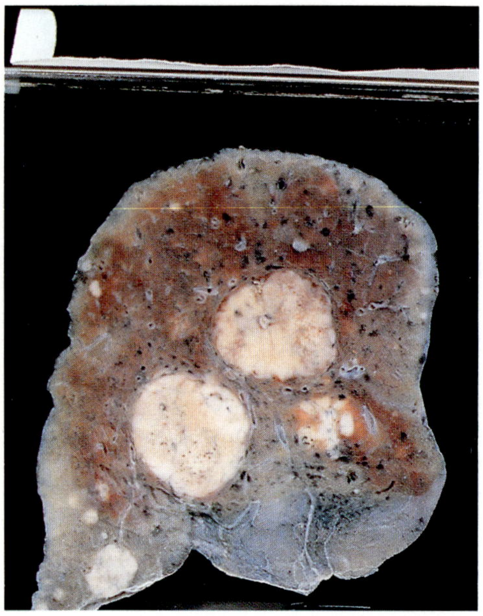

2.76 Metastatic Breast Carcinoma

This is a post-mortem specimen from a 53-year-old woman who was diagnosed as having adenocarcinoma of the left breast with lymph node metastases 2 years previously. At autopsy, metastases were also found in the liver, brain, kidneys and spleen.

A coronal section through the lung shows multiple, pale, discrete nodules of tumour, varying in diameter from 0.3-5cm.

Pulmonary metastases may be found in between 20-30 per cent of all patients dying of malignant disease, almost irrespective of the primary tumour site. However, the commonest sources of pulmonary metastases are carcinomas of the breast, colon, stomach, prostate and the lung itself. The rich and extensive vascular and lymphatic systems in the lung are probably the most important reason for this tendency. Metastases may be single or multiple, small or large, discrete or diffuse; diffuse lymphatic invasion may give rise to lymphangitis carcinomatosa while isolated, large deposits are known as cannon-ball metastases and are characteristically derived from renal or testicular tumours.

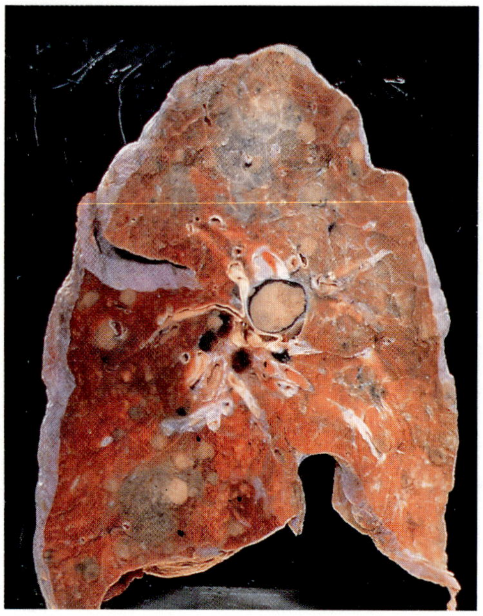

2.77 Metastatic Malignant Melanoma

This is a post-mortem specimen from a 76-year-old woman who had undergone excision of a malignant melanoma arising in the skin of the right side of the neck several years previously.

A coronal section through the lung shows numerous rounded deposits of tumour, varying in diameter from 0.1-1.0cm. Some of these show melanotic pigmentation while others are amelanotic. A deposit is also visible in one of the hilar lymph nodes but the very dark pigmentation of the smaller nodes is purely anthracotic in origin.

Malignant melanoma commonly metastasises, usually by the bloodstream, to the lung and may often be recognised macroscopically by the presence of melanin pigment.

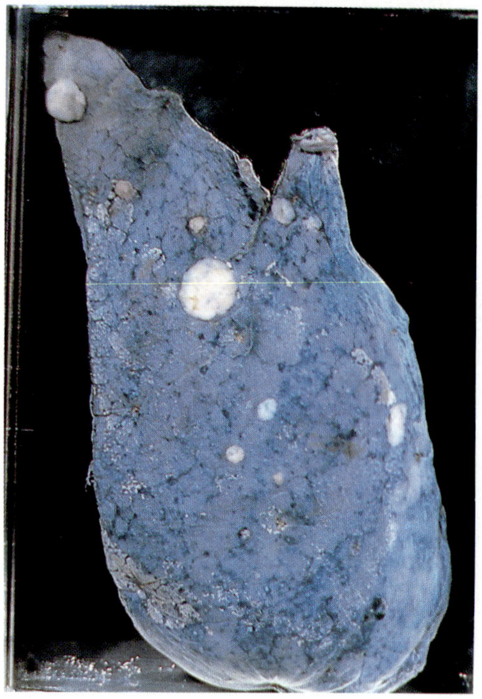

2.78 Metastatic Osteosarcoma

This is a post-mortem specimen from a 65-year-old man who developed an osteosarcoma in the left humerus, having suffered from Paget's disease of the bone for many years.

This lung shows multiple pleural and subpleural deposits of pale tumour, one of which is pedunculated (top left).

The lung is the commonest site of metastases from any sarcoma and this case serves to reiterate that the predominant mode of spread of sarcomas of bone or soft tissue is haematogenous.

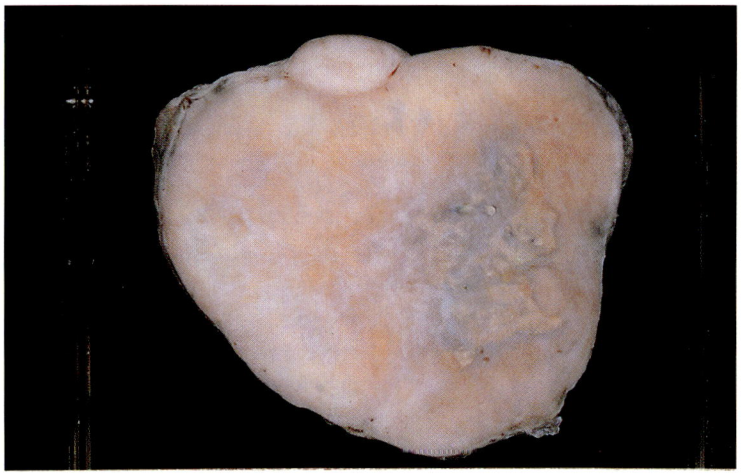

2.79 Fibroma

This specimen was excised from a 58-year-old woman who presented with a cough and dyspnoea but was otherwise well. A chest X-ray revealed a right upper lobe mass. At operation the lesion was found to be compressing the upper lobe bronchus, resulting in distal collapse. However, the mass was readily dissected out without the need to resect the lobe.

The lesion is a smooth, somewhat whorled, pale tumour, measuring 9cm in maximum diameter, and is encapsulated. There is a small focus of necrosis in its upper pole and very small portions of attached lung tissue are visible round the edge of the neoplasm.

Pulmonary fibromas are very rare, benign lesions which may arise either in a bronchial wall or the lung parenchyma. There are no clinical distinguishing features. These tumours not uncommonly show degenerative changes, including necrosis or calcification.

PLEURA AND MEDIASTINUM

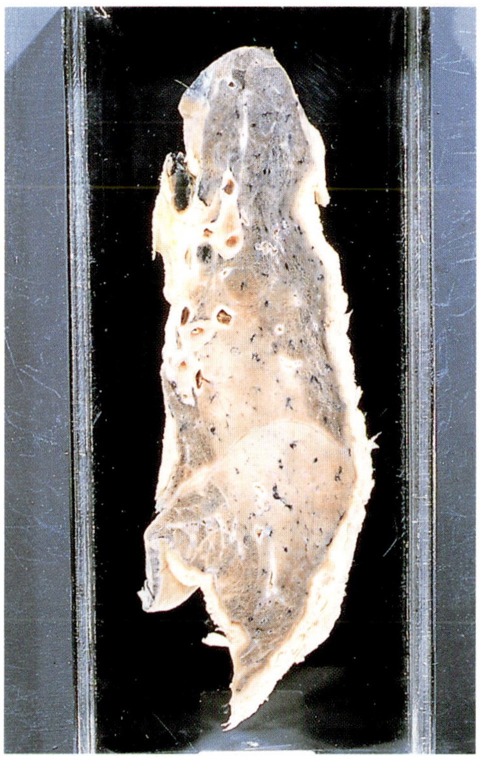

2.80 Pleura: Fibrinous Exudate

This is a post-mortem specimen from a 43-year-old man who died four days after developing pleuritic chest pain.

A coronal section through the left lung shows grey hepatization of the lower lobe, typical of lobar pneumonia (see Legends 2.32 and 2.33). In addition there is a marked fibrinous exudate, up to 0.5cm in thickness, over the visceral pleura.

A pleural fibrinous exudate, with subsequent adhesions, is a common finding in association with an underlying pulmonary inflammatory process, the commonest causes of which are infection or infarction. It simply represents the protein-rich exudate typical of any acute inflammatory process and may or may not be purulent. Organisation of the fibrin leads to the formation of pleural adhesions.

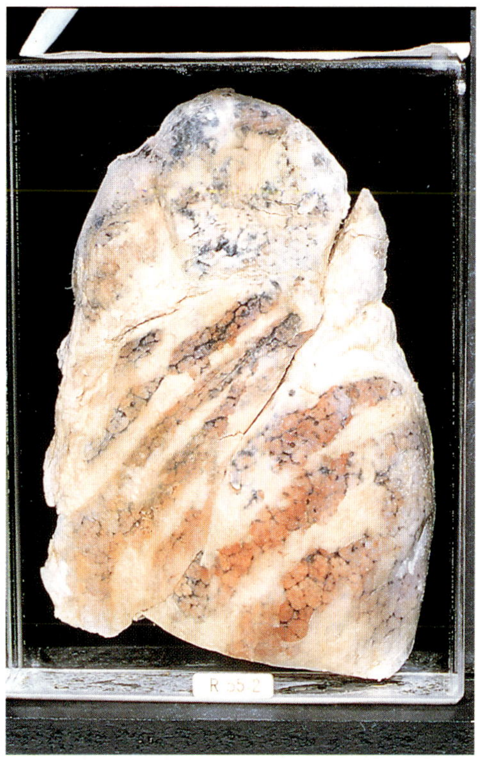

2.81 Pleura: Empyema

This is a post-mortem specimen from a 61-year-old woman who died after developing left-sided lobar pneumonia.

The pleural surface of the left lung is covered in a dense, purulent exudate. The streaked appearance is due to the dense adhesions to the parietal pleura and ribs which were detached during removal of the lung.

An empyema simply represents the presence of copious purulent material in the pleural cavity and may be seen as a complication of many broncho- or lobar pneumonias, tuberculosis or fungal infections.

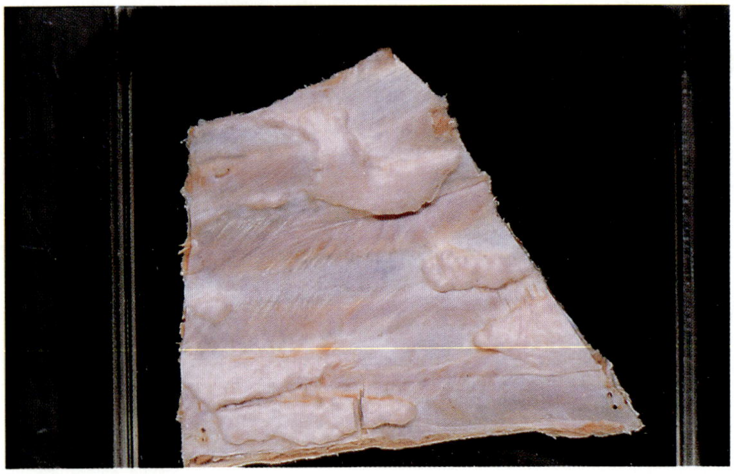

2.82 Pleura: Fibrous Plaques

This was an incidental finding at post-mortem in a 70-year-old man who died of carcinoma of the head of the pancreas.

This is a portion of the chest wall, dissected to show the parietal pleura. The surface of the pleura shows numerous, irregular raised plaques, measuring up to 0.4cm in thickness, which are white in colour.

Fibrous pleural plaques are found in up to 5 per cent of post-mortems and are thought to be a result of asbestos exposure but *not necessarily* asbestosis. The majority of the population are probably exposed at some time in their lives to the inhalation of asbestos fibres, which may migrate through lung tissue to the pleural surface where they initiate a chronic inflammatory, and later fibrotic, process. Clearly, however, diffuse pleural fibrosis and pleural fibrous plaques are commonest in those occupationally exposed to asbestos (see Legend 2.53).

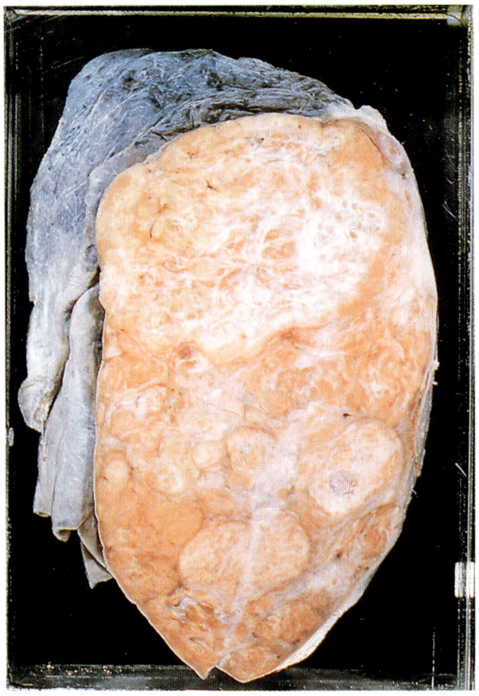

2.83 Pleura: Fibroma

This is a post-mortem specimen from a 50-year-old man who had known quaternary syphilis and died in congestive cardiac failure. He had suffered from increasing dyspnoea for 4 years.

This tumour, which has been bisected, was found to be arising from the posterior parietal pleura and measures 19cm in maximum diameter. A portion of lung tissue, which was adherent to the tumour anteriorly, is also visible. The lesion is well-circumscribed and has a lobulated, somewhat whorled cut-surface.

Pleural fibromas are uncommon, benign lesions which are localised (cf. mesothelioma). They usually arise in adult life in either sex and are slow-growing, often attaining a great size, as in this case. They are frequently associated with a pulmonary osteoarthropathy. Malignant change is extremely rare.

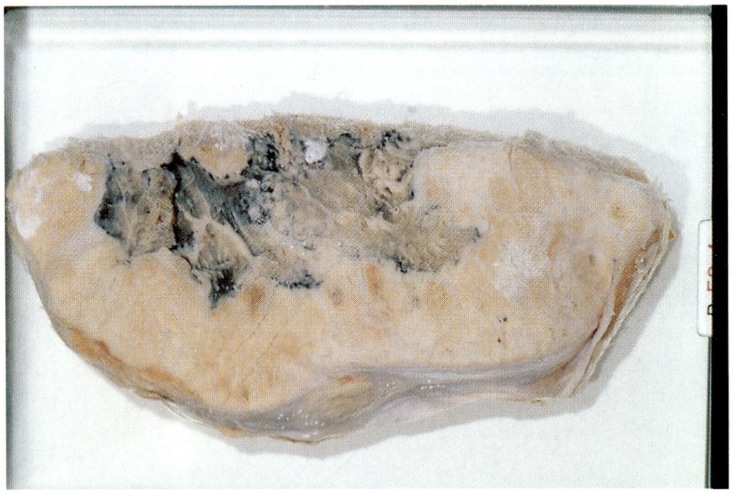

2.84 Pleura: Mesothelioma

This is a post-mortem specimen from a 55-year-old male labourer who had worked for many years in boiler houses. He was diagnosed as having a pleural mesothelioma and, despite intensive chemotherapy, died 11 months later. At autopsy, metastases were found in the liver, adrenals, spleen, peritoneum and bone marrow.

A coronal section through the right lung and pleural cavity shows that the little remaining lung parenchyma is encased in a mass of irregularly infiltrative, pale tumour. The tumour has completely obliterated the pleural cavity.

Mesothelioma is an uncommon malignant neoplasm which arises almost solely in individuals exposed to asbestos from anything between 20-40 years previously. It may arise from either the visceral or parietal pleura and spreads diffusely through the pleural cavity ensheathing and destroying the underlying lung. The prognosis is appalling, there being effectively a 100 per cent mortality within 2 years of presentation. It is an important lesion, which is increasing in incidence, for, in Britain at least, patients so affected or their families are entitled to industrial compensation if occupational exposure to asbestos is proven.

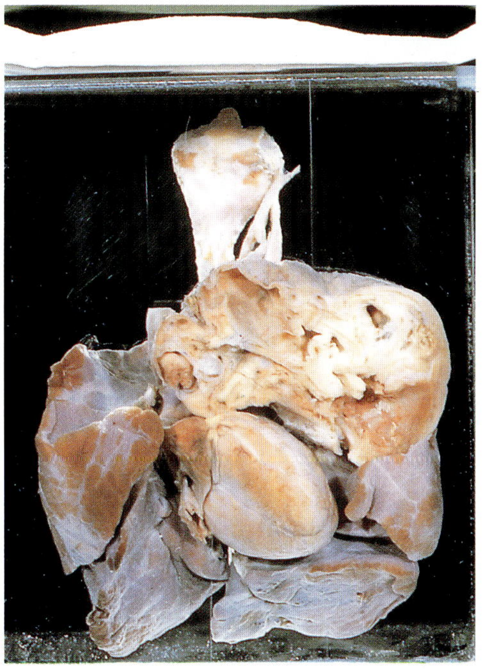

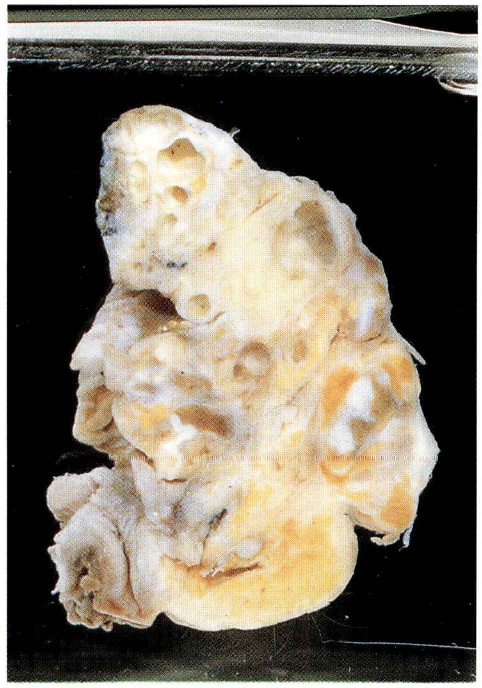

2.85 Mediastinum: Benign (Mature) Teratoma

This is a post-mortem specimen from a 9-month-old male infant who developed increasing dyspnoea with stridor and died.

The posterior aspect of the thoracic viscera is shown. Arising in the superior mediastinum is a large, ovoid, encapsulated tumour, measuring 7 × 4 × 4cm, with its long axis lying transversely. Although not readily visible in this view, the trachea, aorta, upper lobes and both atria have been markedly compressed by the tumour. The cut surface of the lesion is part-solid, part-cystic and focal areas are reminiscent of cerebral tissue. Histologically, the tumour was composed of benign squamous and respiratory epithelium, mucous and serous glands, cerebral and choroid tissue.

Teratomas of the mediastinum are uncommon and reflect the propensity of all germ cell tumours to arise anywhere in the midline. Many such mediastinal tumours appear to arise in the thymus but are in no way related to thymomas. There are two peaks in the age incidence, in the first few years of life and in early adulthood. At least 90 per cent of these lesions are benign (mature) tumours but a small proportion contain malignant elements and have the potential to metastasise.

2.86 Mediastinum: Benign (Mature) Teratoma

This specimen was excised from a 16-year-old girl who presented with a cystic swelling, in the neck, just above the sternal notch. At operation the mass was found to extend into the mediastinum and arose adjacent to the lung hila.

This is a portion of the mass which is principally solid, covered by skin at the bottom right and contains areas of well-formed cartilage and bone.

The wide array of tissues from each of the germ cell layers that may be found in mediastinal teratomas is demonstrated clearly in this example.

3. ALIMENTARY SYSTEM

ORAL CAVITY, PHARYNX AND OESOPHAGUS

Oral Cavity and Pharynx

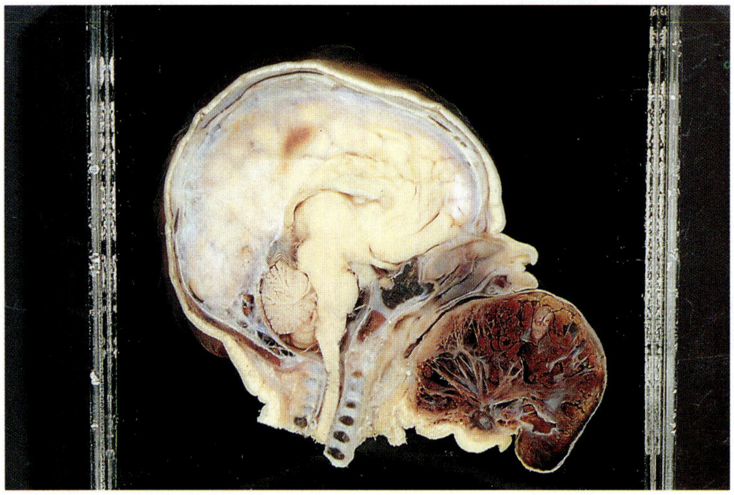

3.1 Tongue: Congenital Haemangioma

This is a post-mortem specimen from a full-term infant who survived for only a few days.

This sagittal section shows massive enlargement of the tongue, which is expanded by a mass composed of large, irregular blood-filled spaces. The thin strands of tissue radiating from the mandibular symphysis represent the vestigial remnants of the tongue's musculature.

Congenital vascular malformations are more common in the oro-facial region than elsewhere and are a frequent cause of macroglossia. However, this case is a particularly gross example. Many would regard these haemangiomas (or lymphangiomas) as hamartomatous in nature. Surgical intervention is made hazardous by the tendency to profuse haemorrhage. Oro-facial haemangiomas, including those of the skin, may occasionally be associated with the Sturge-Weber syndrome, hereditary haemorrhagic telangiectasia (Osler's disease) or Maffucci's syndrome.

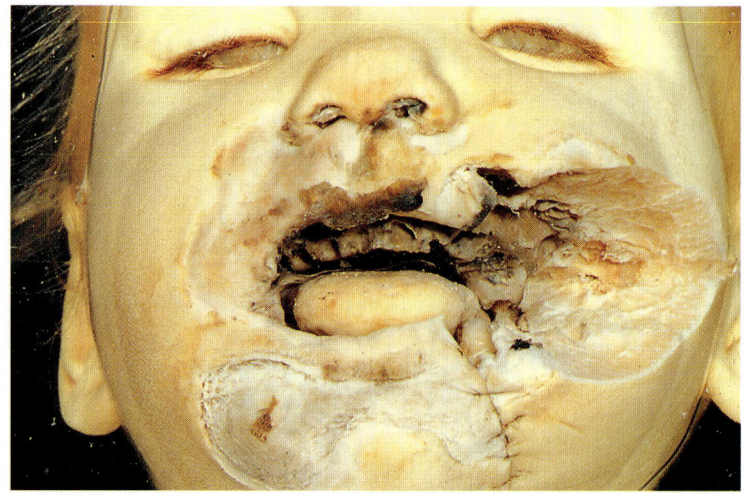

3.2 Face of Child: Necrotising Stomatitis

No clinical details are available.

The face of a child is shown with part of the left cheek removed to expose the oral cavity. The upper lip and adjacent tissue is discoloured and gangrenous. The chin, inner surface of the upper lip and left side of the tongue are ulcerated. The alveolar borders are also necrotic.

Necrotising stomatitis (synonyms: cancrum oris, noma) is now, fortunately, extremely rare in the Western world but may still be seen occasionally in underdeveloped countries. Classically, it has been seen in malnourished children suffering from infectious disease (e.g. measles) but may also occur in those debilitated by malignant disease or cytotoxic treatment. The condition bears some similarity to the lesions of Fournier's gangrene (see Reproductive System volume) and is characterised by a rapidly progressive necrotising cellulitis. The relative contribution of ischaemia or of bacterial infection (various Gram-negative bacilli and anaerobic organisms are frequently isolated) is hard to assess.

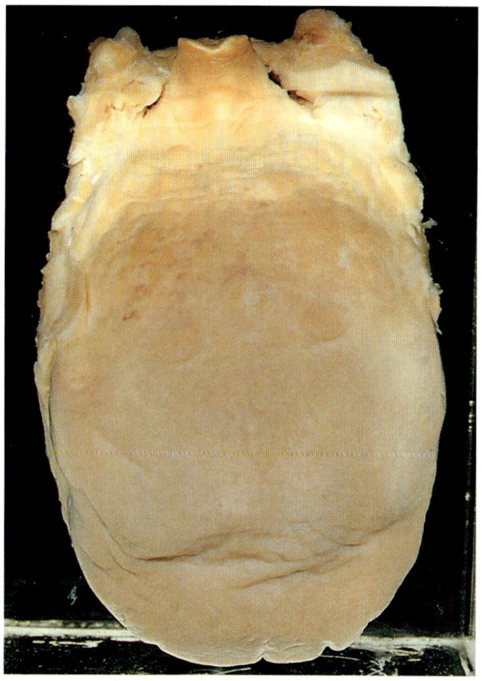

3.3 Tongue: Atrophic Glossitis

This is a post-mortem specimen from an 83-year-old woman with a long history of iron deficiency anaemia. The haemoglobin level was of the order of 8-9g/dl.

The tongue is excessively smooth with marked atrophy of the papillae and the dorsal surface. Note also the pallor of the oral mucous membrane.

Chronic atrophic glossitis is classically seen in cases of longstanding iron deficiency anaemia (e.g. Plummer-Vinson syndrome) but may also be seen in pernicious anaemia, Crohn's disease, coeliac disease and tropical sprue. The precise pathogenesis is unclear. However, since most cases of iron deficiency anaemia with an obscure aetiology are commonly associated with chronic gastritis, it seems likely that disturbance either of vitamin B_{12} or folate metabolism is the most important factor causing impaired epithelial turnover. In a small percentage of cases, squamous carcinoma of the tongue may develop.

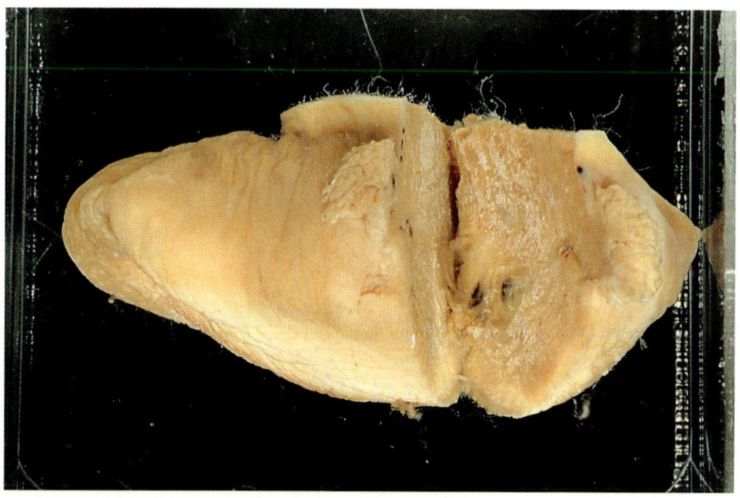

3.4 Tongue: Verrucous Carcinoma

This specimen was excised from a 49-year-old man, whose tongue had been sore for 6 weeks. A small warty lesion was found and a hemiglossectomy performed.

The right half of the tongue, which has been bisected transversely through the lesion, shows a small papillary lesion projecting from the ventral aspect, 4cm from the apex. The cut surface (bottom) demonstrates the superficial nature of this tumour, there being no macroscopical evidence of muscular invasion.

Verrucous carcinoma is a variant of very well-differentiated squamous carcinoma which arises most often in the oral cavity, particularly on the buccal mucosa or gingivae. The elderly are usually affected, with a predominance of males. Aetiologically there is a strong association with tobacco or betel nut chewing and pre-existent foci of epithelial atypia are commonly found. This tumour tends to slow, but extensive, local invasion; however, metastasis to lymph nodes or elsewhere is extremely uncommon.

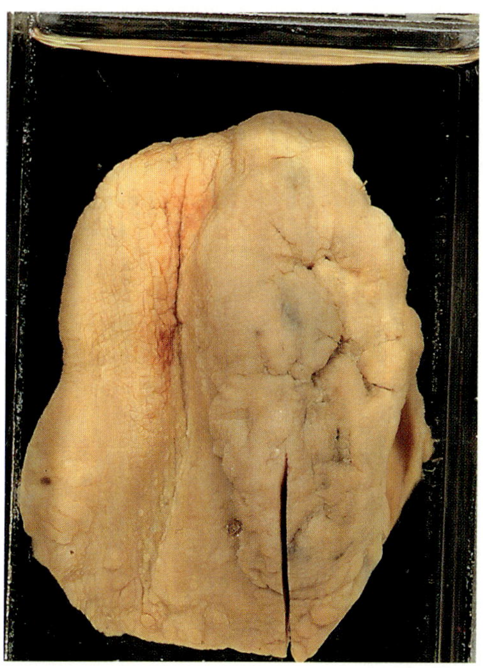

3.5 Tongue: Squamous Carcinoma

This specimen was excised from a 63-year-old man who had noticed an enlarging, painful mass on the right side of his tongue for 8 months. He was known to have had syphilitic glossitis and had numerous carious and infected teeth. Examination also revealed several enlarged, hard submandibular lymph nodes which were also excised.

The dorsal surface of the tongue is shown from which an extensive tumour, measuring 6 × 3 × 1.5cm, projects. The lesion extends posteriorly to the circumvallate papillae and has a nodular, focally ulcerated surface.

Squamous carcinoma of the oral cavity is not uncommon and may arise in the tongue, lips, palate, gingivae or floor of the mouth. The single most important aetiological factor is tobacco smoking but other predisposing causes include excessive intake of alcoholic spirits, betel nut chewing, poor oral hygiene and syphilitic infection. Males are predominantly affected and, while there is a wide age range, these tumours are most common in the 6th and 7th decades. Carcinoma most often arises in the middle third of the tongue and tends to metastasise to lymph nodes early in the course of the disease, having a worse prognosis than squamous carcinoma elsewhere in the oral cavity.

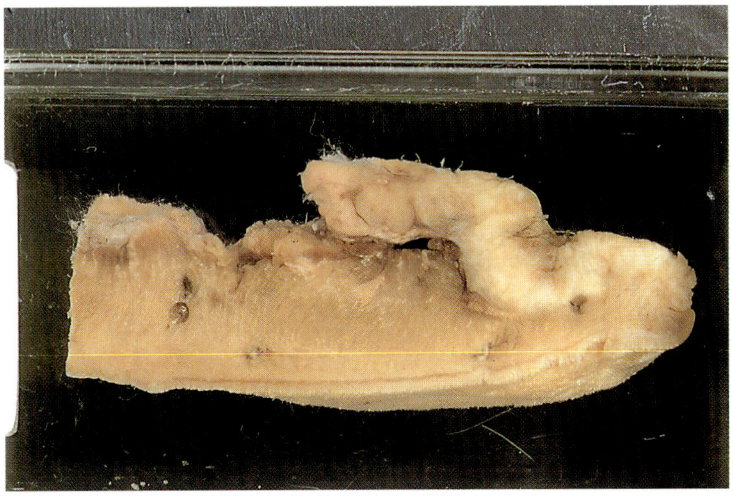

3.6 Tongue: Squamous Carcinoma

This specimen was excised from a 65-year-old male who subsequently died with an inoperable recurrence.

A sagittal section through the tongue shows a pale, infiltrative tumour arising on the ventral surface of the apex. The lesion has spread posteriorly to involve the sublingual salivary glands.

The apex and ventral surface of the tongue are less frequently the sites of origin of carcinoma than the dorsal, middle or posterior thirds. It should be noted that the vast majority of oral squamous carcinomas are histologically well differentiated.

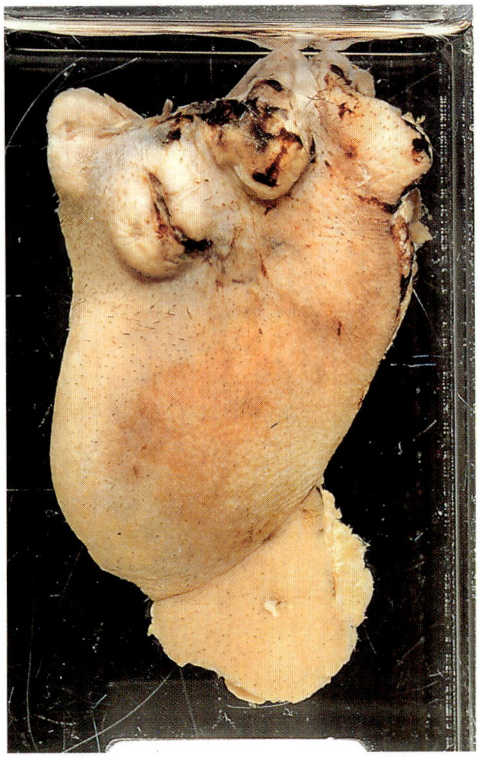

3.7 Lip: Squamous Carcinoma

This specimen was excised from a 74-year-old man who had noticed an ulcer on his lower lip for 6 months.

The specimen consists of the left half of the lower lip with the skin of the chin and subjacent soft tissues. The full thickness of the lip has been destroyed by an ulcerated, pale multinodular tumour, measuring 2.5cm in maximum dimension.

Carcinoma of the lip may also occur due to prolonged exposure to sunlight, in addition to the other factors listed in Legend 3.5. The lower lip is most often involved and the prognosis, in general, is very good, probably because the site of the lesion facilitates an early diagnosis. Untreated cases may show extensive local invasion and tumours of the upper lip, which are comparatively uncommon, are more prone to metastasise than their counterparts in the lower lip.

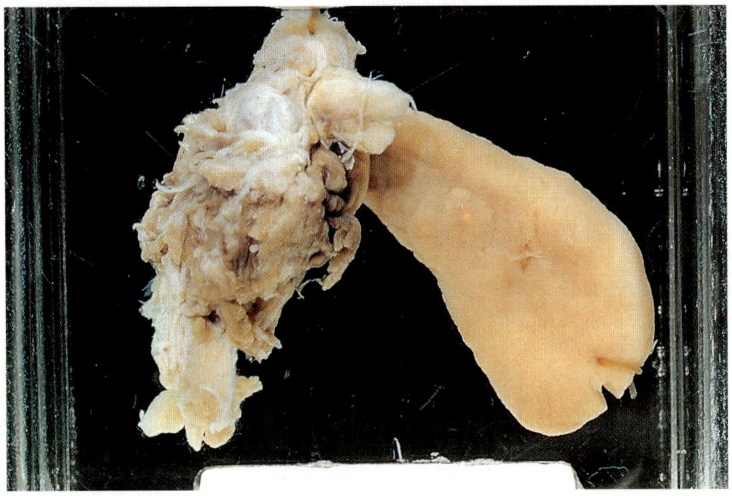

3.8 Oral Mucosa: Fibro-epithelial Polyp

This specimen was excised from a 45-year-old man who had noticed a slow growing polyp at the back of his mouth for 6 years.

The specimen consists of a rather scarred palatine tonsil, from the surface of which a smooth, pear-shaped tumour, measuring 2.5 × 1 × 1cm, projects by a narrow pedicle.

A fibro-epithelial polyp is not uncommon in the oral cavity and is an entirely benign lesion, comparable to the more usual skin tag. It should be noted that most fibrous overgrowths in the oral cavity are not true neoplasms but rather are reactive lesions which tend to arise at a site of irritation either by ill-fitting dentures or repeated chewing or sucking.

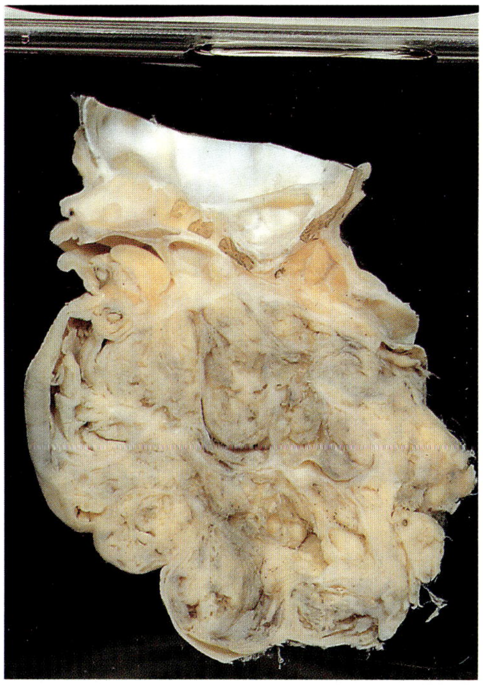

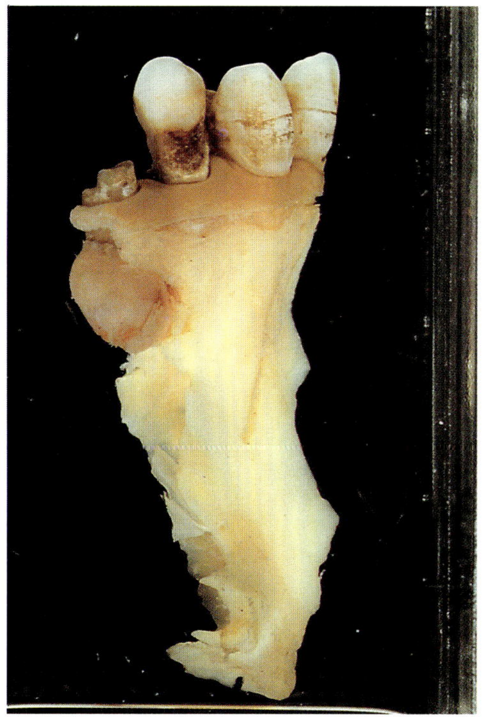

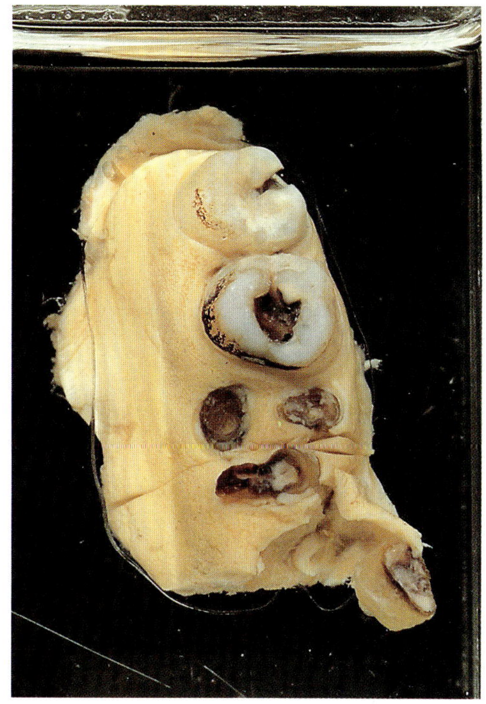

3.9 Floor of Mouth: Benign (Mature) Teratoma

No clinical details are available.

This is a sagittal section though the lower head and neck of a fetus showing a massive, lobulated tumour, measuring 9 × 6 × 6cm, which is occupying the floor of the mouth, pharynx, hyoid and thyroid regions. The precise site of origin is unclear. There are no macroscopical distinguishing features.

Benign teratomas may arise anywhere in the mid-line of the body and are not uncommon, affecting young infants and adolescents particularly or young adults. Lesions of this size are, however, very uncommon and are incompatible with life. When found in a stillborn infant, it is hard to be certain whether they represent true tumours or gross embryonic malformations involving each of the germ layers.

3.10 Upper Jaw: Radicular Cyst

This was an incidental finding at post-mortem in a 48-year-old man.

This is a portion of the left maxilla which shows a cyst in the alveolar process which has developed in connection with the root of the second premolar tooth. Note that the premolar is severely carious.

Radicular cysts (synonyms: apical cyst, dental cyst) are ubiquitous and are the most common type of cyst to develop in association with teeth. They arise at the site of previous chronic inflammation in the pulp, usually as a consequence of infection secondary to caries. Odontogenic epithelium proliferates as a response to infection or inflammation so these cysts usually have a squamous lining. They may remain asymptomatic or become secondarily infected, thus presenting with pain and swelling.

3.11 Upper Jaw: Radicular Cyst

This was an incidental finding at post-mortem in a 28-year-old man who died after undergoing surgery for intestinal obstruction.

Part of the upper jaw is shown. There is severe dental caries and adjacent to one of the roots there is a small cyst, measuring 1cm in diameter.

This case clearly demonstrates the frequency with which radicular cysts are associated with infection, usually as a consequence of dental caries.

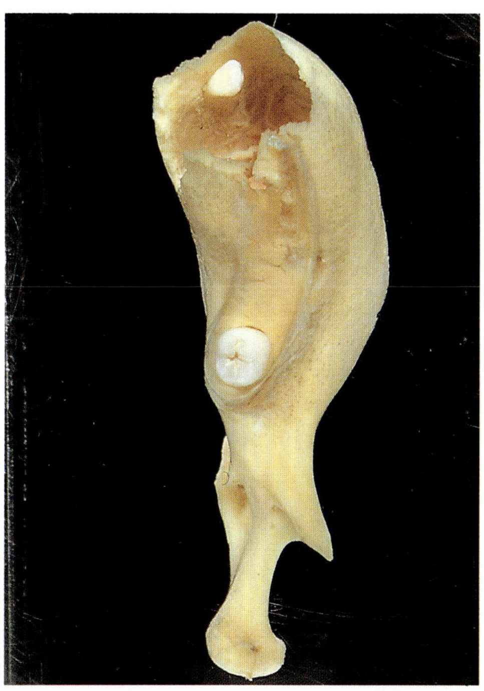

3.12 Lower Jaw: Dentigerous Cyst

This specimen was excised from a 13-year-old girl who had noticed a swelling of the left side of the jaw for 6 months. There was an offensive discharge from the inner surface of the swelling and the teeth were very irregular.

The left half of the lower jaw is shown, the body of which is expanded by an ovoid cyst. The crown of an unerupted canine tooth projects into the lower part of the cyst cavity, which has a granular lining.

Dentigerous cysts (synonym: follicular cysts) are developmental malformations which arise from the enamel organ and are not common. Children and adolescents are most often affected and the cyst forms between the enamel and epithelium of the enamel organ of unerupted teeth, leaving the crown of the tooth protruding into the cyst cavity. There is no inflammatory component (cf. radicular cysts) unless a sinus forms within the oral cavity.

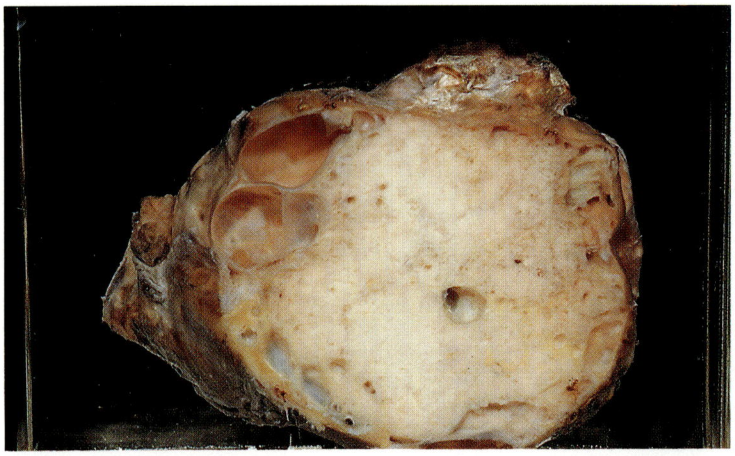

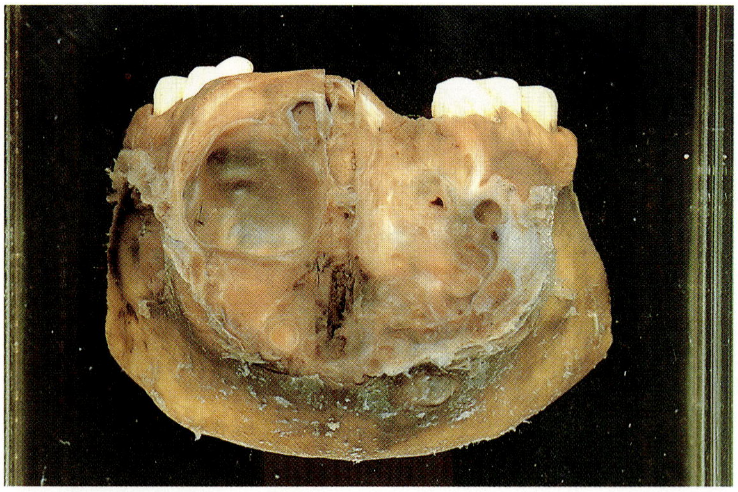

3.13 Lower Jaw: Ameloblastoma

This specimen was excised from a 45-year-old woman who complained of a swelling in the left lower jaw, which had been present for 13 years.

This is a portion of the left mandible which is expanded and distorted by a rounded, well-circumscribed tumour, measuring 8cm in maximum diameter. The cut surface has the typical greyish-white, fibrous appearance, scattered throughout which are cysts of varying size.

Ameloblastomas (synonym: adamantinomas) arise from dental epithelium and originate in the mandible in up to 80 per cent of cases. While there is a wide age range, young adults are most often affected. In the vast majority of cases, these slow-growing tumours are benign but tend to local invasion such that incautious, incomplete excision is often succeeded by local recurrence.

3.14 Lower Jaw: Ameloblastoma

This specimen was excised from a 30-year-old Sudanese man who presented with a gradually enlarging mass in the middle of the lower jaw.

The middle part of the mandible is largely replaced by a mass, measuring 4cm in diameter, containing multiple cysts of varying size.

Extensive cystic change within an ameloblastoma is not uncommon and gave rise to the old-fashioned synonym applied to such cases, the multilocular cyst.

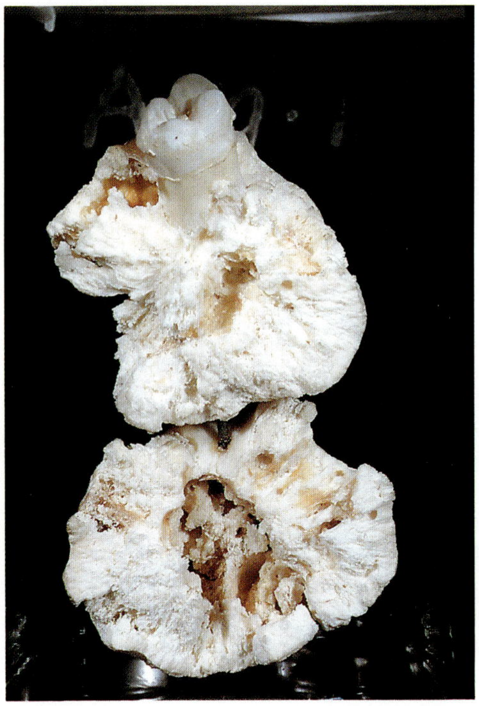

3.15 Molar Tooth: Cementoblastoma

This specimen was excised from a 15-year-old boy who pre-operatively was thought to have a sarcoma of the lower jaw. However, at operation, the tumour was easily shelled out from the surrounding bone.

At the top of the specimen is the second left lower molar tooth, arising from the root of which is a rounded white tumour, measuring 3cm in diameter. The lesion has been bisected to show the cut surface which is composed of bony lamellae, radially arranged around the point of attachment to the tooth.

Cementoblastoma is pathologically very similar to an osteoblastoma and usually arises from one of the molar teeth. Young males are predominantly affected and there may be massive expansion of the jaw. However, this tumour is entirely benign and, as in this case, can usually be enucleated with ease.

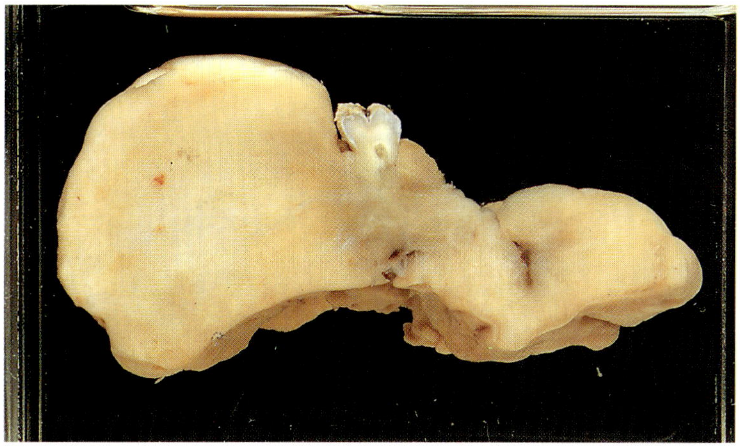

3.16 Maxilla: Cementifying Fibroma

This specimen was excised from a 32-year-old woman who had noticed a swelling of the left upper jaw for 8 years, which she believed to have started adjacent to a tooth. At operation it was extremely firm and extended into the roof of the mouth.

The tumour is lobulated and encapsulated and projects from, and is embedded within, a molar tooth. The cut surface of the lesion has a uniform, pale appearance.

Cementifying fibroma may be classified as a variant of cementoma, being derived from cementum at the dental root. It is usually a solitary lesion, arising most often in the mandible of middle-aged adults, particularly in the molar or premolar region. Long-standing lesions may become heavily calcified and difficult to remove: however, this tumour has no malignant potential.

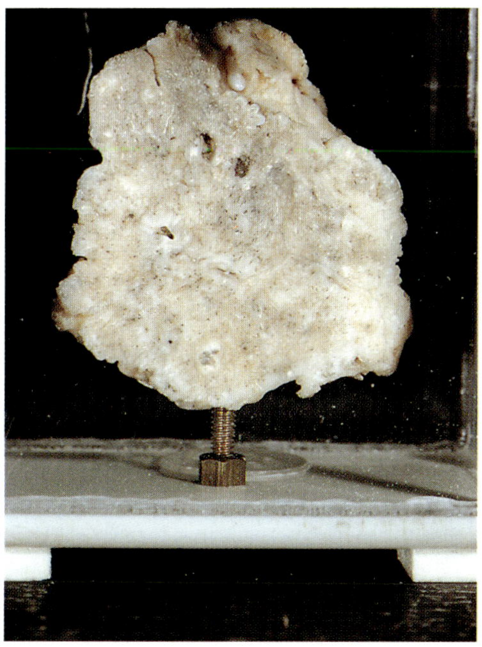

3.17 Lower Jaw: Complex Odontome

This specimen was excised from an 18-year-old girl who presented with an 8 month history of pain in the lower jaw.

The specimen consists of a rounded nodular tumour, measuring 2.5cm in diameter. The cut surface is composed of irregular pulp cavities, dentine and small nodules of enamel.

Odontomes are dental hamartomas and may be divided into two types: compound, composed of several rudimentary teeth and fibrous tissue; and complex, which consists of a patternless mass of dentine, enamel, cementum and periodontal connective tissue. Typically, they present in childhood for at that age they may enlarge; however, growth of these lesions ceases when dentition is complete.

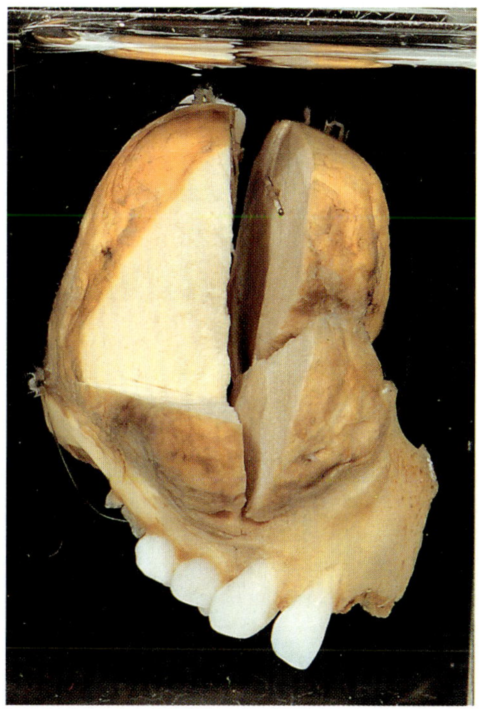

3.18 Maxilla: Monostotic Fibrous Dysplasia

This specimen was excised from an 18-year-old girl.

This is a portion of the right maxilla; a rounded, rather lobulated tumour projects superiorly from the alveolar border. The tumour is encapsulated and has a yellowish cut surface.

The jaw is a common site for a solitary lesion in fibrous dysplasia of bone, but may also be involved in polyostotic disease or Albright's syndrome. While polyostotic disease usually presents in childhood, a solitary jaw lesion may not be detected until bony deformity occurs in adolescence or early adulthood. Females are predominantly affected and, aetiologically, these lesions are thought to be developmental anomalies. Typically they cease to enlarge when skeletal maturity is attained: however, very occasionally, sarcomatous transformation may occur. It should be noted that the case here is unusually well-circumscribed: a degree of fusion with adjacent normal bone is more frequent.

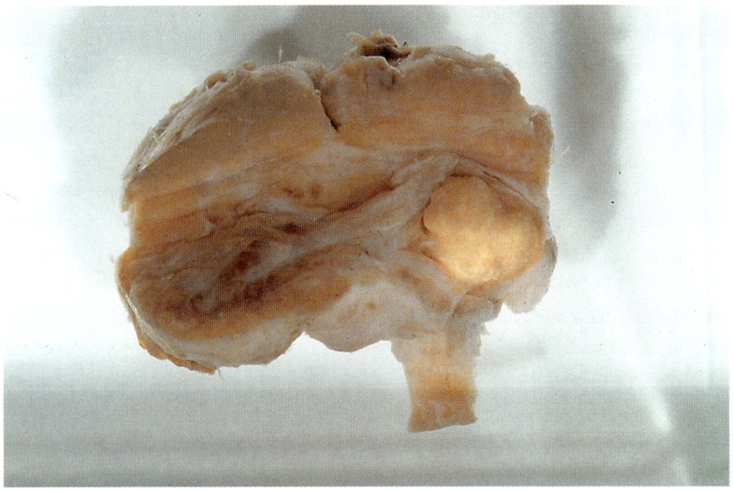

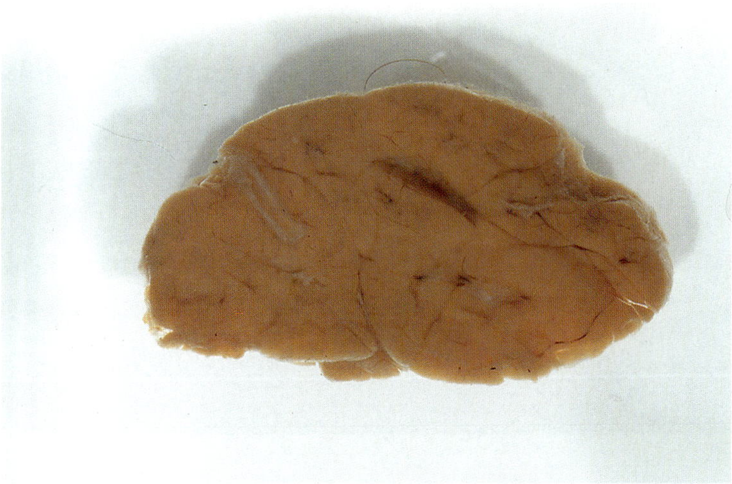

3.19 Submandibular Gland: Calculus

This specimen was excised from a 62-year-old woman who had noticed intermittent swelling beneath the jaw, which became worse after meals, for 10 years. She finally presented with acute sialadenitis and, after antibiotic treatment, the submandibular gland was excised.

The submandibular gland (3.19a) has been bisected to show a yellowish calculus, measuring 1cm in diameter, impacted within one of the ducts. The cut surface of the gland shows diffuse fibrosis. A normal submandibular gland (3.19b) has been mounted for comparison.

Salivary calculi are found most commonly in the submandibular gland and less often in the parotid gland. Elsewhere they are extremely rare. Adults are usually affected, especially men, and the aetiology is unclear. They are composed largely of calcium phosphate and are thought to develop around a fragment of foreign material or inspissated mucus. As a consequence of large duct obstruction, tender swelling of the affected gland at meal times is a common symptom due to the entrapment of mucous secretions. Obstruction also leads to recurrent attacks of inflammation or infection, which may be complicated by fibrosis or abscess formation.

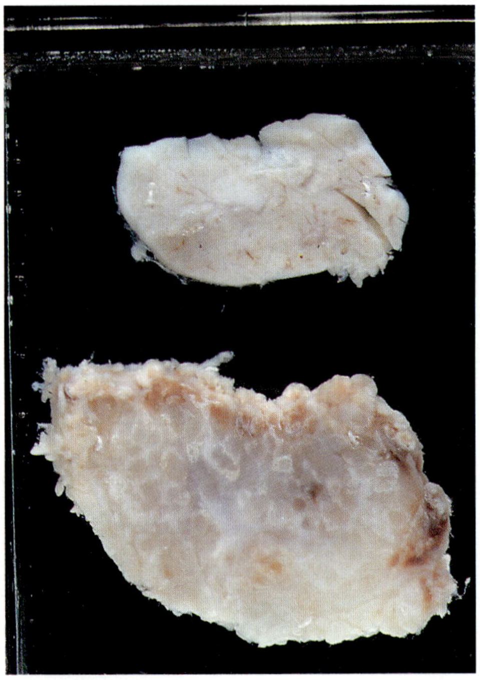

3.20 Parotid Gland: Sjögren's Syndrome

This specimen was excised from a 44-year-old woman, who presented with an 8 year history of bilateral parotid swelling. She also suffered from xerophthalmia, Raynaud's disease and rheumatoid arthritis. A left parotidectomy was performed because of recurrent pain and swelling.

The patient's parotid gland (below) is markedly enlarged when compared to the normal gland mounted above. It also shows less of the normal lobular appearance and the cut surface appears pale and fatty.

Sjögren's syndrome is characterised by swelling of the parotid and/or submandibular glands (sometimes bilaterally), associated with keratoconjunctivitis sicca and xerostomia. Middle-aged adults, particularly females, are typically affected and many patients also suffer from one of the systemic collagen diseases, particularly rheumatoid arthritis. It is an autoimmune disease, histologically typified by a massive lymphocytic infiltrate in the affected salivary gland (the so-called benign lymphoepithelial lesion), and may occasionally be complicated by the development of a salivary non-Hodgkin's lymphoma. (Courtesy of the Gordon Museum, Guy's Hospital Medical School)

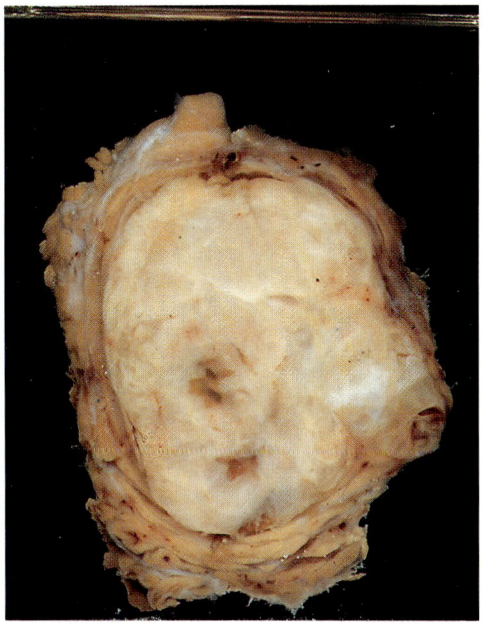

3.21 Parotid Gland: Pleomorphic Adenoma

This specimen was excised from a 36-year-old man who presented with a 4 year history of a swelling near the angle of the left lower jaw.

The parotid gland has been bisected to show virtual replacement by an apparently encapsulated, pale tumour which measures 3.5cm in maximum diameter. The cut surface is multinodular and contains numerous small, translucent foci which have a rather myxoid appearance.

Salivary tumours arise up to 10 times more often in the parotid gland than in the submandibular, sublingual or minor glands. Of such tumours, the pleomorphic adenoma (synonym: mixed salivary tumour) constitutes about 70 per cent. While pleomorphic adenomas have a wide age distribution, young adults are most often affected and there is a marked predominance of females. They are derived from ductular epithelium and the vast majority are entirely benign. However, there is a very marked tendency to local recurrence which can be largely attributed to small nodules or processes of tumour which extend beyond the apparent capsule and are left *in situ* when the tumour is shelled out. For this reason, formal excision with a cuff of normal tissue is preferable but great care has to be taken to avoid damaging the facial nerve which traverses the parotid gland. Usually, true malignancy only occurs in a very small number of either long-standing cases or adenomas that have recurred repeatedly.

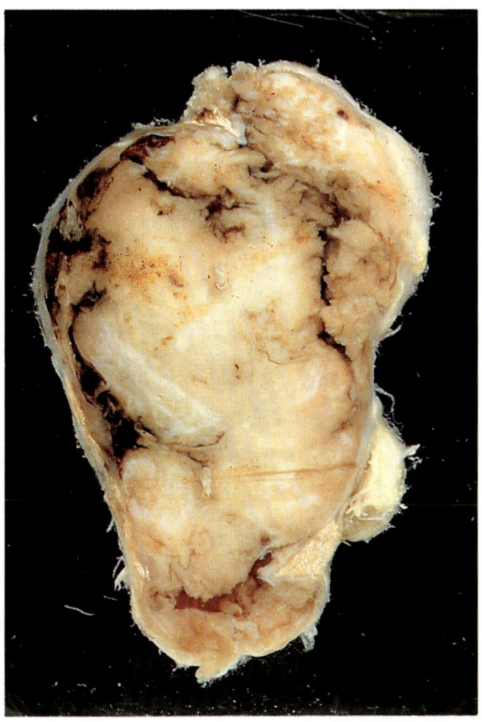

3.22 Parotid Gland: Pleomorphic Adenoma

This specimen was excised from a 45-year-old woman who had first noticed a swelling in front of the left ear 25 years previously.

This ovoid, lobulated tumour, which measures 6 × 4 × 3cm, has a pale cut surface with foci of cystic degeneration and haemorrhage. While appearing to have a well-defined fibrous capsule, at least one nodule (bottom right) lies outside it.

This case demonstrates clearly the irregular multinodularity that these tumours may assume and it is easy to appreciate that small outlying portions of tumour may be inadvertently missed at operation. It is also thought that intra-operative rupture or damage to the tumour may be succeeded by inadvertent local implantation, contributing to the risk of local recurrence.

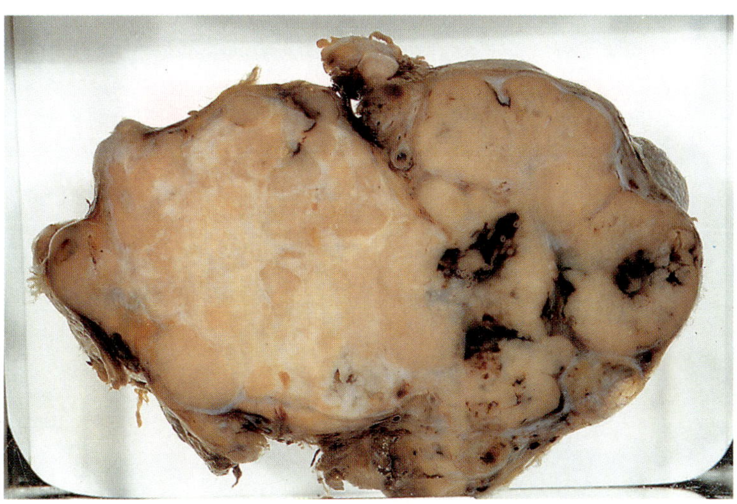

3.23 Submandibular Gland: Carcinoma arising in a Pleomorphic Adenoma

This specimen was excised from a 73-year-old man who had noticed a small lump under the jaw for 25 years. Recently it had increased very rapidly in size, prompting the patient to present to his doctor.

The tumour, which measured 10 × 7 × 6cm in the fresh state has been bisected to show very similar features to a benign pleomorphic adenoma. The lesion appears encapsulated, is multinodular and contains gelatinous and haemorrhagic foci. Histologically, however, there was unequivocal evidence of malignancy.

Approximately 3 per cent of pleomorphic adenomas are thought to undergo malignant change, usually after a latent period of at least 20 years. Almost any microscopical variant of salivary gland carcinoma may develop but, in general, high grade tumours are commonest in this circumstance and fairly rapid metastasis and death is the most frequent result.

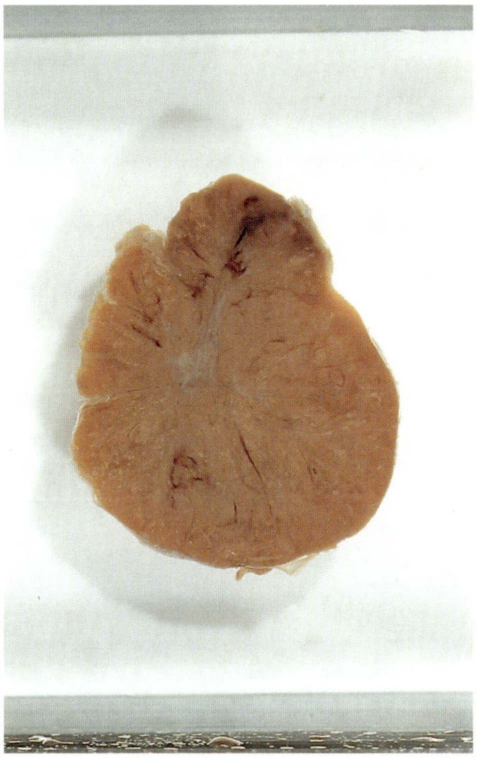

3.24 Parotid Gland: Adenolymphoma

This specimen was excised from a 56-year-old man who had recently noticed a swelling adjacent to the angle of the jaw.

This is a well-circumscribed tumour, with no adjacent normal salivary tissue, which measures 2.5cm in diameter. The cut surface shows fine trabeculae of fibrous tissue and numerous yellowish flecks, representing secretions within glandular spaces.

Adenolymphoma (synonym: Warthin's tumour) accounts for between 5 and 10 per cent of salivary tumours and arises most often in the parotid gland. Patients in the 5th-7th decades are usually affected and there is a marked predominance of males. These tumours are thought to arise from intra-glandular lymph nodes, which contain small foci of salivary tissue; they are not infrequently bilateral or multiple within the same gland, or more than one gland, prompting the unwary to diagnose local recurrence or metastasis. Adenolymphomas commonly show extensive cystic change and are also prone to becoming infected; the development of malignancy, however, is excessively rare. Occasional examples of adenolymphoma arise in lymph nodes outside (but adjacent to) a salivary gland. Ectopic glandular tissue is common in such nodes. It is important that such glands, or an adenolymphoma arising therefrom, should not be mistaken for metastatic tumour.

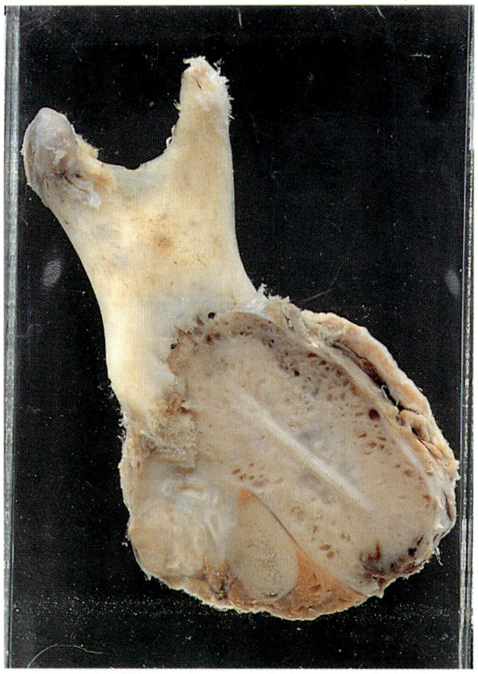

3.25 Minor Salivary Gland: Adenoid Cystic Carcinoma

This specimen was excised from a 60-year-old woman, who presented with a 10 month history of swelling of the right side of her jaw which had rendered her unable to wear dentures. Examination revealed a hard mass extending from the tooth which, on X-ray, showed local destruction of bone. A right hemimandibulectomy was performed but the patient later developed an extensive local recurrence and died.

Arising adjacent to the ascending ramus of the right mandible is a relatively well-circumscribed mass, measuring 5cm in diameter, which has eroded the bone. The cut surface has a lobulated, focally cystic appearance and is brownish in colour. Entrapped within the centre of the tumour is the inferior dental nerve.

Adenoid cystic carcinoma accounts for between 2 and 5 per cent of salivary tumours and arises most often in the submandibular gland. It is commonest in adulthood. This tumour shows a particular tendency to extensive local invasion, especially around nerves, and therefore surgical excision is rarely complete. Local recurrence and, eventually, lymph node and systemic metastases are to be expected in the majority of cases although the time course of this process is extremely variable. (Courtesy of the Gordon Museum, Guy's Hospital Medical School)

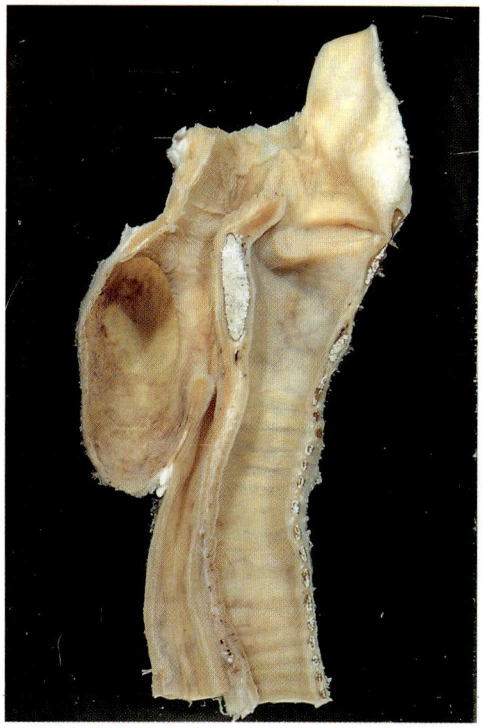

3.26 Pharynx: Diverticulum

This is a post-mortem specimen from a 90-year-old Anglican bishop. He had been aware of the presence of a pouch in his neck for many years; in fact, the pouch used to receive the greater part of the food he swallowed and, when it was filled, he was in the habit of pressing up the side of the neck so as to empty the pouch into the oesophagus.

The larynx, trachea, pharynx and oesophagus have been bisected in sagittal plane. A large ovoid diverticulum, measuring 4cm in diameter, projects from the posterior wall of the pharynx at the level of the cricoid cartilage. The sac, which communicates with the pharynx by a wide aperture, has a smooth lining.

Pharyngeal diverticula, or pouches, arise at Killian's dehiscence, which lies between the upper oblique fibres of thyropharyngeus and the lower transverse fibres of cricopharyngeus. They are pulsion diverticula which occur due to a failure of neuromuscular coordination in the pharyngeal constrictor muscles. If cricopharyngeus fails to relax then the pressure from above is applied directly to the weakest point in the pharyngeal wall, Killian's dehiscence. Such a diverticulum, therefore, projects posteriorly but is usually deflected laterally by the bodies of the adjacent cervical vertebrae. The elderly are typically affected, with males predominating over females.

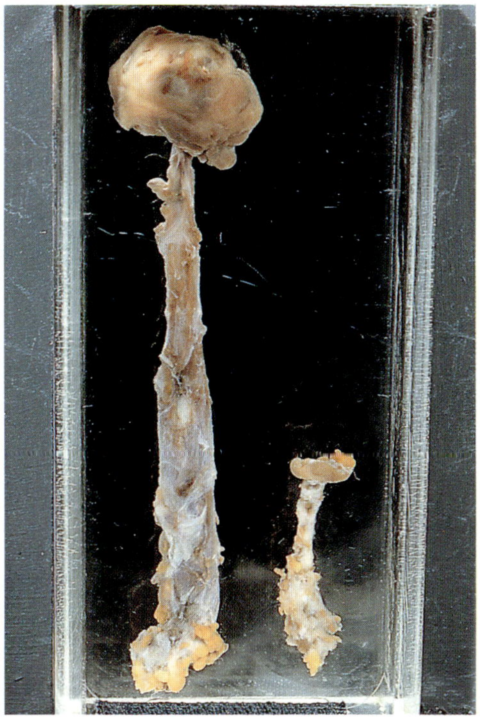

3.27 Neck: Branchial Cleft Fistula and Sinus

These specimens were excised from an 11-year-old girl who had been noted to have a discharging sinus on the right side of the neck since early infancy. She had also developed an intermittently discharging neck sinus on the left. Examination revealed bilateral fistulous openings 3cm above the clavicles. At operation, the left-sided lesion was short and blind-ended while that on the right extended upwards and communicated with the ipsilateral tonsillar bed.

The specimen mounted on the left is 10cm in length and is an epithelial-lined structure extending from the cutaneous opening (bottom) to the right faucial tonsil (above). That on the right is a similar, but blind-ended, sinus tract which measures only 3cm in length.

Branchial fistulae represent persistent, vestigial remnants of the embryonic second branchial cleft. They are epithelial-lined structures which typically open on to the skin in the lower third of the neck, just anterior to the sternocleidomastoid. If complete, they communicate with the pillar of the fauces, adjacent to the tonsils. If incomplete, in strict terminology, they are described as branchial sinuses. They are congenital lesions, which most often present in the first two decades, and may be complicated by infection. A branchial cyst represents a smaller portion of the same vestige which does not communicate with any external surface.

Oesophagus

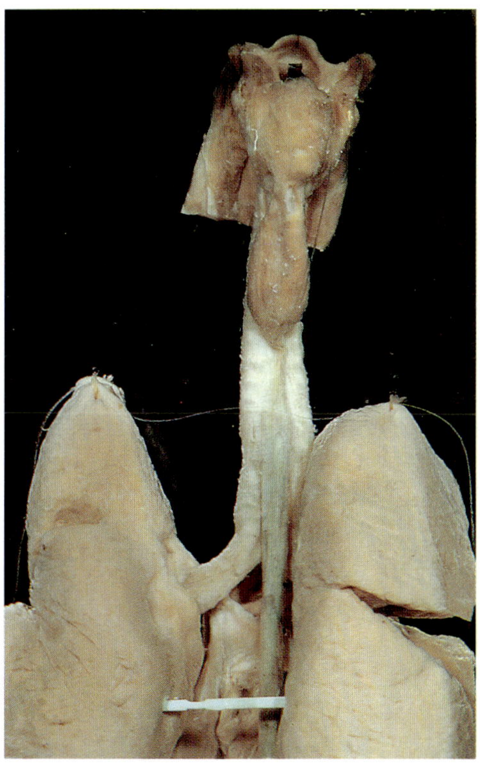

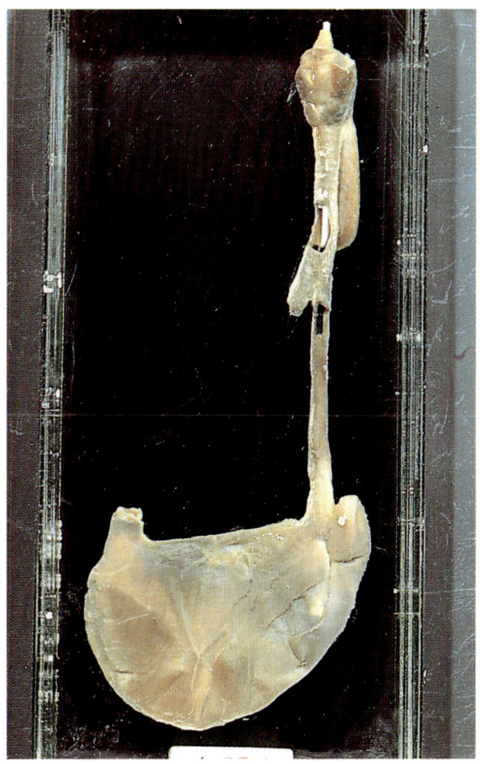

3.28 Oesophagus: Atresia with Tracheo-oesophageal Fistula

These are post-mortem specimens. Figure 3.28a is from a 7-day-old infant. From birth all food was largely regurgitated and there was marked respiratory distress. Figure 3.28b was an incidental finding in a stillborn infant.

The oesophagus, stomach, larynx and trachea are shown (3.28a). The upper 2.5cm of the oesophagus ends blindly just above the level of the tracheal bifurcation. The lower 6cm is in direct continuity with the trachea, which it enters posteriorly just below the blind upper portion. The pharynx, oesophagus, trachea and lungs of the second case are shown in closer view (3.28b). The upper 2cm of the oesophagus again ends blindly at the level of the mid-trachea, while the lower portion opens into the trachea obliquely, just above the latter's bifurcation. The lungs are uninflated, as would be expected in a stillborn infant.

Atresia of the oesophagus, with an associated tracheo-oesophageal fistula, is a not uncommon congenital malformation, occurring in approximately 1 in 1000 live births. Other abnormalities, particularly of the spine, heart, kidneys and anus are often also present. The condition probably arises due to a failure of development or fusion of the septum lying between the trachea and oesophagus. With modern cardiothoracic techniques, surgical reconstruction is usually practical and successful, although subsequent tracheal or oesophageal stenosis is not uncommon.

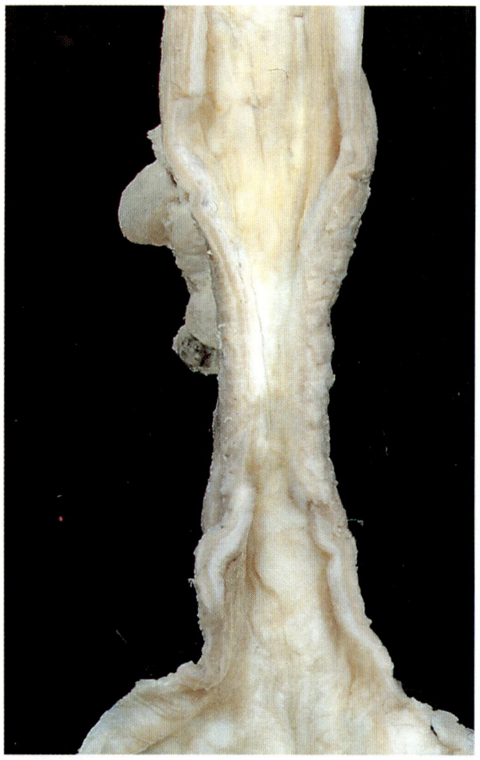

3.29 Oesophagus: Congenital Stenosis

This is a post-mortem specimen from a 10-year-old child. No further clinical details are available.

The oesophagus has been opened to show a narrow stricture measuring 4cm in length, in its middle third. There is associated thickening of the oesophageal wall at this site. Above the stricture, the oesophagus is dilated and hypertrophied, while below it is dilated and atrophic.

Congenital stenosis of the oesophagus is rare in isolation, most often being associated with a tracheo-oesophageal fistula. It simply represents a lesser degree of oesophageal atresia (see Legend 3.28).

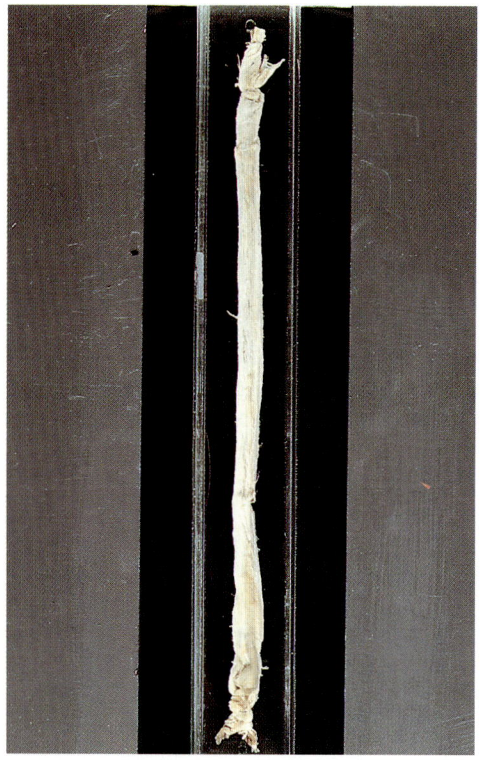

3.30 Oesophagus: Mucosal Cast

This specimen came from a 66-year-old man who had intentionally swallowed a small amount of concentrated hydrochloric acid. Other than some pain, he remained well until 14 days after the initial event, when he brought up this cast after an attack of retching. He subsequently made a full recovery.

The specimen consists solely of the necrotic oesophageal lining which forms a complete cast, measuring 28cm in length.

For a patient to vomit a complete mucosal cast of the oesophagus is excessively rare but may follow the ingestion of a corrosive or very hot liquid: it can also be spontaneous. Very surprisingly, the oesophagus usually heals.

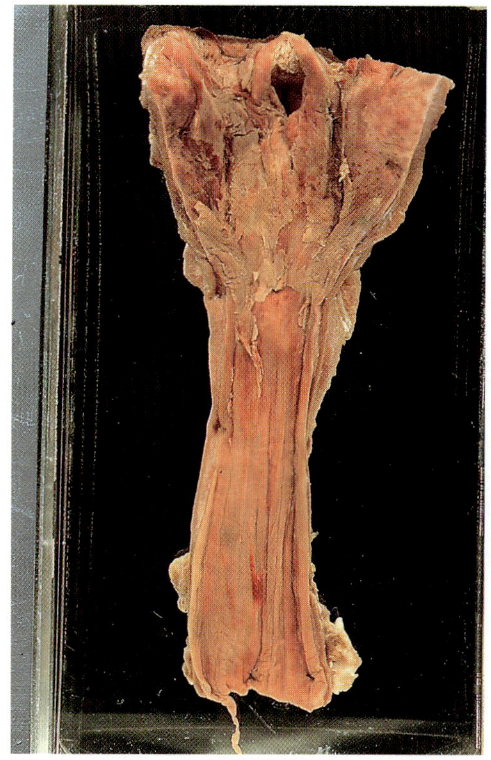

3.31 Oesophagus: Chemical Oesophagitis

This is a post-mortem specimen from a 24-year old male psychiatric patient who had previously attempted to commit suicide 4 times. On this occasion he took a large quantity of mercuric oxide and was admitted to hospital with severe laryngeal oedema and cyanosis. He died soon after.

The oesophagus and pharynx have been opened to show intense mucosal congestion and focal superficial ulceration. Note also the marked swelling of the epiglottis with considerable narrowing of the glottic orifice.

Ingestion of toxic substances, particularly corrosives (including acids and various disinfectants) is a well-recognised cause of acute ulcerative oesophagitis which may often be complicated by the subsequent development of a stricture.

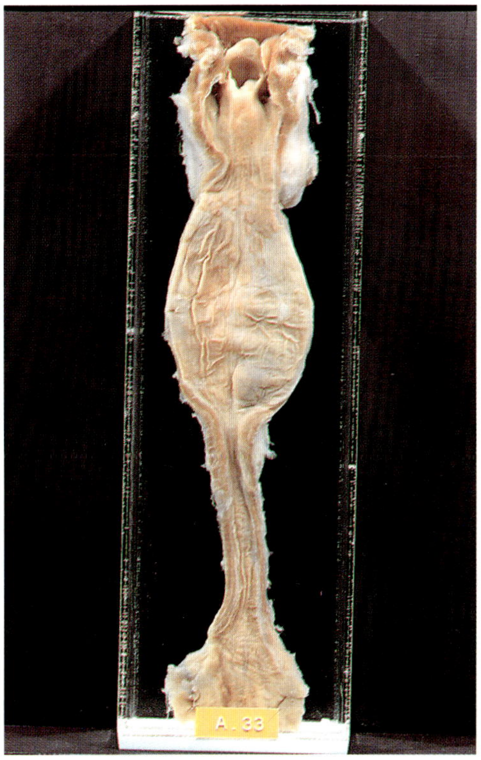

3.32 Oesophagus: Acquired Stricture

This is a post-mortem specimen from a 50-year-old woman who, 6 months previously, had attempted to commit suicide by drinking caustic potash. She was transferred to a psychiatric hospital but symptoms of oesophageal obstruction developed, necessitating performance of a gastrostomy. She died post-operatively of pneumonia.

The oesophagus has been opened to show marked narrowing of its entire distal half, at which site the mucosa appears greyish and scarred. Note the associated muscular hypertrophy of the wall and the proximal dilatation.

The ingestion of corrosive substances may be complicated by the development of an oesophageal stricture. Other causes of an acquired oesophageal stricture include Barrett's ulcer and carcinoma. (Courtesy of the Gordon Museum, Guy's Hospital Medical School)

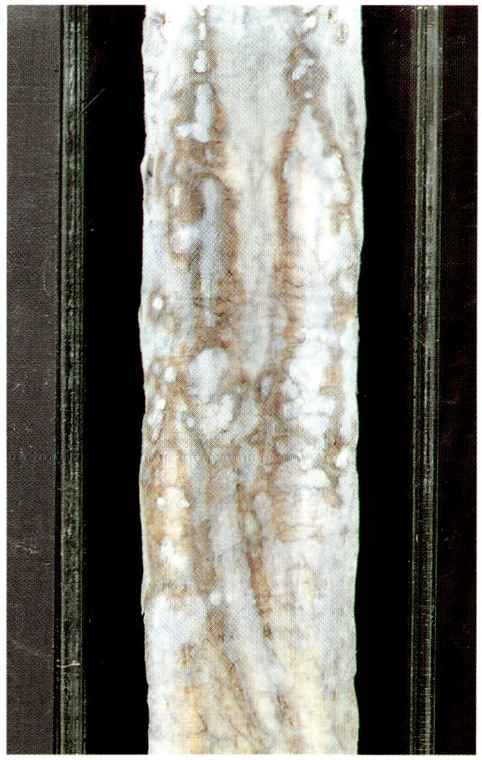

3.33 Oesophagus: Acute Oesophagitis

No clinical details are available.

A portion of the oesophagus has been opened to show the oedematous, opaque mucosal surface with intervening areas of intense congestion and ulceration.

Acute oesophagitis is not uncommon and probably resolves spontaneously without medical attention in many cases. It may be associated with excessive alcohol ingestion, corrosives and many systemic infections. It may also be caused by infection either with *Candida sp.* or *Herpes simplex* Type I, most often in debilitated or immunosuppressed patients.

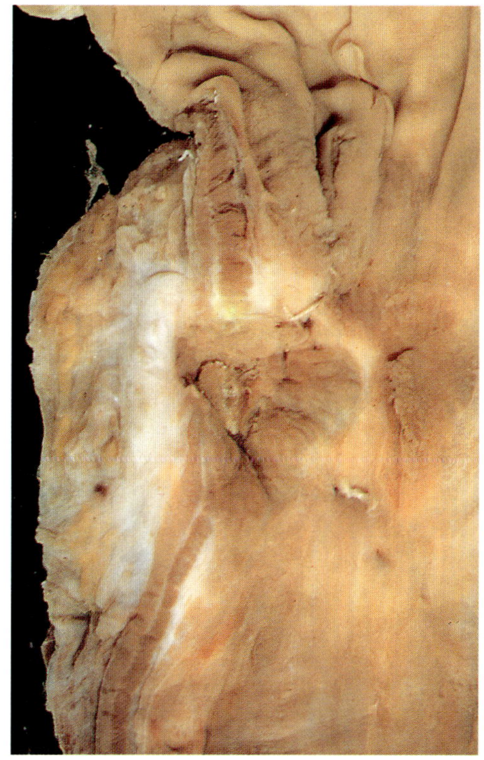

3.34 Oesophagus: Barrett's Ulcer

This was an incidental finding at post-mortem in a 64-year-old woman who died of bronchopneumonia.

The lower end of the oesophagus has been opened and this close-up view shows a punched-out ulcer, measuring 3cm in diameter on the posterior wall just above the oesophago-gastric junction. Note the adjacent mucosal puckering and scarring. The ulcer has also visibly eroded the muscle coat of the oesophagus.

Barrett's ulcer is the term applied to describe peptic ulceration of ectopic gastric mucosa in the lower oesophagus. The commonest origin of this epithelium is gastric metaplasia, occurring as a response to long-standing reflux oesophagitis but true gastric heterotopia is not infrequent. Reflex oesophagitis is therefore the most usual cause of Barrett's ulcers. The features are the same as those of gastroduodenal peptic ulcers (see Stomach section). Adults of either sex are usually affected and possible complications include stricture formation, haemorrhage and, occasionally, perforation.

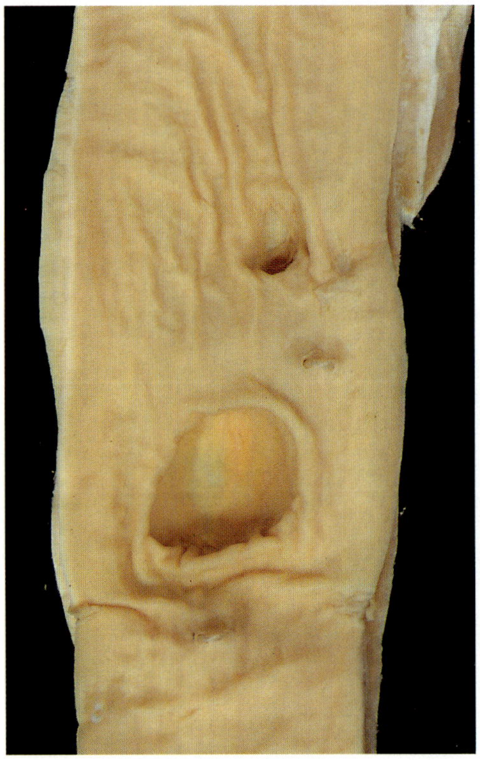

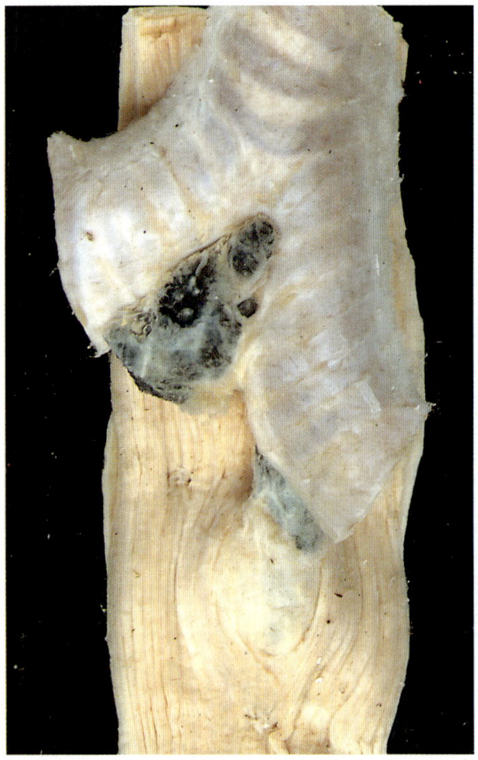

3.35 Oesophagus: Traction Diverticulum

This is a post-mortem specimen from a 62-year-old man. No further clinical details are available.

The middle third of the oesophagus has been opened (3.35a) to show the orifices of two diverticula, the larger measuring 2cm in diameter. The anterior aspect (3.35b) shows the larger diverticulum, the apex of which is adherent to an enlarged, anthracotic lymph node. The smaller diverticulum is similarly adherent but is concealed behind the tracheal bifurcation.

Oesophageal diverticula, which are acquired in the vast majority of cases, may be divided into pulsion and traction types. Pulsion diverticula arise as a consequence of raised intraluminal pressure and might be seen proximal to a stricture or in achalasia. Traction diverticula arise when the oesophagus becomes adherent to an extraneous focus of inflammation. Subsequent scarring and fibrosis result in traction or distortion of the oesophageal wall. Common causes include tuberculous lymphadenitis at the tracheal bifurcation (of which this case is probably a healed example), pleural adhesions or vertebral inflammation. Recognised complications of oesophageal diverticula include epithelial inflammation or ulceration, regurgitation and the very occasional development of carcinoma.

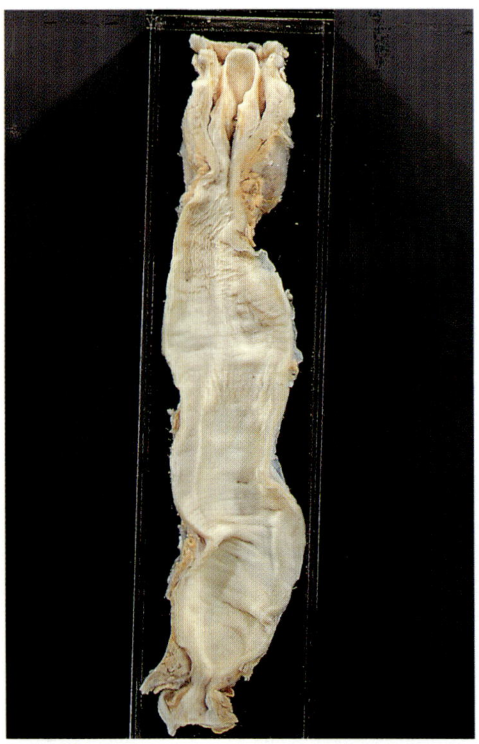

3.36 Oesophagus: Achalasia

This is a post-mortem specimen from a 53-year-old woman who had suffered from dysphagia for the previous 8 years. Barium swallow had revealed a dilated oesophagus with a functional narrowing at the gastro-oesophageal junction. Despite all treatment, the patient suddenly collapsed and died after a fit of coughing.

The oesophagus has been opened to show marked luminal dilatation along almost its entire length, the diameter measuring up to 15cm. The gastro-oesophageal junction, however, appears narrow but there is no evidence of muscular hypertrophy at this site.

Achalasia is a relatively uncommon disorder of oesophageal neuromuscular coordination, characterised by failure of the gastro-oesophageal sphincter to relax during swallowing. Adults are typically affected and the underlying lesion is thought to be a decrease or absence of the non-argyrophilic ganglion cells in the myenteric plexus along the entire length of the oesophagus. Hence peristalsis is by no means normal in the proximal dilated segment either. (Courtesy of the Gordon Museum, Guy's Hospital Medical School)

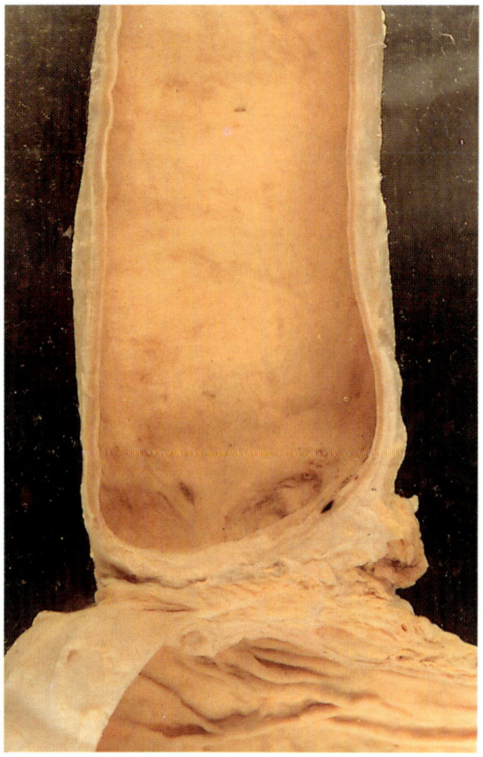

3.37 Oesophagus: Achalasia

This was an incidental finding at post-mortem in a 56-year-old woman who died of disseminated breast carcinoma.

The oesophagus, but not the gastro-oesophageal junction, has been opened to show gross luminal dilatation. Just proximal to the cardia, note the presence of a pulsion diverticulum (left) and a punched-out peptic ulcer (right).

This case demonstrates two of the possible complications of achalasia, of which oesophagitis with ulceration is the more common. Other important complications include aspiration of oesophageal contents (as probably occurred in the preceding case), leading to pneumonia, and the occasional development of squamous carcinoma in the dilated portion. (Courtesy of St. Thomas's Hospital Medical School Museum)

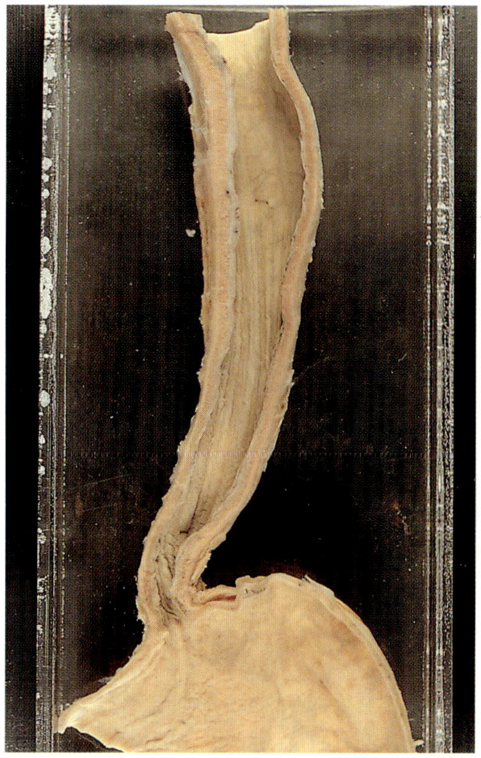

3.38 Oesophagus: Chagas' Disease

This is a post-mortem specimen from a 43-year-old Guyanese man, who had presented with dysphagia and the features of congestive cardiac failure. A presumptive diagnosis of Chagas' disease was made and he died soon after. At autopsy there was marked cardiomegaly with dilatation.

The oesophagus and stomach have been opened to show moderate dilatation of the oesophageal lumen, associated with very marked muscular hypertrophy in the wall.

Chagas' disease (synonym: South American trypanosomiasis) is caused by infection with the protozoon *Trypanosoma cruzi* which is transmitted by insect bites. The organisms tend to multiply in both smooth and cardiac muscle and release a neurotoxin which results in the destruction of ganglion cells. Hence the classical clinical features are cardiomegaly with heart failure, oesophageal dilatation and megacolon. The disease is endemic in Central and South America and, while infection occurs during childhood, the effects are not usually manifest until the 3rd to 5th decades. Many cases pursue a fatal course, largely as a result of cardiac dysfunction. (Courtesy of St. Thomas's Hospital Medical School Museum)

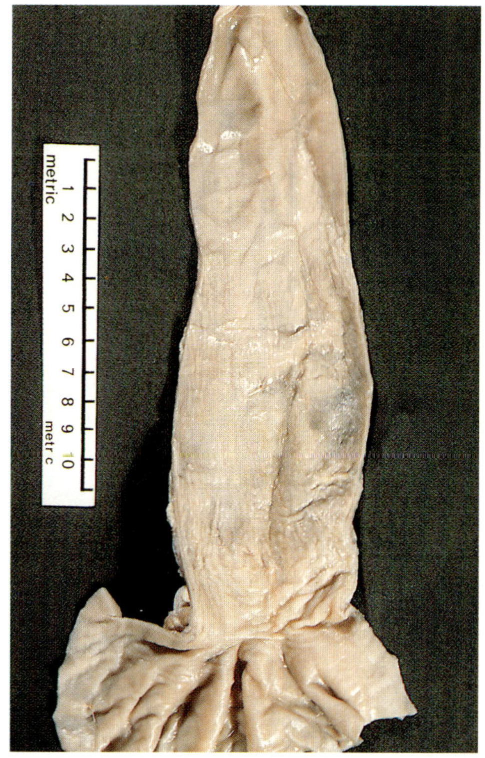

3.39 Oesophagus: Scleroderma

This is a post-mortem specimen from a 55-year-old woman, who died of congestive cardiac failure. She had been forced to give up work as a seamstress 10 years earlier because of severe scleroderma of the fingers. Latterly she had suffered from heartburn, episodic vomiting and anorexia.

The oesophagus has been opened to show marked distal dilatation, extending to the cardio-oesophageal sphincter. Histologically, there was moderate mural fibrosis.

Scleroderma, one of the idiopathic collagen disorders, may affect the oesophagus in isolation or may occur as the commonest visceral manifestation of systemic sclerosis (in which there is principally cutaneous involvement). In either circumstance, this condition is most frequent in middle-aged females. Oesophageal involvement is characterised by mural (particularly submucosal) fibrosis and ischaemic damage. These lead to dysphagia either by disrupting normal peristalsis or by producing a true stenosis. (Courtesy of the Pathology Museum, University of Wales College of Medicine, Cardiff)

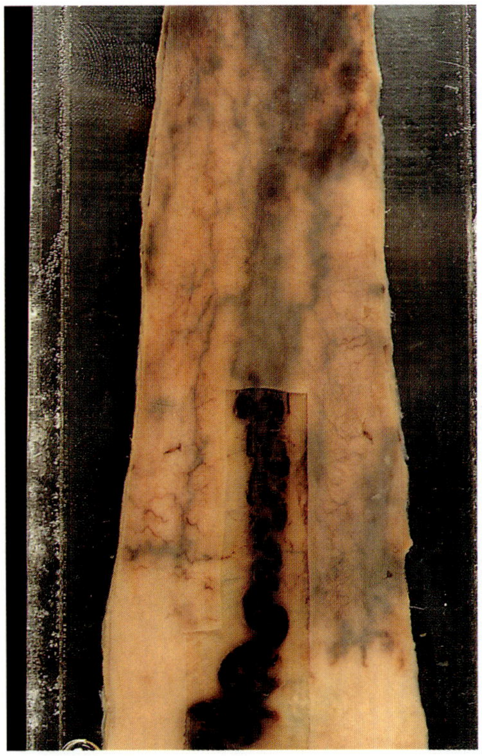

3.40 Oesophagus: Varices

This is a post-mortem specimen from a 68-year-old woman, known to have alcoholic cirrhosis of the liver. She presented with massive haematemesis which was not amenable to conservative treatment. Oesophageal transection with oversewing was performed but she died post-operatively.

The oesophagus has been opened to reveal grossly dilated veins in the submucosa. Only rarely are varices so prominent in an autopsy specimen, as the vessels usually collapse.

Oesophageal varices, which represent tortuous dilated veins, are a complication of portal hypertension (most often due to hepatic cirrhosis). They are typically located distally and because of their superficial location, are prone to ulceration and profuse haemorrhage. Other sites at which varices may develop, as a consequence of portosystemic shunting, are the anterior abdominal wall (caput medusae) and, less frequently, the rectum. (Courtesy of St. Thomas's Hospital Medical School Museum)

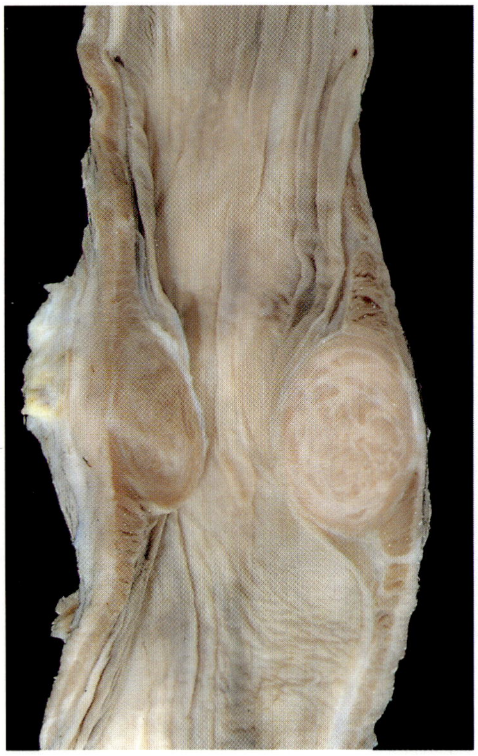

3.41 Oesophagus: Leiomyoma

This was an incidental post-mortem finding in a 76-year-old male murder victim.

The middle third of the oesophagus has been opened, through the lesion, to show a smooth, rounded, well-circumscribed tumour arising in the muscle coat. The tumour measures 2cm in diameter and the cut surface has a characteristically whorled, pale appearance. The overlying mucosa is intact and there is mild proximal muscular hypertrophy, probably due to a degree of stenosis caused by the tumour.

Oesophageal leiomyomas are not uncommon benign tumours of smooth muscle which arise most often in the lower third and show a predilection for males. They may give rise to an intramural nodule or an exophytic mass, typically with surface ulceration, which projects into the oesophageal lumen. Leiomyosarcoma, the malignant counterpart, is comparatively rare.

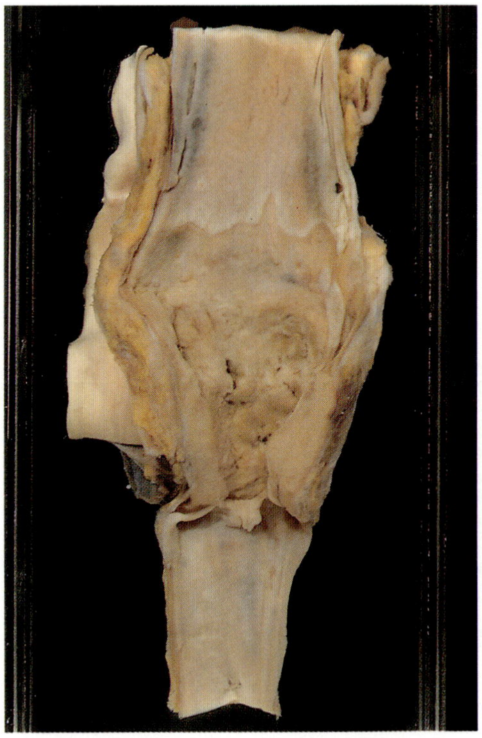

3.42 Oesophagus: Squamous Carcinoma

No clinical details are available.

The middle portion of the oesophagus has been opened posteriorly to show a large, stenosing neoplasm, measuring 6 × 5 × 3cm, which is situated just below the level of the tracheal bifurcation. The luminal surface of the tumour shows focal ulceration and necrosis. Note that the oesophagus above the tumour is dilated.

Carcinoma of the oesophagus accounts for up to 5 per cent of deaths from malignant disease in Britain and may be divided into three topographical subgroups: tumours of the upper third (including post-cricoid carcinoma) which occur predominantly in females (see Legend 3.44); tumours of the middle third, which are the most common, and are usually squamous in nature, and tumours of the lower third (including those at the gastro-oesophageal junction), which are the second most common and are often of glandular origin (adenocarcinoma). Oesophageal carcinoma shows a marked variation in geographical incidence, being particularly common in the Far East, parts of the USSR and Scandinavia: this is attributed to a probable dietary influence. In the United Kingdom, elderly males are most often affected, often in the lower social classes, and recognised aetiological factors include cigarette smoking, ingestion of alcoholic spirits and the pre-existence of a stricture, diverticulum or hiatus hernia. Macroscopically, the tumour most often takes an ulcerating or annular stenosing form: polypoid, exophytic growth (as is often seen in large bowel tumours) is uncommon. Oesophageal carcinoma tends to marked local invasion and, in view of its anatomical location, is frequently inoperable by the time of presentation. Spread of the tumour occurs primarily by lymphatics and death (due to invasion of adjacent structures or cachexia) often occurs before there is evidence of distant haematogenous dissemination. Adenocarcinomas arising in the lower third may represent either origin in a focus of gastric metaplasia (see Legend 3.34) or continuous extension of a gastric lesion arising in the cardia.

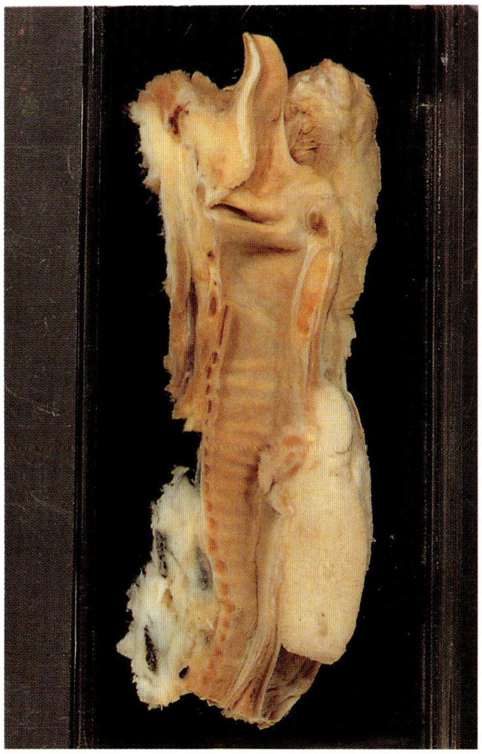

3.43 Oesophagus: Squamous Carcinoma

This is a post-mortem specimen from a 57-year-old man who presented with a short history of dysphagia. A barium swallow revealed neoplastic obstruction of the oesophagus and he died soon after from bronchopneumonia.

This is a sagittal section through the larynx, trachea and anterior wall of the oesophagus (right). Arising in the oesophagus is a solid raised, pale tumour, which measures 6 × 2 × 2cm. Note that the lesion has infiltrated the posterior wall of the trachea and is forming a nodular projection into the tracheal lumen. A mass of adjacent anthracotic, paratracheal lymph nodes are extensively infiltrated by tumour.

This case demonstrates well the way in which oesophageal carcinoma spreads. Local invasion of the trachea, bronchi, lung or even aorta is a common cause of death in such patients, resulting in either aspiration pneumonia or profuse haemorrhage. Oesophageal perforation and mediastinitis may also sometimes occur.

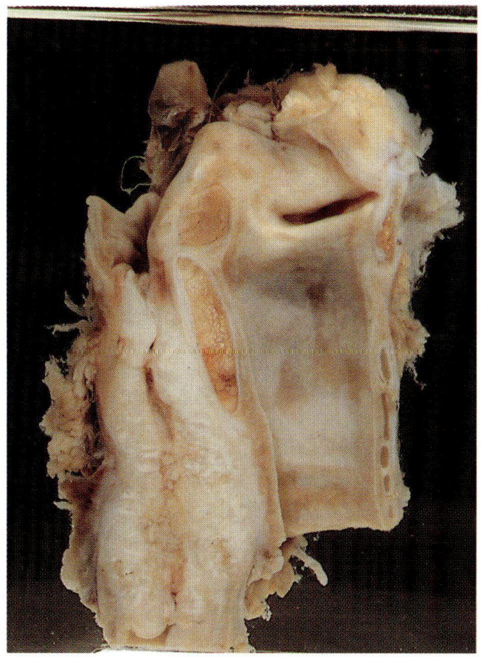

3.44 Oesophagus: Post-Cricoid Carcinoma

This specimen was excised from a 74-year-old woman who presented with dysphagia. She was found to have iron deficiency anaemia with atrophic glossitis and pharyngitis. A diagnosis of Plummer-Vinson syndrome was made and oesophagoscopy revealed an extensive post-cricoid malignant stricture. The larynx and part of the pharynx and oesophagus were excised.

A sagittal section through the larynx with the lower pharynx and upper oesophagus shows an annular stenosing, pale neoplasm, measuring 4cm in length, at the level of the cricoid cartilage. The oesophageal lumen is greatly reduced and there is evidence of early invasion of the posterior laryngeal wall.

Post-cricoid oesophageal carcinoma is always squamous in nature and in the vast majority of cases arises in middle-aged or elderly females suffering from the Plummer-Vinson syndrome. Geographically, there is a markedly increased incidence in Scandinavia. It is thought that dietary factors, in particular deficiency of iron and various vitamins, are aetiologically important. While there is often a coexistent post-cricoid web, its epithelial covering does not show pre-neoplastic or neoplastic changes and it is *not* the site in which the carcinoma develops.

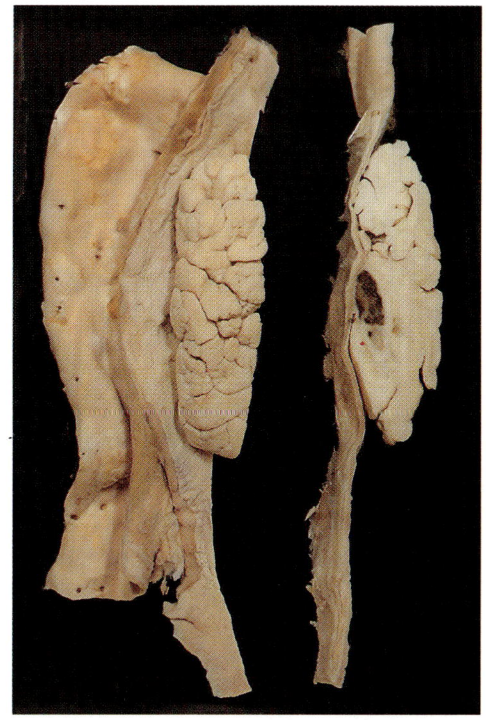

3.45 Oesophagus: Malignant Melanoma

This is a post-mortem specimen from an emaciated 77-year-old woman who had presented with a short history of dysphagia. X-rays and endoscopy confirmed the presence of a lobulated tumour in the mid-oesophagus. She was considered unfit for operation and died 2 weeks later. At autopsy there was no evidence of any metastasis and no primary lesion could be identified in the skin or other muco-cutaneous regions.

On the left a segment of the oesophagus with the thoracic aorta is shown. Projecting into the oesophageal lumen is a pale, coarsely lobulated, rather cerebriform mass, measuring 8cm in maximum diameter, which is pedunculated. On the right, a longitudinal section through the tumour shows a deeply pigmented area in the pedicle.

A malignant melanoma of the oesophagus should always be regarded as metastatic until proved otherwise, despite the fact that normal melanocytes are present in the oesophageal epithelium of a small proportion of the population. However, if there is absolutely no evidence of a tumour elsewhere and there is junctional activity in the oesophagus, then such a case may be classified as an oesophageal primary. Such tumours are extremely uncommon and behave in precisely the same way as their cutaneous counterparts. The prognosis is uniformly poor. Note also that, as in this case, any obstructive oesophageal tumour may cause death by cachexia in the absence of any metastatic spread.

STOMACH

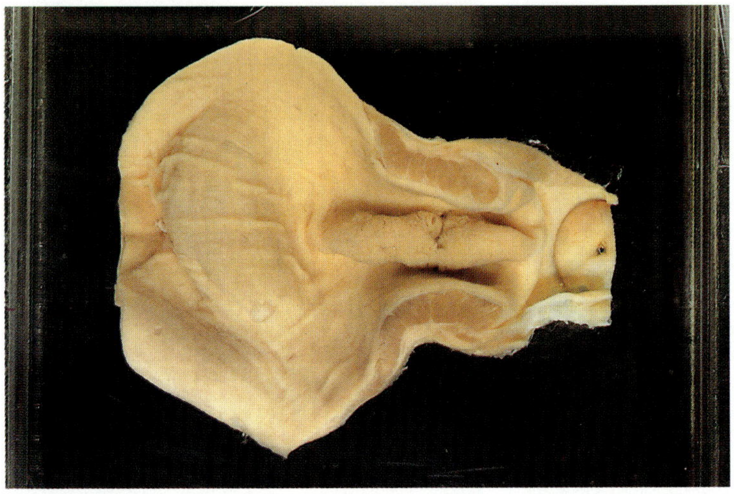

3.46 Congenital Pyloric Stenosis

This is a post-mortem specimen from an 11-week-old infant who had appeared healthy for the first 5 weeks of life. Thereafter persistent vomiting commenced, resulting in marked weight loss and finally death.

The pyloric portion of this infant's stomach has been opened to show a clearly defined region of marked muscular hypertrophy in the wall which encircles the pyloric canal. The overlying gastric mucosa is intact but bulges into the pyloric lumen, as is well demonstrated posteriorly.

Congenital pyloric stenosis occurs in approximately 1 in 350 live births. Up to 80 per cent of cases arise in male infants and first-born children are most often affected. This condition is thought to be inherited by an autosomal recessive gene, there being a marked familial incidence, and results in an as yet unclear primary abnormality of Auerbach's myenteric plexus. As a probable consequence of neuromuscular incoordination, gross hypertrophy of the circular muscularis propria occurs. The functional obstruction which results gives rise to the classical symptom of projectile vomiting and metabolic alkalosis ensues. Prompt relief is afforded by Ramstedt's operation.

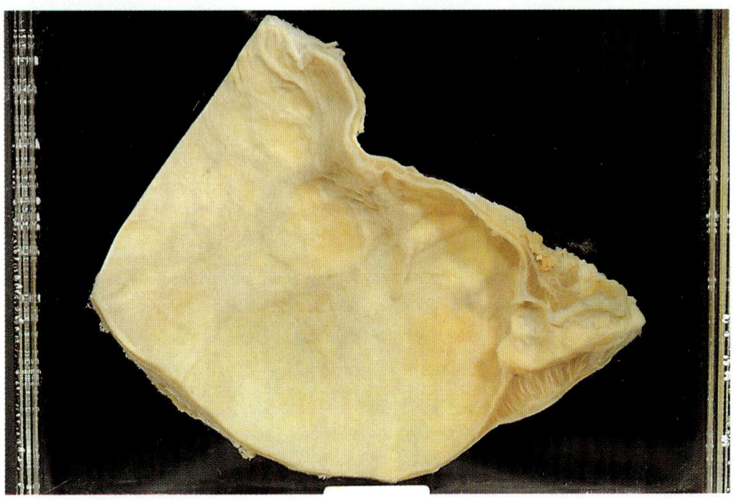

3.47 Adult Hypertrophic Pyloric Stenosis

This specimen was excised from a 45-year-old man who complained of increasingly frequent bouts of dyspepsia and severe vomiting. On examination there was a gastric splash and visible gastric peristalsis. A partial gastrectomy was performed.

The pyloric portion of the stomach has been opened from behind to show very marked hypertrophy of the circular muscle at the pylorus, which is in stark contrast to the thin wall of the proximal dilated stomach. The pyloric canal is markedly stenosed.

Occasional cases are seen in which a milder, or more slowly progressive, degree of congenital pyloric stenosis fails to present until adulthood as here. A congenital web or diaphragm at the pylorus may also be found in adults. However, at this age, secondary causes of pyloric stenosis, including scarring due to peptic ulceration, or obstruction by a carcinoma or a lymphoma, are much more common. Infrequently extrinsic obstruction may also occur.

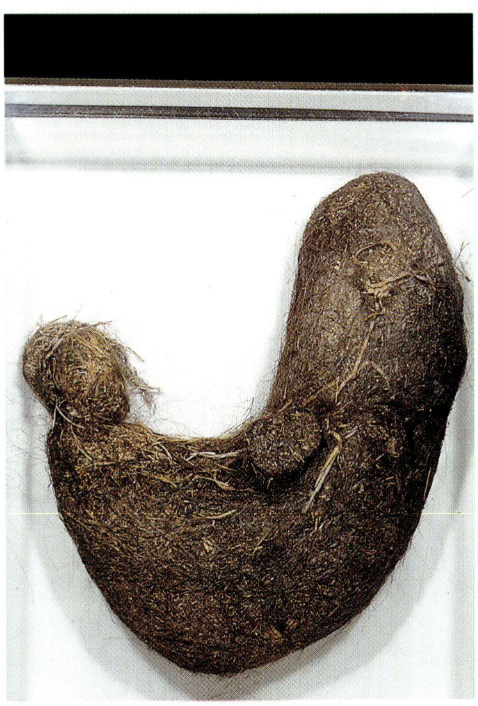

3.48 Trichobezoar

This specimen was removed from a mentally subnormal Arab girl, aged 18, who presented with an abdominal swelling. The swelling was mobile and corresponded to the size and shape of a distended stomach. A gastrotomy was performed.

The specimen consists of a tightly felted mass of hair, mixed with dried grass, which forms a perfect cast of the stomach, including the pyloric antrum and canal.

Trichobezoars, or hair balls, are found most often in the mentally ill or young children, either of whom may show a tendency to chew their hair constantly. Other bezoars (meaning intra-gastric foreign bodies) may be composed of vegetable material, derived from a normal, usually excessively ingested dietary constituent. Surprisingly, total obstruction is comparatively uncommon.

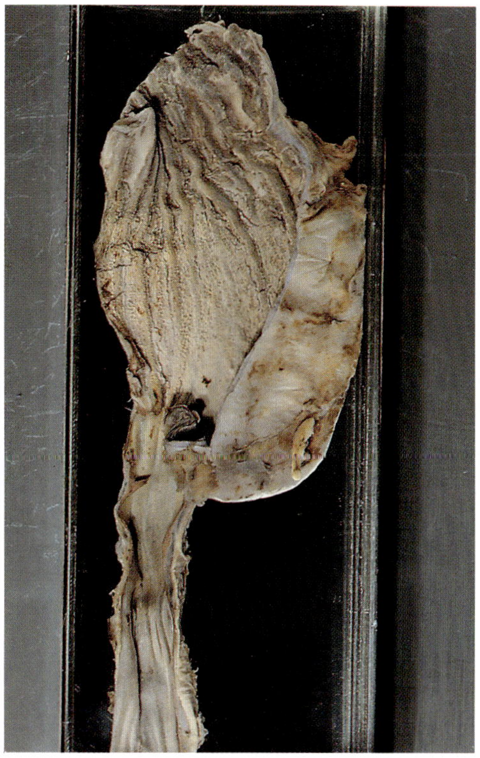

3.49 Lysol Poisoning

This is a post-mortem specimen from a woman who was being treated for depression. She discharged herself from hospital, bought 3 half-litre bottles of lysol and swallowed most of it.

The distal oesophagus and part of the stomach have been opened to show the corrosive effects of lysol. Much of the mucosa is necrotic, dirty grey in colour, and in places has sloughed off the underlying tissue of the gastric wall.

Ingestion of corrosives causes a florid acute gastritis and oesophagitis which may be so severe as to result in total mucosal necrosis.

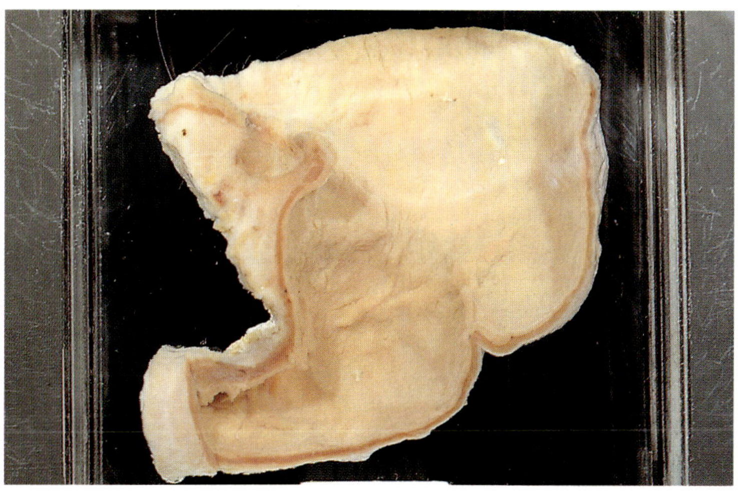

3.50 Chronic Peptic Ulcer

This is a partial gastrectomy specimen from a 47-year-old man who had suffered from long-standing dyspepsia.

The pyloric end of the stomach and the proximal duodenum have been opened to show an irregular ovoid ulcer high on the lesser curve. The ulcer has eroded the full thickness of the stomach wall, as is clearly seen in this view, and is surrounded by dense fibrous tissue.

Benign ulceration in the stomach commonly takes one of three forms: an erosion, an acute peptic ulcer or a chronic peptic ulcer. Gastric erosions and acute ulcers, both of which may be multiple, basically represent progression of an acute gastritis, the former involving the mucosa only and the latter extending into the submucosa. Adults in middle age are typically affected and recognised aetiological factors are as follows: excessive smoking or drinking, a high intake of salicylates or non-steroidal inflammatory drugs, hypovolaemic shock, burns (giving rise to Curling's ulcers) and cerebral injury or neurosurgery (which give rise to Cushing's ulcers). In general, these lesions usually heal with conservative treatment.

Chronic peptic ulcers may be found at a variety of sites which are, in order of frequency, the duodenum, stomach, oesophagus, margins of a gastric stoma, Meckel's diverticulum and the jejunum. In fact the vast majority are found in the duodenum and stomach. While the incidence is declining in the Western world, chronic ulcers are still common, affecting up to 10 per cent of males and 5 per cent of females at some time. Chronic gastric ulcers most often occur in the 5th and 6th decades and are more common in the lower social classes, patients with blood group O and, in some cases, show a familial incidence. Aetiologically, all peptic ulcers result from an imbalance between the acid secretions and mucosal resistance: here gastric and duodenal ulcers differ (see Figure and Legend 3.51). In patients with chronic gastric ulcers there is usually hypochlorhydria and the lesion is usually found in the gastric antrum, particularly on the lesser curve. Factors thought to be important are: an alteration in mucosal blood flow, a local disturbance in the mucosal mucus barrier, duodenal reflux or an impaired gastric emptying rate.

Macroscopically, chronic gastric ulcers are most often sharply punched-out lesions less than 4cm in diameter, which extend into the gastric muscle coat. Adjacent mucosal puckering or scarring is a common feature. Well recognised complications include haemorrhage, perforation, severe scarring leading to pyloric stenosis or an hour-glass stomach and, extremely rarely, the development of gastric carcinoma. Peptic ulcers are *not*, however, regarded as precancerous lesions.

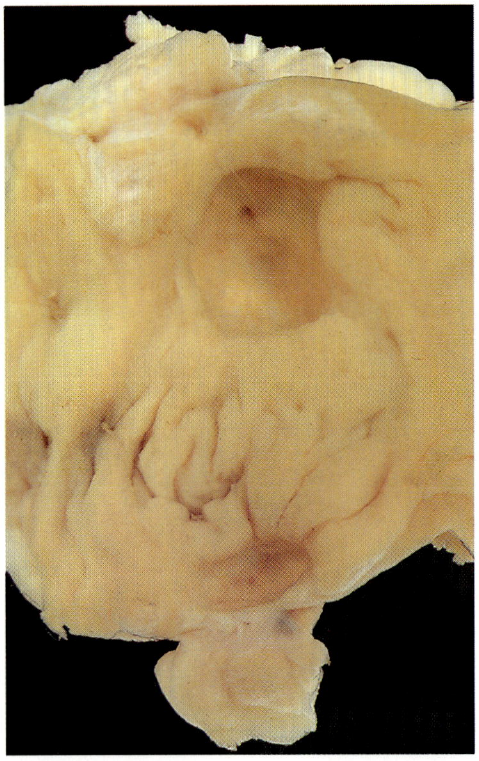

3.51 Duodenum: Chronic Peptic Ulcers

This is a post-mortem specimen from a 46-year-old man who died during anaesthetic induction, prior to undergoing partial gastrectomy. He had suffered recurrent attacks of dyspepsia for nearly 30 years, associated more recently with vomiting. Occult blood was demonstrable in the stools but there had been no haematemesis.

The first part of the duodenum, just distal to the pyloric canal, has been opened to show two chronic ulcers. The larger, situated superiorly, measures almost 2cm in diameter, while the lower lesion is smaller and shows omental adherence to its base.

The duodenum is the single commonest site for chronic peptic ulcers, being at least 4 times more frequently involved than the stomach. The vast majority of ulcers are found in the first part, most especially on the anterior wall. While histopathologically identical to their gastric counterparts and prone to the same complications, the two groups show certain differences.

Duodenal ulcers show no predilection for social class but do show a familial incidence, quite separate from any predisposition to gastric ulceration. As already stated, all peptic ulcers are due to an imbalance between acid secretion and mucosal resistance but, in contrast to gastric ulcers, duodenal lesions are associated with a marked increase in gastric acid secretion. This latter phenomenon may be related to an individual tendency to either increased gastric responsiveness to provocative stimuli or diminished inhibitory pathways. Duodenal ulcers *in no way* predispose to the development of carcinoma: in fact duodenal carcinoma at any site other than adjacent to the ampulla of Vater is extremely rare.

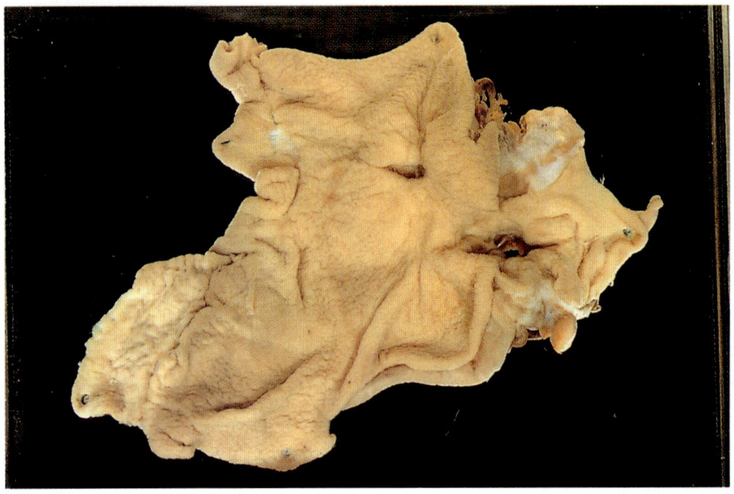

3.52 Stomach and Duodenum: Chronic Peptic Ulcers

This specimen was excised from a 90-year-old woman, who had a long-standing history of indigestion and presented with a perforated ulcer. A Billroth Type I partial gastrectomy was performed.

An irregular portion of the pylorus and the first part of the duodenum have been opened from behind to show an ovoid, almost slit-like, pyloric ulcer, measuring 1cm in length, and two rounded duodenal ulcers, each approximately 1cm in diameter, just distal to the pyloric sphincter. The superior duodenal ulcer has perforated through the bowel wall.

Perforation of a chronic peptic ulcer occurs in about 5 per cent of cases and is especially seen in males. Duodenal ulcers perforate much more often than their gastric counterparts, particularly those situated in the anterior wall, as in this case. Even after partial gastrectomy, up to 50 per cent of patients will develop another ulcer at a later date. It should also be noted that multiplicity of chronic peptic ulcers, as seen in this case, is comparatively uncommon.

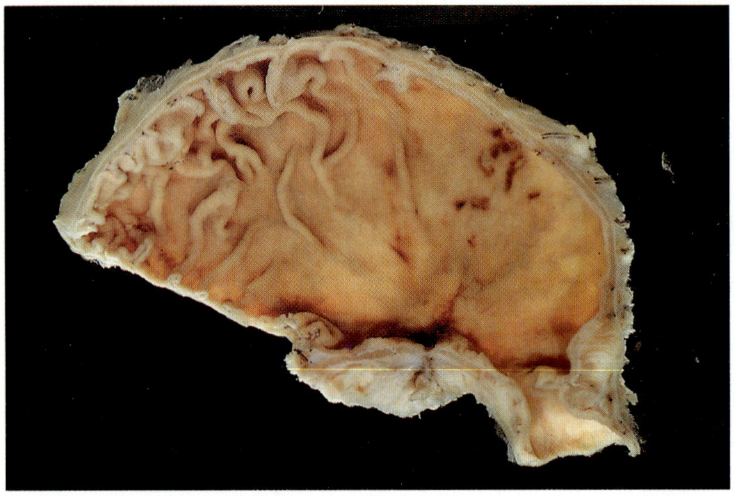

3.53 Chronic Peptic Ulcer and Erosions

This specimen was excised from a 64-year-old man who had suffered 3 previous episodes of melaena which were attributed to a chronic gastric ulcer. On this occasion he presented with profuse haematemesis and melaena of sudden onset and a partial gastrectomy was performed.

The pyloric portion of the stomach has been opened to show an ovoid, chronic ulcer, measuring 1cm in diameter on the lesser curvature. This is seen in cross-section and demonstrates well involvement of the full thickness of the stomach wall, congestion and adjacent fibrosis. Also apparent, near the greater curve, are several very red areas of superficial ulceration, representing gastric erosions which were the sources of the haematemesis.

While a chronic peptic ulcer is the commonest cause of upper gastrointestinal bleeding, up to 30 per cent of cases may be due to an acute ulcer or multiple gastric erosions. Typically, haemorrhage due to erosions is very often preceded by excessive ingestion of salicylates or non-steroidal inflammatory agents. The coexistence of a chronic ulcer, as in this case, may be coincidental or may reflect a predisposing abnormality of the gastric mucosal barrier.

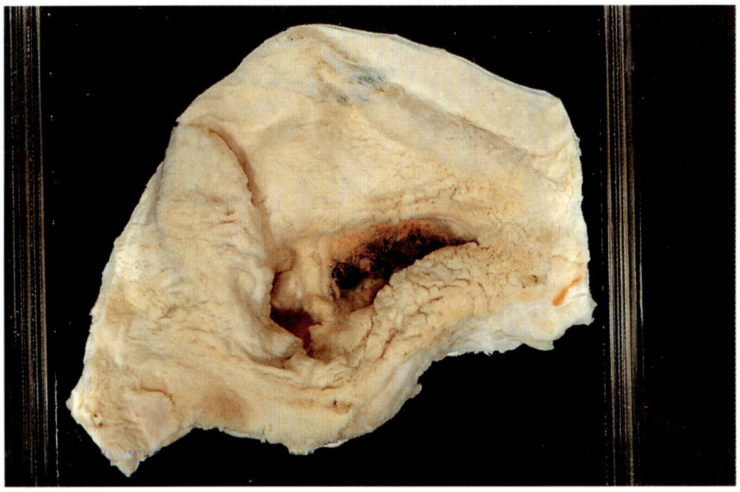

3.54 Haemorrhage due to Chronic Peptic Ulcer

This is a post-mortem specimen from an 88-year-old woman, who had suffered a previous episode of upper gastrointestinal bleeding. Terminally, she collapsed at home with a massive haematemesis and died rapidly.

A portion of the stomach has been opened to show a deep, irregular peptic ulcer, measuring 4 × 2.5 × 1cm. In the floor of the ulcer, a large artery has been eroded and there is adherent blood clot. Note also the copious granulation tissue at the margins of the ulcer.

Massive haemorrhage from a chronic peptic ulcer is most often seen in the elderly and is often preceded by episodes of less significant bleeding. In general surgical intervention is usually necessary since conservative measures often fail to prevent recurrent haemorrhage.

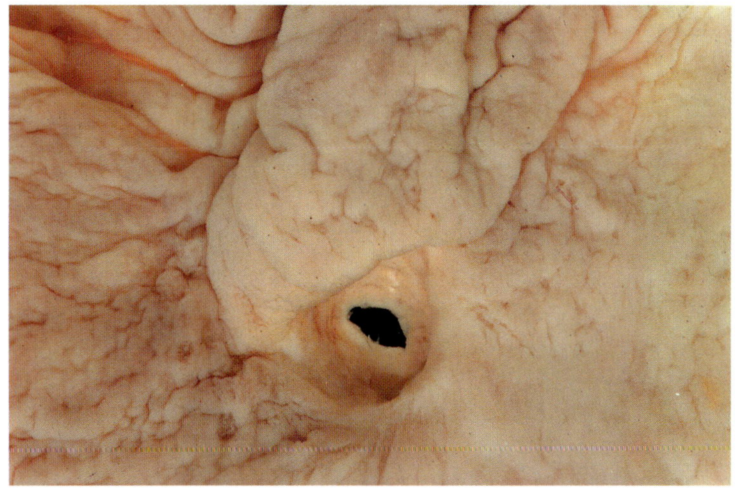

3.55 Perforated Peptic Ulcer

This is a post-mortem specimen from a 54-year-old man, who collapsed after suffering acute epigastric pain for 2 hours. He had an 18 month history of vague dyspepsia and pain after meals.

In the posterior wall of this opened stomach, close to the lesser curvature, is a deeply excavated ulcer, the floor of which is composed of a thin layer of fibrous tissue. The slit-like perforation is self-evident.

Due to their dense fibrous base, chronic peptic ulcers generally perforate less often than their acute counterparts. Anteriorly situated ulcers are more likely to perforate than those in a posterior location since the latter are usually already adherent to adjacent viscera (which may then be eroded). (Courtesy of the Gordon Museum, Guy's Hospital Medical School)

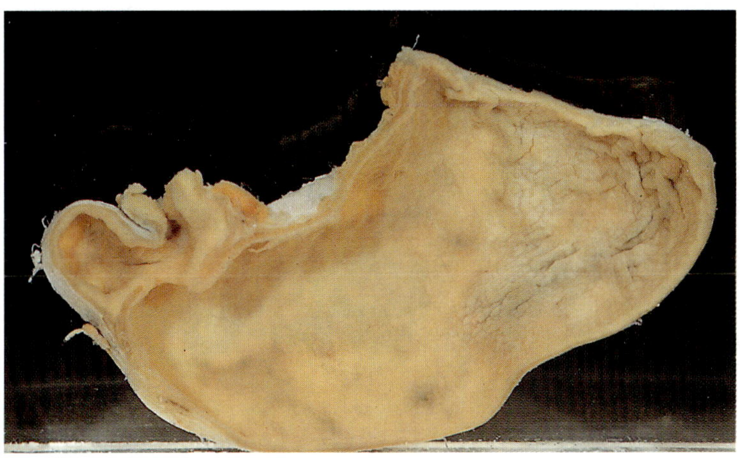

3.56 Pre-stenotic Diverticulum

This specimen was excised from a 42-year-old man who had a 25 year history of dyspepsia. Medical treatment failed to relieve his symptoms and a partial gastrectomy was performed.

The pyloric antrum, canal and proximal duodenum have been opened anteriorly to show dense scarring and stenosis, resulting from previous ulceration, at the junction between the pylorus and duodenum. Just proximally, projecting from the inferior border of the pyloric canal, is a rounded diverticulum, which measures 1.5cm in diameter.

Acquired diverticula are an infrequent complication of peptic ulceration. Most often they occur proximal to an area of stenosis (usually at the pylorus) and are thus pulsion diverticula. They may also occur at the site either of previous ulceration (with little adjacent scarring) or of previous surgery. Congenital diverticula are excessively rare.

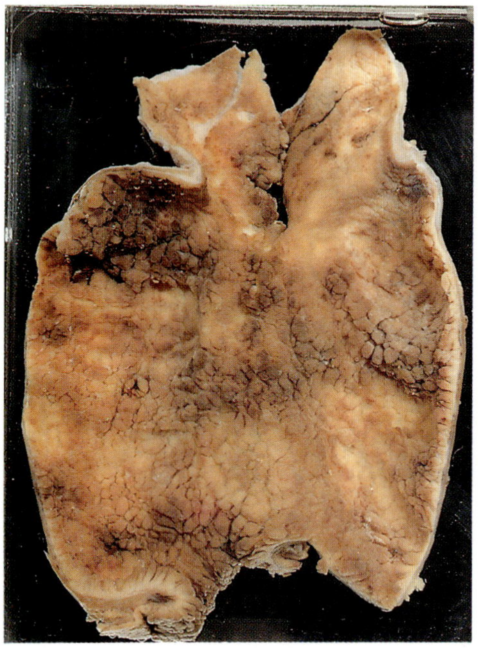

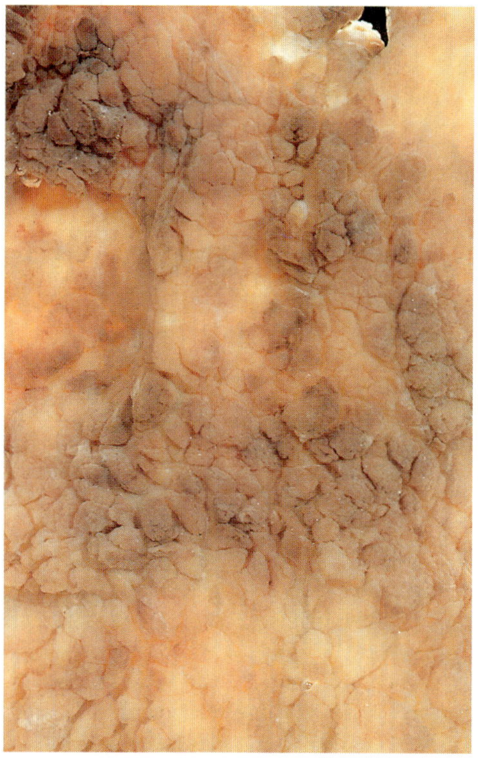

3.57 Peutz-Jeghers Polyposis

No clinical details are available.

The stomach has been opened (3.57a) to show numerous mucosal polyps, some of which are pedunculated, measuring up to 1cm in diameter. The stomach is also moderately dilated. The polyps are more clearly seen in a close-up view (3.57b).

Peutz-Jeghers syndrome comprises gastrointestinal hamartomatous polyp formation and mucocutaneous melanin pigmentation. It is an autosomal dominant inherited condition and is most often recognised in childhood. While the polyps, which are effectively due to proliferation and branching of the muscularis mucosae covered by normal epithelium, are commonest in the proximal small intestine, involvement of the stomach or colon is by no means rare. In the stomach, as elsewhere, they may be complicated by bleeding but, at this site, intussusception is extremely unusual. These hamartomatous polyps have no malignant potential.

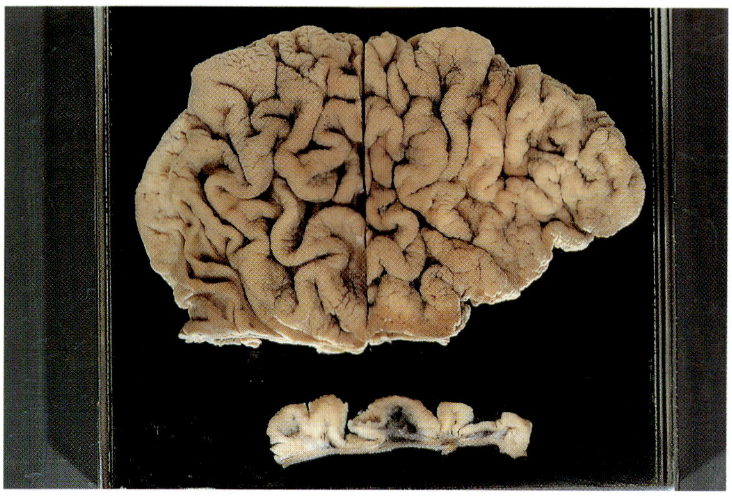

3.58 Ménétrièr's Disease

This specimen was excised from a 35-year-old man who had a 12 year history of abdominal pain and dyspepsia, unrelieved by conservative measures. A subtotal gastrectomy was performed.

The stomach has been opened to show gross exaggeration of the normal mucosal folds in the fundus and body. The antrum is typically spared in this condition. A transverse section, mounted above, demonstrates the rugal hypertrophy to be solely mucosal in origin. The submucosal haemorrhage is an operative artefact. This macroscopic appearance may be confused with the rugal hypertrophy seen in Zollinger-Ellison syndrome (see Figure and Legend 3.59).

Ménétrièr's disease (synonyms: giant rugal hypertrophy, hypertrophic gastritis) is a rare condition of unknown aetiology. Typically it affects males in the 4th-6th decades and may be associated with either increased or decreased gastric acid secretion. A localised form may be seen confined to the greater curvature. Complications include haemorrhage, hypoalbuminaemia (secondary to protein loss) and, occasionally, the development of a gastric carcinoma. Radiological confusion with a carcinoma or polyposis is not uncommon.

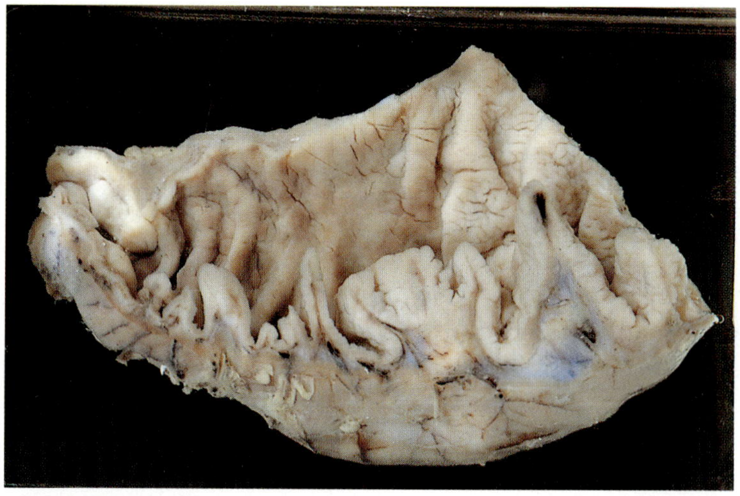

3.59 Zollinger-Ellison Syndrome

This specimen was excised from a 39-year-old man, who had a 2 year history of dyspepsia. He was found to have a duodenal ulcer and hypoproteinaemia and a partial gastrectomy was performed. At operation, in addition to the ulcer, the walls of the stomach seemed unusually thickened.

A portion of the body of the stomach has been opened to show marked hypertrophy of the rugae, particularly well shown in cross-section, adjacent to the greater curvature. Histologically, this is seen to be a result of a greatly increased parietal cell mass.

Zollinger-Ellison syndrome is usually characterised by the presence of a pancreatic gastrin-secreting islet cell tumour, which causes marked gastric hyperacidity and hence peptic ulceration: the latter is often multifocal and may extend as far as the jejunum. A proportion of cases are attributable to hyperplasia of antral gastrin-secreting cells. In either group, some patients develop rugal hypertrophy, as here, which may be confused with Ménétrièr's disease. Unfortunately no further details of this patient are available so the cause, in this case, remains uncertain.

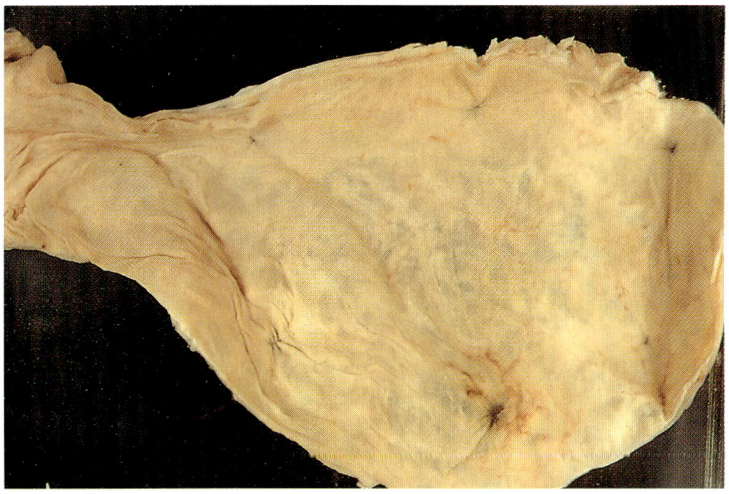

3.60 Pernicious Anaemia

This is a post-mortem specimen from an elderly woman, who had become progressively weaker and finally presented in a moribund condition. Clinically there was marked mucosal pallor; blood and bone marrow examination revealed a profound megaloblastic anaemia.

This opened stomach shows gross mural atrophy such that it now appears almost paper thin. The pylorus (left) is relatively unaffected.

Pernicious anaemia is an autoimmune disease characterised by the development of antibodies to intrinsic factor and gastric parietal cells, hence preventing either the binding or absorption of vitamin B_{12}. This condition is commonest in middle-aged or elderly females and is often associated with other coexistent autoimmune disease, particularly of the thyroid (see Chapter 6). Histologically, affected patients develop atrophic gastritis or severe gastric atrophy (as here), often with intestinal metaplasia of the gastric epithelium. They eventually become achlorhydric. Up to 10 per cent of cases are complicated by the development of a gastric adenocarcinoma. (Courtesy of St. Thomas's Hospital Medical School Museum)

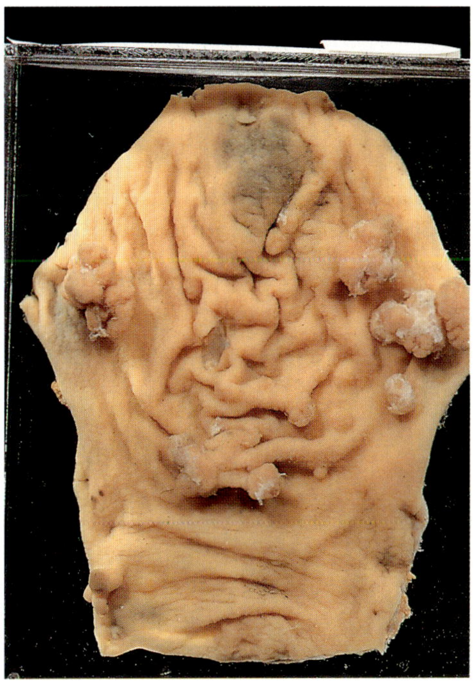

3.61 Multiple Regenerative Polyps

This specimen was excised from a 62-year-old man, who presented with a single episode of haematemesis and melaena. There was no significant history of dyspepsia.

Projecting from the mucosal surface of the body of the stomach are multiple pedunculated and sessile polyps of varying size, some of which are covered in pale mucus.

Regenerative (synonym: hyperplastic) polyps are not uncommon lesions, which are frequently multiple (in contrast to gastric neoplastic polyps) and are of uncertain aetiology. It is likely, however, that they are reactive in nature and are probably related to preceding gastritis. They are not pre-malignant. (Courtesy of the Gordon Museum, Guy's Hospital Medical School)

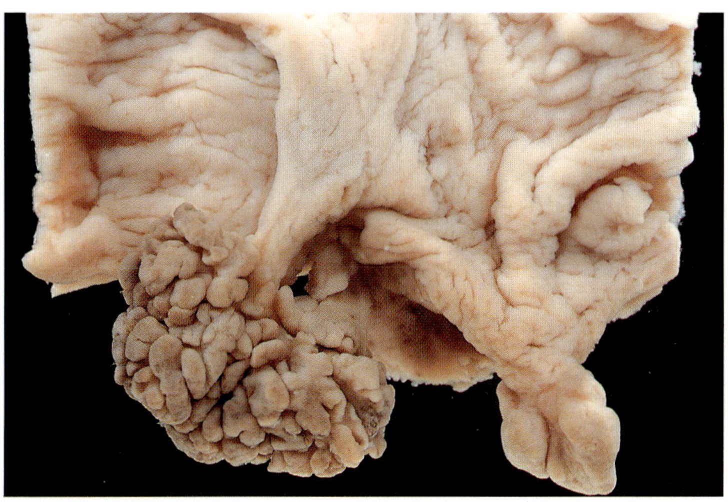

3.62 Tubulovillous Adenoma

This specimen was excised from a 60-year-old man, who was found to have a filling defect in the pyloric antrum on barium meal. Occult blood had been detected in the faeces.

Projecting from the gastric mucosa is a solitary, pedunculated tubulovillous neoplasm, measuring up to 4cm in diameter.

Neoplastic polyps of the stomach are uncommon but are usually found in late adulthood in either sex. They most often adopt a tubulovillous or villous pattern, tubular lesions being quite rare. The majority of lesions are flat and sessile, pedunculation (as here) being relatively unusual. A proportion of cases are associated with pre-existent atrophic gastritis or pernicious anaemia. These polyps have exactly the same pre-malignant potential as their counterparts in the large bowel (see Small and Large Intestines section) and the risk of developing an invasive carcinoma is proportional to polyp size. (Courtesy of the Gordon Museum, Guy's Hospital Medical School)

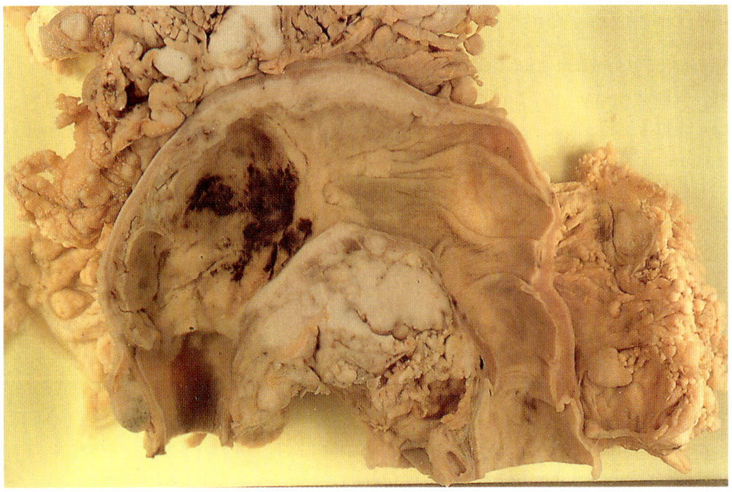

3.63 Adenocarcinoma

This specimen was excised from a 31-year-old man, who presented with weight loss, epigastric pain and a sensation of food 'sticking' in the lower gullet.

The stomach has been opened from behind to reveal a large, nodular, ulcerating neoplasm infiltrating the antrum and proximal pylorus. Invasion of the muscle coat is well demonstrated. The lymph nodes in the mesenteric fat, adjacent to the lesser and greater curves, are replaced by tumour.

Gastric adenocarcinoma is one of the commonest malignant tumours in the Western world but shows a marked geographical variation in incidence. It is particularly common in Japan, Finland and Iceland. Males are affected twice as often as females, most commonly in the 6th and 7th decades. There is a familial tendency and this tumour is more frequent in the lower social classes and those of blood group A. Factors of postulated aetiological importance include nitrosamines, derived from ingested nitrates or nitrites, and dietary intake, particularly smoked food. Recognised predisposing histological lesions are chronic atrophic gastritis with intestinal metaplasia, epithelial dysplasia and uncommonly gastric adenomas: very rarely a chronic peptic ulcer or Ménétrièr's disease may be implicated. While significant progress in detecting early gastric cancer has been made in Japan, very many European cases present with advanced disease, the majority having lymph node metastases at operation. Five-year-survival after gastrectomy is of the order of 10 per cent. (Courtesy of St. Thomas's Hospital Medical School Museum)

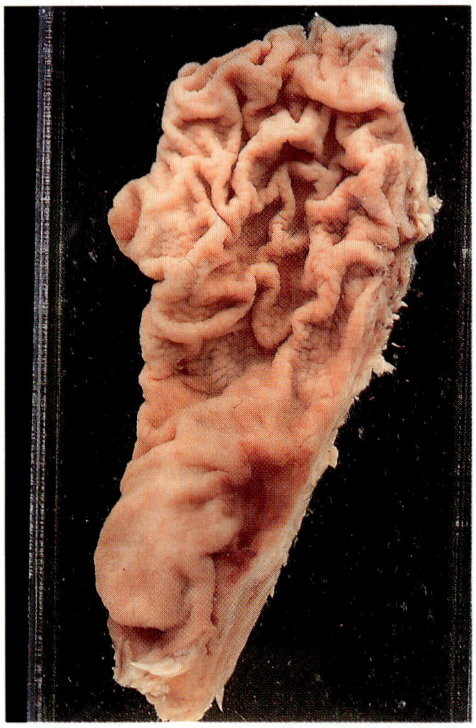

3.64 Adenocarcinoma

This specimen was excised from a 52-year-old man, who had suffered from symptoms of a hiatus hernia for many years. More recently he had become anorexic and had lost 7kg in weight. Barium meal revealed an ulcerated lesion on the lesser curvature and a radical gastrectomy was performed.

Part of the stomach has been mounted to show an irregular ulcer high on the lesser curve. Note that the lesion has a raised, rolled margin, which distinguishes it from a chronic peptic ulcer.

The vast majority of gastric adenocarcinomas are, macroscopically, either nodular and raised or ulcerated. These patterns very often overlap. (Courtesy of the Gordon Museum, Guy's Hospital Medical School)

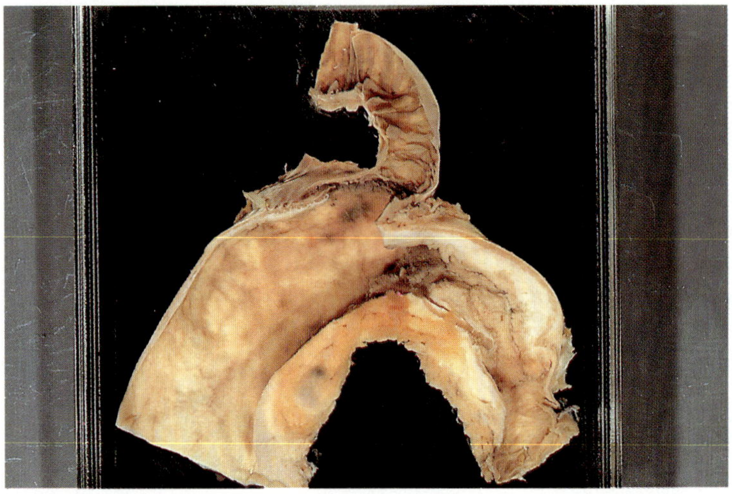

3.65 Stenosing Pyloric Carcinoma

This is a post-mortem specimen from an 84-year-old woman, who presented with a 3 month history of weight loss and was found to be grossly anaemic. A palliative gastroenterostomy was performed 4 days before death.

The distal stomach and pylorus have been opened to reveal a localised, nodular stenosing carcinoma, measuring 6cm in maximum diameter, in the pyloric canal. The tumour shows obvious deep mural invasion but the proximal duodenum is completely unaffected. The gastroenterostomy, 2cm proximal to the tumour, is patent.

Gastric carcinoma is a well-recognised cause of secondary pyloric stenosis in adulthood. In fact adenocarcinomata of the stomach arise most often in the pylorus and pyloric antrum but show a marked tendency to extensive local spread.

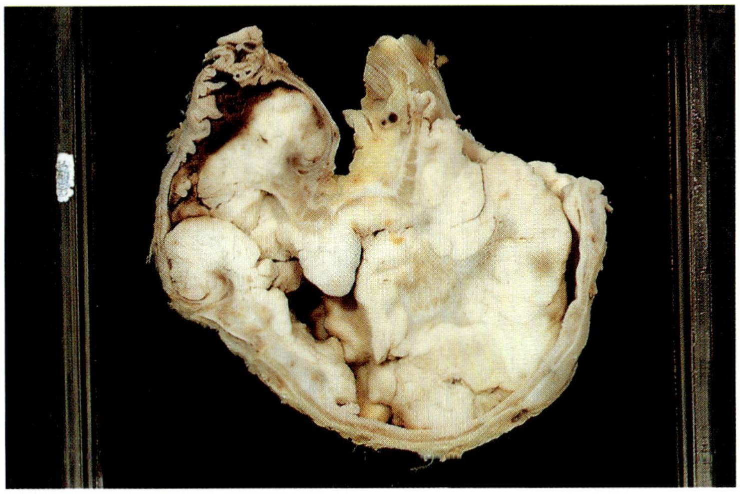

3.66 Polypoid Adenocarcinoma

This specimen was excised from a 62-year-old woman who had a one year history of dyspepsia. A mobile mass was palpable in the epigastrium and a partial gastrectomy was performed.

A portion of the stomach has been opened anteriorly to show a very large, polypoid pale neoplasm, almost filling the gastric lumen. The tumour has arisen on the lesser curvature and can be seen to infiltrate the muscle coat.

This macroscopical variant of gastric carcinoma is very rare.

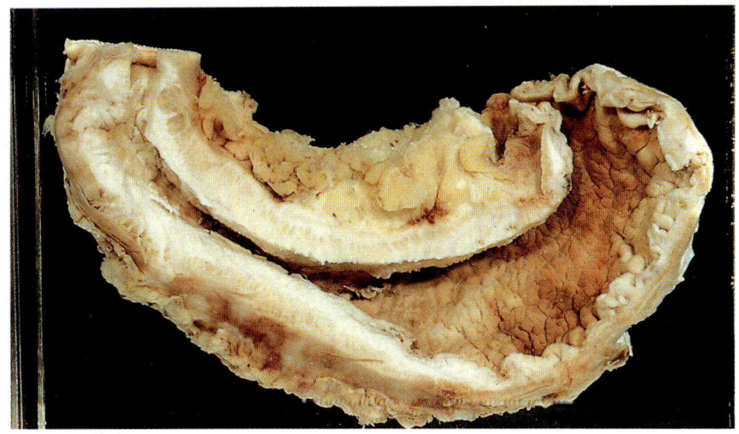

3.67 Diffuse Adenocarcinoma

This specimen was excised from a 64-year-old man who had a 3 year history of dyspepsia. Gastric carcinoma was diagnosed at barium meal and endoscopy: total gastrectomy was performed.

The stomach has been opened anteriorly to show diffuse infiltration of the pylorus and body by a pale neoplasm. While there is marked luminal narrowing, the tumour has no exophytic component. Note also irregular infiltration of the muscle coat.

Diffuse, deeply-spreading gastric carcinoma such as this is known as linitis plastica or 'leather-bottle' stomach and accounts for between 5 and 10 per cent of cases. Much of the pale 'tumour' tissue, in fact, represents submucosal and muscular fibrosis. It should be noted that, while this is a characteristic macroscopical appearance, it does not correspond to any particular histological subtype of gastric carcinoma. However, such diffuse infiltration confers a worse prognosis.

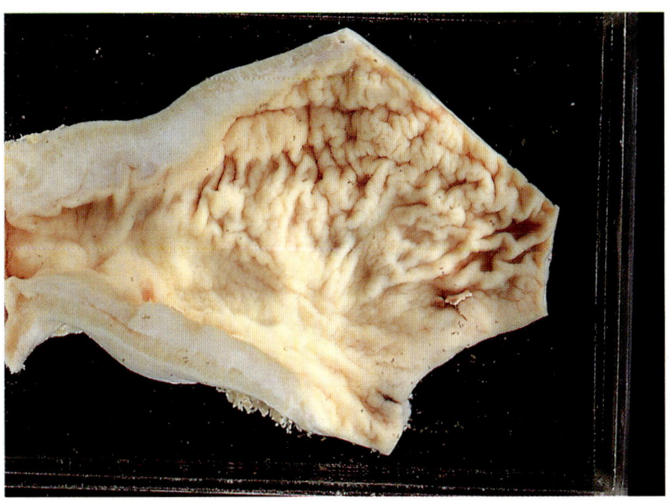

3.68 Superficial Spreading Carcinoma

This specimen was excised from a 45-year-old woman, who presented with a 3 month history of epigastric pain after meals, associated with a feeling of fullness. At laparotomy, the pyloric region was found to be hard and irregular and a subtotal gastrectomy was performed. One year post-operatively she was extremely well with no evidence of tumour.

The pylorus and proximal duodenum have been opened to show diffuse, pale thickening and flattening of the pyloric mucosa. Histologically there was no invasion of the muscle coat and the lymph nodes were not involved.

Superficial spreading carcinoma of the stomach is the least common macroscopical variant, accounting for about 2 per cent of cases. It is most common in the pyloric region and may be difficult to detect either on a barium meal or endoscopically; sometimes it is associated with an adjacent peptic ulcer. This case would be classified as an example of early gastric cancer, in which circumstance the 5-year-survival after gastrectomy should be of the order of 90 per cent. (Courtesy of the Gordon Museum, Guy's Hospital Medical School)

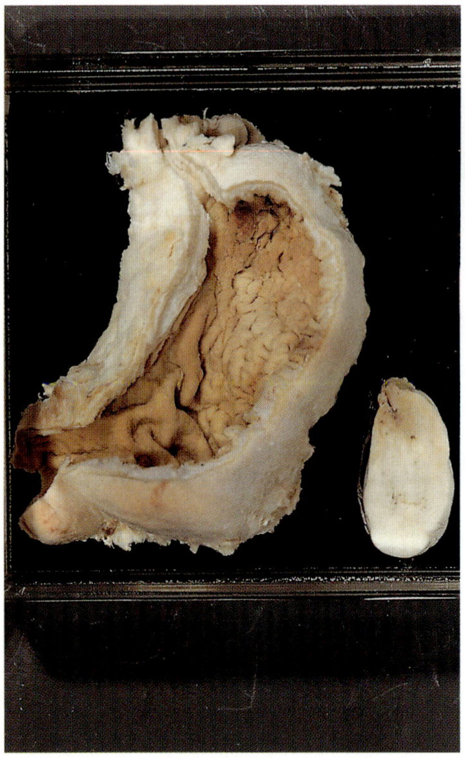

3.69 Adenocarcinoma with Ovarian Metastasis

These specimens were excised from a 65-year-old woman who had a 4 month history of dysphagia. A barium meal showed a tumour of the gastric fundus and oesophagogastrectomy with resection of a right ovarian tumour was performed.

On the left, there is a stenosing diffuse tumour in the fundus of the stomach near the gastro-oesophageal junction. The lumen has been narrowed to 0.4cm in diameter. On the right, the ovary which has been sectioned, shows total replacement by pale tumour. Histologically, the gastric and ovarian lesions were very similar.

Gastric carcinoma has a particular tendency to metastasise to the ovary either transperitoneally or by the bloodstream. When the histological appearance of such a tumour is that of a mucus-secreting signet-ring cell adenocarcinoma, the ovarian moiety is known as a Krukenberg tumour. Ovarian involvement may be bilateral. Other common primary sources of Krukenberg tumours are carcinoma of the breast or colon.

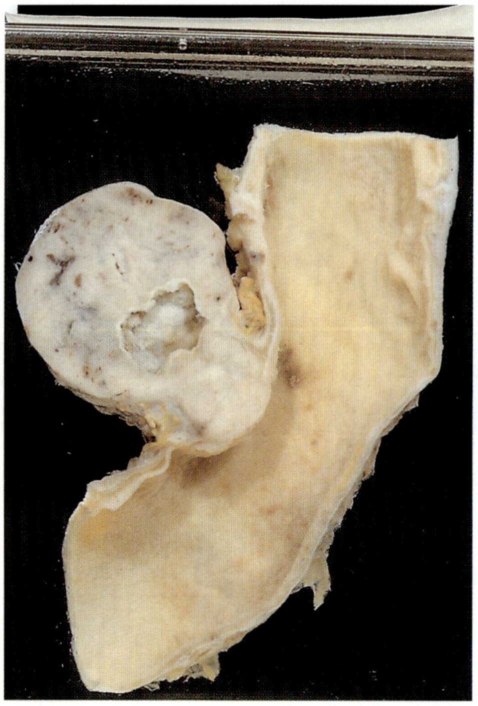

3.70 Leiomyoma

This specimen was excised from a 47-year-old woman who presented with weight loss and a mass in the upper abdomen.

A portion of the stomach has been opened anteriorly to show a pale, well-circumscribed tumour arising in the lesser curvature, which projects both serosally and to a lesser degree, into the gastric lumen. It is covered by attenuated mucosa, which is ulcerated at the apex of the lesion (not visible here). This apical ulcer communicates with the small necrotic cavity, visible on the cut surface.

Gastric leiomyomas are not uncommon, particularly in the elderly, but are usually asymptomatic and may be an incidental finding at post-mortem. They arise from the muscularis propria and may remain intramural or project, either internally or externally. A central apical ulcer is characteristic and may give rise to haemorrhage. Careful application of histological criteria is necessary to distinguish these benign lesions from leiomyosarcoma.

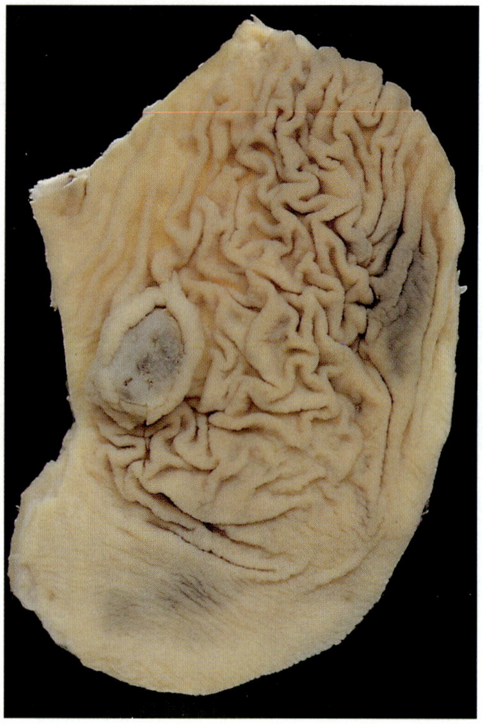

3.71 Epithelioid Leiomyoma

This specimen was excised from a 72-year-old man who presented acutely with haematemesis and melaena. A partial gastrectomy was performed.

A portion of the stomach has been dissected to show a discrete, rounded tumour, measuring 2cm in diameter, the centre of which is extensively ulcerated. Several small arteries are visible in the floor of the apical ulcer.

Epithelioid leiomyoma (synonym: leiomyoblastoma, bizarre leiomyoma, Stout's peculiar tumour) is a histological variant of a gastric leiomyoma and, as such, is not distinguishable macroscopically. Clinically these lesions are most often seen in the 6th and 7th decades and the vast majority behave in a benign fashion.

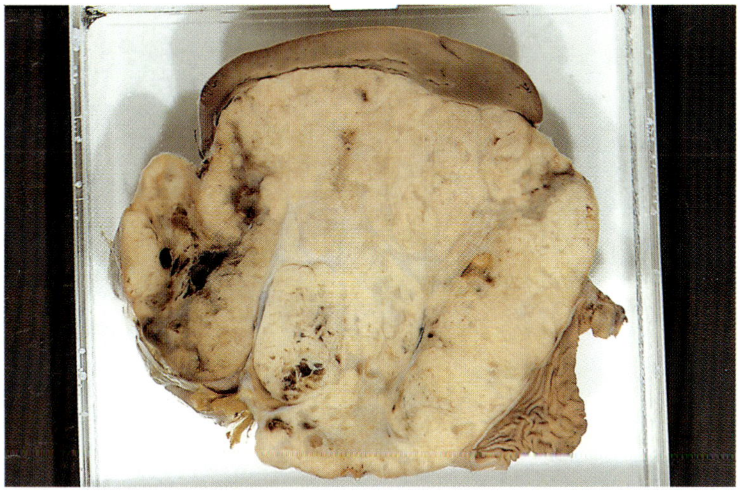

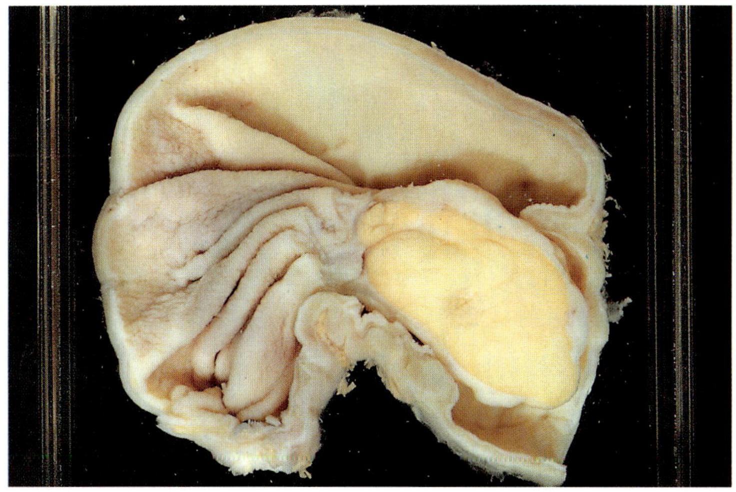

3.72 Leiomyosarcoma

This specimen was excised from a 32-year-old woman who was found to have a large abdominal tumour.

This is a portion of the cardiac end of the stomach; a very large, rounded tumour measuring 20cm in diameter is arising in the stomach wall. The gastric mucosa (left) is stretched over the surface of the neoplasm and there is a shallow apical ulcer, which projects downwards (bottom left). The cut surface of the tumour is pale, whorled and shows irregular foci of haemorrhage and necrosis.

Gastric leiomyosarcoma is uncommon, affects either sex and usually arises in the 5th to 7th decades. In cases when the tumour is as large, haemorrhagic and necrotic as this distinction from a benign leiomyoma (see Figure 3.70 et seq.) is not difficult: however, the only reproducible distinguishing criterion is the degree of mitotic activity seen histologically. Frankly malignant tumours spread by the bloodstream and carry a poor prognosis.

3.73 Submucosal Lipoma

This specimen was excised from a 74-year-old woman who presented with intermittent abdominal pain and vomiting. Barium studies suggested a gastroduodenal intussusception and partial gastrectomy was performed.

The pyloric antrum, canal and proximal duodenum have been opened anteriorly to show a yellow, fatty tumour, arising in the submucosa of the lesser curve, which projects by a pedicle through the pyloric canal. The tumour measures 4cm in maximum diameter and the attenuated, covering mucosa is ulcerated at the apex.

Gastric lipomas are very uncommon and are benign lesions, entirely comparable to their counterparts elsewhere in the body. They usually arise in the pyloric antrum and may be the source of occult haemorrhage if surface ulceration occurs. Pedunculation with or without intussusception, is extremely rare.

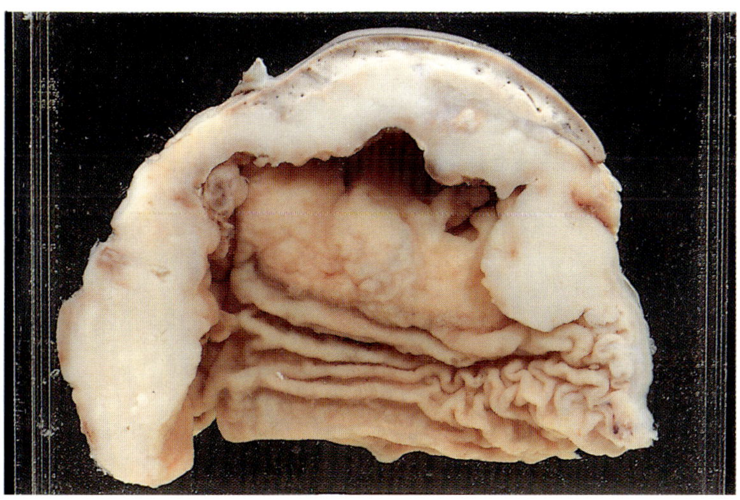

3.74 Non-Hodgkin's Lymphoma

This specimen was excised from a 20-year-old man, who presented with a 3 month history of epigastric pain, more recently associated with increasing dysphagia. Barium meal revealed a large neoplasm involving the distal oesophagus and proximal stomach. At laparotomy the tumour was also invading the liver.

This is part of the gastric fundus, which is extensively infiltrated by a nodular, superficially ulcerated pale neoplasm. The tumour has widely penetrated the serosa and is extending into an excised segment of the left lobe of the liver (top).

Malignant lymphomas account for up to 5 per cent of all gastric neoplasms. While some simply represent involvement by disseminated disease, a significant proportion originate primarily in the stomach. The various classifications of non-Hodgkin's lymphoma are not applicable to extranodal primary neoplasms, but the majority of gastric lymphomas are currently regarded as being of B-cell lineage and were formerly diagnosed as lymphosarcomas. These tumours are most common in middle or late adulthood, typically arise in the body of the stomach and are often large, diffuse lesions (as here). Direct spread into the liver or spleen is a frequent feature. The prognosis is better than that of gastric carcinoma, the overall 5-year-survival being about 50 per cent. (Courtesy of the Gordon Museum, Guy's Hospital Medical School)

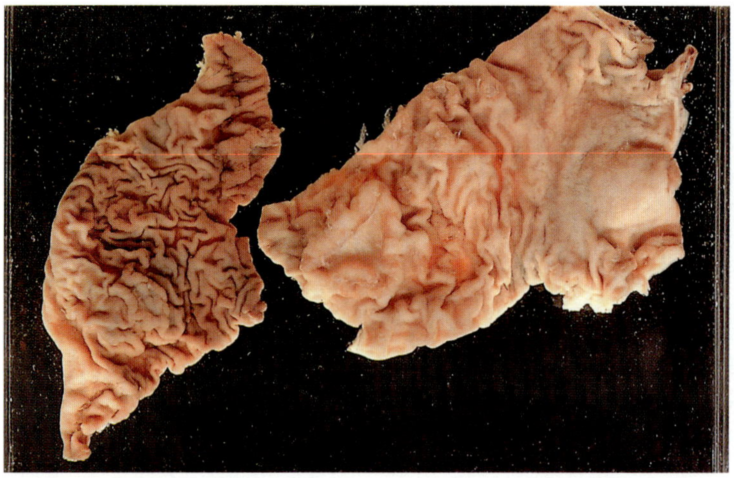

3.75 Non-Hodgkin's Lymphoma

This specimen was excised from a middle-aged woman, who presented with haematemesis and melaena.

Two portions of the stomach have been mounted, each of which shows foci of mucosal ulceration, the margins of which are irregular and rolled.

Gastric lymphomas are often multifocal. They may also simulate a multifocal appearance by spreading extensively in the submucosa, then penetrating the mucosa at topographically separate sites. (Courtesy of the Gordon Museum, Guy's Hospital Medical School)

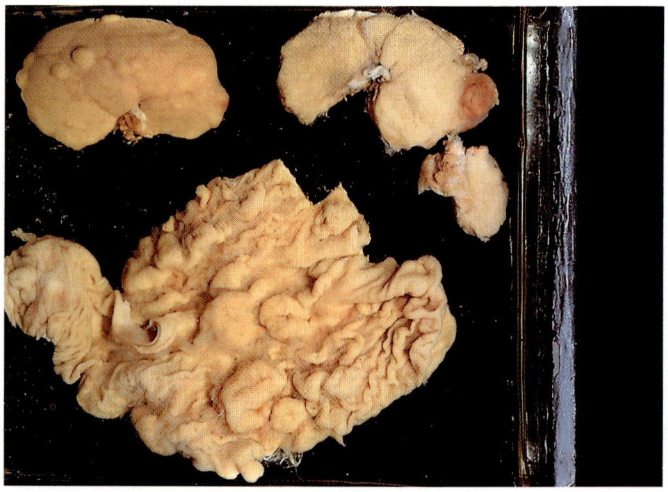

3.76 Acute Lymphoblastic Leukaemia

This is a post-mortem specimen from a 5-year-old girl, who presented with rapidly increasing swelling of the left faucial tonsil. This was soon followed by enlargement of the cervical lymph nodes and anaemia. She died 10 weeks after initial presentation.

The gastric mucosa (right) shows irregular nodular elevation and thickening, due to leukaemic involvement of submucosal and serosal lymphoid tissue. Also mounted are part of one of the tonsils (top left), a group of coeliac lymph nodes (middle left) and one of the kidneys (bottom left), all of which show leukaemic infiltration.

Extensive involvement of visceral tissues in acute leukaemia is much less common than in chronic leukaemia. (Courtesy of the Gordon Museum, Guy's Hospital Medical School)

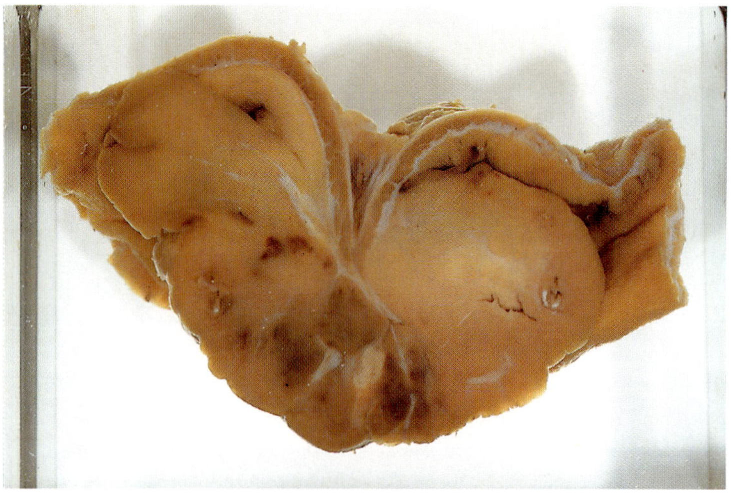

3.77 Solitary Plasmacytoma

This specimen was excised from a 45-year-old man who presented with dyspepsia, weight loss and melaena. Barium meal was suggestive of gastric carcinoma and a partial gastrectomy was performed.

A portion of the stomach has been opened to show a large, mushroom-shaped lobulated tumour projecting into the gastric lumen. The cut surface is pale brownish in colour with foci of haemorrhage and there is superficial ulceration. The underlying muscularis propria has been dragged into the base of the tumour and has been invaded by it.

Solitary plasmacytoma of the gastrointestinal tract is extremely uncommon but seems to occur predominantly in middle-aged males. There is no associated abnormality of plasma or urinary proteins and features of multiple myeloma are absent. Prognosis is dependent upon the presence of lymph node metastases.

SMALL AND LARGE INTESTINES

Small Intestine

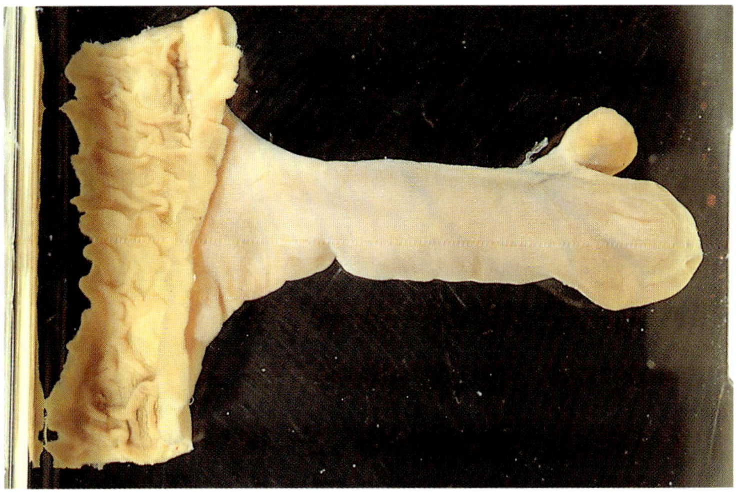

3.78 Ileum: Meckel's Diverticulum

This was an incidental finding at post-mortem in a soldier who died of bacillary dysentery.

Projecting from the free margin of this opened segment of ileum is a saccular diverticulum which measures 5cm in length. A small subsidiary pouch is visible (right) arising adjacent to the blind end of the main diverticulum.

Meckel's diverticulum is the commonest developmental malformation in the alimentary system and occurs in between 2-3 per cent of the population. It represents the proximal vestigial remnant of the vitello-intestinal duct and may, on occasion, remain connected to the umbilicus by either a fibrous vitelline cord or, more rarely, a patent fistulous tract (see Figure and Legend 3.84). The sex incidence is approximately equal and the diverticulum, measuring 2-5cm in length, is usually found on the antimesenteric border of the ileum between 60 and 100cm from the ileocaecal valve. The lumen of the diverticulum is usually narrower than that of the adjacent ileum but luminal continuity between the two is almost always maintained.

Up to 10 per cent of cases present clinically as a result of the complications that may develop within the diverticulum, many of which are represented in the Figures and Legends that follow. One possible complication not represented in this museum collection which should be mentioned is the occasional development of a tumour within such a diverticulum, the commonest being a leiomyoma or carcinoid tumour.

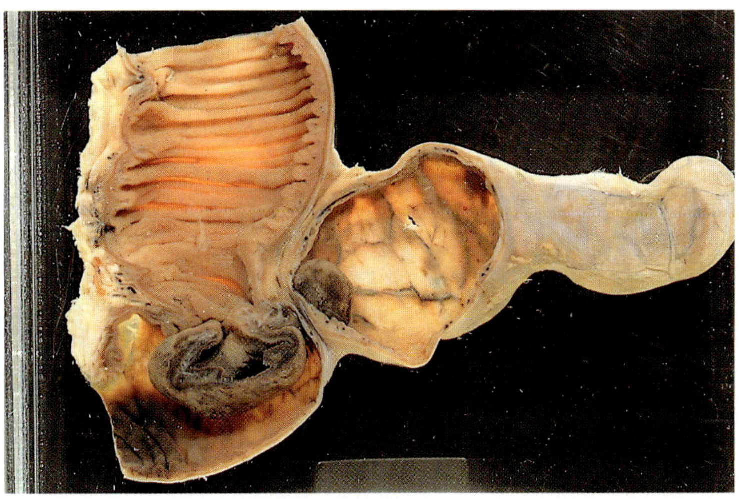

3.79 Ileum: Inflamed Meckel's Diverticulum

This specimen was excised from an 18-year-old youth who presented with a 5 day history of increasing abdominal pain, vomiting and abdominal distension. Laparotomy was performed.

The diverticulum, which measures 6cm in length, and neighbouring ileal mucosa are markedly inflamed; mucosal congestion and a purulent exudate are clearly evident. The opening of the diverticulum is very narrow and is further obstructed by a fragment of sloughed, necrotic mucosa.

Acute or chronic inflammation in a Meckel's diverticulum lined by normal small intestinal mucosa is quite common and probably results from impaction or stagnation of faecal material within the lumen with the development of superadded sepsis.

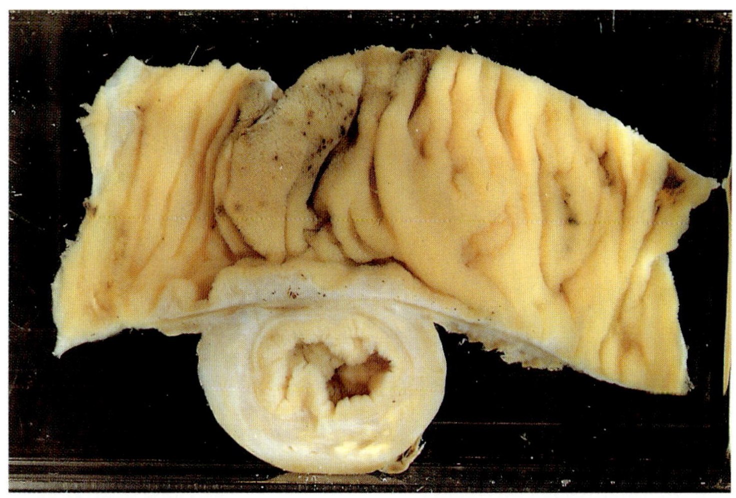

3.80 Ileum: Meckel's Diverticulum with Heterotopic Gastric Mucosa

This specimen was excised from a 3-year-old boy who presented with a 4 month history of intermittent abdominal pain associated with diarrhoea and melaena. A perforated Meckel's diverticulum was found at laparotomy.

The diverticulum, which measures 3cm in diameter, is lined by thick, rugose, gastric-type mucosa. The wall is oedematous but the site of perforation is not apparent in this view.

Epithelial heterotopia of various types, including gastric, colonic or duodenal, is quite common in Meckel's diverticula. Gastric heterotopia is the most frequent variety seen and may give rise to peptic ulceration (see below).

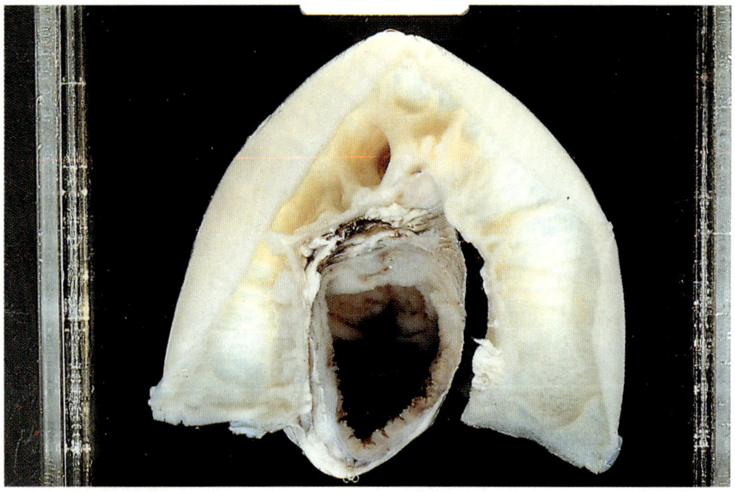

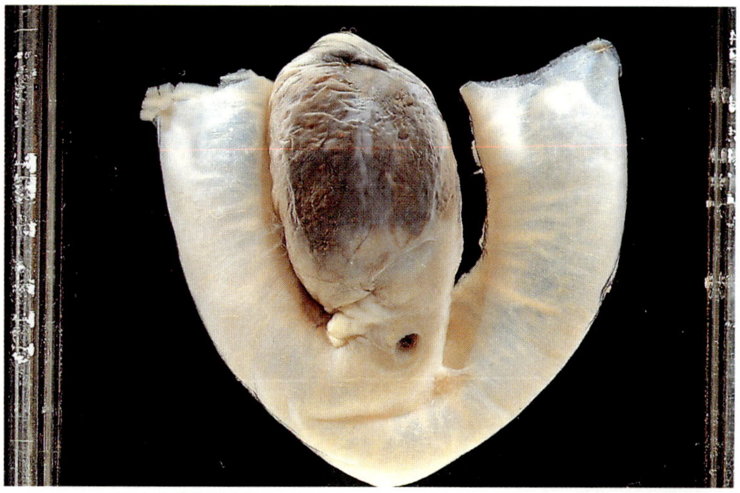

3.81 Ileum: Meckel's Diverticulum with Perforated Peptic Ulcer

This specimen was excised from a 16-year-old boy who had a long history of post-prandial indigestion. He presented acutely with severe lower abdominal pain.

The diverticulum (3.81a), measuring 5cm in length, is lined by thick haemorrhagic mucosa and, in the fresh state, the lumen was distended by blood clot. The opening of a small perforated ulcer in the neck of the sac is seen on the reverse of the specimen (3.81b).

The presence of heterotopic gastric epithelium, which is usually focal, within a Meckel's diverticulum may occasionally result in peptic ulceration of the adjacent unprotected small intestinal type mucosa. If the entire diverticulum is lined by gastric mucosa, the ulceration usually develops in the adjacent distal portion of ileum. The complications of peptic ulceration at this site are the same as in the stomach or duodenum (see Stomach section).

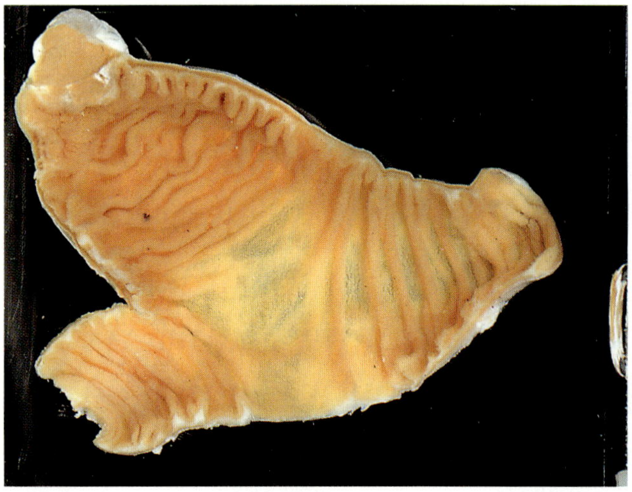

3.82 Ileum: Meckel's Diverticulum with Heterotopic Pancreatic Tissue

This specimen was excised from a 22-year-old man who had suffered repeated attacks of melaena over the previous 2 years. Exploratory laparotomy revealed a Meckel's diverticulum containing blood. Post-operatively he made an uninterrupted recovery.

At the apex of this wide-necked diverticulum, measuring 6cm in length, is a rounded nodule of solid, tan-coloured tissue. The adjacent mucosa, which is focally ulcerated, was shown histologically to be gastric in type.

Nodules of heterotopic pancreatic tissue are also common in the wall of Meckel's diverticula but rarely give rise to symptoms themselves. This patient's symptoms were attributable to peptic ulceration of the coexistent gastric epithelium.

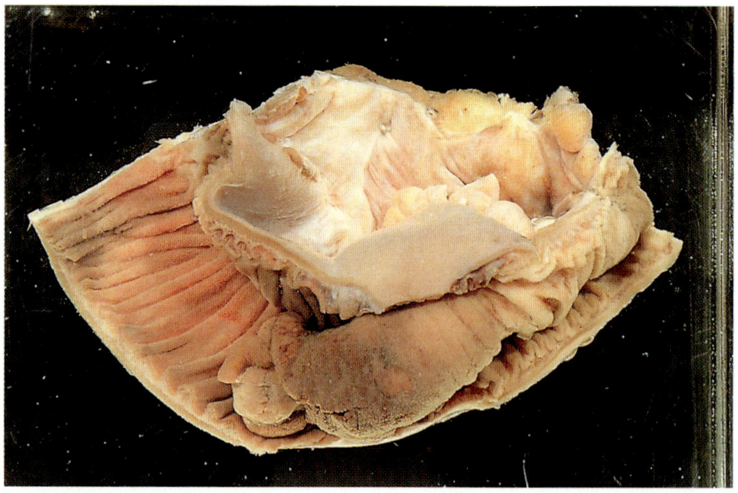

3.83 Ileum: Meckel's Diverticulum with Intussusception

This specimen was excised from a 37-year-old man who had suffered recurrent attacks of colicky abdominal pain for 6 months. Occult blood was detected in the faeces and exploratory laparotomy revealed a chronic ileal intussusception.

This segment of ileum has been opened anteriorly to show an invaginated Meckel's diverticulum, measuring 6 × 2 × 1.5cm, obstructing the bowel lumen. The distal portion of the intussuscepted diverticulum is intensely congested and oedematous.

While intussusception of a Meckel's diverticulum into the ileal lumen itself is a well-recognised complication, there is also an increased risk of ileo-ileal intussusception at the site of such a diverticulum.

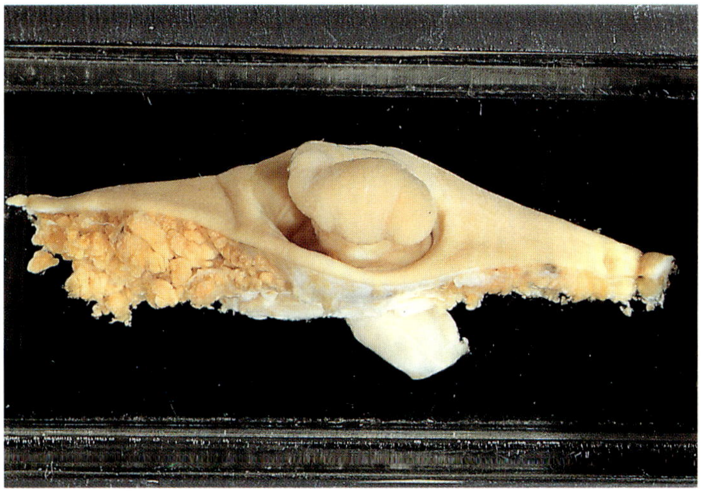

3.84 Umbilicus: Persistent Vitello-intestinal Duct

This specimen was excised from an 8-month-old infant, whose mother had noticed that the child had had a persistently discharging sinus at the umbilicus since birth.

The specimen consists of a peri-umbilical ellipse of skin and subcutaneous tissue. On the external surface, in the umbilical orifice, there is a rounded protrusion, measuring 1cm in diameter, which is covered by pale, velvety mucosa. A small opening at its base communicates with a thin-walled, duct-like structure (right) which, *in vivo*, communicated with the ileal lumen approximately 20cm proximal to the ileocaecal valve.

Complete persistence of the vitello-intestinal duct (also known as Meckel's fistula) is much less common than a simple Meckel's diverticulum (see Legend 3.78). Foci of ectopic gastric epithelium or pancreatic tissue may be found anywhere along the length of the duct, as in the more usual diverticulum (see Legend 3.80 et seq.).

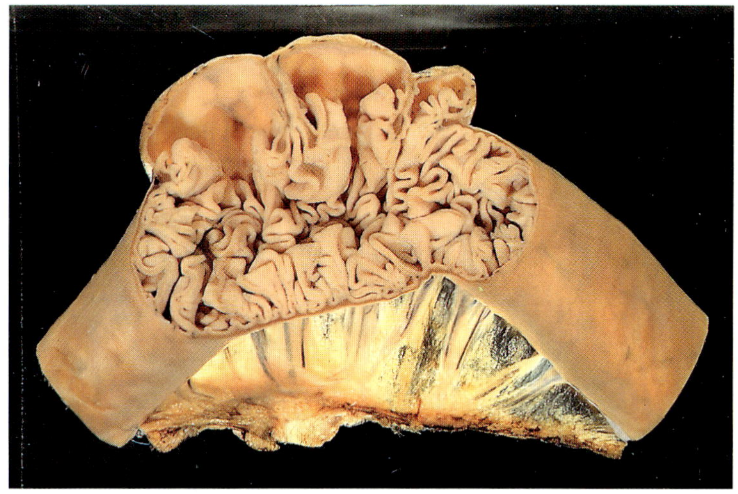

3.85 Jejunum: Congenital Diverticulum

This specimen was excised from a 41-year-old woman, who presented with a long history of intermittent left-sided abdominal pain associated with occasional vomiting and constipation. At laparotomy, a diverticulum was identified approximately 4cm distal to the duodeno-jejunal flexure. Excision led to complete relief from her symptoms.

The excised loop of jejunum has been opened to show a trilocular, smooth-walled diverticulum projecting from the anti-mesenteric border.

Diverticula, other than Meckel's, are relatively uncommon in the small bowel, particularly if compared to the occurrence of such lesions in the large bowel. The majority are acquired, due to a failure of peristaltic muscular coordination, and may be a cause of malabsorption. Congenital small intestinal diverticula are most often ileal in origin. Those arising in the duodenum or jejunum are sometimes associated with vertebral anomalies and, like enterogenous cysts, they may represent partial persistence of the neuro-enteric canal.

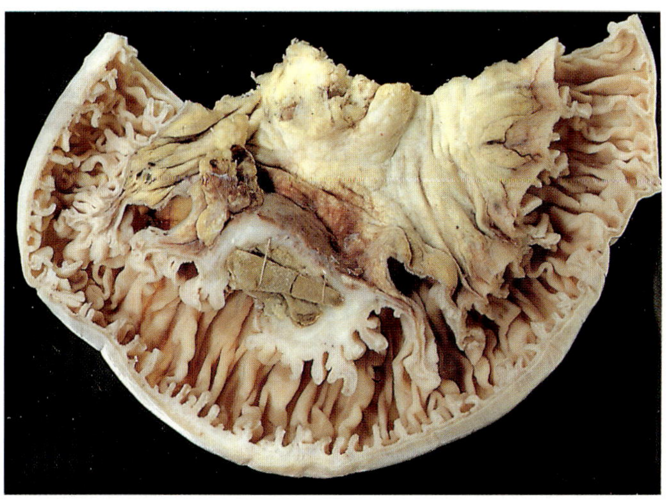

3.86 Jejunum: Diverticulitis

This specimen was excised from a 49-year-old man who presented with acute abdominal pain and melaena. Laparotomy was performed.

Multiple diverticula are evident in this loop of small bowel, one of which is particularly large and has a fibrotic thickened wall. Contained within its lumen is a bile-stained fragment of bone (presumably ingested at some time in the past) which has ulcerated through the diverticular wall, giving rise to a florid peritonitis.

It is comparatively unusual for small bowel diverticula to present as a consequence of inflammation, in contrast to those in the large bowel.

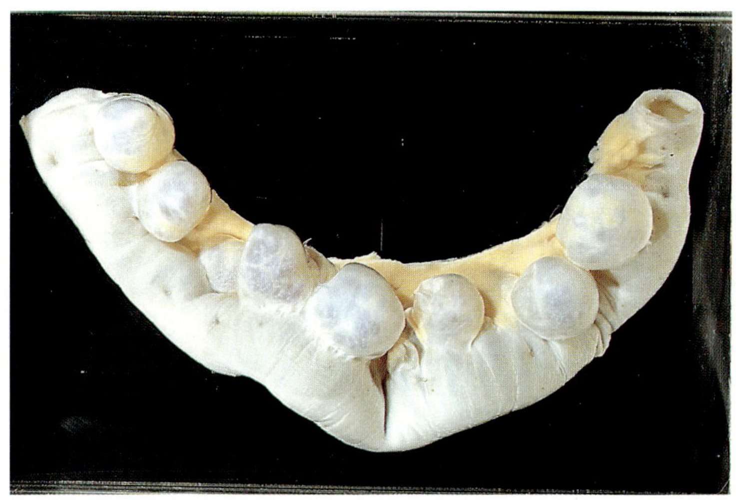

3.87 Ileum: Diverticular Disease

This was an incidental post-mortem finding in a 66-year-old man who died of congestive heart failure.

This segment of ileum shows a chain of thin-walled diverticula projecting from the mesenteric border. There is no evidence of inflammatory change.

These are probably acquired diverticula, induced by incoordinate peristalsis. Such diverticula may be distinguished from the congenital variant by the lack of a circular muscle coat in the former, while the latter usually has a full thickness bowel wall.

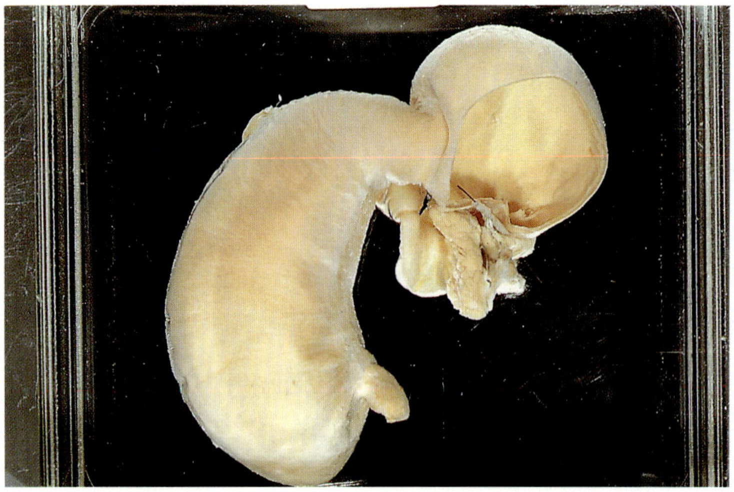

3.88 Duodenum: Congenital Atresia

This is a post-mortem specimen from a neonate. No other clinical information is available.

The specimen consists of the stomach and duodenum of an infant. The duodenum is grossly dilated and shows complete blind-ended occlusion, proximal to the insertion of the common bile duct.

Small intestinal atresia or stenosis is seen in approximately 1 in 5000 live-born infants, atresia being distinctly more common than stenosis. The commonest sites affected are the ileum and duodenum and known clinical associations include Down's syndrome and the presence of a single umbilical artery. Mothers of affected fetuses may commonly develop hydramnios in the last trimester of pregnancy. Atresia may take one of three forms, comprising either an imperforate septum between the two portions of bowel, connection of the two by a vestigial fibrous cord, or complete separation, as shown here.

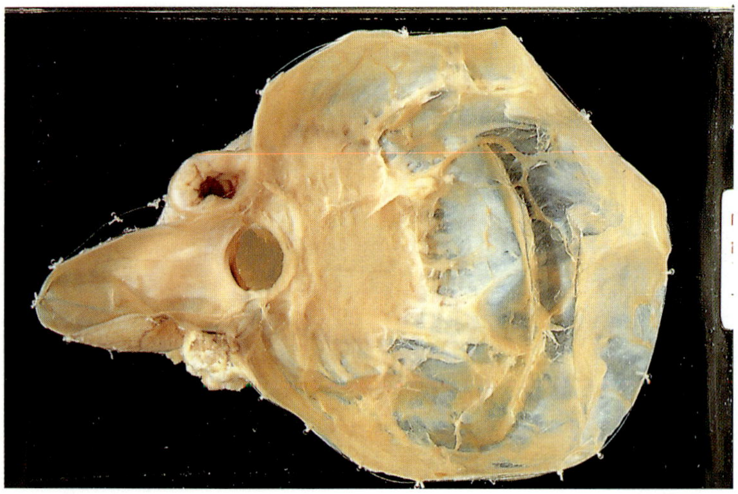

3.89 Jejunum: Enterogenous Cyst

This specimen was excised from a 5-year-old girl who presented with abdominal pain and dysuria. A mass was palpable in the lower abdomen which, at laparotomy, proved to be a large cyst in the region of the jejunum and its mesentery.

This is a large bilocular cystic structure with the jejunum (now cut in cross-section) passing through the centre. The portion of the cyst above the jejunal lumen is much smaller than the lower moiety. The cyst is thin-walled, translucent and embedded in mesenteric fat.

Enterogenous cysts are comparatively rare congenital malformations which may arise within any of the layers of the bowel wall or within its mesentery. There is rarely any communication with the true bowel lumen but these cysts are characteristically lined by mature intestinal epithelium. They may represent some form of persistence of the neuro-enteric canal and are occasionally seen in the mediastinum or adjacent to the vertebral column.

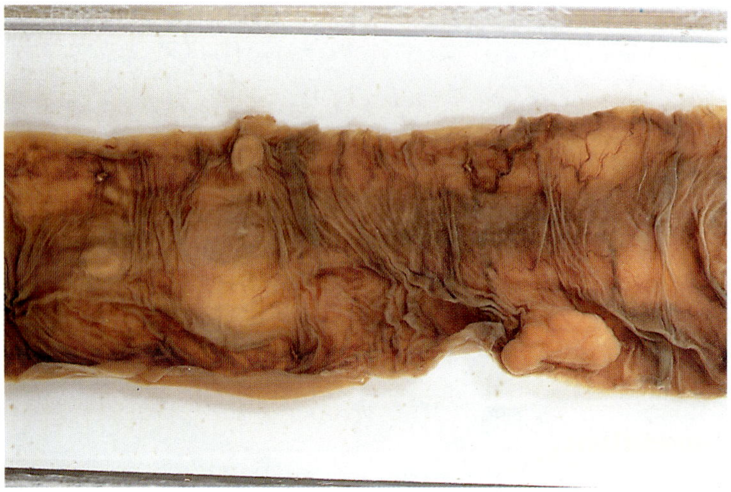

3.90 Jejunum: Lymphatic Cysts

These lesions were an incidental finding at post-mortem in a 72-year-old man who died of a massive pulmonary embolism.

A length of rather congested jejunum has been opened to show 3 yellowish nodules, the largest (bottom right) measuring 1cm in diameter. Other similar lesions, when sectioned, were composed of cystic spaces filled with yellowish material.

Lymphatic cysts of the small intestine are fairly uncommon developmental malformations which are typically multiple. They are of no clinical significance.

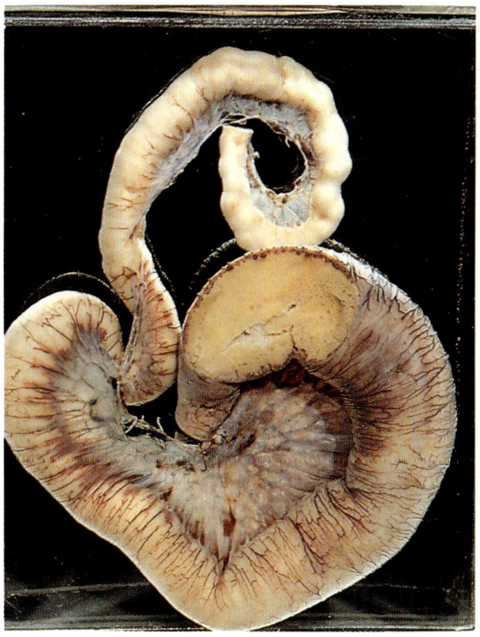

3.91 Ileum: Meconium Ileus

No clinical details are available.

The proximal portion of this loop of ileum is grossly distended and the lumen is completely obstructed by inspissated meconium. Prolonged fixation and preservation of the specimen has altered the colour of the meconium from greenish-black to yellow.

Meconium ileus is a condition of neonates in whom it is one of the most common causes of intestinal obstruction. It is typically seen in infants with cystic fibrosis (mucoviscidosis), of whom up to 10 per cent will suffer this complication. It results from the adherence of unusually viscid or tenacious meconium to the bowel wall, followed by obstruction and sometimes perforation. Occasional sporadic idiopathic cases, unassociated with cystic fibrosis, are seen which are rarely followed by any other problems.

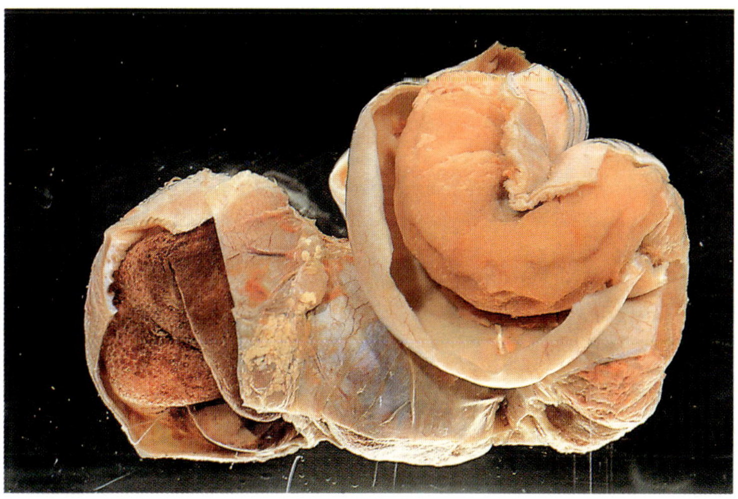

3.92 Ileocaecal Intussusception

This specimen was excised from a 4-month-old male infant who presented with a 2 day history of vomiting. He was pyrexial and had passed a large quantity of bright red material per rectum. A mass was palpable in the right iliac fossa and, at laparotomy, the intussusception was found to be irreducible and was therefore resected.

The distal ileum (right) and the proximal caecum (left) have been opened to show an extensive intussusception of the more proximal ileum. The apex of the intussusceptum has passed through the ileocaecal valve (which remains unopened) and is extremely congested. The intussuscipiens is markedly dilated.

Intussusception is defined as invagination of a portion of bowel into the lumen of the adjacent bowel, usually being proximal into distal. This condition is most often seen in childhood (particularly in the first year of life), shows a predilection for males, and is most commonly ileocaecal or ileo-ileal. The incidence is approximately 2 cases per 1000 live births. Pathogenetically, swelling of Peyer's patches, possibly as a result of viral infection, is thought by many to provide the necessary mucosal protrusion that predisposes to intussusception. Very few cases are seen in adulthood and such examples usually show a causative mural or mucosal lesion (see Figure and Legend 3.94).

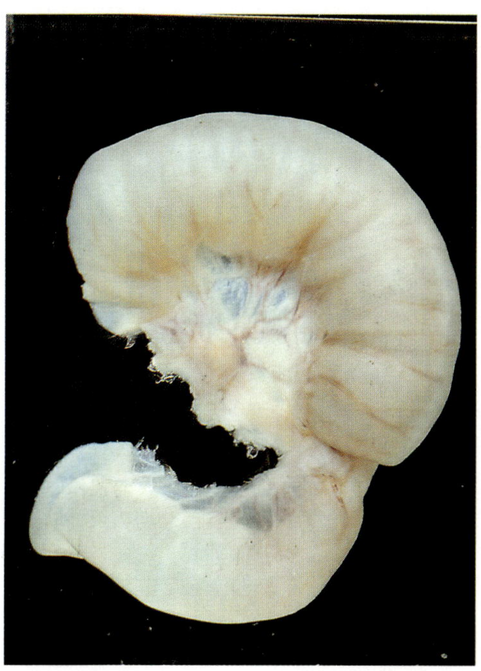

3.93 Ileum: Agonal Intussusception

This was an incidental finding at post-mortem in an infant who died of bronchopneumonia.

The specimen consists of a short segment of ileum, the distal portion being on the left. There is a short retrograde intussusception, which shows no associated oedema or inflammation.

Intussusception, as an agonal event in small infants, is comparatively common and of no significance. It is thought to occur near the actual time of death as a result of abnormal peristalsis and therefore no vital reaction is to be expected.

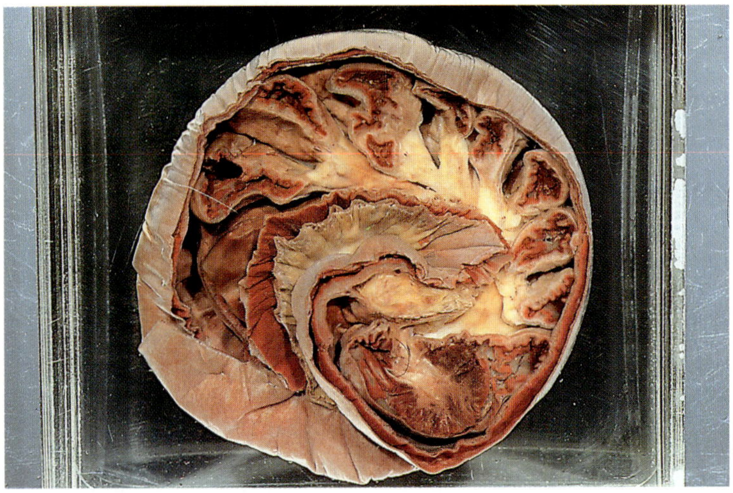

3.94 Jejunum: Intussusception with an Adenomatous Polyp

This specimen was excised from a 19-year-old man who presented with acute epigastric pain and vomiting. Clinically there were signs of peritonitis and a sausage-shaped mass was palpable just below the umbilicus. At laparotomy an irreducible jejuno-jejunal intussusception was found and resected.

A loop of dilated, markedly congested jejunum is shown into which a proximal segment has intussuscepted. The intussusceptum is completely infarcted and at its apex (bottom right) there is a large, solid polypoid tumour.

As already mentioned (Legend 3.92), intussusception in adulthood is almost always associated with an obstructive mechanical cause such as a foreign body or a polypoid tumour (as in this case). Very occasionally, colo-colic intussusception may be seen in adults at the site of an exophytic large bowel adenocarcinoma (see Figure 3.156).

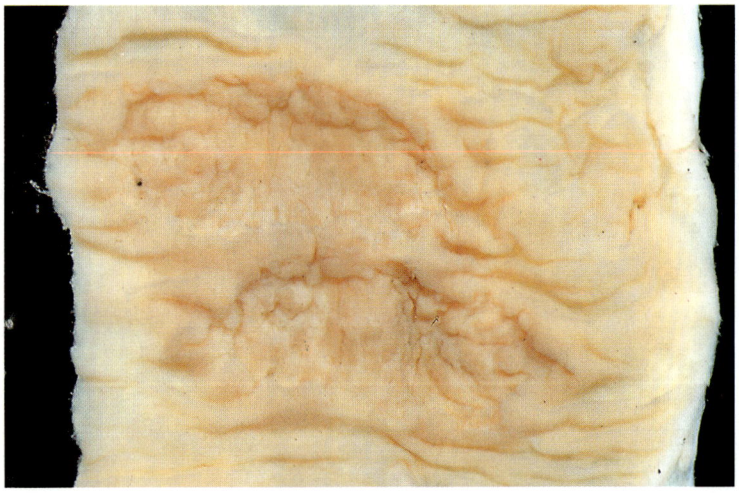

3.95 Small Intestine: Tuberculosis

No clinical details are available.

A close-up view of this small intestinal mucosa reveals characteristic irregular ulcers, with undermined edges, which are orientated in the *transverse* axis of the bowel wall (i.e. perpendicular to the direction of the lumen).

Small intestinal tuberculosis, now fairly uncommon in the Western world, may take either of two forms. It may be due to primary infection by *Mycobacterium bovis*, which is classically ingested in unpasteurised cow's milk, this type being characterised by inflammatory changes predominantly in the mesenteric nodes. Alternatively, secondary infection may occur, which results from the swallowing of sputum infected with *Mycobacterium tuberculosis* in patients already suffering from pulmonary disease. It is the secondary form which is most often responsible for the ulcerative enteritis which ensues. While the inflammatory changes may commence in Peyer's patches, circumferential spread in the lymphatics of the bowel wall soon occurs and it is this mode of spread which accounts for the transverse orientation of the ulcers (cf. typhoid). Recognised complications include perforation, fibrosis with stricture formation and secondary malabsorption.

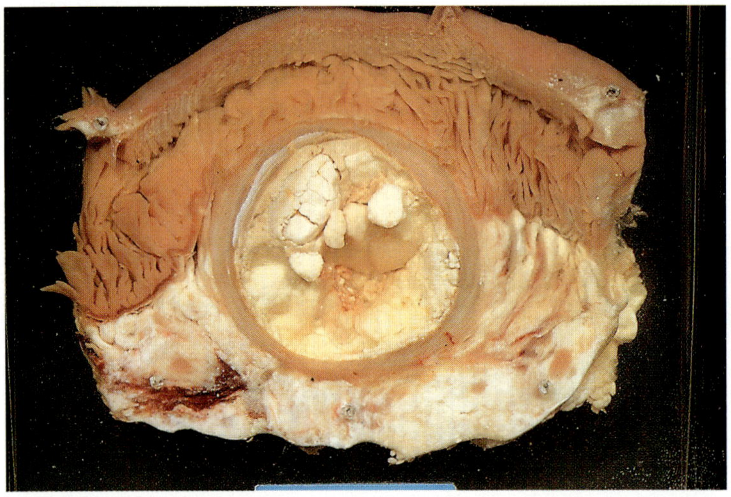

3.96 Mesenteric Lymph Node: 'Burnt Out' Tuberculosis

This specimen was excised from a 50-year-old woman who complained of intermittent abdominal pain. A tender mass was palpable below the umbilicus and, at laparotomy, an inflammatory mass centred upon a tuberculous node was found which had caused adhesions between the ileum and sigmoid colon.

A loop of ileum is seen stretched over a rounded nodule, measuring 4cm in diameter, in the mesentery. The nodule is composed of thick, yellowish caseous material, foci of dystrophic calcification and a dense fibrous pseudocapsule. No recognisable lymphoid tissue remained histologically, and there was no evidence of active tuberculosis.

This is the typical appearance of obsolescent primary intestinal tuberculosis with no evidence of bowel damage and solely the features of healed infection in a lymph node. Nodes such as this are (or were at one time) a common source of distracting, calcific opacities on plain abdominal X-rays.

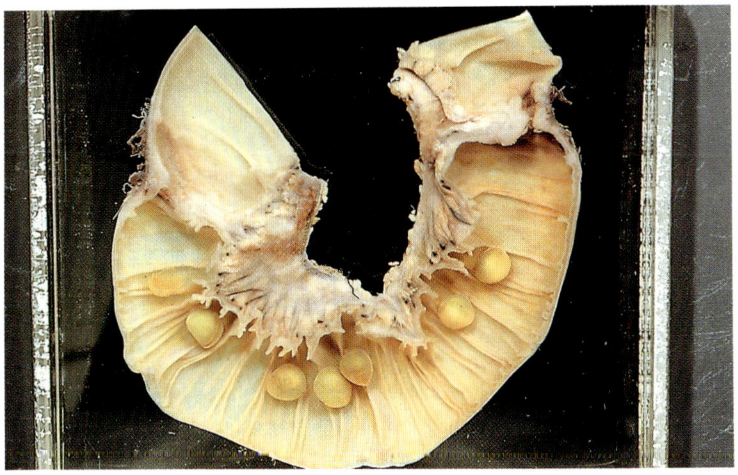

3.97 Ileum: Tuberculous Stricture

This specimen was excised from a 30-year-old woman who presented with a 9 month history of colicky lower abdominal pain associated with intermittent vomiting and abdominal distension. At laparotomy two ileal strictures just proximal to the ileocaecal valve were revealed.

This loop of ileum has been opened to show two tight fibrous strictures, just proximal to each of the resection margins. At the site of each stricture there are friable tags of fibrinous exudate on the serosal surface.

Healing of intestinal tuberculous ulcers, usually secondary in nature (see Legend 3.95), is often succeeded by dense reparative fibrosis with consequent luminal narrowing leading to symptoms of intestinal obstruction.

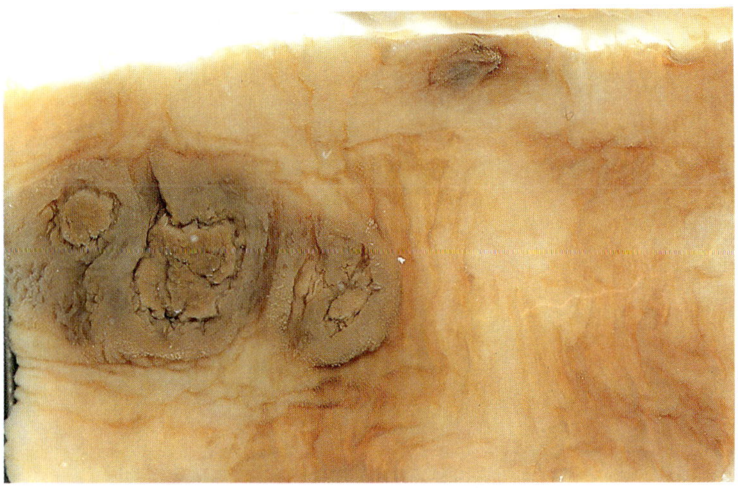

3.98 Ileum: Typhoid Fever

This is a post-mortem specimen from a young soldier who died following removal of a perforated appendix during an attack of typhoid fever. Pure cultures of *Salmonella typhi* were isolated from the appendix, gall bladder and spleen.

A close-up view of the ileal mucosa shows intense focal congestion, oedema and ulceration, which is orientated in the *longitudinal* axis (parallel to the bowel wall) and corresponds to one of Peyer's patches.

Typhoid (or enteric) fever is now fairly rare in the Western world but remains endemic in parts of Asia and Africa. It results from ingestion of the Gram-negative bacillus *Salmonella typhi* in contaminated food or drink. The typhoid bacilli penetrate the small intestinal mucosa, are taken up in the lymphoid tissue of the Peyer's patches and then enter the bloodstream where they multiply. This produces a septicaemic illness, characterised by pyrexia and mental confusion, and is followed (usually 1-2 weeks later) by the typical gastrointestinal symptoms when the organisms are re-excreted into the bowel through the biliary system. It is at this stage that the characteristic longitudinal ulceration of Peyer's patches occurs. Well-recognised complications of this ulceration include profuse bleeding and perforation. Systemic manifestations include splenomegaly, hepatic necrosis or Zenker's degeneration of the abdominal wall musculature (see Chapter 9).

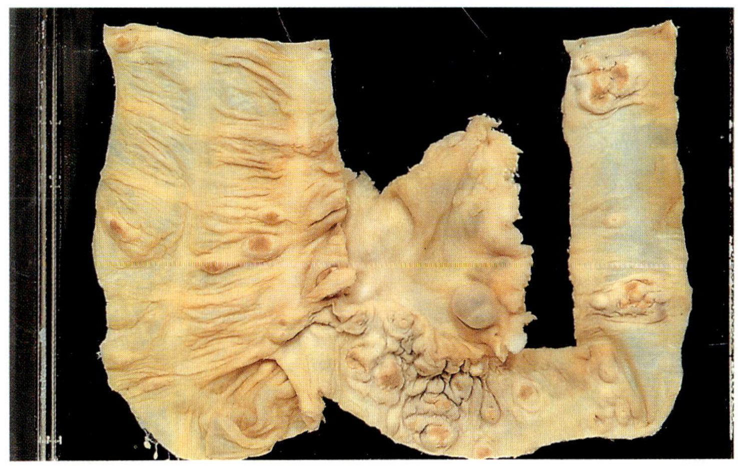

3.99 Ileocaecal Junction: Typhoid Fever

This is a post-mortem specimen from a 34-year-old soldier, posted in Egypt, who presented with a 6 week history of headache, pyrexia and, later, diarrhoea. Blood cultures were positive for *Salmonella typhi* and there was splenomegaly. Delirium rapidly developed and the patient died.

The terminal ileum and caecum have been opened to show pronounced swelling and ulceration of both Peyer's patches and smaller lymphoid follicles in the large bowel. The typical longitudinal orientation of the lesions is not so apparent here. Note also the enlarged, congested mesenteric lymph nodes.

This case demonstrates that involvement of large bowel lymphoid tissue also occurs in a small proportion of cases.

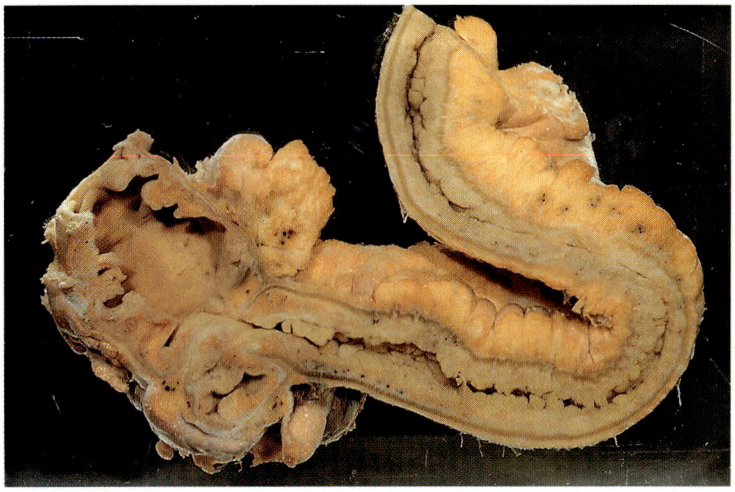

3.100 Ileum: Crohn's Disease

No clinical details are available.

The terminal ileum, measuring 20cm in length, and the proximal caecum are shown. The walls of the ileum are greatly thickened and fibrotic with consequent diffuse luminal narrowing, giving rise to the classical 'hose-pipe' appearance. Just proximal to the ileocaecal valve, irregular mucosal ulceration is visible.

Crohn's disease is a chronic granulomatous inflammatory condition which may affect *any* part of the alimentary tract and typically develops in young adults of either sex. The terminal ileum seems to be predominantly affected. The aetiology is unknown but the disease is thought to represent some form of hypersensitivity reaction to an environmental antigen. Some cases show an undoubted genetic predisposition.

Macroscopically the condition is characterised by discontinuous zones of inflammation in the bowel, known as 'skip' lesions (cf. ulcerative colitis), which may be manifest as mucosal ulceration, a 'cobblestone' appearance (due to mucosal fissuring with adjacent oedema) or by stricture formation of variable length and number. Since the inflammatory process involves the full thickness of the bowel wall (cf. ulcerative colitis), fibrous thickening extending to the serosal surface is typical. Serosal involvement in turn predisposes to the development of adhesions, both between loops of bowel and between the bowel and other intra-abdominal organs. Recognised clinical associations include ankylosing spondylitis, iritis, sclerosing cholangitis and skin lesions such as pyoderma gangrenosum and erythema nodosum. Local complications attributable to the disease process include malabsorption, intestinal perforation, the formation of fistulae, anal fissures and, rarely, the later development of intestinal adenocarcinoma.

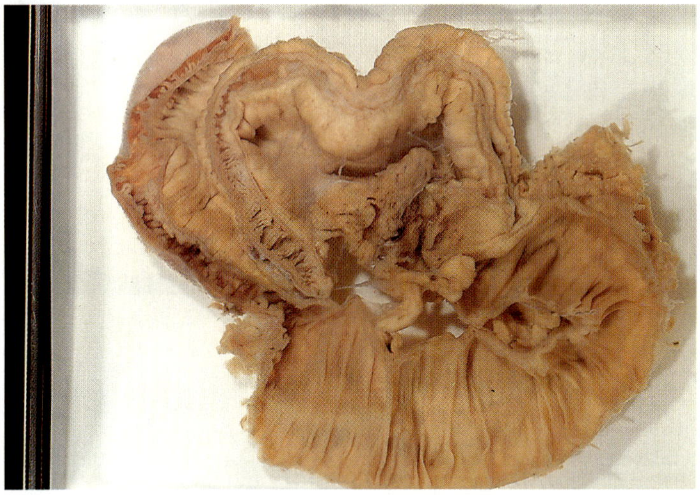

3.101 Ileum: Crohn's Disease

This specimen was excised from a 58-year-old man who had first presented 3 years earlier with intermittent intestinal obstruction. Crohn's disease was diagnosed and an ileo-colostomy performed to isolate the affected segment. However, 2 years post-operatively, chronic intestinal obstruction developed so the ascending colon and terminal ileum were resected.

The distal ileum, caecum and ascending colon are shown. The terminal 30cm of the ileum have been isolated and the proximal portion anastomosed to the side of the colon. The walls of the isolated loop are markedly thickened and fibrotic and the lumen is reduced to a narrow slit. The proximal portion of ileum show less advanced disease, the walls being congested and oedematous and the mucosa superficially ulcerated.

This case demonstrates well that any form of surgical intervention in Crohn's disease is commonly followed by the development of new lesions in previously uninvolved bowel. As a consequence, repeated intestinal operations may become necessary, carrying with them the attendant risk of ever-increasing adhesions, fistula formation and malabsorption (due to simple loss of surface area).

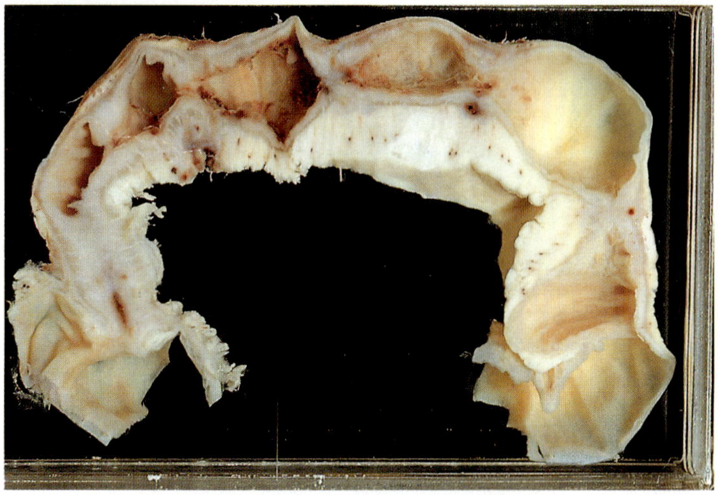

3.102 Ileum: Crohn's Disease

This specimen was excised from a 32-year-old woman with a 2 year history of intermittent diarrhoea and fever. A tender mass was palpable in the right iliac fossa and a laparotomy was performed.

The distal ileum and a tiny portion of caecum are shown. The bowel wall is irregularly thickened and fibrotic, particularly at the ileocaecal valve where the lumen is almost obliterated. Proximally there are 5 separate tight stenoses, between which the short segments of bowel are markedly dilated and the mucosa attenuated.

This case clearly demonstrates the typical patchy distribution of Crohn's disease. Subacute intestinal obstruction due to stricture formation is one of the more common ways in which this disease may present.

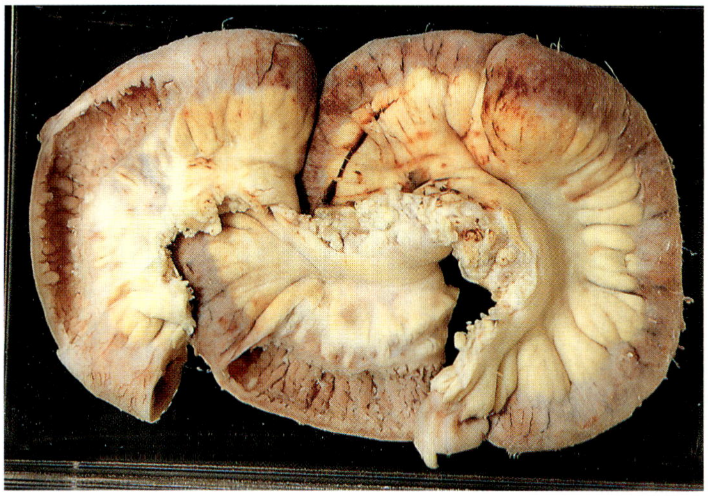

3.103 Ileum: Crohn's Disease

This specimen was excised from a 28-year-old man who, after a 3 month history of ill-defined 'indigestion', presented acutely with right iliac fossa pain and diarrhoea. A laparotomy was performed.

This portion of terminal ileum shows intense mucosal and serosal congestion, associated with moderate thickening of the bowel wall. Patchy mucosal ulceration is also evident. Note also the mesenteric oedema and enlarged lymph nodes.

This case probably represents an example of acute diffuse Crohn's ileitis, an early stage of the disease. This appearance, having no features of chronicity, is rarely seen as most such cases are now managed medically.

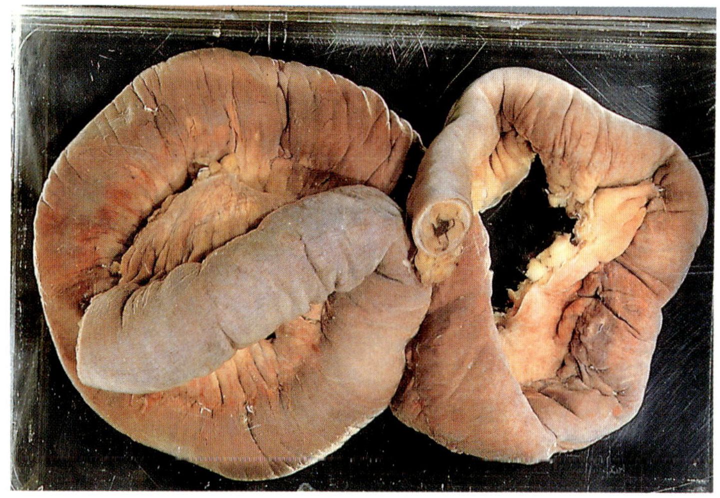

3.104 Small Intestine: Mesenteric Venous Thrombosis

This specimen was excised from a 52-year-old man, who complained of increasingly severe acute epigastric pain. He developed signs of peritonitis and, at laparotomy, almost 1m of the proximal small intestine was found to be intensely congested and swollen. The arterial supply was demonstrably intact and excision of the affected loops with end-to-end anastomosis was performed.

This length of small intestine is deeply congested and oedematous. The serosal surface appears roughened and lustreless. Numerous thrombosed veins were identified in the mesentery (not apparent in this view).

Mesenteric venous thrombosis is much less frequently responsible for small intestinal ischaemia than is arterial occlusion. Well-recognised causes include external compression of the superior mesenteric vein (e.g. by tumour), retrograde spread of thrombus in the portal vein (see Hepatobiliary System section), the presence of intra-abdominal sepsis with portal pyaemia and any cause of hypercoagulability. Haemorrhagic infarction of the affected bowel results and may be complicated by the secondary development of bacterial necrotising enteritis.

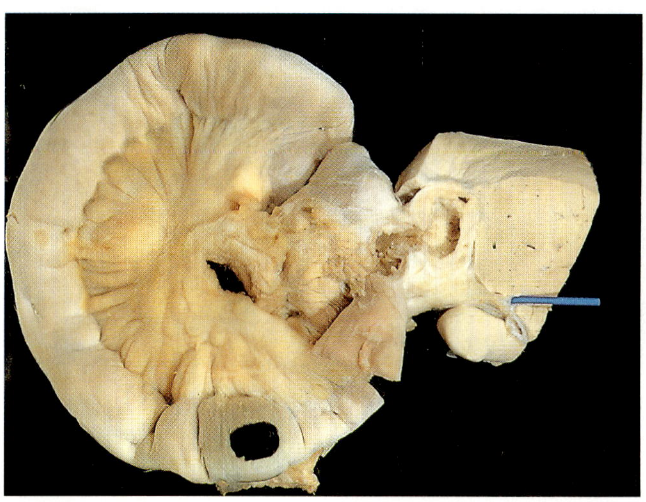

3.105 Jejunum: Obstruction by Gall Stone

This is a post-mortem specimen from a 77-year-old woman who had presented acutely with symptoms of upper intestinal obstruction. At laparotomy she was found to have a gall stone impacted in the jejunum, associated with dense adhesions between the gall bladder and the duodenum. A second larger stone was palpable in the gall bladder. Following removal of the jejunal stone it was decided to delay cholecystectomy until the patient had recovered from this acute episode. However, she was readmitted as an emergency 5 weeks later with signs of acute peritonitis and shock, and died 8 hours later.

A portion of the liver with the gall bladder, duodenum and jejunum are shown. The gall bladder, which has been opened, is markedly shrunken, has a thick fibrotic wall and is firmly adherent to the duodenum, into which it opens through a wide fistula. The duodenum and proximal jejunum are dilated and 30cm along the jejunum an opening has been made to show the lumen completely obstructed by a large pigmented gall stone, measuring 4.5cm in diameter. The jejunum had perforated through the fold just proximal to the stone.

Obstruction of the small bowel by a gall stone is a relatively uncommon complication of cholelithiasis (see Hepatobiliary System section) but is most often seen in elderly females and usually follows long-standing, low-grade cholecystitis associated with ulceration of a stone into the adherent duodenum. Obstruction usually occurs in the terminal ileum, but when the stone exceeds 2-3cm in diameter, it may become impacted more proximally (as here). Very occasionally, stones may also ulcerate into the ascending or transverse colon but this is less likely to give rise to intestinal obstruction.

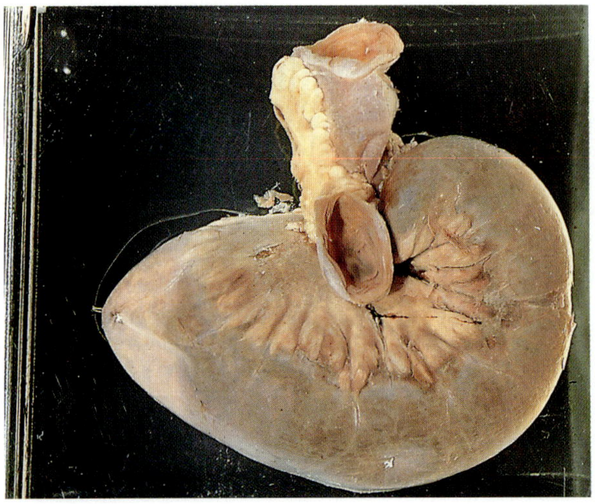

3.106 Ileum: Volvulus

No clinical details are available.

The central portion of this loop of small bowel, measuring 30cm in length, has rotated upon itself, causing gross dilatation and strangulation. The serosal surface is intensely congested.

Volvulus of the small bowel is comparatively rare but may occur in two distinct circumstances; in the neonate it may complicate a failure of rotation in which the caecum remains on the left side; in the adult it is most often due to the presence of adhesions.

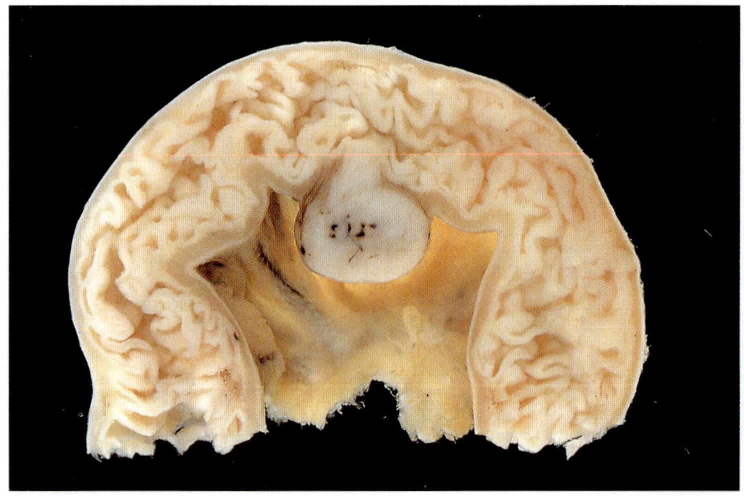

3.107 Ileum: Leiomyoma

This was an incidental finding at post-mortem in an adult male who died of a coronary thrombosis.

A pale tumour, arising from the muscle coat, and showing some central degeneration projects from the mesenteric border of this loop of ileum. Only a small intraluminal moiety, covered by normal mucosa is present.

Small intestinal leiomyomas, which arise from the muscle coat of the bowel wall, are not uncommon lesions of adulthood. The extent to which they project intraluminally or extramurally varies from case to case and many remain asymptomatic. Since, on histological grounds, it can be extremely difficult to distinguish between benign and malignant intestinal smooth muscle tumours, careful follow-up is mandatory as approximately 30 per cent of cases eventually metastasise.

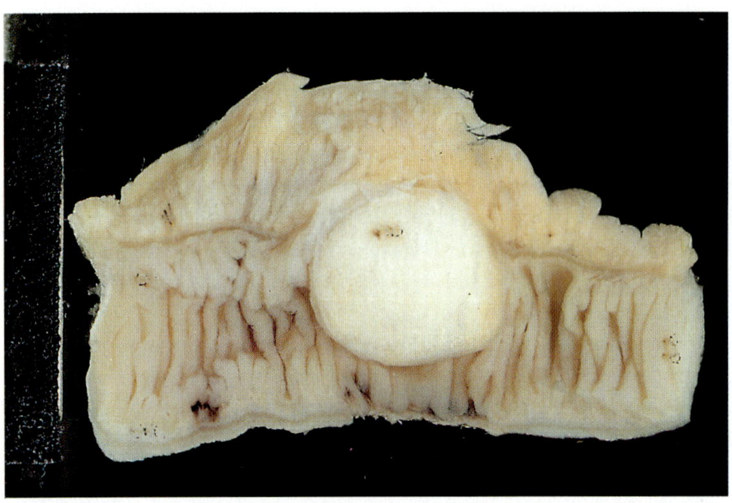

3.108 Ileum: Submucosal Lipoma

This was a coincidental finding at post-mortem. No further clinical details are available.

This segment of small bowel has been opened to show a discrete, rounded, pale, fatty tumour projecting into the lumen. The surface is covered by an attenuated layer of normal mucosa.

Lipomas of the small bowel are uncommon benign lesions, which are usually submucosal in origin. While they are most often asymptomatic, large pedunculated lesions may give rise to obstruction or intussusception.

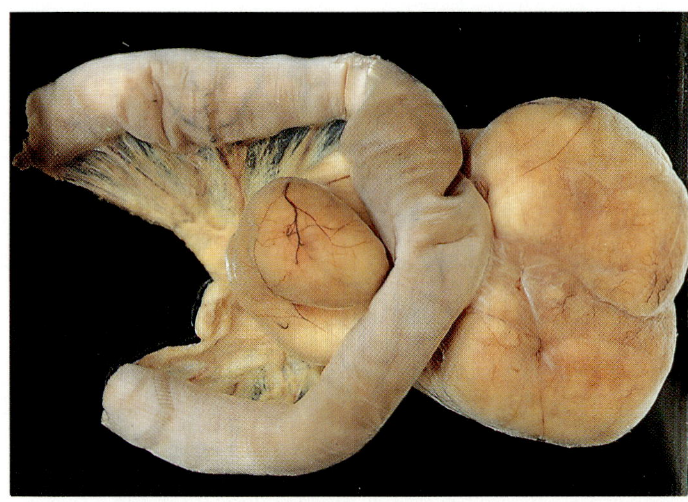

3.109 Ileum: Subserosal Lipoma

This was an incidental finding at post-mortem in a 76-year-old woman who died from a chronic subdural haematoma.

Projecting in a dumb-bell fashion from the serosal surface of this loop of ileum is a large, well-circumscribed fatty tumour, measuring 8cm in maximum diameter.

Subserosal lipomas are less common than their submucosal counterparts but are less likely to give rise to complications.

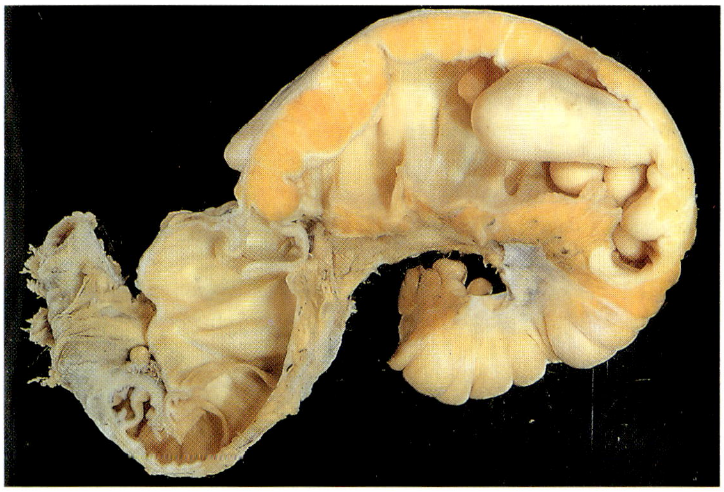

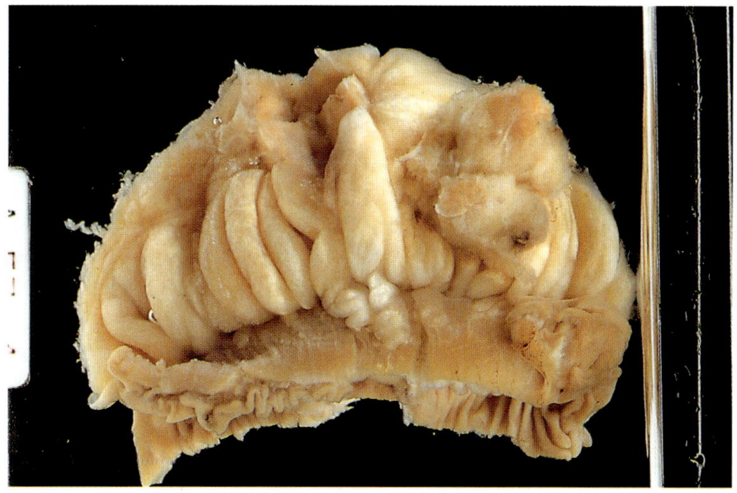

3.110 Ileum: Lipomatosis

This specimen was excised from a 48-year-old obese woman who had complained of abdominal discomfort and a variable bowel habit for many years. A soft indefinite mass was palpable in the right iliac fossa. Laparotomy was performed.

The specimen consists of terminal ileum and a portion of caecum (left). The ileal lumen is markedly dilated and the wall is diffusely infiltrated with fat as far as the ileocaecal valve. In addition there are several submucosal lipomata, measuring up to 6cm in diameter, projecting into the lumen.

Lipomatosis in the region of the ileocaecal valve is extremely rare but a nevertheless well-recognised entity. Whether it represents a hyperplastic or hamartomatous process is uncertain.

3.111 Ileum: Carcinoid Tumour

No clinical details are available.

This segment of small bowel (right) has been opened longitudinally to reveal a small, stenosing neoplasm, the cut surface of which is yellow in colour. In the mesenteric fat, there are several enlarged lymph nodes (left) which are replaced by similar tumour.

Carcinoid tumours (synonym: argentaffinomas) of the small intestine are about half as common as those of the appendix (see Figure and Legend 3.130). They arise most often in the distal ileum, show a predilection for males and typically present between the ages of 50 and 70. While the clinical course may be very indolent, the majority of these neoplasms eventually metastasise to lymph nodes or the liver; as a consequence, some authorities feel that all small intestinal carcinoid tumours should be regarded as malignant (cf. those of the appendix). These lesions secrete 5-hydroxytryptamine, which is normally metabolised in the liver and therefore has no systemic effects. However, the development of liver or other systemic metastases circumvents this metabolic process and the carcinoid syndrome may then ensue.

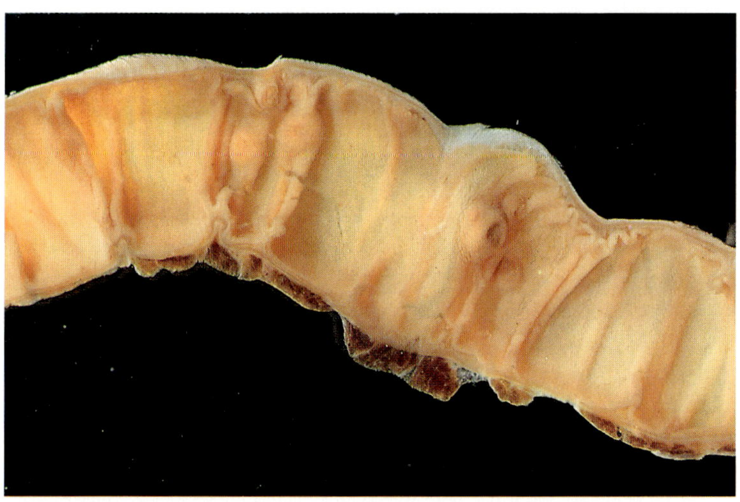

3.112 Ileum: Multiple Carcinoid Tumours

This specimen was excised from a 35-year-old woman who presented with central abdominal pain associated with anorexia and an altered bowel habit. At laparotomy numerous small nodules were found extending over a 1m length of the ileum.

A segment of the affected ileum has been opened longitudinally to show multiple, small, yellowish mucosal tumours, one of which shows superficial ulceration.

Multiplicity of gastrointestinal carcinoid tumours is not uncommon and may occasionally be associated with the development of a heterotopic intestinal adenocarcinoma. This appearance should not be mistaken for intraluminal metastases which are very rare.

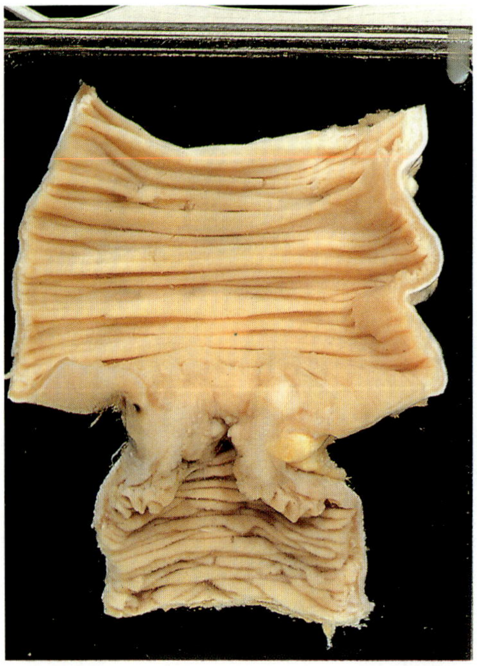

3.113 Jejunum: Adenocarcinoma

This specimen was excised from a 75-year-old woman who presented with a 6 week history of profuse vomiting. A barium meal was unhelpful and laparotomy was performed.

A segment of jejunum has been opened to show an annular, stenosing tumour, which extends over a length of 1.5cm and has infiltrated the full thickness of the bowel wall. Proximal to the obstruction, the intestine is markedly dilated and shows muscular hypertrophy.

Primary small intestinal carcinoma is very uncommon but most often arises in the proximal jejunum, duodenum or terminal ileum. Patients of either sex in the 5th and 6th decades are typically affected and there is a significant association with pre-existent Crohn's disease or coeliac disease (gluten enteropathy). The macroscopical appearances and pattern of metastasis are much the same as those seen in the more common large intestinal carcinomas (see Figure and Legend 3.164 et seq.).

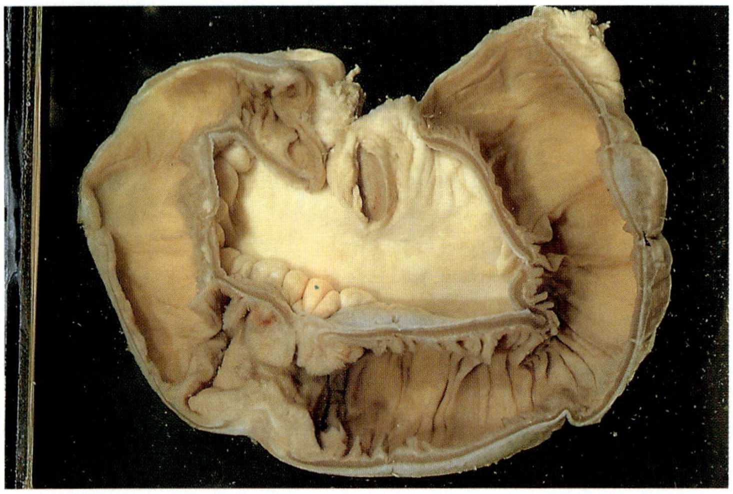

3.114 Ileum: Adenocarcinoma

This specimen was excised from a 54-year-old man who presented acutely with colicky abdominal pain. A tumour was palpable below the umbilicus and laparotomy was performed.

This loop of ileum has been opened to show an annular, stenosing tumour extending over a length of 3cm. At the tumour site the lumen is reduced to 0.5cm in diameter and the proximal bowel (right) is dilated. At the apex of the attached mesentery an enlarged lymph node infiltrated by pale tumour is visible.

Despite the fact that both examples of small intestinal carcinoma shown here are stenosing lesions, the polypoid macroscopical variant is more usual. These lesions frequently present with intestinal obstruction or intussusception.

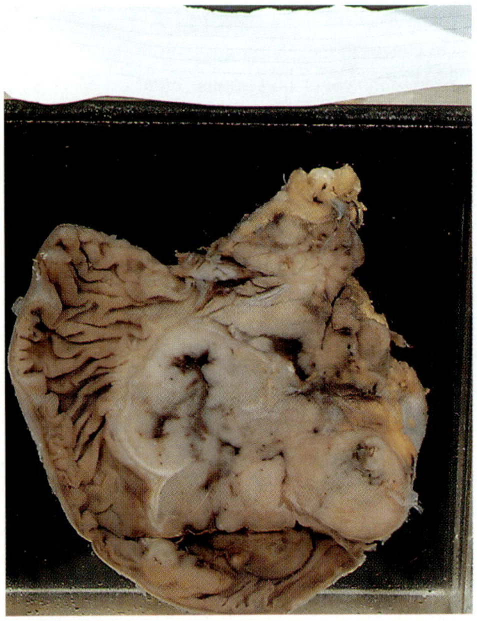

3.115 Duodenum: Leiomyosarcoma

This specimen was excised from a 38-year-old man who presented with a 4 year history of intermittent melaena. He had undergone previous partial gastrectomy for presumed peptic ulceration. On this occasion gastroscopy was negative and at laparotomy a duodenal tumour was found which was invading the head of the pancreas.

A loop of duodenum and the head of the pancreas have been dissected to show a pale, focally haemorrhagic tumour arising from the duodenal wall (below). It extends both superiorly into the pancreas, where it forms a lobulated mass 5cm in diameter, and intraluminally, where it is deeply ulcerated.

As already stated (see Legend 3.107), distinction between benign and malignant gastrointestinal smooth muscle tumours can be very difficult since the clinical features of the two groups are very similar. The presence of extensive local invasion, metastasis, and prominent abnormal mitotic activity are the only reliable pointers to malignancy. The overall 5-year-survival of patients with true sarcomas is about 50 per cent.

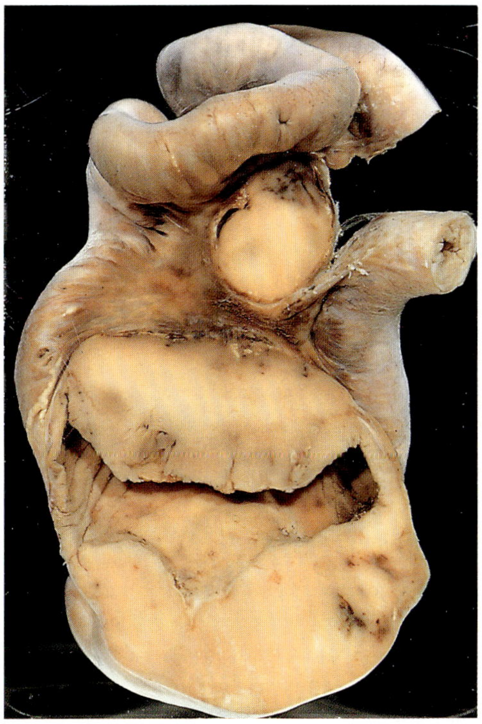

3.116 Ileum: Non-Hodgkin's Lymphoma

This specimen was excised from a 6-year-old boy who presented with a short history of right iliac fossa pain. Laparotomy revealed a tumour in the terminal ileum and enlarged mesenteric nodes. Four months later there was a massive local recurrence.

This loop of small bowel is completely enveloped by a pale tumour mass, measuring 8cm in diameter. The intestinal mucosa is completely replaced by focally necrotic neoplastic tissue. Note the mesenteric lymph node replaced by similar tumour.

This tumour was classified as a lymphoblastic lymphoma (Kiel) and might have been called reticulum cell sarcoma in the past. Primary lymphomas of the small bowel are largely non-Hodgkin's in type and typically arise in the terminal ileum of middle-aged adults. Such tumours are rare in children, with the exception of Burkitt's lymphoma in Africa. Well-recognised predisposing conditions include coeliac disease and alpha-heavy chain disease. In general the prognosis is poor, there being very few 5-year-survivors.

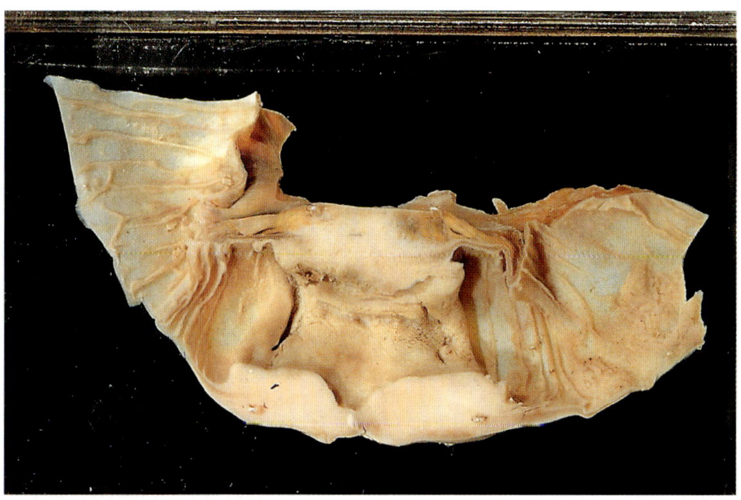

3.117 Ileum: Non-Hodgkin's Lymphoma

This is a post-mortem specimen from a 49-year-old man who presented with increasing weakness. Examination revealed hepatomegaly and, at laparotomy, multiple tumours were found along the length of the small bowel. The patient died post-operatively and, at autopsy, disseminated tumour was also found in the lungs, brain, vertebrae, kidneys and adrenals.

This loop of ileum has been opened to show diffuse infiltration of the full thickness of the bowel wall by a pale, ulcerated neoplasm, which extends over a length of 5cm.

This case represents secondary involvement of the bowel by disseminated lymphoma, which clearly presented at a late stage. It was classified histologically as lymphoplasmacytoid in type (Kiel). Secondary spread to the alimentary tract is much more common in non-Hodgkin's lymphoma than in Hodgkin's disease and is seen most frequently in Burkitt's lymphoma. The presence of multiple tumours (as here) is characteristic.

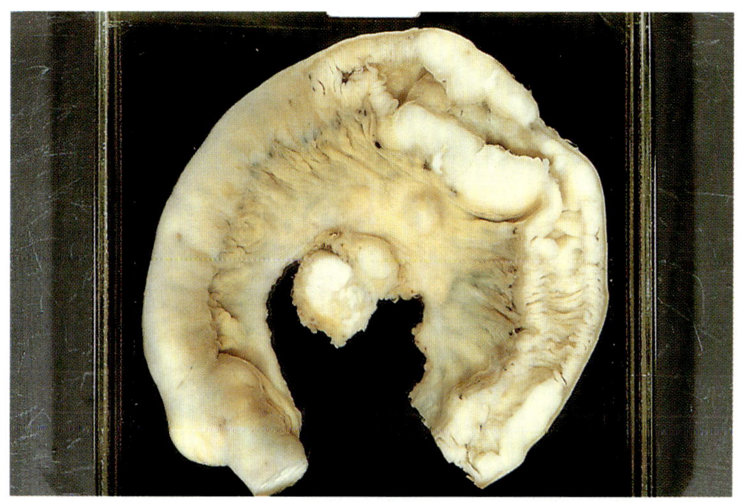

3.118 Ileum: Metastatic Amelanotic Malignant Melanoma

This specimen was excised from a 60-year-old man, who presented with a very variable bowel habit, weight loss and frequent vomiting. Numerous investigations were unhelpful but signs of intestinal obstruction developed and a laparotomy was performed. No details of this patient's primary tumour, which was not detected pre-operatively, are available.

This partly opened loop of small bowel shows 3 separate pale, infiltrative deposits of tumour, along with several enlarged mesenteric nodes which are replaced by further metastases.

The propensity of malignant melanoma to metastasise to almost any site is well known. Such lesions, when amelanotic, may easily cause confusion both clinically and pathologically: the case here was thought initially to be a multicentric lymphoma. In general metastasis of any tumour to the small bowel is uncommon.

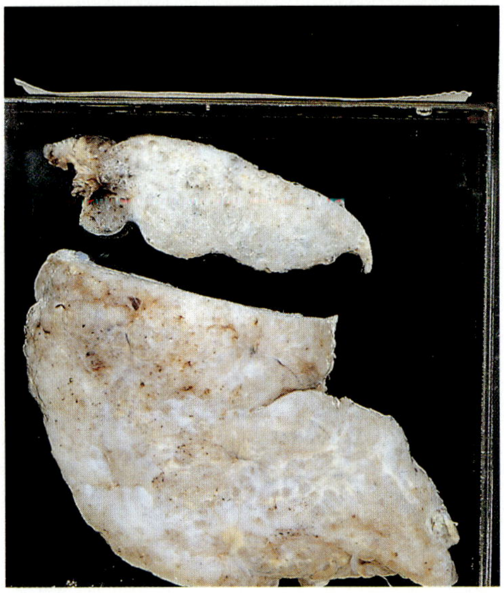

3.119 Greater Omentum: Pseudomyxoma Peritonei

This specimen was excised from a 32-year-old woman who had undergone resection of a large mucinous cystadenoma of the left ovary one year previously. At that time small gelatinous nodules were noted in the omentum and there was free mucoid fluid in the peritoneal cavity. More recently, she had developed increasing abdominal swelling and signs of renal failure. At laparotomy a mass of jelly-like material was found to be replacing the omentum and occupying the entire pelvis. This was excised and she made a complete recovery.

Two portions of the greater omentum show marked thickening and replacement by cystic, grey, myxoid material.

Pseudomyxoma peritonei (characterised by masses of gelatinous material within the peritoneal cavity) is a well recognised complication following rupture of an ovarian mucinous cystadenoma or cystadenocarcinoma (see Chapter 5), a mucocele of the appendix, or any intra-abdominal carcinoma showing florid mucin secretion. It is important to note that this occurrence does not imply *per se* dissemination of a malignant lesion.

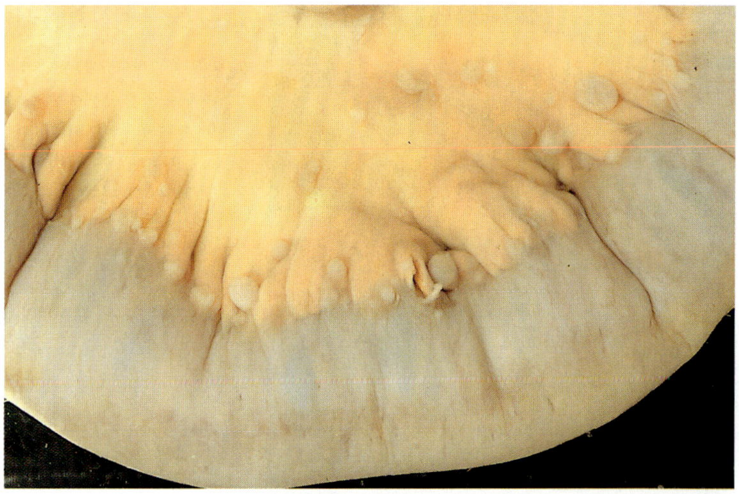

3.120 Mesentery: Secondary Carcinoma

This is a post-mortem specimen from an elderly woman who presented with a 2 month history of altered bowel habit, anorexia and weight loss. She was found to have ascites and there was a palpable pelvic mass. At laparotomy there was carcinomatosis peritonei, associated with large masses of secondary tumour in the omentum and pouch of Douglas. She died 2 weeks later.

On the peritoneal surface of this segment of small intestinal mesentery are multiple small, pale nodules of tumour.

Multiple intra-abdominal metastases, representing extensive trans-coelomic spread are common and most often originate from a primary visceral malignancy, particularly a carcinoma of the large bowel, stomach or ovary. However, almost any cancer may be responsible and, in this case, the histological appearances were highly suggestive of dissemination from an occult adenocarcinoma of the breast.

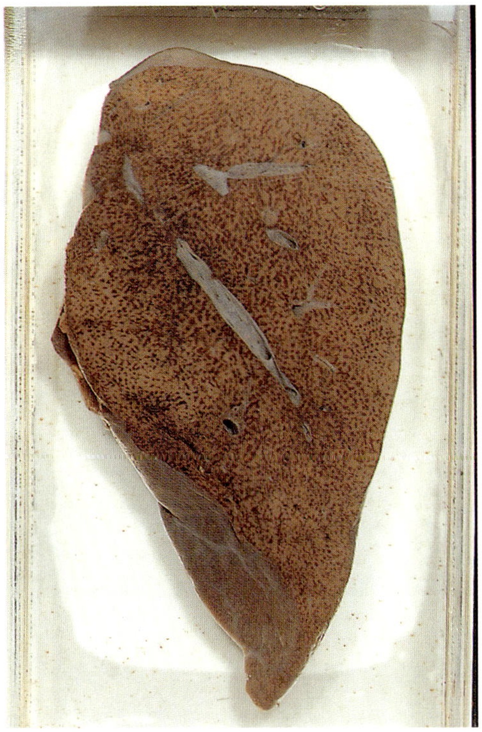

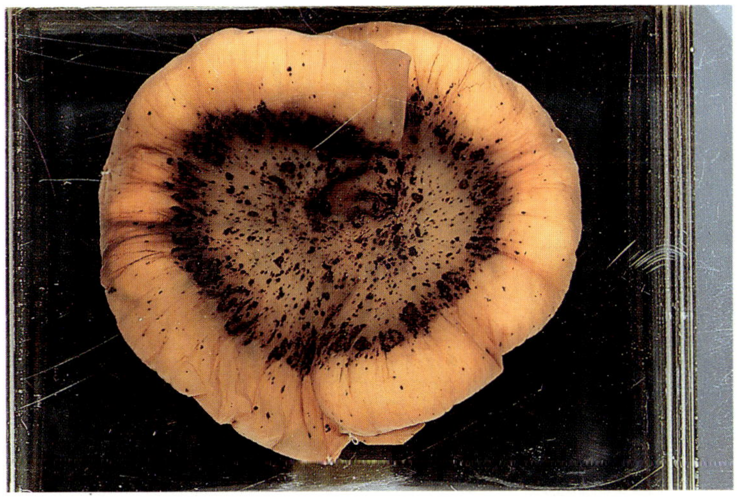

3.121 Greater Omentum and Mesentery: Secondary Malignant Melanoma

These are post-mortem specimens from a 57-year-old woman who had undergone wide excision of a malignant melanoma arising in the skin of the left arm 3 years previously. Over the succeeding period she developed local recurrence, followed by lymph node and cutaneous metastases. She later developed melanomatous infiltration of the bladder and increasing abdominal pain with distension.

The lower margin of the stomach and a segment of transverse colon are shown (3.121a) with attached greater omentum which is massively infiltrated by heavily pigmented metastatic melanoma. A loop of small bowel with its mesentery (3.121b) shows similar changes although the intestinal serosa is less severely involved.

It is well known that malignant melanoma may pursue a relentless course with extensive metastases to almost any site.

Appendix

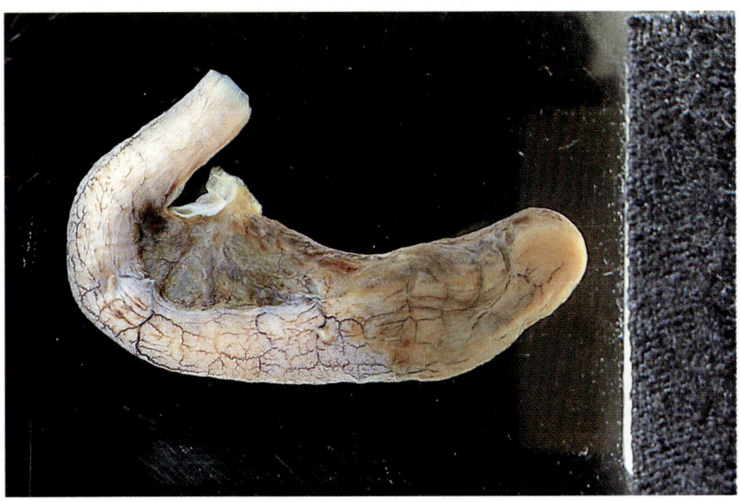

3.122 Appendix: Acute Appendicitis

This specimen was excised from an 8-year-old boy who presented with a 24 hour history of right iliac fossa pain, associated with vomiting and a loose bowel action. Appendicectomy was performed.

The serosal surface of this unopened appendix shows acute congestion proximally and is covered by a yellowish fibrinopurulent exudate distally.

These are the typical macroscopic appearances of 'early' acute appendicitis. Acute appendicitis remains extremely common in the Western population, particularly between the ages of 10 and 30 years. It is, however, a very unusual condition in parts of Africa and Asia and this is thought to reflect dietary differences. The precise aetiology is uncertain but it is widely believed that luminal obstruction (due either to faecoliths or localised lymphoid hypertrophy) results in distal oedema, mucosal damage and subsequent secondary bacterial inflammation. Thereafter florid suppuration commonly ensues and well-recognised complications include perforation, abscess formation, appendiceal gangrene, suppurative thrombophlebitis, and the development of a mucocele.

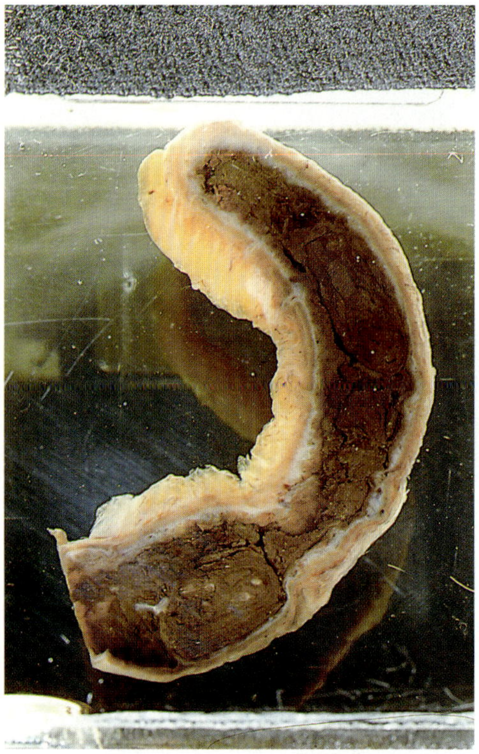

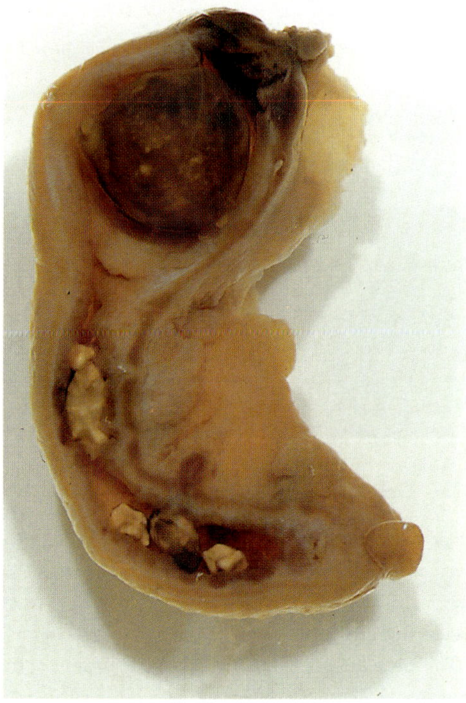

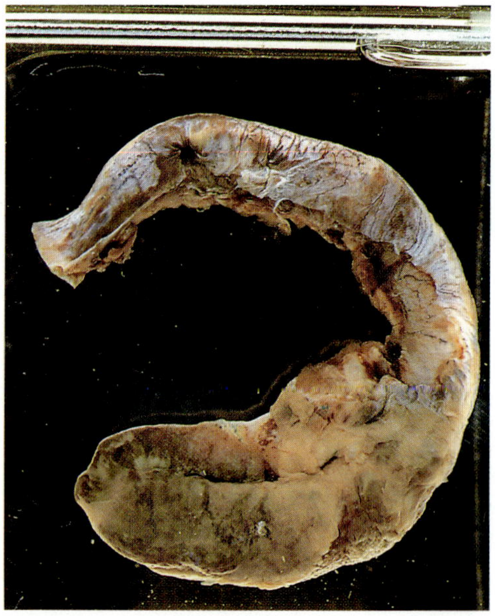

3.123 Appendix: Acute Appendicitis

This specimen was excised from a 61-year-old man who presented with a classical history of acute appendicitis. Appendicectomy was performed.

The appendix is markedly oedematous and shows obvious mucosal necrosis. Proximally, the lumen is occluded by 3 dark faecoliths.

Intraluminal faecoliths, often completely obstructing the lumen, can be found in up to two-thirds of acutely inflamed appendices and as such they are probably the most common initiating factor.

3.124 Appendix: Acute Appendicitis

This specimen was excised from a 45-year-old man who presented with a 12 hour history of severe pain in the right iliac fossa. Appendicectomy was performed.

The lumen of this oedematous, congested appendix is occluded proximally by a large faecolith, measuring 1.7cm in diameter, which shows small yellowish foci of dystrophic calcification. Several smaller faecoliths situated distally are more obviously calcified.

Progressive laminar enlargement and subsequent dystrophic calcification are very common features of faecoliths.

3.125 Appendix: Acute Appendicitis

This specimen was excised from a 16-year-old boy who developed acute abdominal pain associated with frequency of micturition. At operation free pus was present in the pelvis. Appendicectomy was performed.

This appendix is swollen, congested and becoming gangrenous. *In vivo* a small perforation was apparent on the antimesenteric border approximately 2cm from the tip.

Perforation remains a life-threatening complication of acute appendicitis, although the advent of effective anti-anaerobic antibiotics has lessened the seriousness of this occurrence. Perforation may lead to a generalised peritonitis and localised or distant abscess formation. Intestinal adhesions develop very commonly thereafter.

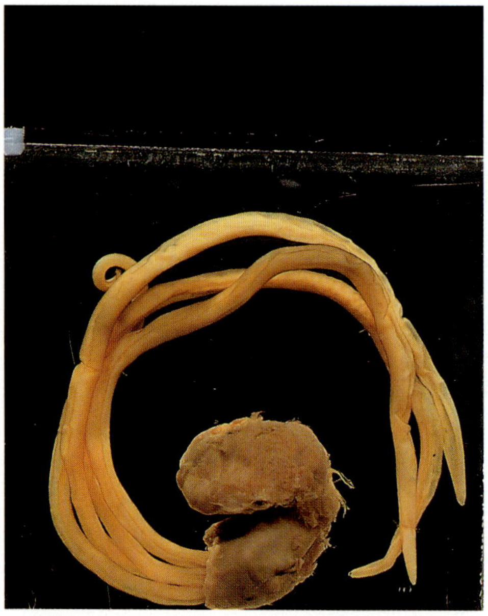

3.126 Appendix: Acute Appendicitis with Roundworms

This specimen was excised from a 7-year-old Iranian child, who presented with a typical history of acute appendicitis. At laparotomy, the caecum was also full of roundworms which were removed.

The appendix (bottom) is markedly oedematous and congested. Projecting from its base are 4 large roundworms.

Roundworms of which *Ascaris lumbricoides* is the commonest to parasitise humans, are acquired through ingestion of their ova in contaminated food. The adult worms then typically inhabit the small bowel, where they give rise to local symptoms if they reach a sufficient number to cause obstruction. They may, however, migrate into the biliary and pancreatic ducts or portal venous system, thence giving rise to much more serious illness. Appendiceal or large bowel involvement is very uncommon. (Courtesy of the Gordon Museum, Guy's Hospital Medical School)

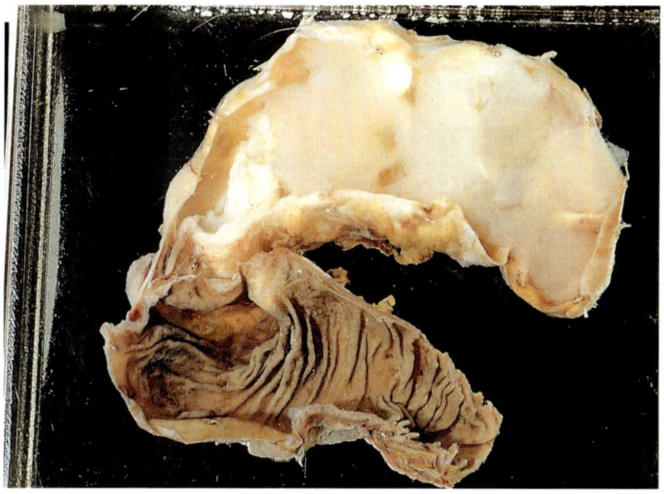

3.127 Appendix: Mucocele

This specimen was excised from a 72-year-old man who had suffered an episode of severe abdominal pain several weeks previously. A mass was palpable in the right iliac fossa and laparotomy was performed.

A portion of the caecum and ascending colon is shown from which is suspended a massively dilated appendix measuring 12 × 6 × 3cm. The appendiceal wall is attenuated and the lumen is distended by viscid, pale mucinous material.

Mucoceles of the appendix are not uncommon, presenting most often in middle age, and are thought to be a sequela of low-grade appendicitis with luminal obstruction. They may be complicated either by rupture, giving rise to pseudomyxoma peritonei (see Legend 3.119), or by suppurative inflammation which results in the formation of an empyema. It should be noted that mucinous cystadenomas and cystadenocarcinomas of the appendix may have a very similar macroscopic appearance.

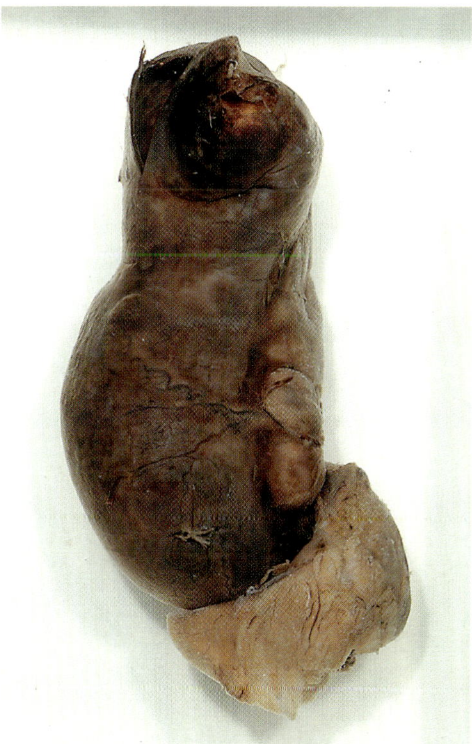

3.128 Appendix: Mucocele with Torsion

This specimen was excised from a 63-year-old woman who presented with a short history of colicky abdominal pain, associated with vomiting and constipation. Laparotomy was performed.

The entire appendix is distended and gangrenous. The tip has become torted and has undergone haemorrhagic infarction. In the fresh state the appendiceal lumen was distended by copious bloodstained mucinous material.

It would appear, in this unusual case, that distal torsion has brought to light a pre-existent mucocele.

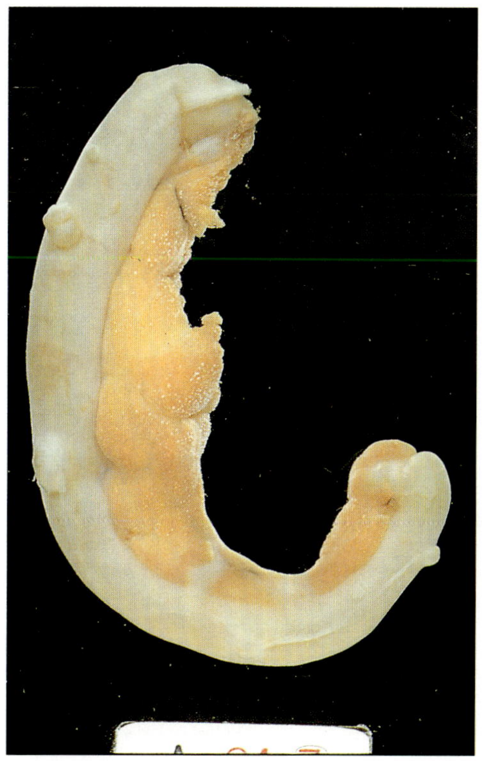

3.129 Appendix: Diverticulosis

This was an incidental finding at post-mortem in a 73-year-old woman who died of cerebral infarction.

Projecting from the antimesenteric border of this otherwise normal appendix are a number of small, rounded diverticula.

In the majority of cases, diverticular disease of the appendix is an acquired lesion, entirely analogous to the same condition seen in the colon. In fact, appendiceal diverticula, which are not rare, are almost invariably associated with similar lesions in the more distal large bowel and the aetiology and complications are the same at both sites (see Figure and Legend 3.149 et seq.). Occasionally, appendiceal diverticula can be congenital in nature, being distinguished from the acquired form by their diminished tendency to become inflamed and the presence of a normal, full thickness intestinal wall.

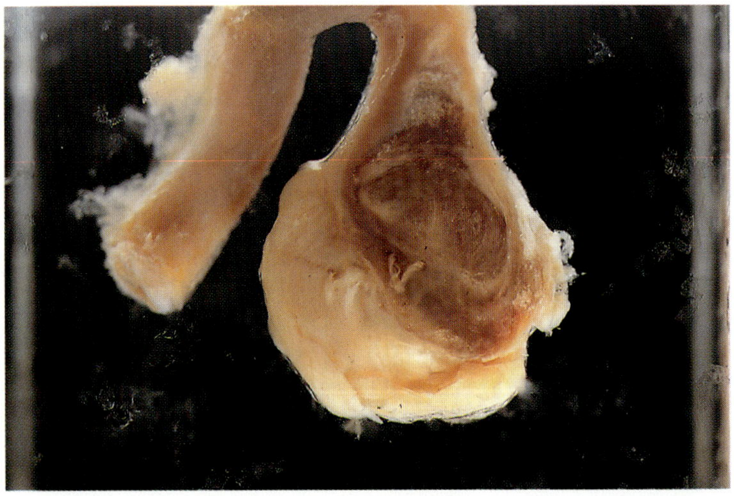

3.130 Appendix: Carcinoid Tumour

This specimen was excised from a 59-year-old woman in whom it was found incidentally during the course of a routine cholecystectomy.

The appendix has been mounted to show a pear-shaped, yellow-brown tumour at its distal end, which measures 2.5cm in length.

The appendix is the single most common primary site of gastrointestinal carcinoid tumours (argentaffinomas), the ileum being second in frequency (see Figure and Legend 3.111). Appendiceal lesions are typically seen in young adults and usually pursue a benign course, in contrast to those arising in the small bowel. As a consequence, the carcinoid syndrome is a rare complication of appendiceal lesions.

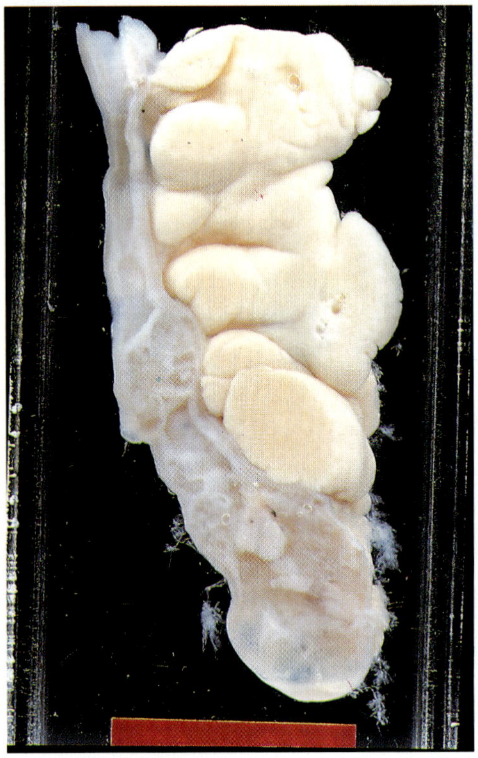

3.131 Appendix: Mucinous Cystadenocarcinoma

This lesion was found at post-mortem in an 83-year-old man who died with carcinomatosis peritonei. The primary tumour site had not been identified prior to death.

The appendix is diffusely expanded by a multilocular, cystic tumour, composed largely of pale mucinous material.

Adenocarcinoma of the appendix is extremely rare but is most often of the histological type seen in this case. The elderly are typically affected and may present with symptoms of acute appendicitis. The clinical behaviour and prognostic features are the same as those of conventional colonic adenocarcinoma (see Legend 3.164). These tumours may occasionally give rise to pseudomyxoma peritonei. (Courtesy of the Gordon Museum, Guy's Hospital Medical School)

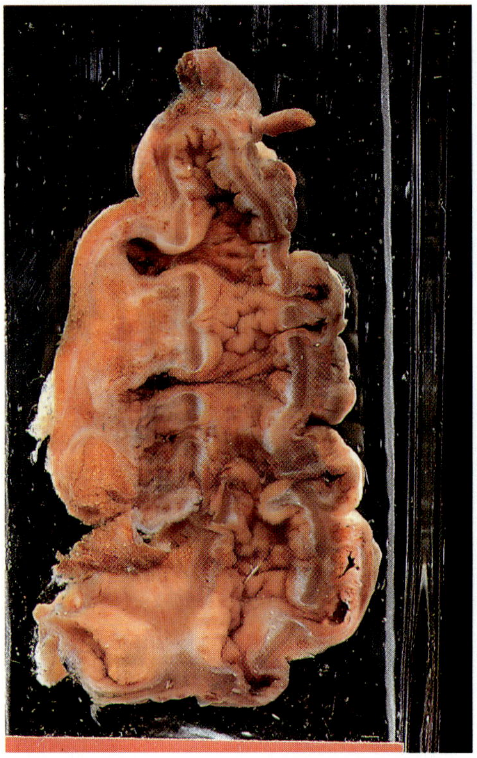

3.132 Appendix: Adenocarcinoma and Diverticulitis

This specimen was excised from a 41-year-old man who presented with a 2 day history of the symptoms of acute appendicitis. He had suffered a similar attack of abdominal pain one year previously.

The most conspicuous abnormality in this appendix is the presence of numerous diverticula, some of which are congested and inflamed. In addition, however, at the base of the appendix (top) there is a small, annular stenosing neoplasm composed of solid whitish tissue.

Histologically, this is an example of an uncommon type of appendiceal carcinoma which is very similar to conventional colonic adenocarcinoma. The prognosis is the same as that of mucinous cystadenocarcinoma. (Courtesy of the Gordon Museum, Guy's Hospital Medical School)

Large Intestine

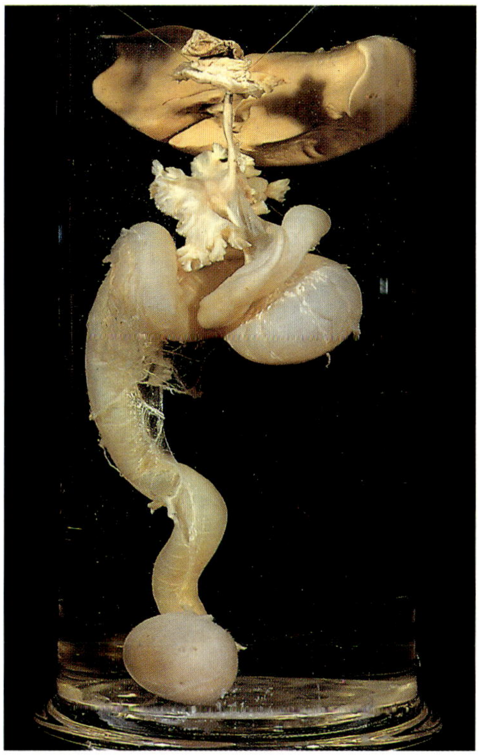

3.133 Colon: Congenital Atresia

No clinical details are available.

The terminal ileum, large intestine and liver (above) of a neonate are mounted along with the vessels passing to the umbilicus. The colon (below) is markedly distended and terminates as a blind sac. The rectum was completely absent.

Congenital atresia or stenosis of the colon is extremely rare but represents a hindgut anomaly. Similar lesions of the anus or rectum are, however, more common, affecting approximately 1 in 5000 live-born infants.

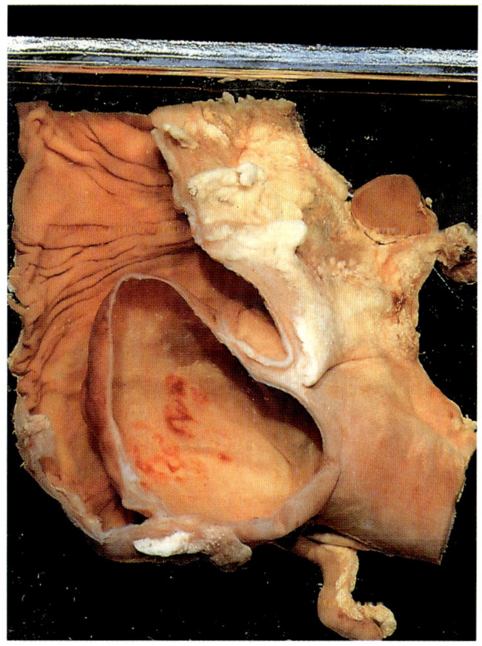

3.134 Caecum: Enterogenous Cyst

This specimen was excised from a 22-year-old woman who presented with a 6 week history of severe intermittent lower abdominal pain. A mass was palpable in the right iliac fossa and laparotomy was performed.

The terminal ileum, caecum and part of the ascending colon are shown. The caecum has been opened to reveal a thin-walled cyst, measuring 7cm in diameter, arising at its lower pole just distal to the obstructed ileocaecal valve. The mucosa of the cyst and adjacent bowel are inflamed and reactive lymph nodes are visible in the mesentery.

Enterogenous cysts are even more rare in the large bowel than in the small intestine but are thought to arise by the same congenital mechanism (see Legend 3.89).

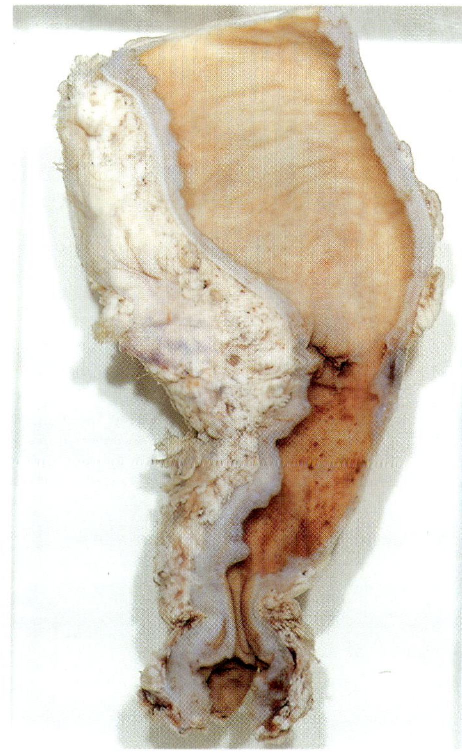

3.135 Colon: Hirschsprung's Disease

This specimen was excised from a 9-year-old boy who had suffered from abdominal pain, associated with intermittent abdominal distension and a very variable bowel habit, since birth. He finally presented with acute large bowel obstruction and, following formation of a colostomy, a rectosigmoidectomy was performed.

The lower sigmoid colon and rectum have been opened to show the dilated proximal normal bowel (above) with an abrupt transition to the narrow, diseased rectum below.

Hirschsprung's disease is an uncommon congenital disorder which typically presents in infancy and particularly affects boys. This condition is characterised by an absence of ganglion cells in both the myenteric and submucosal plexuses of the affected segment of bowel, associated with marked hypertrophy of the autonomic nerve fibres. The aganglionic bowel, which *always* extends proximally from the anus, is therefore narrow and fails to transmit peristalsis. The length of bowel involved varies from case to case but most often includes only the rectum and sigmoid colon. Those cases affecting the transverse colon, or extending even more proximally, are known as 'long-segment' Hirschsprung's. Complications include complete intestinal obstruction and failure to thrive.

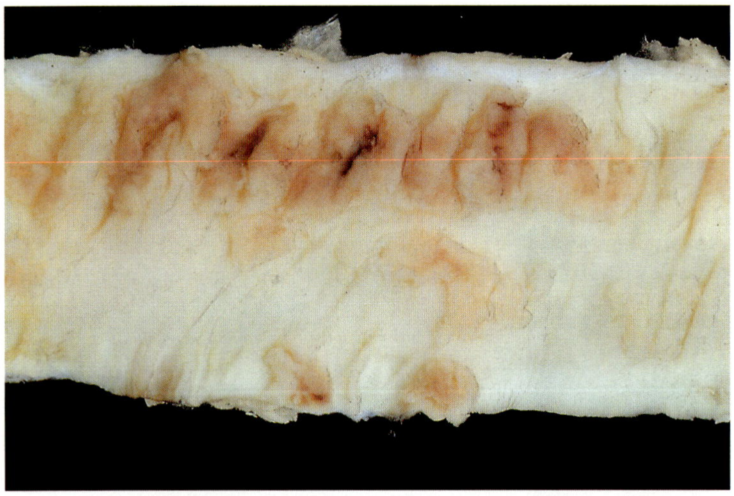

3.136 Colon: Ischaemic Ulceration due to Malignant Hypertension

This is a post-mortem specimen from a 77-year-old woman who presented with severe iron deficiency and chronic renal failure. She developed malignant (accelerated) hypertension and died.

A portion of the colon has been opened to show multiple, raised areas of haemorrhagic ulceration. Histologically, the features were those of haemorrhagic infarction and many of the submucosal arterioles showed marked fibrinoid necrosis.

Malignant hypertension is a relatively uncommon cause of what is simply acute ischaemic colitis. The most frequent cause is arterial obstruction due to either atheroma of one of the mesenteric arteries (with or without superadded thrombosis) or to systemic emboli, usually from the left side of the heart. Other causes include venous occlusion, hypotension or primary vascular disorders. The region of the splenic flexure and proximal descending colon are at greatest risk, since this region has the poorest blood supply (being at the 'watershed' between the superior and inferior mesenteric vessels). While the macroscopic appearances shown here are typical, with predominantly mucosal involvement, some cases show infarction of the full thickness of the bowel wall, giving rise to a florid necrotising colitis. Some lesions are rapidly fatal, others require resection of a segment of infarcted bowel while others resolve, at least partially, to undergo fibrosis and formation of an ischaemic stricture (see Figure 3.138).

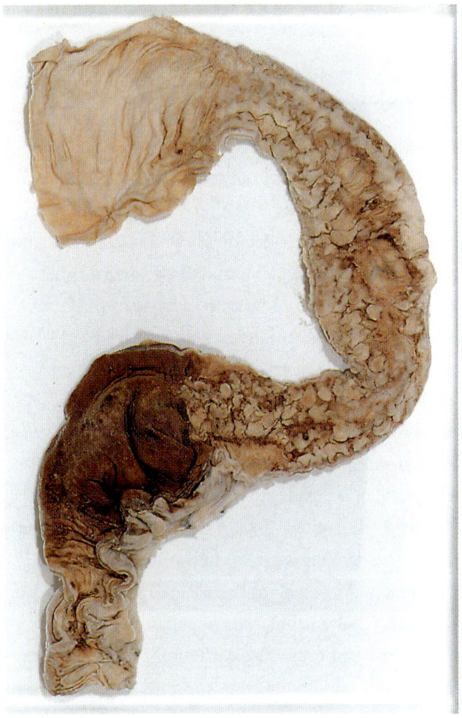

3.137 Colon: Acute Ischaemic Colitis

This is a post-mortem specimen from a 75-year-old man who developed acute severe lower abdominal pain vomiting and bloody diarrhoea. He was admitted to hospital in profound hypotensive shock and was found to have suffered a silent acute myocardial infarct. He rapidly developed acute renal failure, repeated episodes of cardiac arrest and died.

The descending colon, sigmoid colon and proximal rectum have been opened to show florid acute ischaemic changes. Much of the bowel shows ulceration and multifocal necrosis and, distally, there is an area of complete haemorrhagic infarction.

This is a much more typical history of acute ischaemic colitis than that in Legend 2.136. The macroscopic features are characteristic.

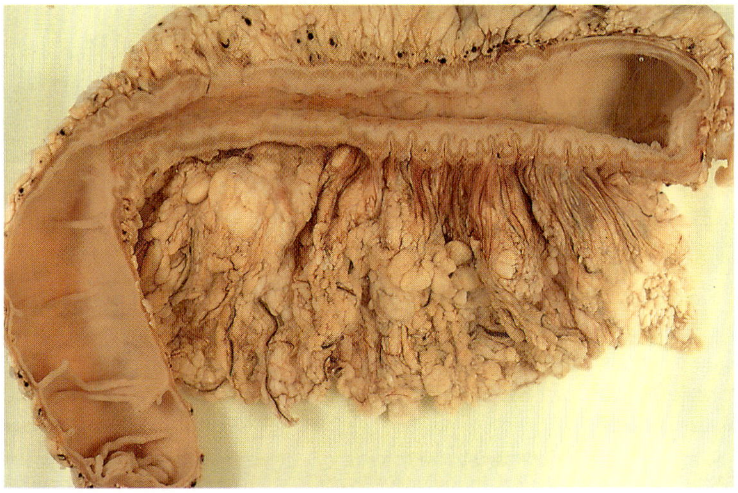

3.138 Colon: Chronic Ischaemic Colitis

This specimen was excised from an elderly male, who presented with colicky abdominal pain and constipation. Some months earlier, he had suffered a brief, self-limiting episode of acute abdominal pain associated with diarrhoea. Barium enema revealed a stricture in the distal transverse colon and laparotomy was performed.

The distal transverse colon and splenic flexure have been opened from behind to show an obvious, discrete stricture. At the affected site, there is very marked submucosal fibrosis but the muscularis propria is relatively preserved.

Chronic ischaemic colitis is a consequence either of a prolonged or an acute episode of diminished blood flow, without full thickness infarction, which has led to complete mucosal necrosis and consequent submucosal inflammation and fibrosis. As would be expected (see Legend 3.136), the region of the splenic flexure is most often affected. Patients with this condition tend to be elderly and often have widespread atheromatous vascular disease. (Courtesy of St. Thomas's Hospital Medical School Museum)

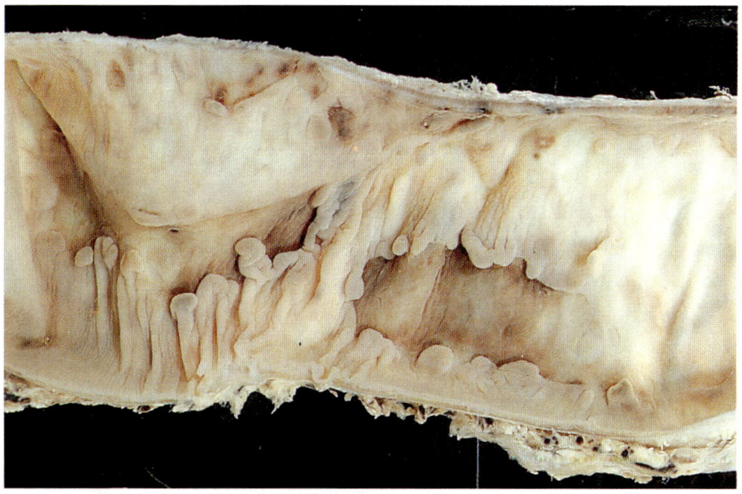

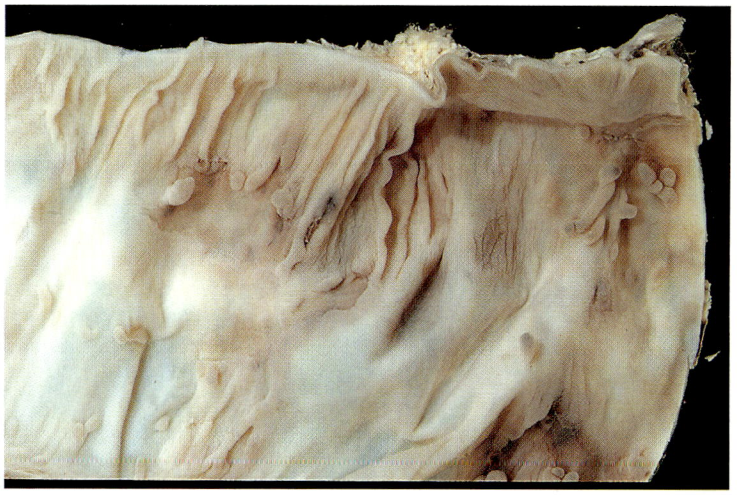

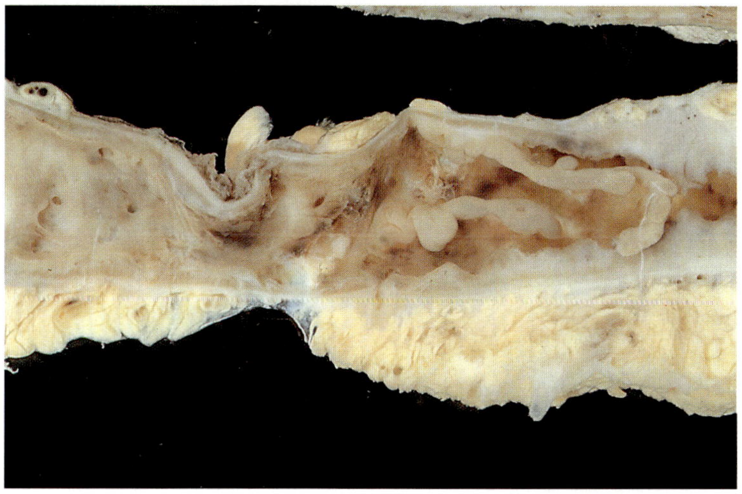

3.139 Colon: Ulcerative Colitis

This specimen was excised from a 22-year-old man who had a 2 year history of increasingly severe abdominal pain, weight loss and diarrhoea. Two exploratory laparotomies revealed diffuse inflammation of the large bowel with enlarged mesenteric nodes but no localised lesion. Two years after first presentation, and as a consequence of his persistent symptoms, a total colectomy was performed.

Three segments of the large bowel have been opened to show the typical mucosal lesions of ulcerative colitis. There is linear, superficial mucosal ulceration (3.139a), with associated hyperaemia and focal hyperplasia of the adjacent epithelium. Note that the ulcers have undermined edges. A partially healed segment (3.139b) shows irregular areas of mucosal flattening, with loss of the haustral pattern, and several small inflammatory mucosal tags are present. A further segment (3.139c) shows thickening of the bowel wall with obvious mucosal inflammatory pseudopolyposis, forming mucosal bridges: the haustral pattern is completely effaced.

Ulcerative colitis is an idiopathic, chronic inflammatory disorder of the large bowel which *always* involves the rectum (with or without proximal spread) and is characterised by predominantly mucosal involvement. It presents most often in young adults and shows a slight predilection for females. There is an inconsistent familial tendency, an association with HLA-B27 and an increased incidence in individuals having a 'neurotic' or particularly 'sensitive' personality.

Important macroscopic features, other than those detailed here are:
1) the presence of anatomically continuous mucosal involvement (cf. Crohn's disease), extending proximally from the rectum, sometimes into the terminal ileum (so-called 'backwash ileitis');
2) shortening of the bowel with loss of the normal haustral pattern (giving rise to a 'hosepipe' appearance on barium enema), and
3) the presence of rather smooth, granular mucosa, unassociated with submucosal fibrosis.
Stricture formation (in the absence of neoplasia) is *not* a feature of the disease.

Complications include acute fulminant colitis (leading to toxic megacolon), a significant risk of developing colonic adenocarcinoma (between 5-10 per cent of affected patients), sclerosing cholangitis, chronic hepatitis, arthritis (often resembling ankylosing spondylitis), iridocyclitis and skin lesions, such as pyoderma gangrenosum.

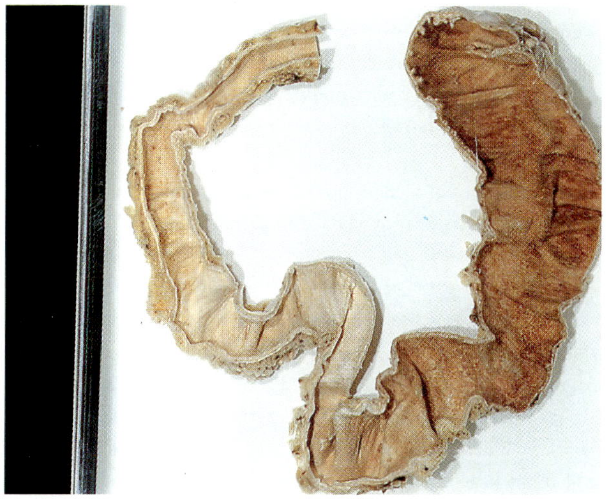

3.140 Colon: Ulcerative Colitis

This specimen was excised from a 17-year-old boy who had a 2½ year history of abdominal pain, watery diarrhoea and iron-deficiency anaemia. A barium enema revealed typical colitic changes, extending from the rectum to the caecum. He was treated with steroids, sodium cromoglycate and sulphasalazine, which led to a marked improvement in his condition. However, symptoms recurred and a panprotocolectomy was performed.

The entire large bowel has been opened. The rectum and descending colon (right) show a smooth, rather pale mucosal appearance and there is obvious bowel shortening. In contrast, the caecum and ascending colon show superficial ulceration, the mucosa having a hyperaemic, granular surface.

These are the appearances of ulcerative colitis in partial remission, there being no evidence of *active* disease in the distal bowel, although the typical features of healed colitis are apparent.

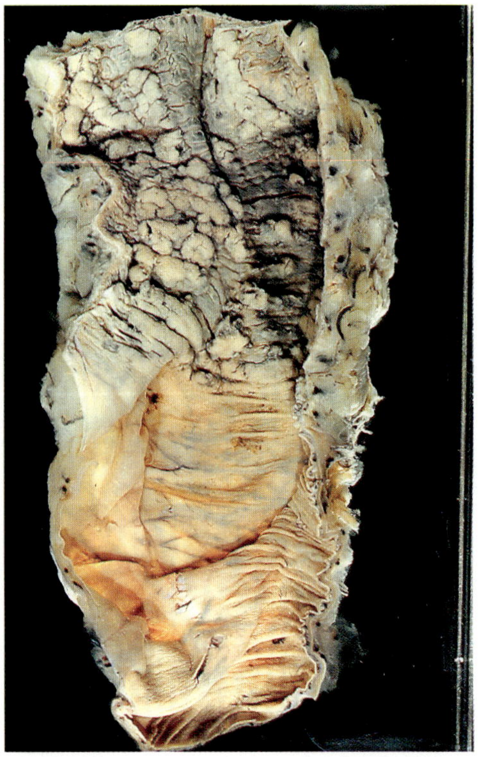

3.141 Colon: Ulcerative Colitis with Toxic Megacolon

This specimen was excised from a 27-year-old man who presented with a 9 week history of severe diarrhoea (passing up to 13 stools per day). He was found to be anaemic and a barium enema revealed the typical features of ulcerative colitis in the distal colon and rectum. While in hospital he developed acute abdominal distension, with signs of large bowel obstruction, and at laparotomy the colon was markedly dilated and extremely friable. A total colectomy was performed.

A portion of the descending colon has been opened to show obvious luminal dilatation and severe, diffuse mucosal ulceration distally. Irregular islets of elevated, surviving mucosa are apparent, although even they appear lustreless and devitalised when compared with the proximal, relatively normal bowel.

Acute fulminant inflammation develops in up to 10 per cent of patients with ulcerative colitis and may sometimes be the presenting feature. It is characterised by marked luminal dilatation, usually of the transverse colon, associated with attenuation of the bowel wall. Toxic megacolon is a life-threatening complication, often leading to colonic perforation, and surgical intervention is always necessary.

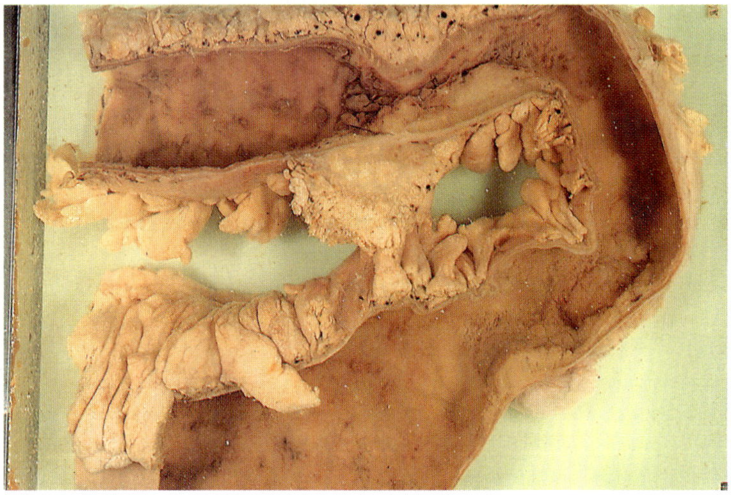

3.142 Colon: Ulcerative Colitis complicated by two Carcinomas

This specimen was excised from a 47-year-old woman, who had suffered from ulcerative colitis for many years.

This length of large bowel has been opened to show general luminal dilatation, with a mainly smooth, rather pale mucosal surface, representing quiescent ulcerative colitis. Several small inflammatory pseudopolyps are apparent (top left). In addition, there are two separate raised neoplasms arising in the mucosa (top middle and bottom right), both of which are infiltrating the bowel wall.

As already stated, colonic adenocarcinoma develops in up to 10 per cent of patients with ulcerative colitis. Factors that increase this risk include early age at onset of the colitis, duration of the disease, and severity (and topographical extent) of the inflammatory process. In general, it is held that the increased incidence of neoplasia is apparent after a minimum of 10 years preceding colitis, but that thereafter the risk is 30 times that of the normal population. It should be noted that patients with ulcerative colitis who develop an adenocarcinoma tend to fare worse than those with a carcinoma unassociated with inflammatory bowel disease. (Courtesy of St. Thomas's Hospital Medical School Museum)

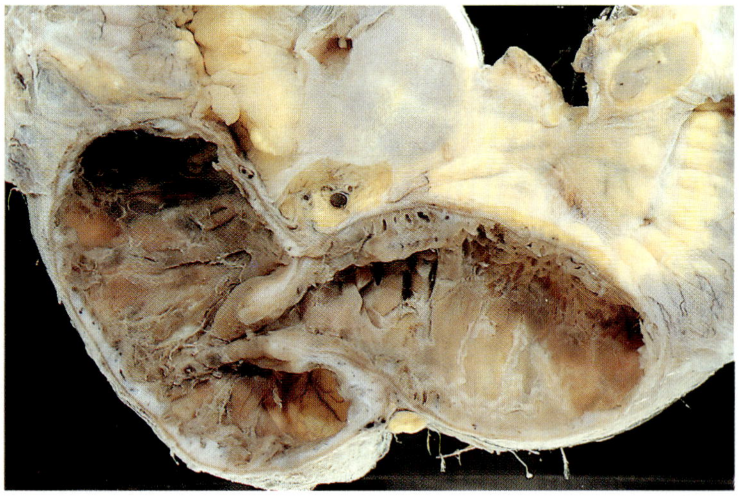

3.143 Ileocaecal Junction: Crohn's Disease

This specimen was excised from a 12-year-old boy who presented with a 4 week history of weight loss, rectal bleeding and abdominal pain. Laparotomy revealed oedema and congestion of the terminal ileum, suggestive of acute Crohn's disease, and the abdomen was closed. However, the symptoms persisted and 6 months later a right hemicolectomy was performed.

The ileocaecal junction has been opened to show florid inflammation, mucosal ulceration and fissuring of both the small and large bowel components. The adjacent mesenteric lymph nodes (above) are markedly swollen.

The pathogenesis and typical features of Crohn's disease, which is commonest in the small intestine, have already been discussed (see Legend 3.100 et seq.). At least 30 per cent of affected patients have large bowel disease, either in isolation or in association with small intestinal involvement. As in small bowel disease, multifocal, discontinuous ulceration and inflammation of the bowel wall is characteristic, although the classical 'cobblestone' appearance is much less common in the large bowel. The association with adenocarcinoma of the large bowel is less convincing than that with similar tumours in the small bowel.

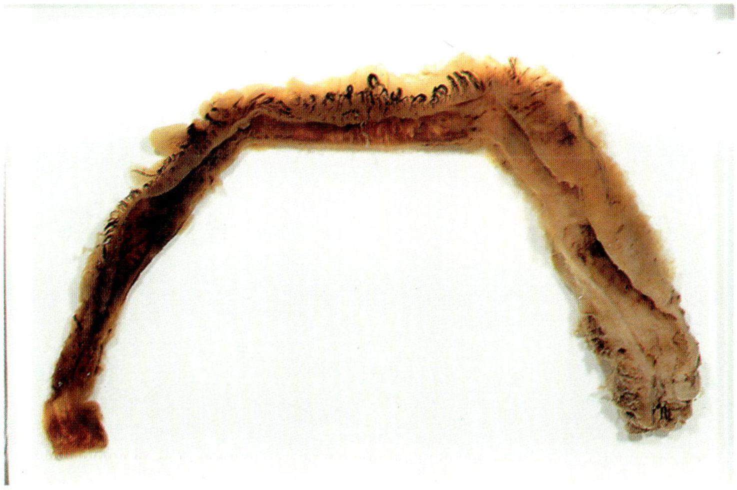

3.144 Sigmoid Colon and Rectum: Crohn's Disease

This specimen was excised from a 55-year-old woman who had suffered 2 previous attacks of 'colitis'. On this occasion she presented with a 3 week history of bloody diarrhoea and weight loss. Proctoscopy revealed a granular mucosa, exuding pus, which bled on contact. She was given systemic steroids and steroid enemata; the latter, however, were noted to discharge through the vagina. The patient became pyrexial and progressively more anaemic, and consequently a total colectomy was performed.

The sigmoid colon and rectum have been opened to show diffuse ulceration, particularly distally, with small irregular areas of relatively unaffected mucosa. The bowel lumen is markedly narrowed. In the fresh state, the entire colon showed multiple, similarly diseased segments with foci of sparing as seen proximally here.

Crohn's disease of the large bowel may take a variety of forms, ranging from small localised foci of inflammation with stricture formation to diffuse involvement of most of the intestine. The latter may be clinically and macroscopically confused with ulcerative colitis. Diffuse disease confined to the rectum is also a well-recognised variant.

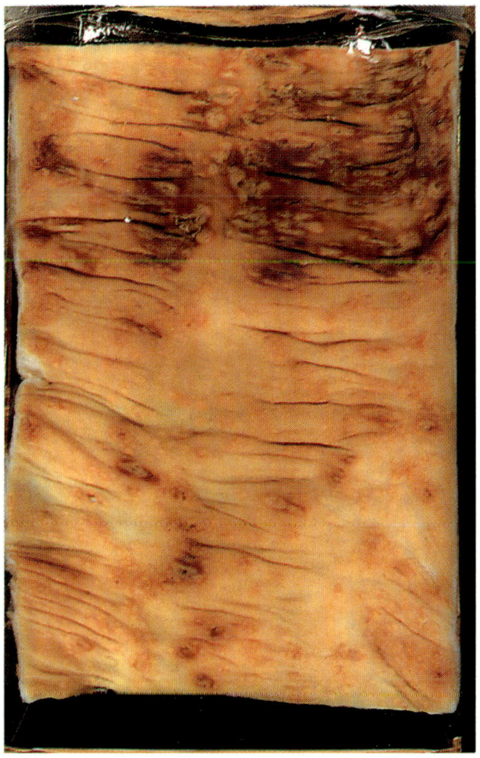

3.145 Colon: Bacillary Dysentery

No clinical details are available.

This segment of large bowel has been opened to show multiple discrete and confluent, haemorrhagic mucosal ulcers, some of which are covered by purulent exudate.

Bacillary dysentery is most often due to infection with *Shigella sonnei* although other *Shigellae* or *Salmonellae* are not infrequently responsible. This condition is usually seen in small outbreaks either in institutions or in patients with crowded living conditions. Poor standards of hygiene and contamination of food are important aetiological factors. Small intestinal involvement is extremely uncommon and most cases pursue a self-limiting course. There is, however, a recognised mortality in infants and, occasionally, adults may develop chronic infection. Other possible complications include the development of a liver abscess, myocarditis and splenic infection.

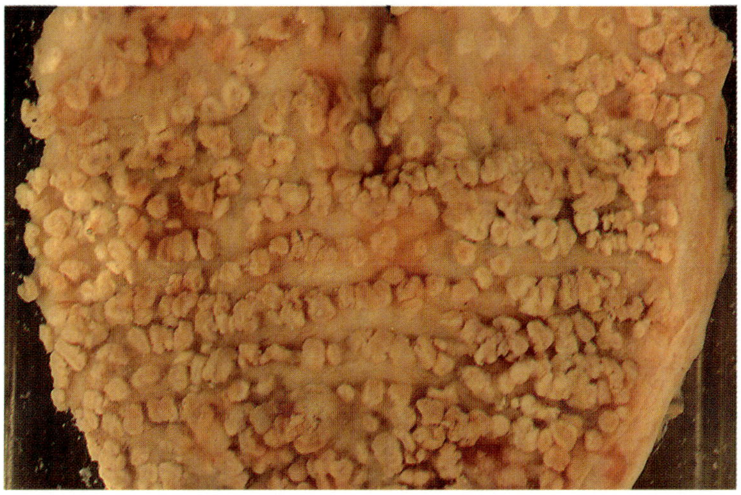

3.146 Colon: Pseudomembranous Colitis

This is a post-mortem specimen from a 73-year-old diabetic woman. She had suffered from repeated urinary tract infections, which had been treated with several courses of antibiotics. Latterly she developed intractable diarrhoea and died.

This segment of large bowel has been opened to show numerous raised yellowish plaques, measuring up to 2mm in diameter, adherent to the mucosal surface. In places these are becoming confluent.

Pseudomembranous colitis is a relatively recently delineated entity, although it has been recognised for over 50 years. The disease typically follows either antibiotic treatment or major abdominal surgery, either of which may alter the natural colonic bacterial flora or the colon's susceptibility to bacterial colonisation. In either circumstance, the patient's bowel is then colonised by *Clostridium difficile*, the exotoxin of which leads to mucosal erosions or necrosis with an overlying fibrinopurulent exudate, hence the diarrhoea. While clindamycin and lincomycin were the principal causative antibiotics originally implicated, cases of pseudomembranous colitis have now been attributed to a very wide variety of such drugs. Vancomycin, which has never been implicated, remains the treatment of choice. (Courtesy of St. Thomas's Hospital Medical School Museum)

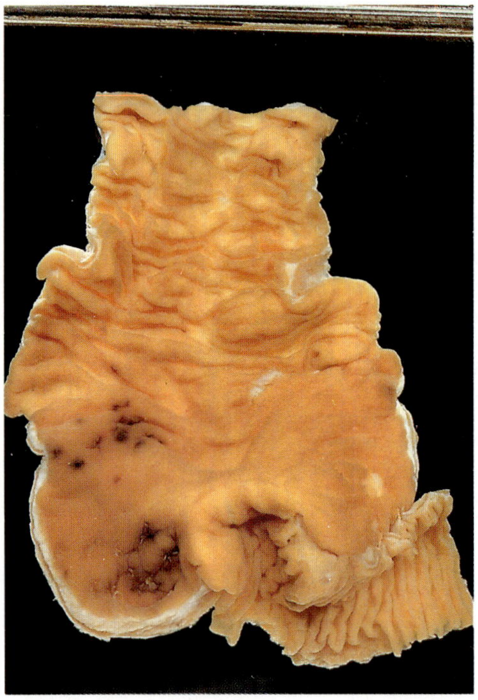

3.147 Caecum: Amoebiasis

This specimen was excised from a 67-year-old male missionary who presented with a 2 week history of bleeding per rectum. At laparotomy the caecum was found to be grossly thickened and oedematous.

The terminal ileum, caecum and part of the ascending colon have been opened to show small, yellowish raised lesions. Superficial and deep mucosal ulcers, some of which are haemorrhagic, are also visible. The bowel wall is markedly thickened.

Amoebiasis is caused by the protozoon *Entamoeba histolytica* and predominantly affects the large bowel; infection is spread via the oro-faecal route. While this disease is particularly common in tropical countries, isolated cases are sometimes encountered in more temperate Western climes. Macroscopically, amoebiasis is characterised by yellowish foci of mucosal necrosis and flask-shaped (or undermined) ulcers which may occur anywhere in the large bowel but are predominant in the rectum or caecum. Severe diffuse involvement is uncommon but life-threatening. Complications include involvement of the peri-anal skin, intestinal perforation, involvement of the portal venous system (leading to amoebic 'abscesses' in the liver or elsewhere), and chronic infection, which may result in a fibrotic pseudotumour, the 'amoeboma'.

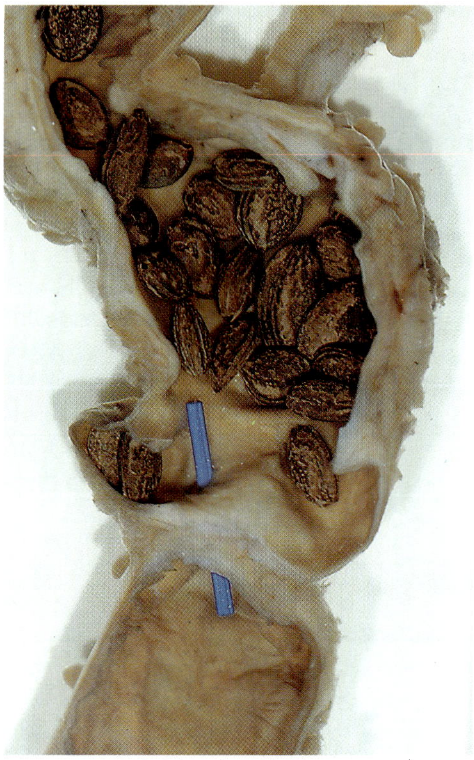

3.148 Colon: Tuberculous Stricture

This specimen was excised from a 67-year-old woman who presented with a long-standing history of right-sided abdominal colicky pain. Plain abdominal X-ray revealed a group of oval opacities in the right iliac fossa. Laparotomy was performed, at which 27 fruit stones were found in the caecum proximal to the stricture.

The caecum and part of the ascending colon have been opened to reveal a tight stricture (marked with a blue probe) proximal to which numerous fruit stones have accumulated. Histologically the bowel and adjacent lymph nodes showed evidence of healed tuberculous infection.

The pathogenesis and typical appearances of intestinal tuberculosis have already been discussed in the small bowel (see Legend 3.95 et seq.). The ileum is the most commonly affected site, but the caecum is frequently involved. Tuberculous infection of the large bowel distal to the caecum is, however, very uncommon. The macroscopical changes are classically more localised than in Crohn's disease, which is the principal differential diagnosis. Healing by fibrosis often leads to stricture formation.

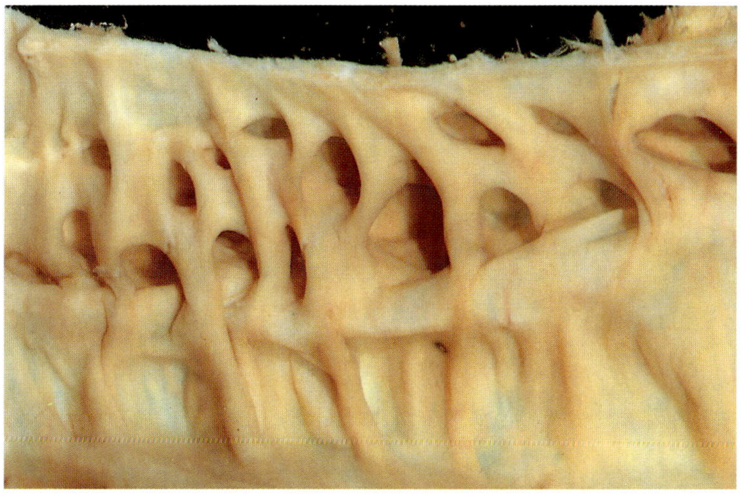

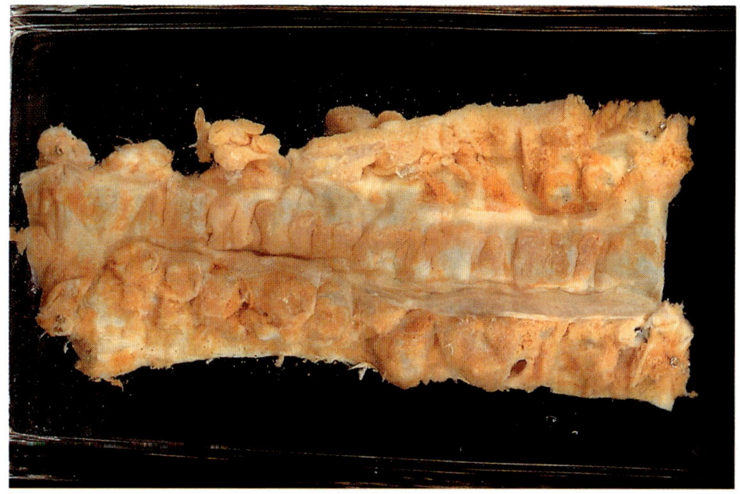

3.149 Colon: Diverticular Disease

No clinical details are available.

This segment of large bowel (3.149a) has been opened to show multiple, wide-mouthed diverticula, which measure up to 1cm in diameter, opening on the mucosal surface. Posteriorly (3.149b) these project through the muscle coat to form thin-walled, hemispherical sacs on the serosal aspect.

Diverticular disease of the large bowel is ubiquitous in the Western world and increases in incidence with age. The diverticula are of acquired (pulsion) type and herniate through the muscle coat, most often in 2 rows between the taeniae coli (the points of weakness where vessels enter the bowel wall). They are most common in the sigmoid colon but may be seen anywhere in the large bowel.

Aetiologically, diverticular disease is significantly related to the ingestion of a low fibre (roughage) diet. This results in the production of small, hard faeces which require increased, and sometimes incoordinate, segmental peristalsis to move them along the bowel lumen. This, in turn, leads to a marked elevation in intraluminal pressure with consequent extrusion of the mucosa at points of weakness.

Complications include acute or chronic inflammation, which may give rise to perforation, pericolic abscess formation or the development of fistulae. Chronic low-grade blood loss is a common feature but occasionally massive haemorrhage, usually rectal in origin, results from erosion of a submucosal artery. Diverticular disease *does not* predispose to carcinoma of the colon. The two conditions may, however, coexist in the same patient as both commonly occur in the same population.

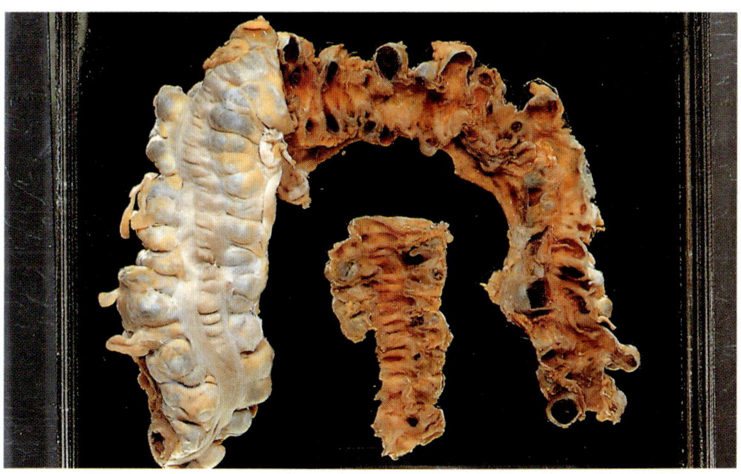

3.150 Colon: Diverticular Disease

This was an incidental finding at post-mortem in a 73-year-old man who died of a coronary thrombosis.

The entire colon is mounted and all but the caecum and ascending portion has been opened. The most distal portion has been opened separately (in a different plane) to demonstrate anatomical continuity between the diverticula and bowel lumen. Many of the diverticula in the larger opened segment contain inspissated faeces, while proximally, similar lesions can be seen protruding in rows either side of the taenia.

This case demonstrates the classical features of diverticular disease; while involvement of the sigmoid colon is invariable, and often localised, changes affecting the entire large bowel may occur.

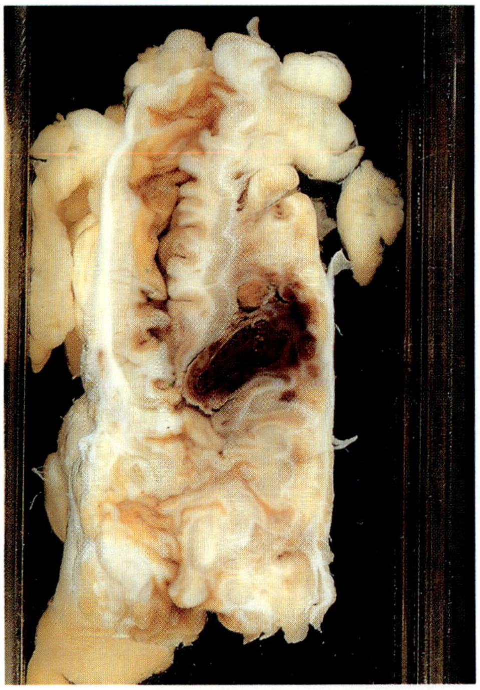

3.151 Colon: Diverticulitis

This specimen was excised from an elderly man who presented with fresh bleeding per rectum. At laparotomy, in addition to florid diverticulitis of the sigmoid colon, there was a perforation of the bowel wall.

This opened segment of sigmoid colon shows obvious diverticular disease. In addition, there is mucosal congestion and an area of serosal haemorrhage (middle left), just above which there is a faecolith outside the bowel wall, indicative of recent perforation.

Episodes of inflammation in diverticular disease are very common, resulting from mucosal damage by inspissated faeces within the diverticula. Perforation is much less frequent but carries a significant mortality as a result of the faecal peritonitis which ensues.

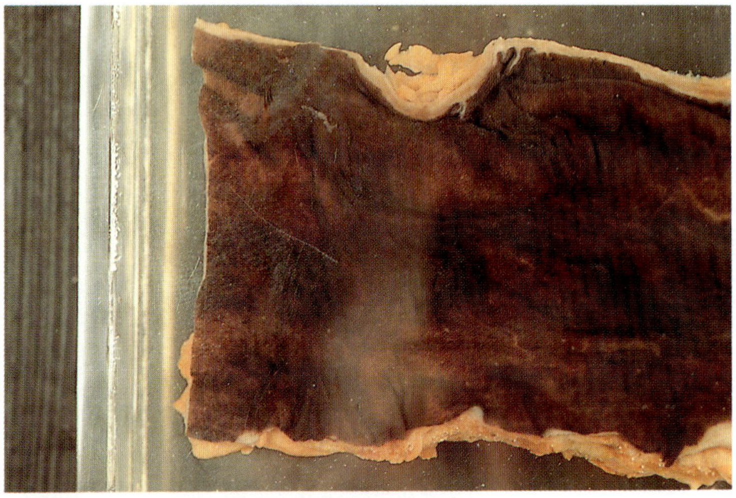

3.152 Colon: Melanosis Coli

This was an incidental finding at post-mortem in 76-year-old woman, who died of pancreatic carcinoma.

This segment of large bowel has been opened to show deep brownish-black pigmentation of the mucosa.

Melanosis coli is a harmless consequence of repeated, long-term use of anthracene purgatives. It is less common now than 50 years ago, but is typically more marked in the caecum and ascending colon. The pigment represents lipofuscin, derived from cellular degradation products, which is taken up by macrophages: it is *not* melanin. Occasionally, prolonged use of purgatives may lead to diarrhoea with potassium and water loss, sometimes with steatorrhoea. This condition, known as cathartic colon, is typified macroscopically by melanosis coli and an unusual 'snake skin' mucosal appearance. In such cases, there is demonstrable damage to neurons in the myenteric plexus. (Courtesy of St. Thomas's Hospital Medical School Museum)

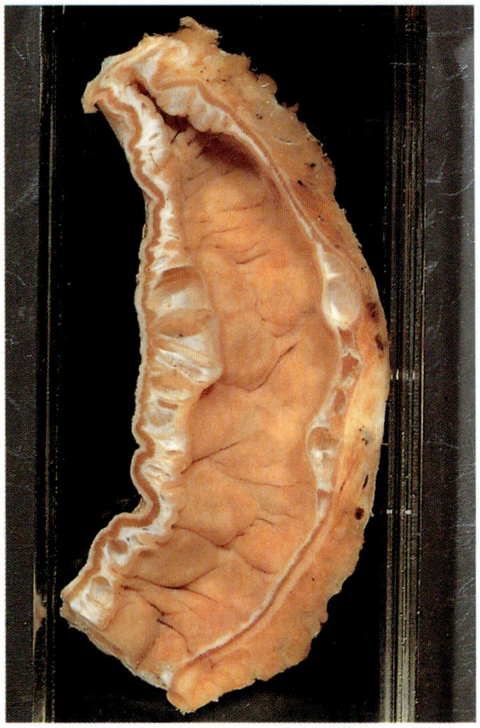

3.153 Colon: Pneumatosis

This specimen was excised from a 56-year-old man who presented with a 10 month history of mild intermittent abdominal pain associated with the passage of blood and mucus per rectum.

Part of the sigmoid colon has been opened to show numerous, thinwalled cysts, measuring up to 1.5cm in diameter, situated predominantly in the submucosa. Elevation of the mucosa by the underlying cysts, which in the fresh state were filled with air, gives a rather cobblestone appearance.

Pneumatosis coli, a condition characterised by gas-filled cysts in the colonic submucosa or serosa, is very uncommon, although identical lesions arising in the small bowel are less rare. The aetiology is unknown but these lesions may be found in childhood (often associated with an episode of necrotising enterocolitis) or in middle-aged adults (often in patients with chronic respiratory disease). While usually asymptomatic, damage to the overlying attenuated mucosa may give rise to rectal bleeding or diarrhoea.

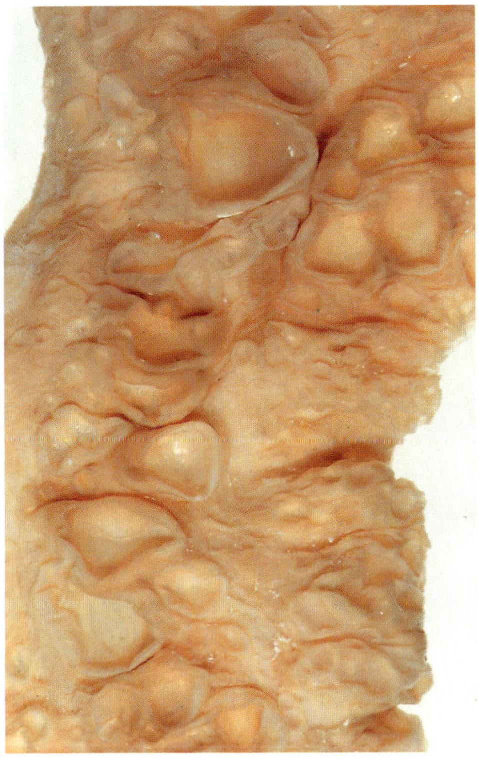

3.154 Colon: Pneumatosis

This was an incidental finding at post-mortem in a 79-year-old man who died of bronchopneumonia.

A segment of the descending colon has been opened to show numerous submucosal cysts (now collapsed), measuring up to 2cm in diameter.

This typical mucosal pattern may sometimes be mistaken for polyposis or Crohn's disease on radiological examination.

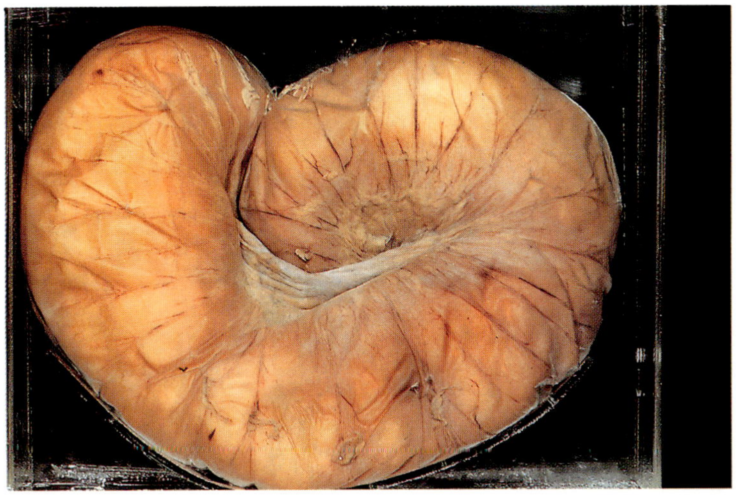

3.155 Sigmoid Colon: Volvulus

This specimen was excised from an 89-year-old man who presented with a one week history of abdominal pain, constipation and increasing distension. A clinical diagnosis of sigmoid volvulus was confirmed by X-ray examination and a laparotomy was performed at which the affected segment was untwisted and resected.

The unopened sigmoid colon, which is much longer than normal, is grossly distended, measuring up to 13cm in diameter. The serosal vessels are engorged but there is no evidence of ischaemic damage.

Large intestinal volvulus, in which the bowel becomes twisted, is fairly uncommon in the Western world but most often affects the sigmoid colon or caecum. Secondary ischaemia due to obstruction of the venous return is not unusual. The most frequent predisposing factor is the presence of an unusually long or mobile segment of bowel but this condition is also more common in the elderly, the chronically constipated or the mentally ill (for which there is no explanation). The principal complications are those of ischaemia (including gangrene), due to vascular obstruction in the twisted mesentery.

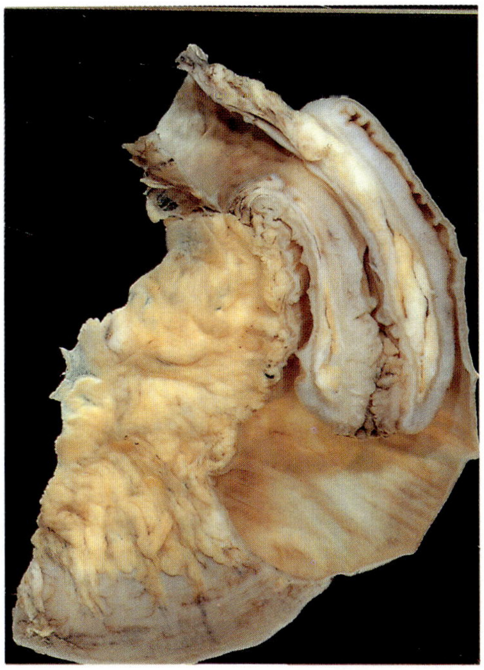

3.156 Colon: Intussusception due to a Carcinoma

This specimen was excised from a 40-year-old woman who presented with a brief history of colicky abdominal pain, diarrhoea and one episode of bleeding per rectum. A mobile mass was palpable in the epigastrium, and the caecum and ascending colon were distended. Laparotomy was performed.

Part of the transverse colon has been opened to show a partially reduced intussusception. A papillary neoplasm located at the apex of the intussusception is obstructing the bowel lumen. The intussuscipiens is markedly oedematous.

Intussusception occurs much less frequently in the large than in the small bowel, although mechanically it is directly comparable (see Legend 3.92 et seq.). However, cases in childhood account for a much smaller percentage and, in adults, a mucosal or mural neoplasm is almost always the predisposing cause (as here).

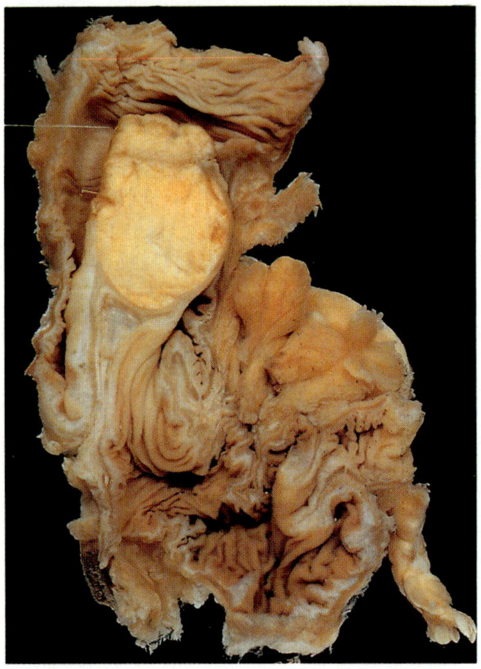

3.157 Colon: Intussusception due to a Lipoma

No clinical details are available.

The caecum and ascending colon have been opened to show an intussusception. The intussusceptum, which measures 9cm in length, has arisen from the lateral wall and contains a well-circumscribed, submucosal lipoma.

Lipomas are the commonest benign colonic tumours to initiate an intussusception, although neoplastic polyps and leiomyomas are sometimes responsible.

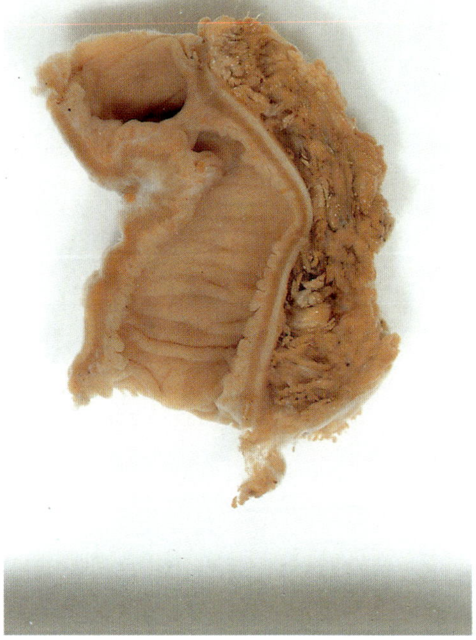

3.158 Colon: Endometriosis

This specimen was excised from a 42-year-old woman, who presented with a 6 month history of non-specific abdominal pain associated with frequency of defaecation and the occasional passage of mucus or blood per rectum. Laparotomy revealed a stricture in the sigmoid colon which was excised.

This segment of large bowel has been opened to show a tight stricture at the site of a fibrous scar (right) and an area of serosal haemorrhage (left).

Endometriosis (see Chapter 5) is only seen in women of reproductive age and is characterised by the presence of ectopic endometrial tissue outside the uterus. Pelvic structures, including the intestines, are most often affected and local adhesions are a common complication. Occasionally a small, rather fibrous mass ('endometrioma') is formed, as in this case, and obstruction may result.

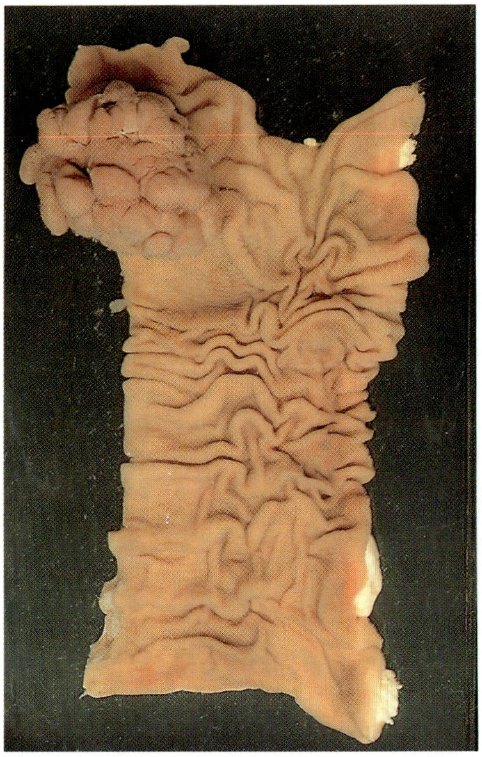

3.159 Colon: Tubular Adenoma (Neoplastic Polyp)

This specimen was excised from an adult male who presented with a 2 month history of rectal bleeding and an altered bowel habit. At laparotomy a polypoid lesion was found in the sigmoid colon and was resected.

A segment of the sigmoid colon has been opened to show a rounded, pedunculated neoplasm, which measures 3cm in diameter, projecting from the mucosa. The surface of the polyp has a smooth, nodular appearance.

Neoplastic polyps of the large bowel (synonym: adenomatous polyps) may be divided into 3 types: tubular, tubulovillous and villous, of which the mixed tubulovillous variant is the most usual. They are extremely common, particularly with advancing age, in the Western population. The true incidence is uncertain as many remain asymptomatic. The aetiology is thought to parallel that of colonic adenocarcinoma (see Legend 3.164).

The polyps may be solitary or multiple; only when they exceed approximately 100 in number is the diagnosis of familial polyposis suggested (see Figure and Legend 3.162 et seq.). They arise at any site in the large bowel but the largest (and more often symptomatic) lesions tend to be situated in the left side of the colon. An important feature, which all 3 types have in common, is the invariable presence of epithelial dysplasia which amounts, quite often, to carcinoma-in-situ and as such they are all premalignant.

Factors which are thought to increase the risk of true invasive malignant change are:

1) increasing polyp size (particularly if greater than 2cm in diameter);
2) the severity of epithelial dysplasia, and
3) the histological type of polyp, villous being more dangerous than tubular.

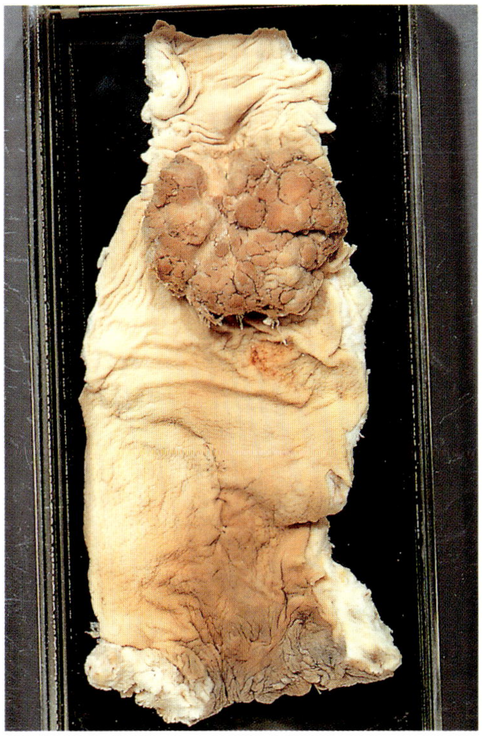

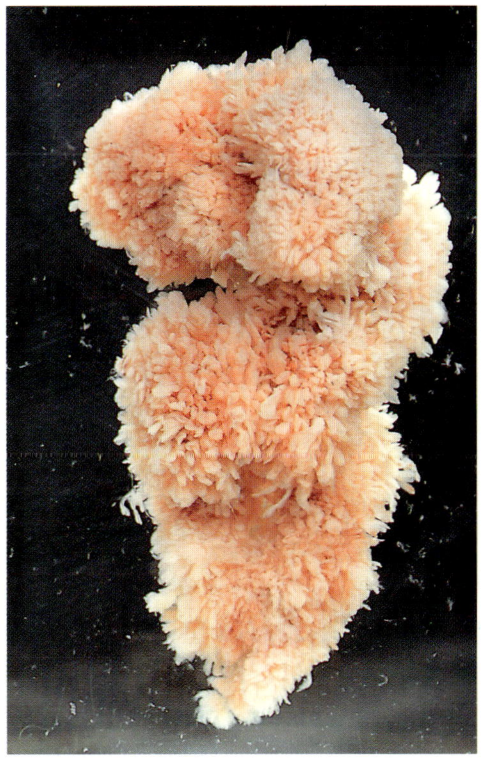

3.161 Rectum: Villous Adenoma (Neoplastic Polyp)

This specimen was excised from a 48-year-old man, who presented with a 5 month history of intermittent rectal bleeding. Examination revealed a villous tumour in the posterior rectal wall, which was histologically proven to be benign, and local excision was performed.

The specimen consists of a typical villous neoplasm, measuring 7 × 3 × 0.5cm. The numerous frond-like processes are particularly well shown in this case.

Recognised complications of neoplastic polyps, other than the development of carcinoma, include rectal bleeding, hypokalaemia (usually due to excessive mucus secretion from a large villous adenoma) and intussusception.

3.160 Rectum: Villous Adenoma (Neoplastic Polyp)

This specimen was excised from a 76-year-old woman who underwent an abdominoperineal resection for removal of this large rectal tumour.

The distal rectum is distended by a large, sessile (broadbased), villous (papillary) neoplasm, which measures 8cm in diameter. The surface of the tumour is composed of numerous frond-like processes. Histologically there was no evidence of invasion.

Villous adenomas (synonym: villous papillomas) account for only about 10 per cent of neoplastic polyps. They are typically large, broad-based and ill-defined lesions which show a predilection for the rectum. As a consequence of their large size, broad base and the presence of severe dysplasia, they are particularly prone to progress to true adenocarcinoma: the risk of such a change is estimated to be approximately 40 per cent.

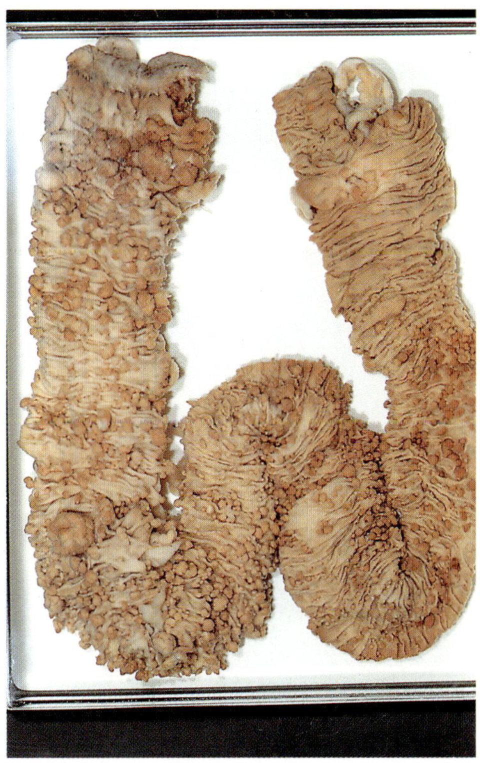

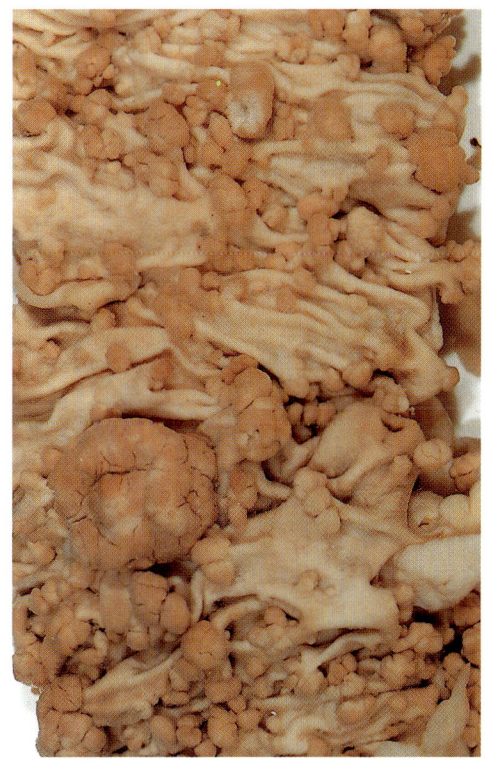

3.162 Colon: Familial Polyposis with two Adenocarcinomas

This specimen was excised from a 36-year-old man who presented with a 2 week history of diarrhoea and vomiting, associated with lower abdominal pain. Barium enema showed multiple filling defects throughout the entire colon, compatible with polyposis, and biopsy of a broad-based lesion in the rectum revealed invasive adenocarcinoma. On careful questioning the patient had a strong family history of colonic carcinoma.

The entire large bowel has been opened to show numerous tubular adenomas projecting from the mucosa, the majority of which measure less than 1cm in diameter (3.162a). Note that the polyps are larger and more numerous in the distal colon, while the caecum and ascending colon are relatively spared. In addition, in the distal rectum there is a larger, more nodular lesion from which the biopsy was taken and a similar lesion, seen in close-up (3.162b), just beyond the splenic flexure was also shown to be a carcinoma.

Familial polyposis coli is an autosomal dominantly inherited condition, characterised by the development of hundreds (or even thousands) of neoplastic polyps in the large bowel. These polyps, which tend mainly to be tubular or tubulovillous in type, seem to appear in the 2nd or 3rd decades but are not present in early childhood. The principal importance of familial polyposis coli is that every affected individual, if left untreated, will eventually develop large intestinal adenocarcinoma, often at multiple sites. The latent period between polyp formation and progression to carcinoma seems to be of the order of 10 years; as a consequence it is recommended that all patients with familial polyposis should undergo prophylactic panproctocolectomy.

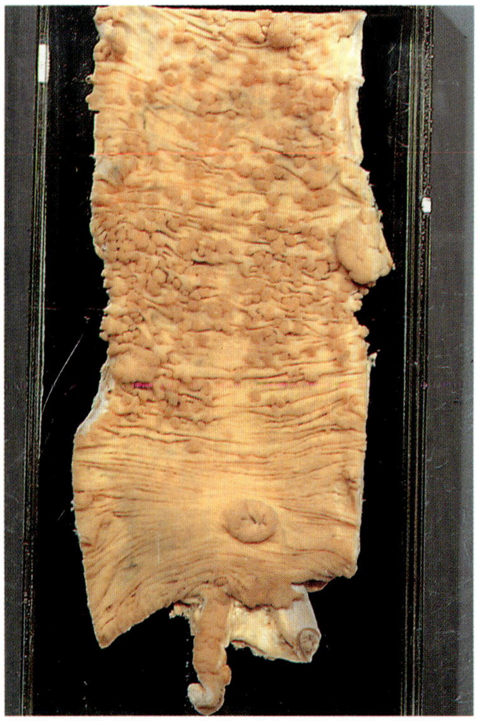

3.163 Colon: Familial Polyposis Coli

This specimen was excised from a 29-year-old man who presented with a 2 month history of rectal bleeding. Barium enema revealed multiple polyps and a rectal adenocarcinoma. An anterior resection was carried out. Thereafter he remained well and 6 and 18 months later, left and right prophylactic hemicolectomies were performed.

This opened caecum and ascending colon, with attached appendix, shows multiple tubular adenomata which increase in number distally. The rounded structure visible in the proximal caecum is the orifice of the ileocaecal valve.

It is typical in familial polyposis coli to find that the number and size of the adenomata present increase progressively from the caecum to the rectum.

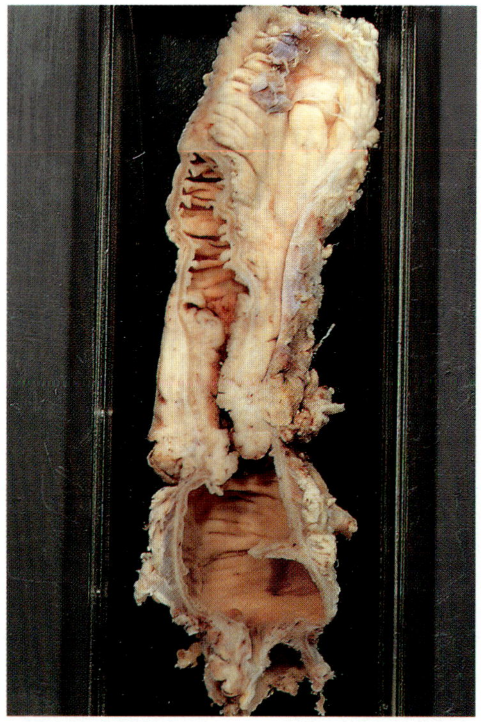

3.164 Rectum: Adenocarcinoma

This specimen was excised from a 59-year-old man who, having suffered episodic diarrhoea, presented with large bowel obstruction. An abdominoperineal resection was performed.

The rectum and distal sigmoid colon have been opened to show a fungating, pale neoplasm arising in the proximal rectum. The tumour has virtually occluded the bowel lumen and has visibly penetrated the full thickness of the bowel wall. An enlarged lymph node, replaced by metastatic tumour, is apparent in the adjacent mesenteric fat.

Carcinoma of the large bowel is the second most common cause of death from malignant disease in Britain and is very common in the Western world. It most often presents in the 6th and 7th decades and shows a moderate predilection for males (except in the caecum, see Legend 3.167). Epidemiologically, the incidence is highest in Westernised countries, this tumour being very rare in parts of Africa and Asia. The following may be important aetiological factors:
1) a low fibre diet (increased intestinal transit time allows prolonged contact with carcinogens);
2) a high fat diet, or
3) a diet-induced alteration in intestinal bacterial flora (leading to impaired degradation of bile salts, which may be carcinogenic).
Recognised predispositions include a positive familial tendency and an association with pre-existent colonic adenomata, familial polyposis, ulcerative colitis and ureterosigmoidostomy. Topographically, the majority of these tumours arise in the left side of the large bowel, particularly the rectum (corresponding to the sites at which neoplastic polyps are most common). Interestingly, in low incidence areas, carcinoma is more frequent in the right colon and tends to present in younger individuals. Up to 5 per cent of patients, either synchronously or asynchronously, develop more than one colonic cancer.

The 5-year-survival correlates well with the degree of histological differentiation (being approximately 60 per cent for moderately differentiated lesions which are the most common) and with the Dukes' system of pathological staging. At operation approximately half the cases are already Dukes' stage C, for which the 5-year-survival is approximately 30 per cent. In up to 15 per cent of cases, careful histological examination reveals transition from a neoplastic polyp to invasive adenocarcinoma, underlining the premalignant nature of such polyps.

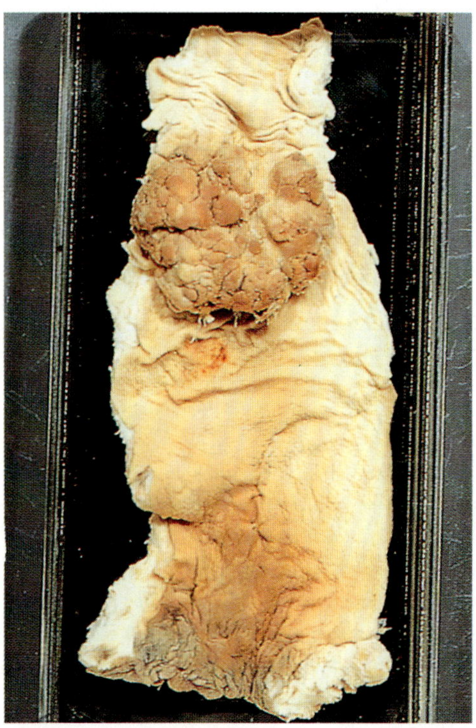

3.165 Rectum: Adenocarcinoma

This specimen was excised from an 81-year-old woman who had been passing bright red blood per rectum for the previous 6 months. Examination revealed a polypoid tumour in the lower rectum; biopsy revealed invasive adenocarcinoma. An abdominoperineal resection was performed.

In the distal rectum, 11cm proximal to the anal margin, a fungating, multinodular neoplasm is present. In the fresh state, the tumour was confined to the bowel wall macroscopically and was very well differentiated histologically.

Macroscopically, the majority of colonic cancers are exophytic in appearance, although they very commonly show central ulceration. A significant proportion, however, show an annular stenosing pattern (see Figures 3.166 and 3.168). In contrast to gastric lesions, diffuse scirrhous tumours are extremely unusual. It is interesting to note that, in the very elderly, colonic adenocarcinoma is often very well differentiated (as here) and often carries a comparatively good prognosis.

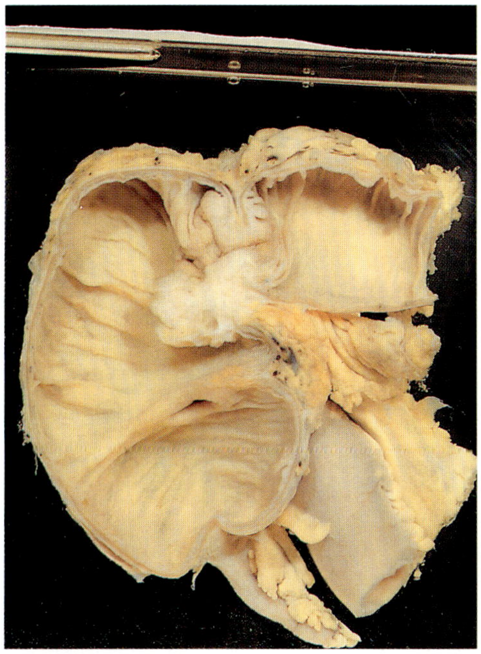

3.166 Ascending Colon: Adenocarcinoma

This specimen was excised from a 57-year-old man who presented with a one year history of right upper quadrant abdominal pain. Examination revealed a tender mass beneath the right costal margin and barium enema showed a tumour just proximal to the hepatic flexure. A right hemicolectomy was performed.

The distal ileum, caecum and ascending colon have been opened to show an annular stenosing neoplasm at the hepatic flexure; the bowel lumen has been reduced to a narrow cleft. Proximally, there is obvious dilatation of the intestine with some associated muscular hypertrophy.

Carcinomas of the transverse colon and either hepatic or splenic flexures account for approximately 10 per cent of the total cases, being rather less common than caecal neoplasms and much less frequent than recto-sigmoid tumours. The annular stenosing appearance, which may be seen at any site, is facilitated by circumferential spread of the tumour in submucosal (or serosal) lymphatic channels.

Large bowel obstruction, is the commonest complication of colonic carcinoma and may lead to proximal stercoral ulceration or perforation. Obstruction is the principal reason for the fact that up to 30 per cent of cases present as a surgical emergency. Other complications include iron-deficiency anaemia, hypokalaemia (particularly associated with large villous rectal lesions) and intussusception in adults.

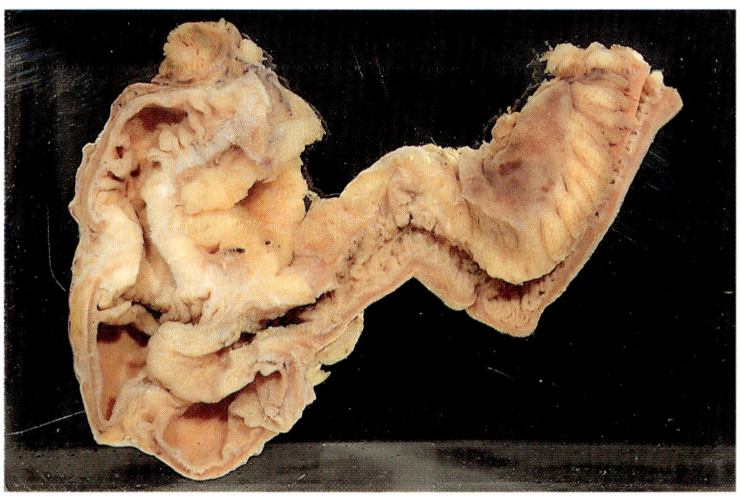

3.167 Caecum: Adenocarcinoma

This specimen was excised from a 68-year-old woman, with a long history of iron-deficiency anaemia, who presented with a one month history of increasing tiredness and a lump in the lower right abdomen. A mass was palpable in the right iliac fossa and barium enema revealed a caecal carcinoma. An extended right hemicolectomy was performed.

The terminal ileum and caecum have been opened to show an annular, pale neoplasm arising just distal to the ileo-caecal valve. The tumour has visibly penetrated the full thickness of the bowel wall.

Adenocarcinoma of the caecum accounts for about 10-15 per cent of all large bowel cancers and, in contrast to the majority, is most common in females. Owing to the distensibility of the caecum (which diminishes the risk of obstruction) and the fact that any bleeding will be altered before its passage per rectum, these tumours often remain asymptomatic for some considerable time, thus very often being Dukes' stage C at operation. A common mode of presentation is as long-standing or refractory iron-deficiency anaemia.

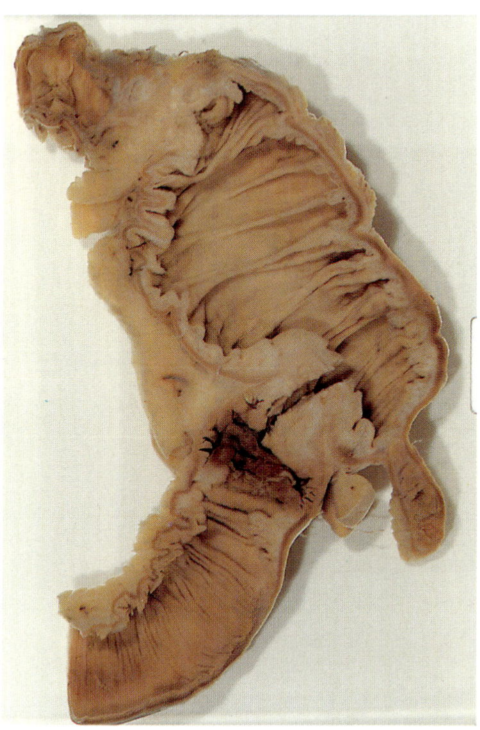

3.168 Ascending Colon: Adenocarcinoma

This specimen was excised from a 70-year-old man who presented with a one month history of colicky abdominal pain associated with anorexia and weight loss. On examination, intermittent visible peristalsis was apparent in the right iliac fossa and there was a palpable mass. A right hemicolectomy was performed.

The distal ileum, caecum and ascending colon have been opened to show an annular stenosing neoplasm, measuring 3cm in length, that has almost completely occluded the bowel lumen. The proximal large bowel is distended and shows prominent muscular hypertrophy.

This is a particularly good example of an obstructive annular carcinoma. Tumours of the hepatic flexure or transverse colon, by virtue of extensive local invasion, may occasionally form fistulae with the duodenum or stomach.

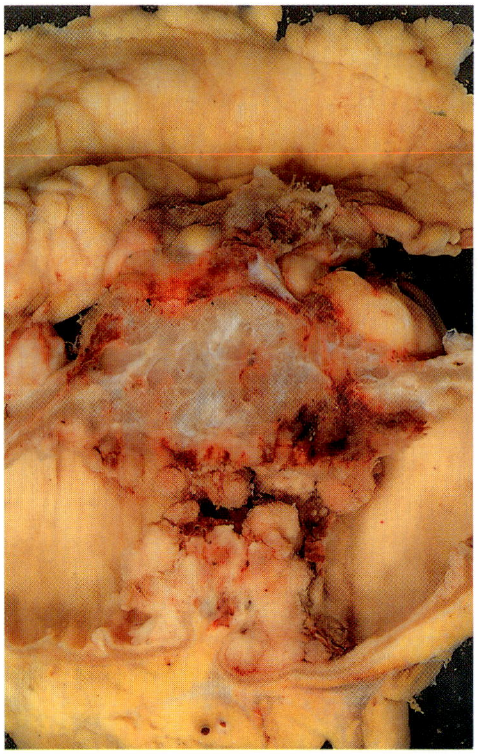

3.169 Transverse Colon: Colloid Carcinoma

No clinical details are available.

This segment of large bowel has been opened to show an exophytic neoplasm which has clearly infiltrated through the full thickness of the bowel wall into the greater omentum. Note the pale gelatinous appearance of the bulk of the tumour.

Approximately 10 per cent of colonic cancers show copious mucus secretion, rendering the tumour soft and myxoid in nature. Such tumours tend to arise in relatively younger individuals and peritoneal spread or perforation may sometimes give rise to pseudomyxoma peritonei (see Figure and Legend 3.119).

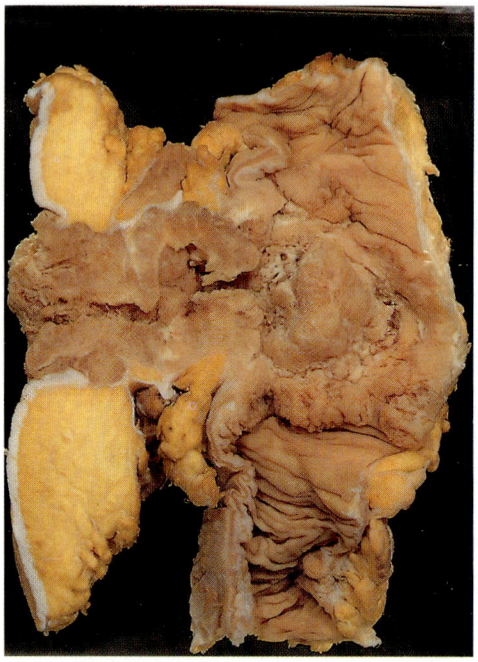

3.170 Transverse Colon: Adenocarcinoma with Extensive Local Invasion

This specimen was excised from a 40-year-old woman who presented with a short history of a supra-umbilical mass associated with a discharging sinus: this had been preceded by 3 weeks of nausea and peri-umbilical pain. Examination revealed an abscess cavity in the anterior abdominal wall and a biopsy was diagnosed as adenocarcinoma. Laparotomy was performed.

Part of the transverse colon, with overlying subcutaneous fat and skin, has been dissected to show an ulcerated neoplasm which, having penetrated the bowel wall, has extended as a fistulous track (lined by tumour) to the skin surface.

Local invasion by colonic cancer, while most often confined to the bowel wall above and below the tumour, may sometimes be extensive, particularly in poorly differentiated or pelvic neoplasms. It should also be noted that adenocarcinoma of the large bowel is particularly prone to 'implantation' metastasis i.e. the seeding of metastases by cells shed intra-operatively into the wound or adjacent viscera.

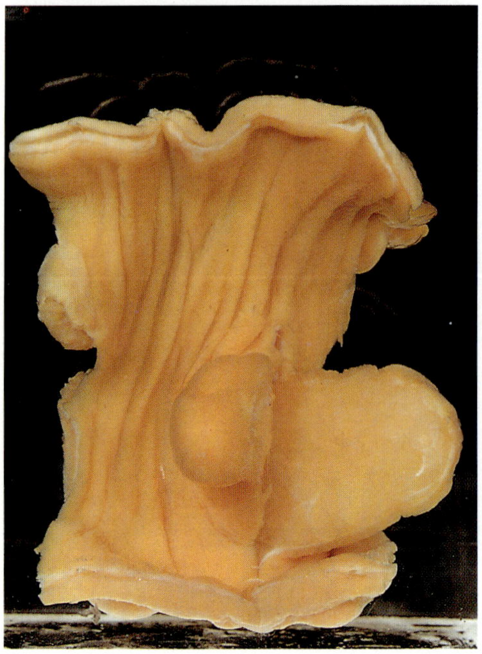

3.171 Colon: Submucosal Lipoma

This specimen was excised from a 46-year-old woman who presented with acute abdominal pain. Laparotomy revealed a retrograde colonic intussusception, at the apex of which was a palpable mass.

This segment of large bowel has been opened to show a broad, pedunculated, fatty tumour, measuring 2.5 × 2 × 1.5cm, which arises in the submucosa. The cut surface (right) shows that the lesion is covered by a layer of normal mucosa.

Lipomas arising in the large bowel are relatively rare benign lesions which most often present either by precipitating an intussusception (as here) or by giving rise to rectal bleeding as a result of superficial ulceration. They are most often submucosal in origin.

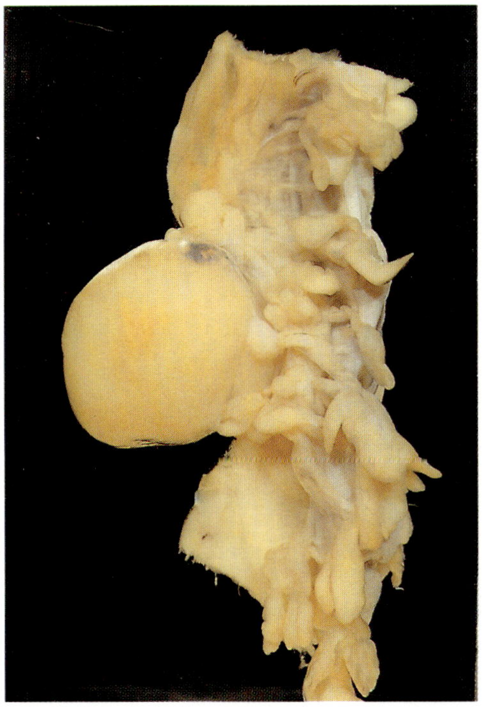

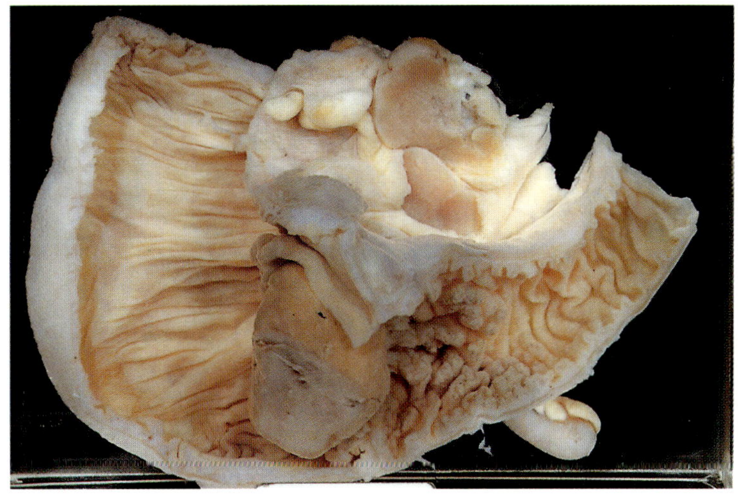

3.173 Caecum: Non-Hodgkin's Lymphoma

This specimen was excised from a 10-year-old girl, who presented with a 6 week history of intermittent colicky abdominal pain. The pain became more continuous and localised to the right iliac fossa and a laparotomy was performed.

Arising in the caecum, just distal to the ileocaecal valve, is a large, polypoid neoplasm, measuring 4 × 4 × 3cm, which has resulted in almost complete luminal obstruction. Note the adjacent enlarged mesenteric nodes.

Primary lymphomas (nearly always non-Hodgkin's in type) of the large bowel are less common than those in the small intestine but most often arise in the caecum. The case here was classified as diffuse centroblastic (Kiel). Macroscopically, annular, locally infiltrative lesions are more common than the intraluminal growth seen here. Predisposing conditions include ulcerative colitis and various malabsorptive conditions. The prognosis is very variable.

3.172 Colon: Subserosal Lipoma

This was an incidental finding at post-mortem in a 66-year-old man who died of a coronary thrombosis.

Arising from the serosal surface of this portion of large bowel is a pedunculated, fatty tumour which is covered by the visceral peritoneum.

Subserosal lipomas of the large bowel very often remain asymptomatic.

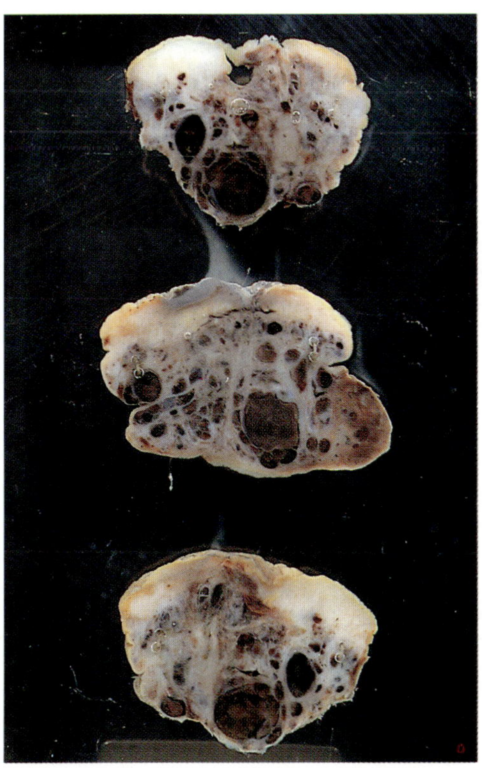

3.174 Anal Canal: Haemorrhoids

No clinical details are available.

Three excised haemorrhoids have been sectioned to show a large number of dilated vascular spaces beneath the surface epithelium, many of which are thrombosed.

Haemorrhoids represent dilated venous plexuses, derived from the superior rectal vein, which are usually situated in the submucosa just above the dentate line. They are ubiquitous, and are usually asymptomatic. Possible causes include chronic straining at defaecation or micturition, a muscular abnormality of the anal sphincter, the erect posture and a familial tendency. Secondary causes may include pregnancy or an adjacent rectal carcinoma. In long-standing cases, similar lesions, distal to the dentate line, may arise from the anal submucosa. Complications include bleeding, thrombosis, strangulation, prolapse and infection.

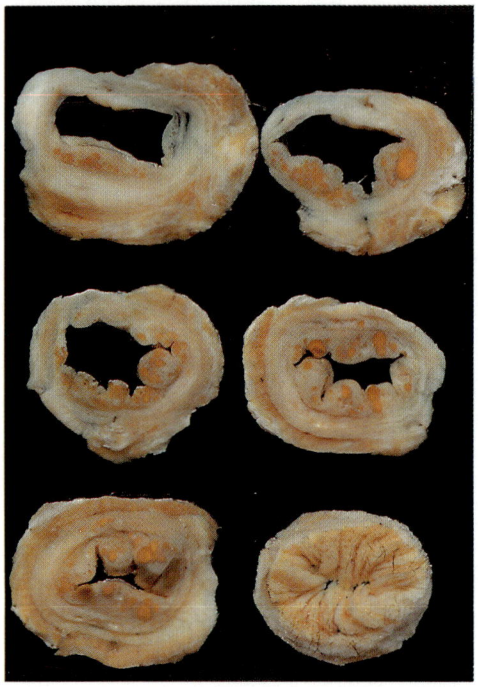

3.175 Anal Canal: Haemorrhoids

No clinical details are available.

These are a series of transverse sections through the anal canal which show symmetrical submucosal swellings. Owing to the extreme age of the specimen (being collected in 1867), thrombi within the ectatic venous plexuses appear yellowish in colour.

When viewed from the lithotomy position, haemorrhoids are typically distributed in the 3, 7 and 11 o'clock positions in the anorectal canal, corresponding in location to the terminal divisions of the superior rectal vein. However, smaller lesions commonly distort this distribution by presenting in between these 3 principal sites.

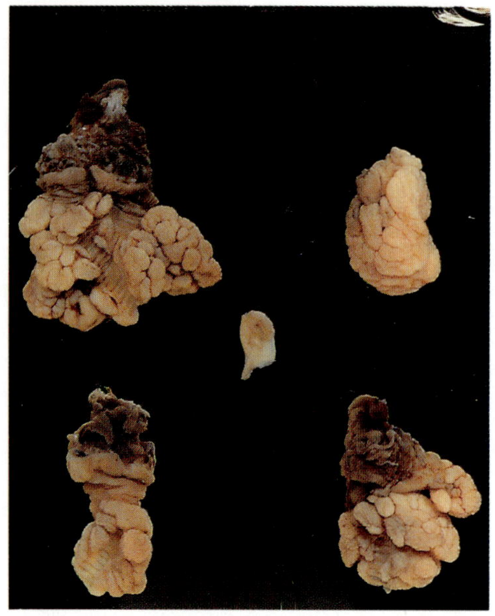

3.176 Anal Canal: Haemorrhoids Complicated by Viral Warts

These specimens were excised from a 46 year-old man who presented with a 5 day history of rectal bleeding. Examination revealed a cluster of anal warts and, at operation, the patient was also found to have prolapsed piles, some with warts developing on them.

Three haemorrhoids, showing marked submucosal congestion (top and bottom left, bottom right) and two simple warts are shown. Each piece of tissue shows exuberant, papilliferous overgrowth of the surface epithelium.

Viral (venereal) warts (synonym: condylomata acuminata) arise from anal or perianal skin; since the surface of long-standing haemorrhoids may undergo squamous metaplasia, warts may also present at that site. Such viral warts are extremely common and are due to infection by one of the human papillomaviruses. It is thought that they may, on occasion, predispose to the development of verrucous carcinoma (a well-differentiated variant of squamous carcinoma). They should be distinguished clinically from condylomata lata, which are syphilitic in origin and tend to be more pedunculated with a smooth, moist surface.

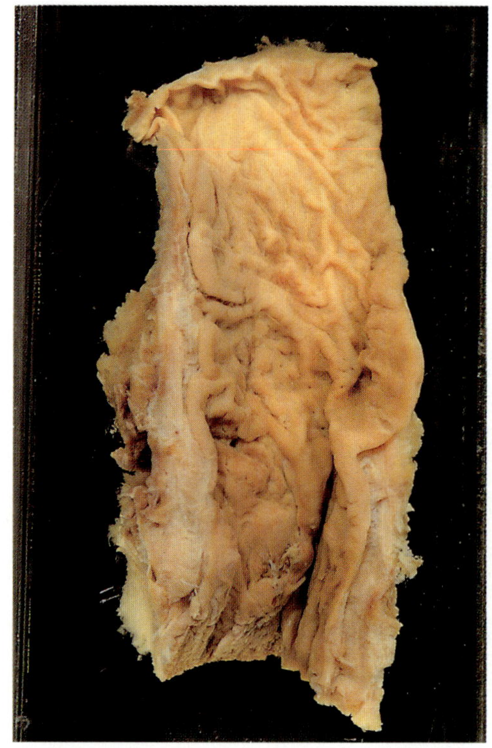

3.177 Anorectal Junction: Adenocarcinoma

This specimen was excised from a 64-year-old man who presented with a 3 month history of passing frequent, small stools. A small tumour was palpable in the anal canal and biopsy revealed an adenocarcinoma. Abdominoperineal resection was performed.

The distal rectum and anal canal have been opened to show an ulcerated neoplasm, measuring 3cm in diameter, which has arisen above the anorectal junction but has spread by local infiltration to involve the anal mucosa.

While this case should be classified as a colonic adenocarcinoma (see Figure and Legend 3.164 et seq.), it is worth noting that poorly differentiated rectal tumours do occasionally show extensive intramural spread (either upward or downward), thus sometimes presenting as an anal neoplasm. This type of spread is, however, comparatively unusual in large bowel cancers, in contrast to gastric adenocarcinoma.

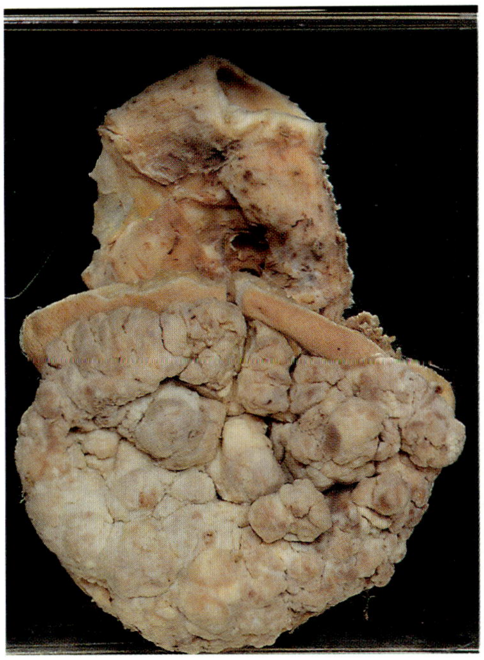

3.178 Anus: Squamous Carcinoma

This specimen was excised from a 56-year-old vagrant who gave a 5 year history of increasingly severe anal ulceration, for which he had never previously sought treatment. An abdominoperineal resection was performed.

The distal (unopened) rectum, anus and perineal skin are mounted to show a very large, ulcerated and polypoid neoplasm completely obscuring the anal orifice. The tumour, which measures 12cm in diameter, shows extensive perineal involvement.

Squamous carcinomas of the anus are divided into those tumours arising in the anal canal (most often above the dentate line) and those arising in skin at the anal margin. Both are comparatively uncommon, being at least 20 times less frequent than rectal adenocarcinoma. The aetiology is uncertain, although lack of personal cleanliness or anal intercourse may be implicated. Tumours of the anal canal, which are 3 times as common as those at the anal margin, tend to proximal rectal spread and dissemination predominantly to intrapelvic lymph nodes; the 5-year-survival is about 50 per cent. In contrast, squamous cancers arising at the anal margin tend to be slow-growing neoplasms which metastasise to inguinal nodes and have a 5-year-survival of approximately 70 per cent.

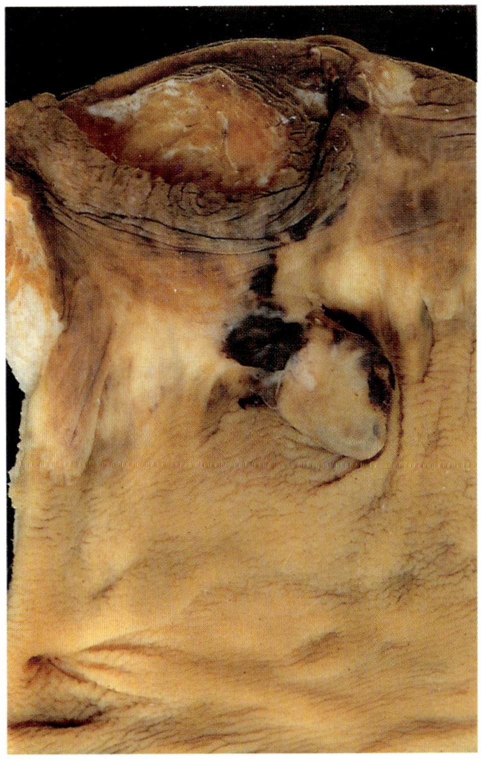

3.179 Anus: Malignant Melanoma

This specimen was excised from a 74-year-old woman who presented with a brief history of episodic rectal bleeding. A hard mass was palpable in the lateral wall of the anal canal and an abdominoperineal resection was performed.

The anal canal has been opened to show a flattened, ovoid nodule, measuring 2cm in diameter, arising at about the level of the dentate line. The edge of the tumour shows obvious melanotic pigmentation and an irregular streak of pigment extends from the nodule to the anal margin.

Anal malignant melanoma, like squamous carcinoma, can be divided into two types; those tumours arising in the anal canal and those arising from anal skin. The latter group are entirely comparable to conventional cutaneous malignant melanomas (see Chapter 8). Malignant melanoma of the anal canal is fairly rare and tends to present in late adulthood in either sex. It shows a predilection for extensive local invasion and early lymph node metastasis such that 5-year-survival is virtually nil and most patients die within a year.

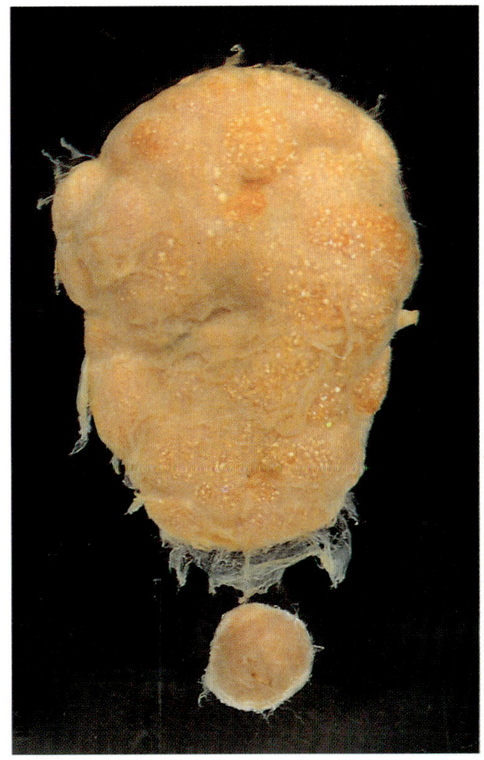

3.180 Peritoneum: 'Loose Bodies'

These were coincidental findings at laparotomy in an obese patient.

Two approximately spherical masses of fatty tissue, the larger measuring 4.5cm in maximum diameter, are shown. The latter shows fine granular calcification over its peritoneal surface.

Peritoneal loose bodies are very common and are thought to represent colonic appendices epiploicae (i.e. pouches of the visceral peritoneum filled with fat) which have separated from the bowel wall, usually by aseptic necrosis. The latter may occasionally undergo torsion and present with acute abdominal pain, but most often their dislocation from the bowel is entirely asymptomatic.

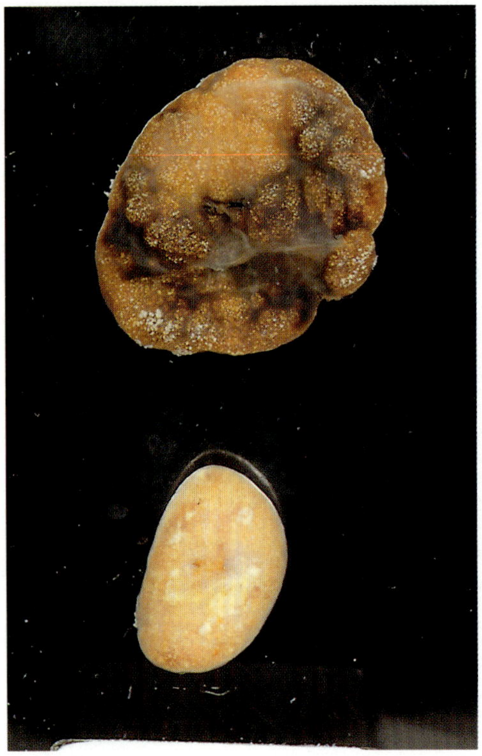

3.181 Peritoneum: Torted Appendix Epiploica and 'Loose Body'

These specimens were removed from a 32-year-old man who presented with lower abdominal pain and a fever. At laparotomy, a gangrenous appendix epiploica was removed from the rectosigmoid junction and a loose body was found in the pelvis.

Above, the torted appendix epiploica shows obvious haemorrhagic necrosis; below, the loose body shows extensive calcification.

Following necrosis, loose bodies (also known as peritoneal 'mice') commonly undergo fibrosis, hyalinisation and dystrophic calcification, such that they may even become apparent on a plain abdominal X-ray.

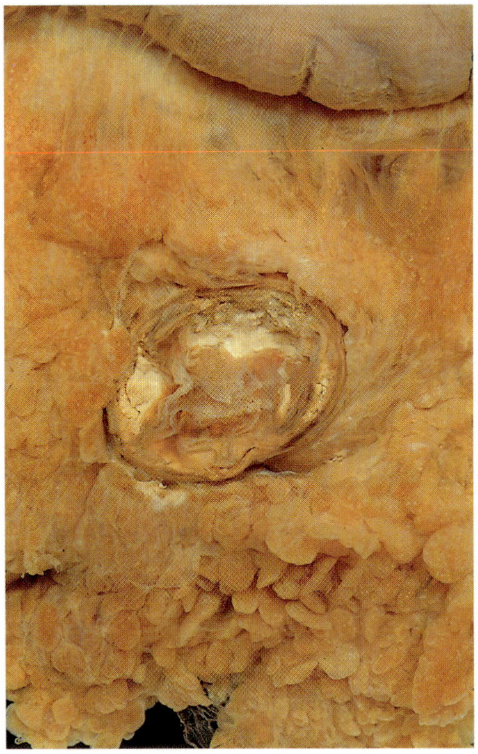

3.182 Greater Omentum: Hydatid Cyst

This was a coincidental finding at post-mortem in a 47-year-old woman from Australia.

Within the omental fat, beneath the transverse colon, is an ovoid cyst, measuring 3.5cm in diameter. Within its cavity, a compressed, folded hydatid membrane is apparent and there is extensive dystrophic calcification.

Hydatid disease is caused by ingestion of the ova of the tapeworm *Echinococcus granulosus* and is most often seen in sheep farming communities, usually being transmitted by dogs which act as the intermediate host. The organisms invade the portal venous system and are thence carried to all parts of the body. The cysts are typically multilocular, containing numerous daughter cysts within which the brood capsules are formed. The case here shows little evidence of disease activity, being apparently 'burnt out'. The diagnosis may be made by demonstration of cutaneous hypersensitivity to hydatid antigen, the Casoni test.

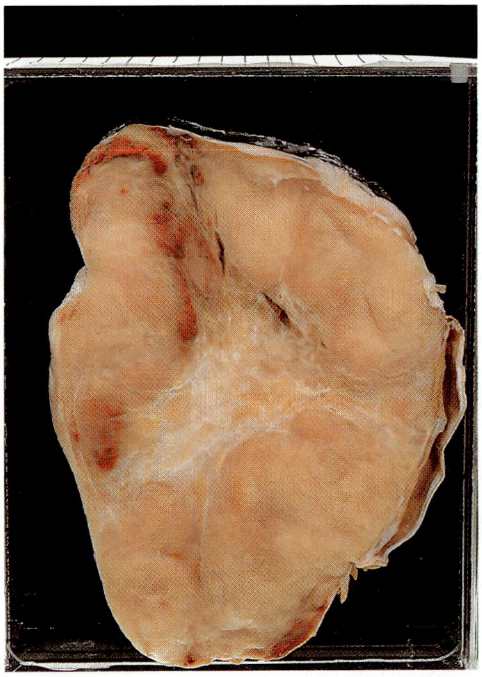

3.183 Mesocolon: Metastatic Myxoid Liposarcoma

This specimen was excised from a 68-year-old woman who had undergone resection of a myxoid liposarcoma from the right thigh only a few weeks previously. She represented with an abdominal mass and a metastasis in the left breast.

A section through this secondary deposit of tumour shows it to be pale and rather well circumscribed; in the fresh state it was gelatinous in consistency. Note a compressed segment of large bowel on the right.

Liposarcoma is typically a tumour of late adulthood which most often arises in the limbs (particularly the thigh) or the retroperitoneum. There are 4 principal histological subtypes, well-differentiated, myxoid, lipoblastic and pleomorphic, of which the myxoid variant is most common. All have a tendency to recur and up to 50 per cent metastasise, especially the lipoblastic and pleomorphic subtypes. While myxoid liposarcoma usually tends to a relatively better prognosis, it should be noted that this patient had noticed the primary thigh tumour for 6 years and did not present until it had ulcerated through the skin.

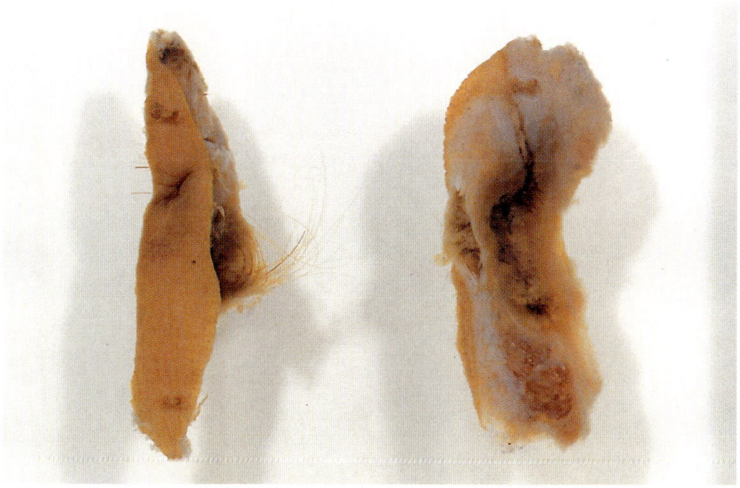

3.184 Natal Cleft: Pilonidal Sinus

This specimen was excised from a 44-year-old man who had noticed an infected lesion between his buttocks. On examination there was a small cutaneous sinus over the tip of the coccyx, from which a tuft of hair projected. Excision was performed.

The affected skin and subcutaneous tissue has been bisected to show a loculated abscess cavity (right), which opens onto the skin surface through a narrow sinus. On the left, the opposite portion of the cavity is seen to contain a small mass of matted hair.

Pilonidal sinuses are common, acquired lesions which result from the impaction of shed hairs in skin or sebaceous glands. Males are predominantly affected, particularly in the 3rd decade of life and the natal cleft is by far the most common site. They may also, however, be seen in the axilla and the interdigital clefts of hairdressers. Impaction of the hair or hairs leads to local suppurative inflammation with abscess formation and the development of ramifying sinus tracks.

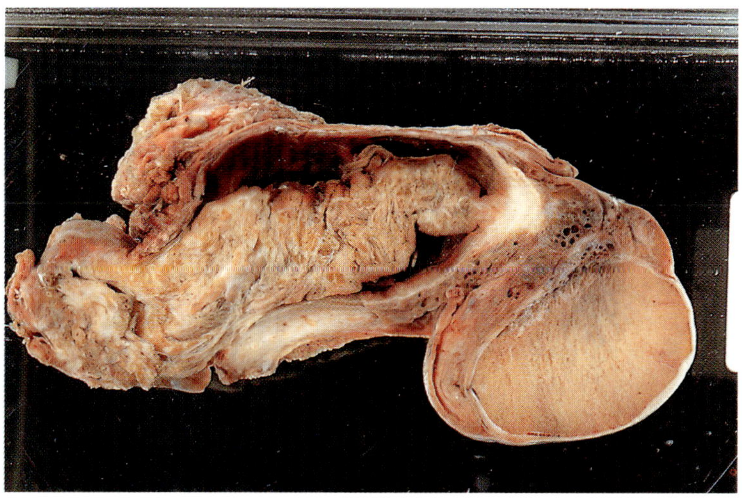

3.185 Indirect Inguinal Hernia

This specimen was excised from a 68-year-old man who had suffered from an inguinal hernia since childhood.

A longitudinal section through the hernial sac, with attached testis, shows it to be filled with a portion of incarcerated omentum. The grey areas in the omental fat, when examined histologically, were found to be metastatic deposits of adenocarcinoma, derived from a gastric cancer which had been resected 4 months previously.

Indirect inguinal herniae, which are extremely common, are thought to develop within the sac of a persistent processus vaginalis and therefore pass down the inguinal canal. Males are most often affected but, in contrast to direct herniae, presentation may be at any age, and frequently in childhood. The most important complication is strangulation of the entrapped contents, be they bowel, mesentery or omentum.

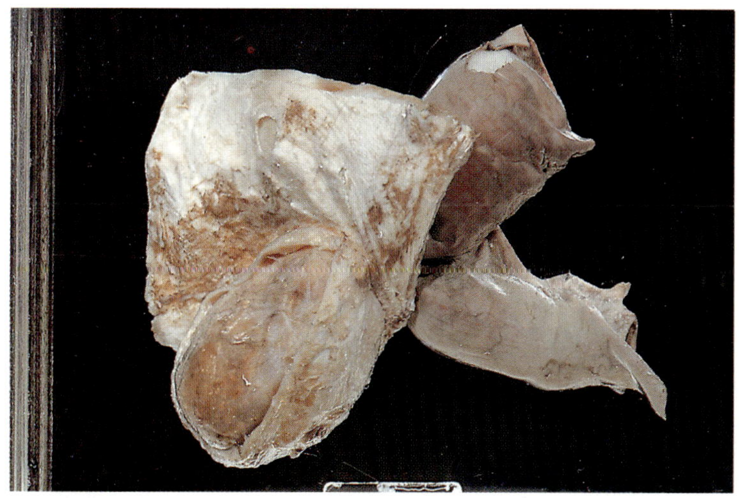

3.186 Direct Inguinal Hernia

No clinical details are available.

A loop of discoloured small bowel, covered in serosanguinous exudate, can be seen protruding through a gap in the transversalis fascia. The proximal bowel (top right) is dilated and markedly congested.

About 15 per cent of inguinal herniae are direct in type. They are commonly bilateral, arise almost exclusively in males and develop due to a congenital or acquired weakness or a gap in the transversalis fascia in the posterior aspect of the inguinal canal. Heavy lifting, a chronic cough, or straining at stool are predisposing factors. Strangulation, as here, is relatively unusual.

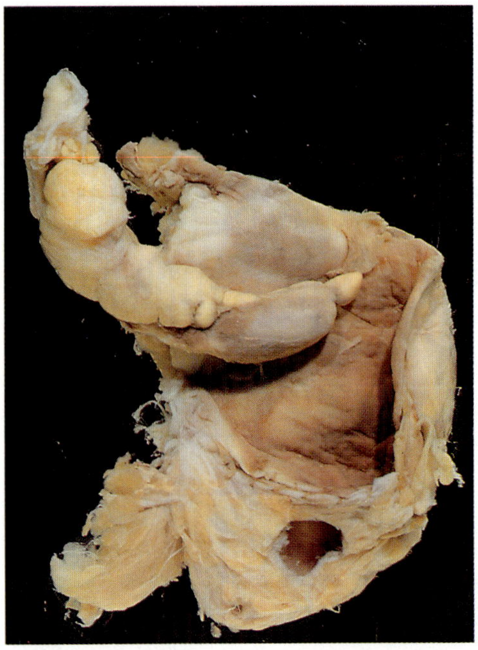

3.187 Femoral Hernia

This specimen was excised from a 45-year-old woman who had noticed a swelling in the right groin for 20 years. She presented with a brief history of severe abdominal pain. Examination revealed a tender femoral hernia, measuring 8cm in length, which at operation, was found to contain an acutely inflamed appendix.

The hernial sac, which is markedly congested, has been opened to show that it contains the distal portion of the appendix, the tip of which is gangrenous.

Femoral herniae are less common than the inguinal or incisional types but are seen most often in middle-aged females. They represent protrusion of intraperitoneal tissues into the femoral canal, are most common on the right and are frequently bilateral. Because of the tight femoral ring they are at a very significant risk of becoming strangulated.

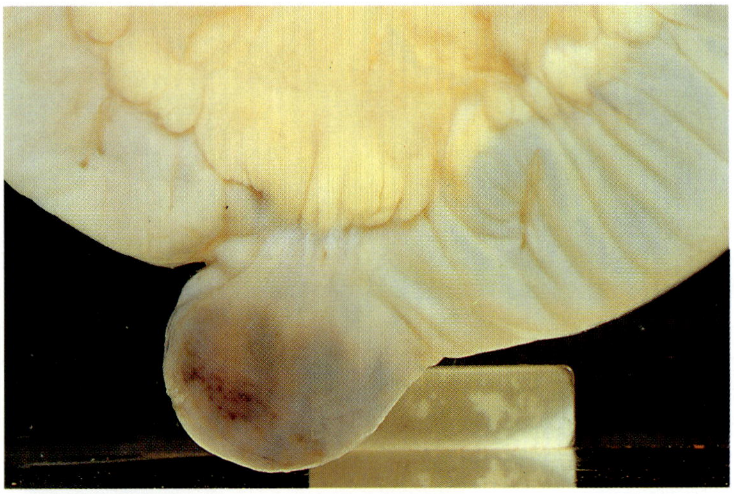

3.188 Ileum: Richter's Hernia

This is a post-mortem specimen from a 64-year-old female patient from a long-term psychiatric hospital. After apparently being constipated for only a short time she rapidly developed profuse vomiting with hypotension and died.

The specimen consists of a loop of ileum; a portion of the wall is gangrenous, having become strangulated in a hernial sac. Although only about two-thirds of the bowel circumference is involved, the lumen is completely obstructed.

Richter's hernia, in which only part of the bowel circumference becomes entrapped, is most often seen as a complication of a femoral hernia. Symptoms and signs are often non-specific such that paralytic ileus or strangulation may supervene before the true nature of the condition becomes apparent.

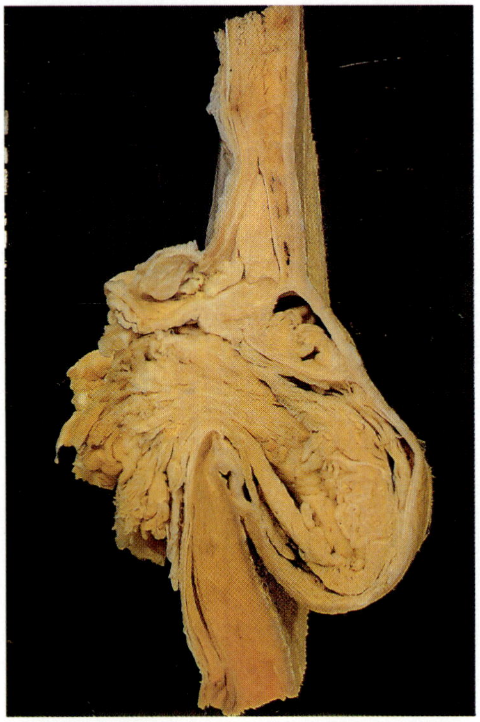

3.189 Umbilical Hernia

No clinical details are available.

A sagittal section through a portion of the anterior abdominal wall shows a hernial sac filled with omentum projecting through the abdominal musculature in the umbilical region.

Umbilical herniae may be of 3 types. They may be characterised by protrusion of part or all of the midgut, a congenital malformation known as exomphalos; they may be acquired during early childhood through a weak umbilical scar (often seen in cretinism), or they may be acquired lesions of adulthood, which are actually para-umbilical, arising through a weakness in the linea alba.

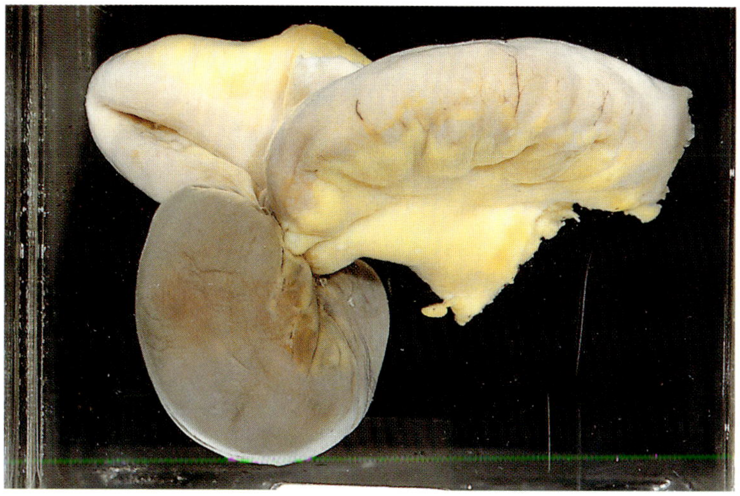

3.190 Ileum: Strangulated Internal Hernia

This is a post-mortem specimen from a 77-year-old woman who died after suffering non-specific gastrointestinal symptoms for one week. At autopsy, a portion of ileum was found to have passed through a fenestration in the mesenteric arterial arcades and to have become strangulated.

The specimen consists of a length of ileum, the central position of which, measuring 8cm in length, has undergone torsion. The proximal unaffected portion is mildly congested.

Internal hernias are relatively uncommon but are a well-recognised cause of intestinal obstruction, often in the absence of strangulation. The most frequent orifices through which such hernias occur are the foramen of Winslow, a gap in the mesentery or mesocolon, or one of the retroperitoneal fossae.

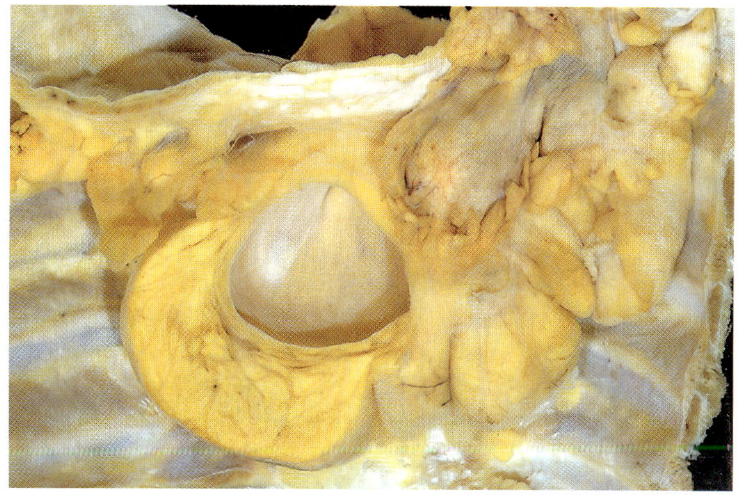

3.191 Diaphragmatic Hernia

This was an incidental finding at post-mortem in a 63-year-old woman who died post-operatively after undergoing a bowel resection.

The anterior wall of the thorax, with the diaphragm, is viewed from behind. Immediately posterior to the sternum, a hernial sac, measuring 8cm in diameter, projects through a diaphragmatic defect. The fundus and lateral aspect of the sac are covered by a thick layer of fat. In the fresh state it was possible to demonstrate that the hernia had occurred through the space between the sternal and costal origins of the diaphragm (the foramen of Morgagni).

Diaphragmatic herniae may be congenital or acquired, passing either through the foramen of Morgagni (as above), the foramen of Bochdalek (the pleuroperitoneal canal), the oesophageal hiatus, or a weakness in the dome of the diaphragm. They may also follow any thoraco-abdominal operation or severe trauma. In childhood, such herniae are frequently associated with ipsilateral pulmonary hypoplasia but, even in the absence of this coexistent feature, respiratory embarrassment may occur.

HEPATOBILIARY SYSTEM

Liver

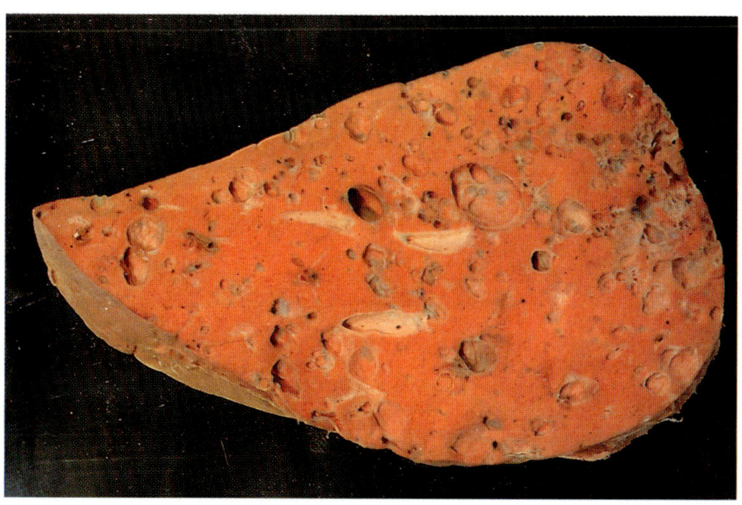

3.192 Liver: Polycystic Disease

This was an incidental finding at post-mortem in an 85-year-old woman who died of bronchopneumonia. There was no history whatever to suggest abnormal hepatic function.

A section through the liver reveals numerous, smooth-walled cysts, measuring up to 1.5cm in diameter, scattered throughout the parenchyma.

Hepatic polycystic disease is an uncommon autosomal dominantly inherited condition which is usually detected in middle or late adulthood. The condition is of little clinical significance, having little or no effect on liver function. However, in up to 50 per cent of cases, it is associated with adult-type polycystic renal disease (see Chapter 4); in such patients diminishing renal function will determine the prognosis.

Cerebral artery aneurysms are known to be associated with adult renal polycystic disease and therefore may also commonly accompany a polycystic liver. Other recognised co-phenomena include cysts in the pancreas and, less often, the lungs or spleen.

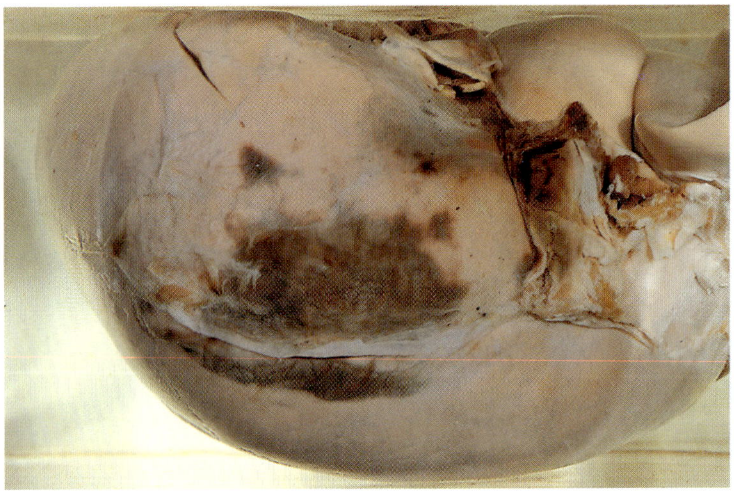

3.193 Liver: Subcapsular Haematoma

This is a post-mortem specimen from a 9-year-old girl who died after sustaining multiple injuries in a road traffic accident.

The liver shows a localised haematoma beneath the capsule, extending over the upper surface of the right lobe. There is no evidence of rupture onto the free surface.

Subcapsular haematomas such as this represent the result of intraparenchymal shearing stresses that result in the tearing of a vessel or vessels in the liver substance. This appearance is usually associated with trauma and may give rise to tender, palpable hepatomegaly. In neonates, it is also a well-recognised complication of particularly difficult obstetric delivery by instrumentation.

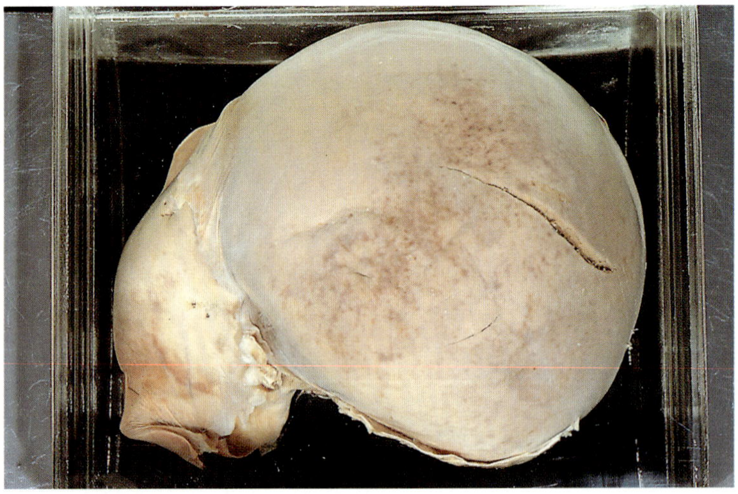

3.194 Liver: Rupture

This is a post-mortem specimen from a 46-year-old woman who suffered a cardiac arrest 4 days after undergoing an operation for a duodenal ulcer. Prolonged attempts at resuscitation including external cardiac massage were unsuccessful. At autopsy death was found to be due to a massive pulmonary embolism, however, it was also discovered that the resuscitative measures had resulted in 10 fractured ribs and rupture of the liver, there being 2l of free blood in the peritoneal cavity.

The liver shows an oblique linear tear, measuring 8.5cm in length, in the antero-lateral surface of the right lobe. There is a further, smaller tear higher up on the same surface. Note also that the organ is very pale, being virtually exsanguinated.

Hepatic rupture is a major surgical emergency and almost always results from a crushing injury or force applied antero-posteriorly. The right lobe is most often affected as it is larger than the left and relatively immobile. This is a classical injury seen in car drivers who, if involved in a serious accident, are struck by the bottom end of the steering wheel.

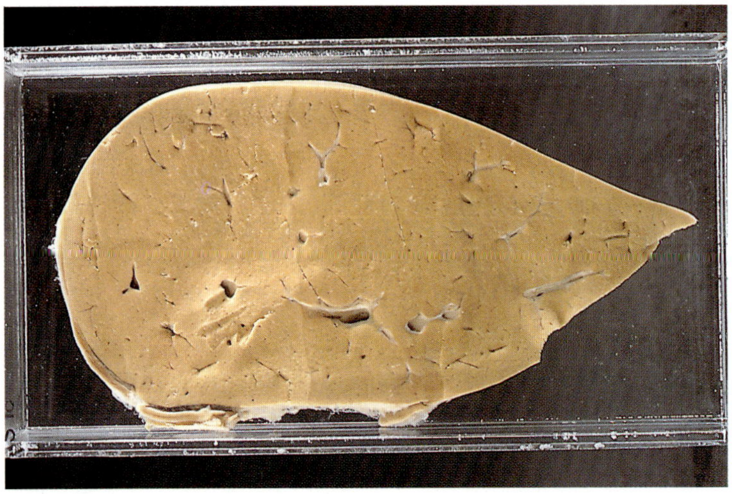

3.195 Liver: Fatty Change

This is a post-mortem specimen from a 23-year-old woman, who died of ulcerative colitis.

The cut surface of this enlarged fatty liver is rather paler than normal, being orange-brown in colour. There is no evidence of scarring.

Hepatic fatty change is due to the excessive accumulation of neutral fat in the cytoplasm of parenchymal cells and results from alterations in lipid metabolism (due to any cause) in which the liver plays an important role. The commonest predisposing factors are chronic passive venous congestion (leading to relative hypoxia), alcohol abuse, obesity and diabetes mellitus, severe systemic illness (usually neoplastic or infective) and malnutrition (in particular kwashiorkor). Other less frequent causes include various toxic chemicals (e.g. carbon tetrachloride), some of the glycogen storage diseases, Reye's syndrome and, very rarely, pregnancy. (Courtesy of the Pathology Museum, Royal Free Hospital Medical School)

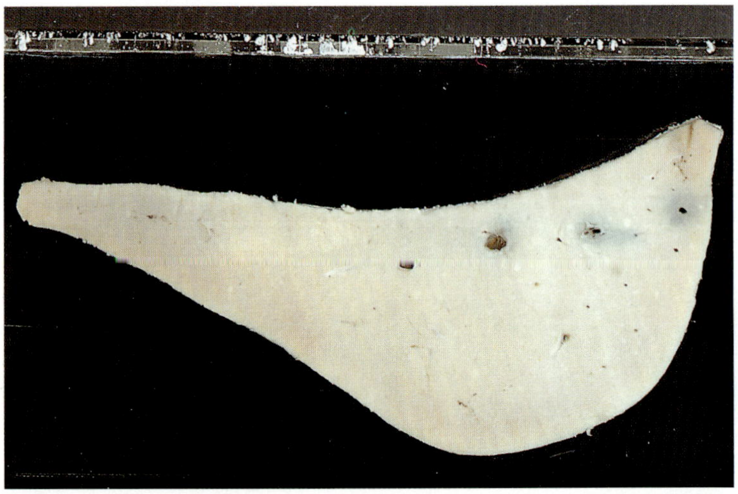

3.196 Liver: Amyloidosis

No clinical details are available.

The cut surface of this liver shows a uniform, waxy, semi-translucent pallor.

The liver is more often affected in secondary amyloidosis than in the primary or myeloma-associated forms. The ß-pleated sheets of fibrillary protein deposited in the space of Disse are therefore usually composed of serum amyloid A protein, a normal acute phase reactant. Frequent predisposing causes include chronic infection (e.g. bronchiectasis or tuberculosis) and chronic inflammatory diseases, such as Crohn's disease or rheumatoid arthritis. There is rarely any impairment of hepatic function.

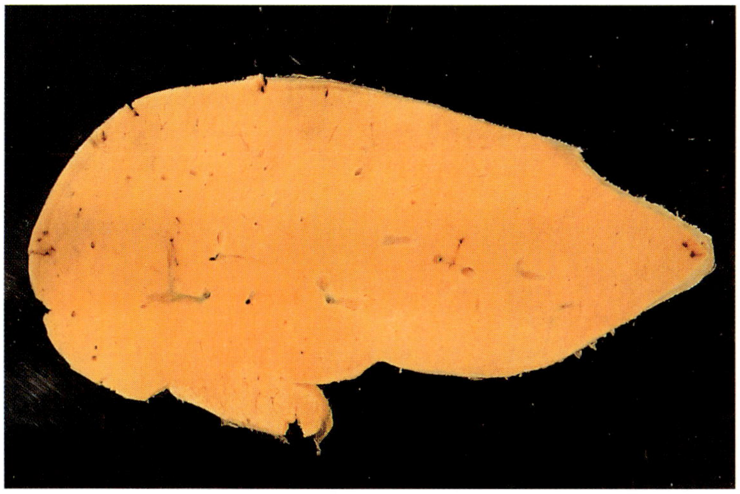

3.197 Liver: Secondary Amyloidosis

This is a post-mortem specimen from a 13-year-old boy who had suffered from florid tuberculous osteomyelitis with discharging sinuses for 5 years.

This section of liver has been stained with Lugol's iodine solution, which stains the amyloid material a yellow-brown colour.

The affinity of amyloid proteins for iodine solutions was responsible for the introduction of the term 'amyloid', since it was thought that the substance deposited was in some way related to starch.

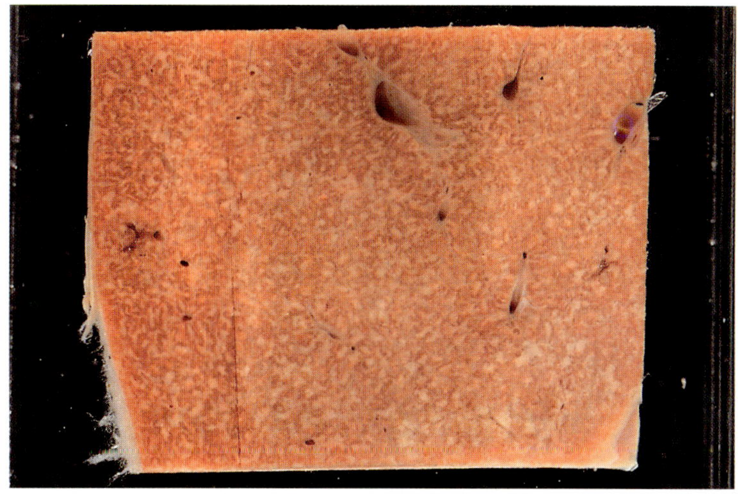

3.198 Liver: Amyloidosis

No clinical details are available.

This portion of hepatic tissue has been stained using Congo Red to reveal fairly diffuse deposition of amyloid. The pale areas represent the remaining normal liver parenchyma.

The Congo Red technique may be used for detecting the presence of amyloid both macroscopically and microscopically; in the latter, apple green birefringence of the positively stained material is pathognomonic. (Courtesy of the Gordon Museum, Guy's Hospital Medical School)

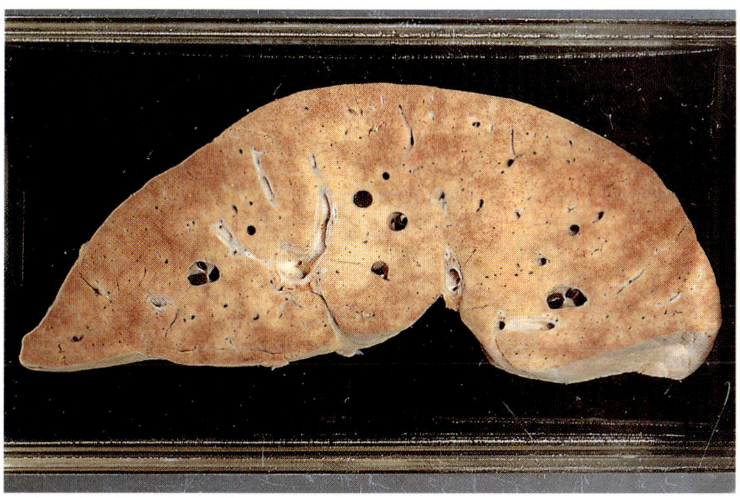

3.199 Liver: Passive Venous Congestion

This is a post-mortem specimen from an elderly male who died in severe congestive cardiac failure 5 years after suffering extensive myocardial infarction.

The cut surface of the hepatic parenchyma has a mottled 'nutmeg' appearance, characterised by small areas of reddish congestion surrounded by areas of yellow discolouration.

This nutmeg appearance (typical of passive venous congestion due to congestive cardiac failure) results from the combination of centrilobular venous engorgement associated with a degree of atrophy and fatty change in the surrounding hepatocytes. This appearance may also be seen as a result of occlusion of the major hepatic veins (see Figure and Legend 3.7). It should be noted that chronic passive venous congestion may lead to a progressive increase in the amount of fibrous tissue around centrilobular veins. When extensive, this has been labelled as 'cardiac cirrhosis', a very dubious term since disruption of the hepatic architecture and nodular regeneration are not, *per se*, features of a long-standing nutmeg liver.

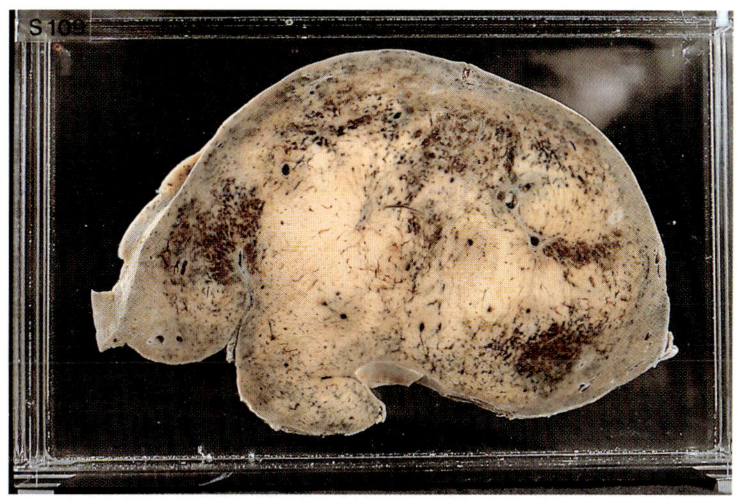

3.200 Liver: Budd-Chiari Syndrome

This is a post-mortem specimen from a 45-year-old adult, who had been diagnosed as having polycythaemia rubra vera 3 years previously. At autopsy there were extensive thromboses within the efferent hepatic veins.

The cut surface of this liver shows irregular areas of intense congestion and mottling, separated by rather pale, brownish-yellow parenchyma. Many of the veins are visibly occluded by thrombus, some of which is organised.

Budd-Chiari syndrome results from occlusion of the major hepatic veins, most often by thrombus, which leads to an appearance similar to that of passive venous congestion. While many cases remain idiopathic, recognised causes include any coagulopathy (particularly polycythaemia rubra vera), occlusion of major hepatic veins or the inferior vena cava by tumour, thrombophlebitis of the hepatic veins and various drugs or chemical toxins. Veno-occlusive disease, which is endemic in the West Indies and is often attributable to the ingestion of plant alkaloids, gives rise to similar features but is characterised by multifocal occlusion of small centrilobular or sublobular hepatic veins. (Courtesy of the Pathology Museum, Royal Free Hospital Medical School)

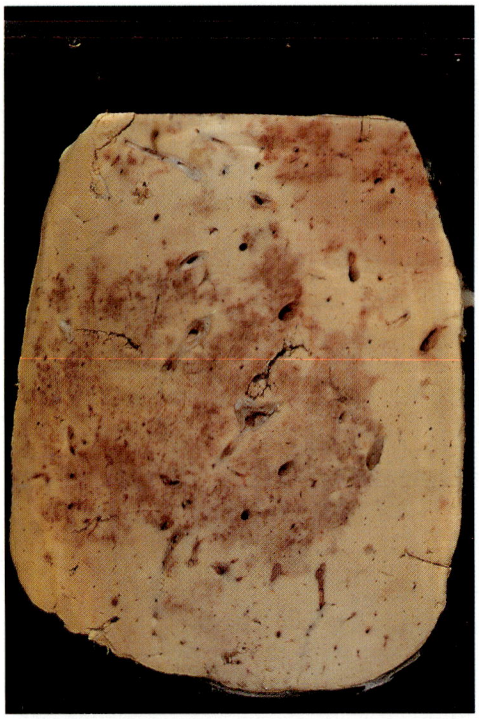

3.201 Liver: Eclamptic Necrosis

This is a post-mortem specimen from a 33-year-old woman who had developed albuminuria in the 28th week of pregnancy. Thereafter hydramnios was noted and her blood pressure rose progressively to 160/120mmHg by the 34th week. It was decided to induce labour but, before anything could be done, she began to vomit and died.

The cut surface of the hepatic parenchyma shows extensive haemorrhagic necrosis. In the fresh state, the liver was soft with capsular wrinkling and the necrosis was predominantly located in the subcapsular area.

Multifocal hepatic necrosis associated with sinusoidal thrombosis is a common feature in patients dying of eclampsia.

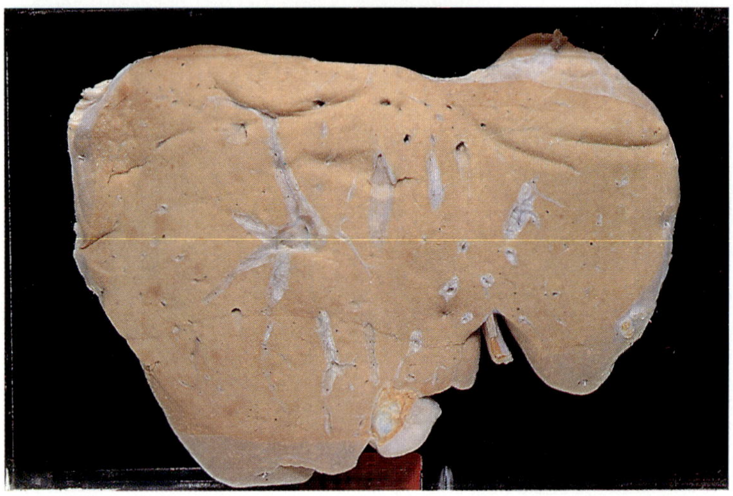

3.202 Liver: Acute Fulminant Viral Hepatitis with Massive Necrosis

This is a post-mortem specimen from a 56-year-old man who presented with a 2 week history of jaundice. He was already known to have renal disease with hypertension. His condition deteriorated rapidly and he died of hepatic failure.

The cut surface of the liver is notably pale, representing almost total necrosis with a few islands of viable hepatic parenchyma remaining as brownish foci on the left. The surface of the liver appears wrinkled. In the fresh state the liver was reduced in size, weighing only 670g.

Acute viral hepatitis is divided into 3 principal types: A, B and non-A non-B; less common causes include infection with cytomegalovirus, herpes simplex, rubella or yellow fever virus. Hepatitis A is spread by the orofaecal route, has an incubation period of 2-6 weeks and is very common world-wide, being endemic in some underdeveloped countries. It usually pursues a mild clinical course, very rarely leading to massive hepatic necrosis, and long-term infection with consequent chronic hepatitis does not occur. Hepatitis B, in contrast, is spread largely in blood, blood products or certain secretions such as semen, has an incubation period of 2-6 months and, while universally common, is most prevalent in tropical countries and Eastern Asia. The acute illness is often severe, being fatal in up to 10 per cent of cases, and a proportion of patients become carriers of infection or may develop chronic hepatitis, cirrhosis or hepatocellular carcinoma. Hepatitis non-A non-B is clinically similar to the type B infection but serum or tissue markers of the latter (such as hepatitis B surface antigen) are absent. (Courtesy of the Gordon Museum, Guy's Hospital Medical School)

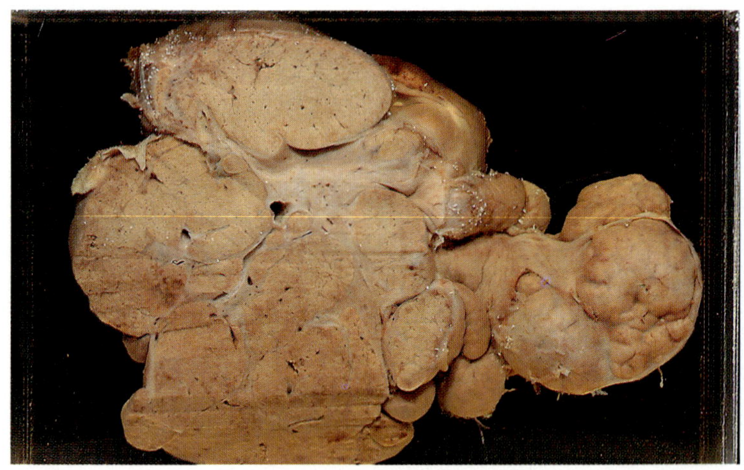

3.203 Liver: Chronic Active Hepatitis and Cirrhosis

This is a post-mortem specimen from a 45-year-old man, who had suffered an attack of viral hepatitis 26 years previously. He had represented with features of cirrhosis and oesophageal varices at the age of 37 and, latterly he developed progressive jaundice and ascites and died.

The cut surface of the liver shows an obvious, irregular macronodular cirrhosis (see Figure and Legend 3.213). Histologically there was additional evidence of active hepatitis with piecemeal necrosis.

Chronic hepatitis, which most often complicates hepatitis B infection, may be divided into active (aggressive) and persistent types. Rarer causes include drugs (such as methyldopa) and so-called lupoid (auto-immune) hepatitis. Chronic active hepatitis usually represents a particularly aggressive host response to type B, or non-A non-B infection. Its significance lies in the fact that changes in the lobular liver architecture lead to cirrhosis in 50 per cent or more of patients. Chronic persistent hepatitis is a milder disease, unassociated with parenchymal destruction, which does not usually progress to cirrhosis. (Courtesy of the Gordon Museum, Guy's Hospital Medical School)

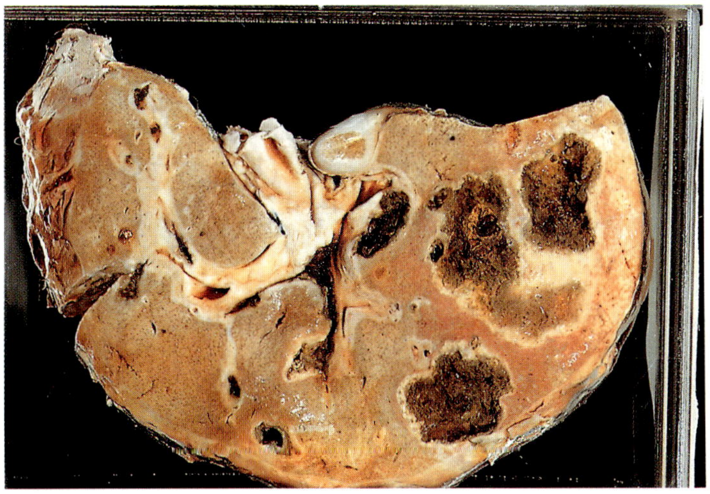

3.204 Liver: Multiple Pyogenic Abscesses

This is a post-mortem specimen from a 68-year-old man who, 2 months after undergoing a Polya gastrectomy for a perforated peptic ulcer, developed severe epigastric pain and vomiting. The polymorphonuclear white cell count was markedly elevated and laparotomy revealed a large abscess in the upper part of the right lobe of the liver which was subsequently drained. However, the patient died 5 weeks later with unremitting sepsis.

The liver has been sliced to reveal a number of large, irregular abscess cavities located predominantly in the right lobe and filled with bile-stained necrotic debris.

True suppurative abscesses in the hepatic parenchyma are usually a complication of portal pyaemia, ascending biliary infection (often in the presence of obstruction) or systemic septicaemia. When portal pyaemia develops secondary to diverticulitis or appendicitis, the infective organisms are usually Gram-negative *Enterobacteriaceae* or anaerobes; bacillary dysentery is also a well-recognised cause. Any source of bacterial peritonitis may, however, be responsible and in this case it seems most likely that the perforated gastric ulcer was the initiating factor.

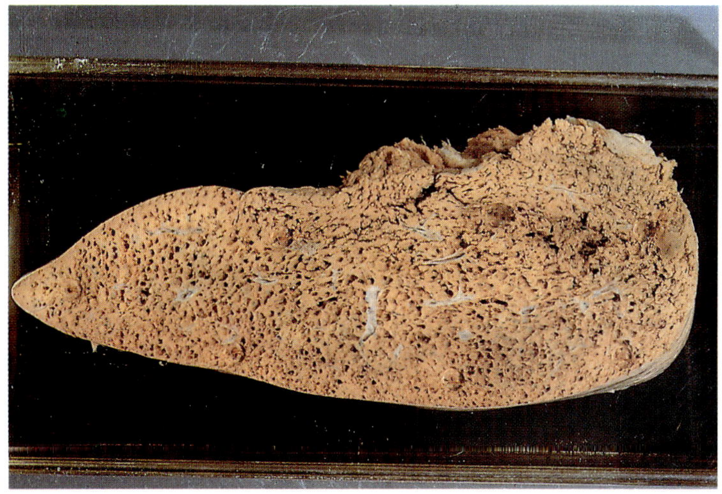

3.205 Liver: Gas Gangrene

This is a post-mortem specimen from an adult male who, following a long history of a right-sided aural discharge, presented in a semicomatose state. A radical mastoidectomy was performed at which pus was found over the transverse sinus. He developed extensive gas gangrene of the soft tissues in the head and neck, from which *Clostridium perfringens* was cultured, and died rapidly.

The liver parenchyma has a honeycomb appearance throughout, known as 'foamy' liver, which is a result of profuse gas formation by the clostridial organisms.

This appearance may be seen following bacteraemia or septicaemia due to infection by *Clostridium perfringens* (*welchii*). The organism produces its often lethal effects by the liberation of a variety of toxins which cause haemolysis and extensive tissue necrosis. Gas formation, which occurs in devitalised tissues *in vivo*, is often much more pronounced in post-mortem specimens.

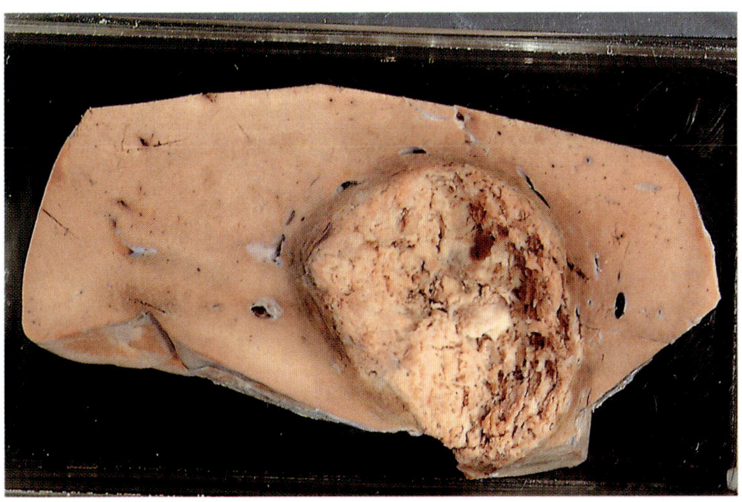

3.206 Liver: Amoebic 'Abscess'

This is a post-mortem specimen from a soldier who, following one week of slight diarrhoea and abdominal pain, developed profuse intestinal haemorrhage and died rapidly. At autopsy there was florid colonic ulceration and 2 hepatic abscesses were present.

Part of the right lobe of the liver has been sectioned to show an 'abscess' cavity in the lower pole. The cavity contains yellowish-pink material and the rim of adjacent hepatic parenchyma is markedly congested.

Amoebiasis, due to infection by the protozoon *Entamoeba histolytica*, is predominantly a disease of the colon (see Small and Large Intestines section) but spread of organisms, via the portal venous system, to the liver occurs in up to one-third of affected patients. The mature trophozoites induce liquefactive necrosis in the hepatic parenchyma but true suppuration does not occur, hence the designation 'abscess' is inaccurate. Hepatic amoebic 'abscesses', particularly if untreated and long-standing, are well known occasionally to rupture into the right pleural cavity, lung, an adjacent viscus, or even subcutaneously.

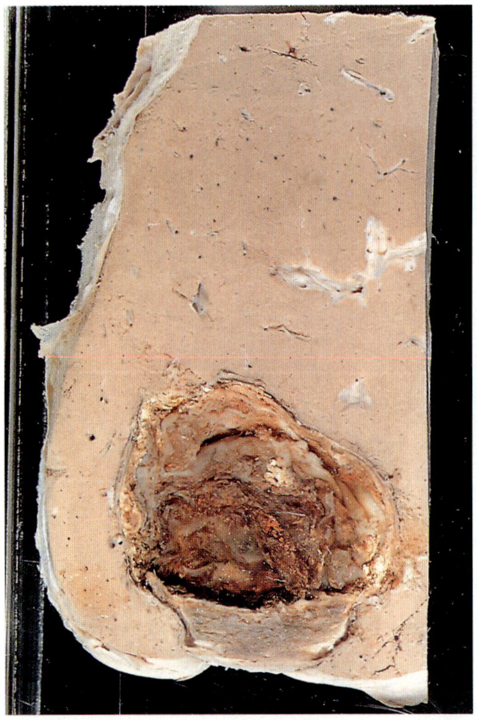

3.207 Liver: Hydatid Disease

This was an incidental finding at post-mortem in a 68-year-old Australian man who died following rupture of an abdominal aortic aneurysm. No evidence of hydatid disease had been detected during life.

A section through the right lobe of the liver shows a cystic structure, measuring 6cm in diameter, near the superior surface. The cyst, which is rather shrunken, is packed with folded hydatid membrane and shows evidence of previous haemorrhage and dystrophic calcification. The disease, in this case, appears 'burnt out'.

Hydatid disease is due to infestation by the tapeworm *Echinococcus granulosus* and is seen most often in rural, particularly sheep farming, communities. The definitive host is the dog and transmission occurs by the oro-faecal route to intermediate hosts such as farm animals and man. The worm itself parasitises the small intestine most often, but the cestode ova invade the adjacent small blood vessels from whence they are carried principally to the liver. As a result, up to 60 per cent of human cases show hepatic involvement. Hydatid cysts in the liver are usually solitary and are located in the right lobe in the vast majority of cases. The diagnosis may be made *in vivo* by demonstration of cutaneous hypersensitivity to hydatid antigen, the Casoni test. Calcification is a common feature of effete hydatid cysts and should be remembered as an occasional source of unexplained calcific lesions found on X-ray.

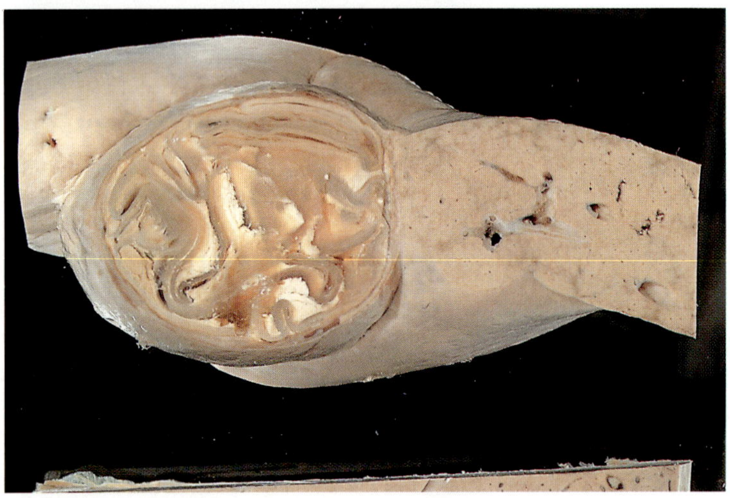

3.208 Liver: Hydatid Disease

This was an incidental finding at post-mortem in a 47-year-old Australian woman who died of unrelated causes. At autopsy there were cysts in the liver, omentum and uterus.

A section through the liver shows a shrunken obsolescent cyst which demonstrates particularly well the complex, folded hydatid membranes. These membranes represent the remnants of cyst capsules.

When 'active', hydatid cysts contain large amounts of fluid and pale, so-called hydatid 'sand', the latter representing free scolices and capsules. However, during the course of involution, the fluid component is reabsorbed, leaving only the membranes as shown here.

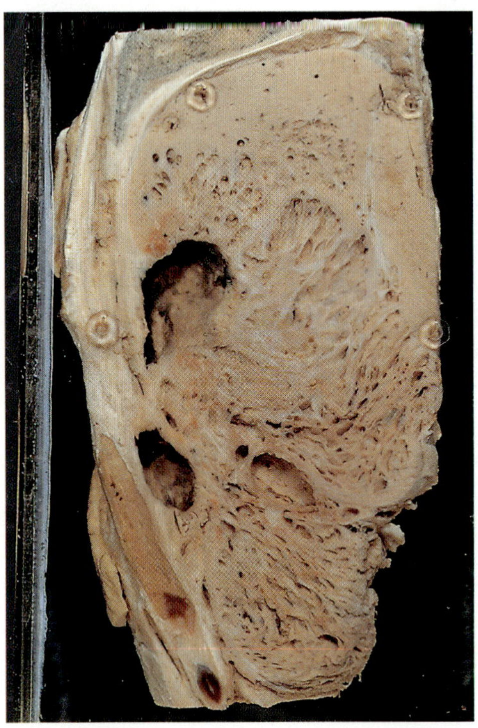

3.209 Liver: Actinomycosis

This is a post-mortem specimen from an adult male who, following a period of malaise, weight loss and night sweats, presented with a subcutaneous abscess over the right 8th rib in the mid-axillary line. More than 2l of fluid were drained from the abscess but a persistent sinus developed and the patient gradually deteriorated over the ensuing year and died.

This is a coronal section through the right lobe of the liver with the adjacent diaphragm, lung base, ribs and subcutaneous tissue. The hepatic parenchyma is replaced by numerous inter-communicating abscess cavities of varying size, which have penetrated through the full thickness of the chest wall (left). Note also the dense adhesions between the liver, diaphragm and lung base.

Actinomycotic infection of the liver is almost always a result of portal venous spread from a primary focus in the ileocaecal region. Honeycomb abscesses, as seen here, are characteristic. Primary intestinal infection is commonest in young adults, particularly males, and typically induces chronic suppuration with extensive sinus formation.

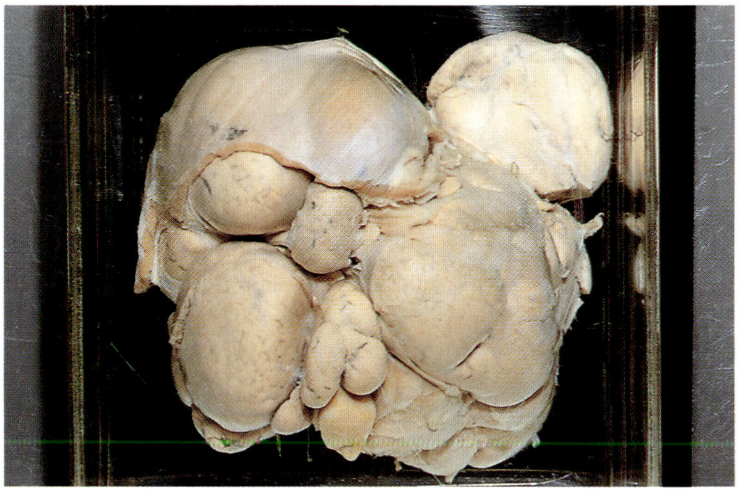

3.210 Liver: Tertiary Syphilis

This is a post-mortem specimen from a 69-year-old woman who had developed a perforating ulcer of the palate 4 years previously. She was found to have a strongly positive Wassermann reaction and she eventually died following rupture of a syphilitic aortic aneurysm.

The liver, with part of the diaphragm, is shown. It is markedly shrunken and shows an irregular, multinodular appearance, each nodule being separated by a deep fibrous fissure. This appearance is known as hepar lobatum.

Hepatic involvement in syphilis is usually a feature of the tertiary stage of the disease and is characterised by the development of gummata. Healing commonly leads to dense scarring, the cause of the lobulation seen in this liver.

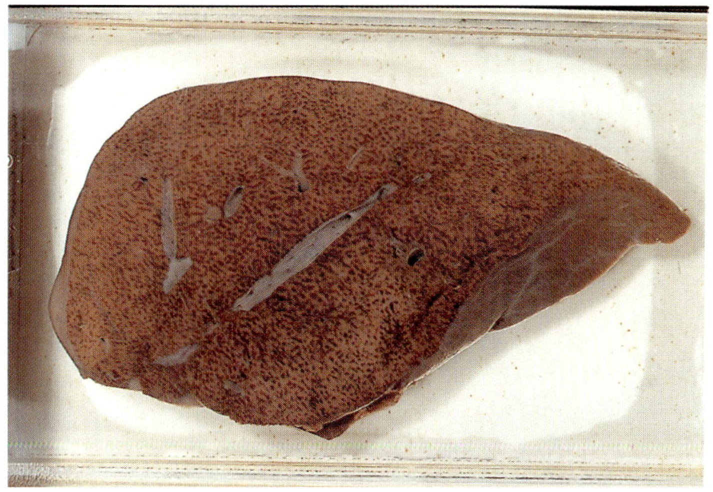

3.211 Liver: Parenchymal Necrosis due to Paracetamol

This is a post-mortem specimen from a female adult who suffered from depression and committed suicide by taking an overdose of over 40g of paracetamol. She died 9 days after admission to hospital.

The liver has a 'nutmeg' appearance, not dissimilar to that of chronic venous congestion, characterised by alternating red and yellow mottled areas.

This appearance is the result of extensive centrilobular necrosis, the characteristic feature of paracetamol poisoning. Less often, massive confluent hepatic necrosis may be seen. Other chemical agents which cause centrilobular necrosis are chloroform and carbon tetrachloride.

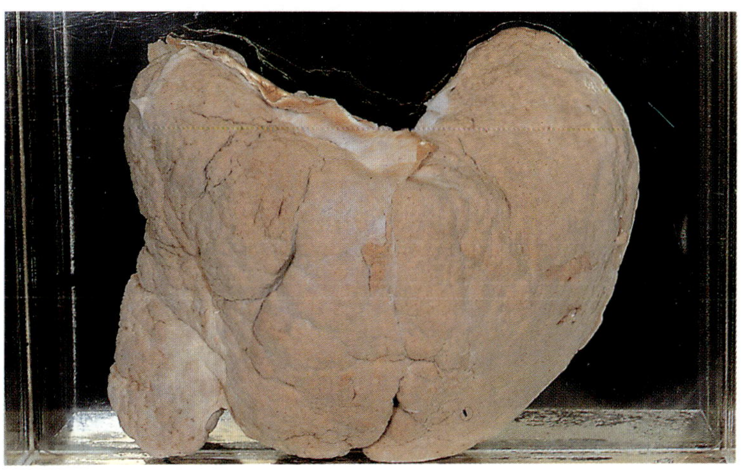

3.212 Liver: Alcoholic Micronodular Cirrhosis

This is a post-mortem specimen from a 64-year-old woman, a known alcoholic for the previous 12 years, whose condition gradually deteriorated and she later died.

The capsular surface of this liver is irregularly scarred and shows fine, diffuse, nodularity, the nodules varying from 1-3mm in diameter. Note also the yellowish-brown discoloration.

Hepatic cirrhosis is defined as a diffuse, irreversible condition characterised by the presence of nodular regeneration, a disordered parenchymal architecture and fibrosis. It may be subclassified on the basis of the size of nodules; less than 3mm (1cm in the USA) being micronodular, and those larger than 3mm, varying up to 5cm in diameter, being macronodular. In fact there is most often a mixed pattern, such that the terms micronodular and macronodular are of very limited value. The main classification of cirrhosis is by cause.

The most common cause of this condition is alcohol abuse, which accounts for approximately 50 per cent of cases, or more in the Western world. However, up to one-third may follow extensive hepatocellular necrosis due to hepatitis B or non-A non-B. In Africa and Asia, hepatitis is by far the commonest cause. Other important aetiological factors are biliary disease (primary or secondary), haemochromatosis and Wilson's disease. Less than 15 per cent of cases would now be classified as idiopathic. Alcoholic cirrhosis is increasing in incidence, is predominantly seen in middle-aged adults of either sex, and is typified by a micronodular pattern initially. Complications of cirrhosis include portal hypertension (with associated splenomegaly, ascites and oesophageal varices), decreased synthesis of albumin and various clotting factors, gonadal atrophy, encephalopathy, or renal failure, and the development of hepatocellular carcinoma in up to 15 per cent of cases (particularly in those due to hepatitis).

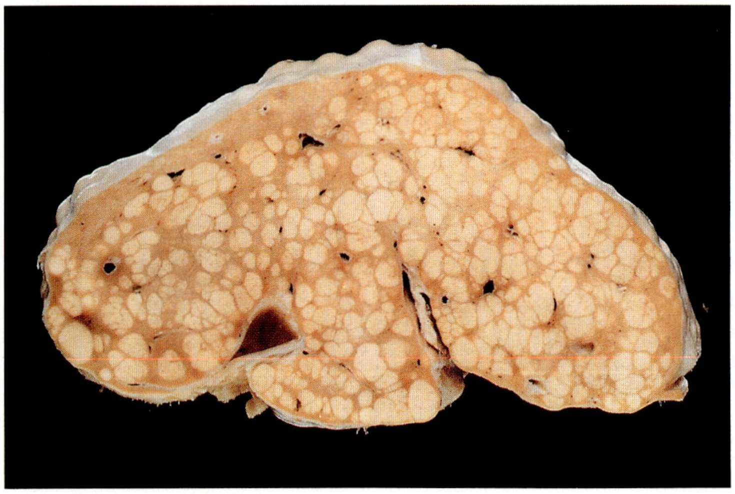

3.213 Liver: Macronodular Cirrhosis

This is a post-mortem specimen from a 32-year-old woman who died following massive haemorrhage from oesophageal varices.

The liver is shrunken (weighing only 1020g at autopsy) and the cut surface shows numerous large, pale nodules (measuring up to 2.5cm in diameter), separated by bands of greyish fibrous tissue.

The aetiology in this case was not apparent. However, the commonest cause of macronodular cirrhosis is preceding viral (B or non-A, non-B) hepatitis. Other important causes include so called 'lupoid' (idiopathic autoimmune) hepatitis, various drugs (e.g. methyldopa), Wilson's disease (see Figure and Legend 3.216) and α_1-antitrypsin deficiency. A macronodular pattern is also common in the later stages of alcoholic cirrhosis. The percentage of patients with hepatitis B or non-A non-B who develop cirrhosis is uncertain since, in many cases, the initiating viral infection goes undetected clinically. However, in patients in whom this occurs there is an intervening phase in which they develop chronic active (aggressive) hepatitis, the pathogenetically important phase of the disease. As already stated, patients with postviral cirrhosis are at particular risk of developing hepatocellular carcinoma.

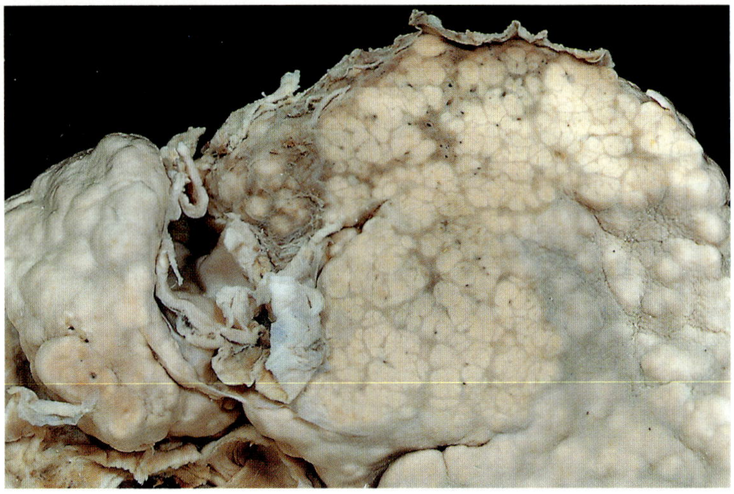

3.214 Liver: Mixed Micro- and Macronodular Cirrhosis

This was an incidental finding at post-mortem in an 80-year-old woman who died of congestive cardiac failure.

The liver is irregularly shrunken and the cut surface shows the characteristic, pale, multinodular pattern. The nodules, which are separated by bands of fibrous tissue, vary in diameter from about 2mm to over 1cm.

Many cirrhotic livers, particularly if long-standing, will show a mixed pattern of nodule sizes, as shown here. It is believed that the majority of true mixed micro- and macronodular cases represent the late stages of an originally micronodular lesion. However, distinction from pure macronodularity (characterised by a wide variation in nodule size) may only be possible by the identification of regenerative nodules less than 3mm in diameter (1cm in the USA).

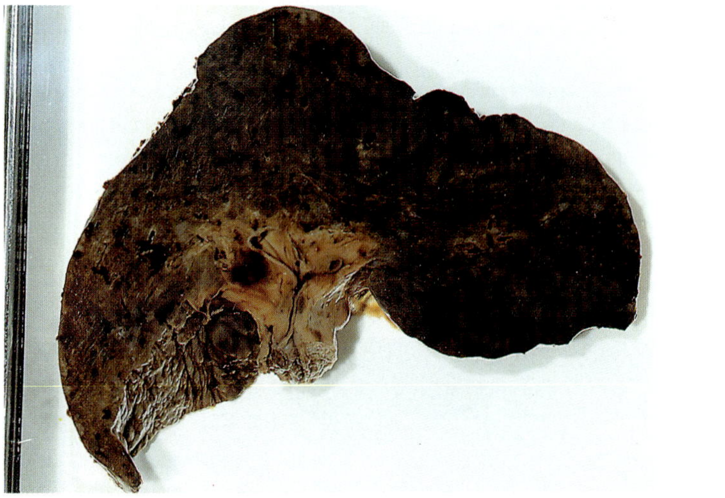

3.215 Liver: Primary Biliary Cirrhosis

This is a post-mortem specimen from a 60-year-old woman who had suffered from jaundice for 2 years. The biochemical picture suggested an obstructive cause but exhaustive investigations failed to identify an organic obstruction. She died following a pathological femoral fracture, which was attributed to hypovitaminosis D and osteomalacia consequent upon prolonged obstructive jaundice.

The liver has been sectioned to show deep bile-staining associated with a nodular parenchymal pattern and fine fibrosis.

Primary biliary cirrhosis is a relatively uncommon idiopathic condition which occurs primarily in middle-aged females and is characterised by the gradual onset of what appears to be obstructive jaundice for which no cause can be found. Itching may be a prominent symptom in the early stages. An autoimmune pathogenesis is currently favoured and is supported by the presence of anti-mitochondrial antibodies in at least 90 per cent of patients, raised levels of serum immunoglobulin M, and a frequent clinical association with Hashimoto's disease and Sjögren's syndrome.

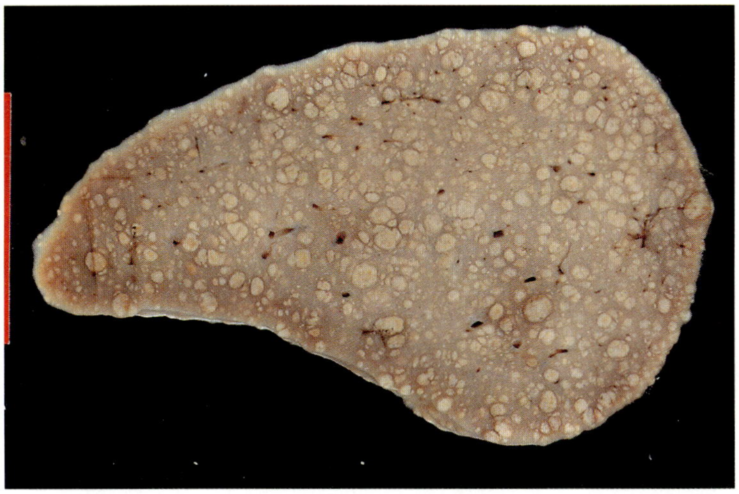

3.216 Liver: Cirrhosis due to Wilson's Disease

No clinical details are available.

The cut surface of this liver is greyish in colour and shows a mixed macro- and micronodular cirrhosis.

Wilson's disease is a rare autosomal, recessively inherited condition, characterised by abnormally high storage of copper in the tissues associated with decreased levels of serum caeruloplasmin. The disease presents in early or middle adulthood either with neurological dysfunction (due to copper deposition in the lentiform or caudate nuclei) or with the features of abnormal liver function. Typically a macronodular cirrhosis develops in many patients but hepatocellular carcinoma is an extremely rare complication (cf. haemochromatosis). (Courtesy of the Gordon Museum, Guy's Hospital Medical School)

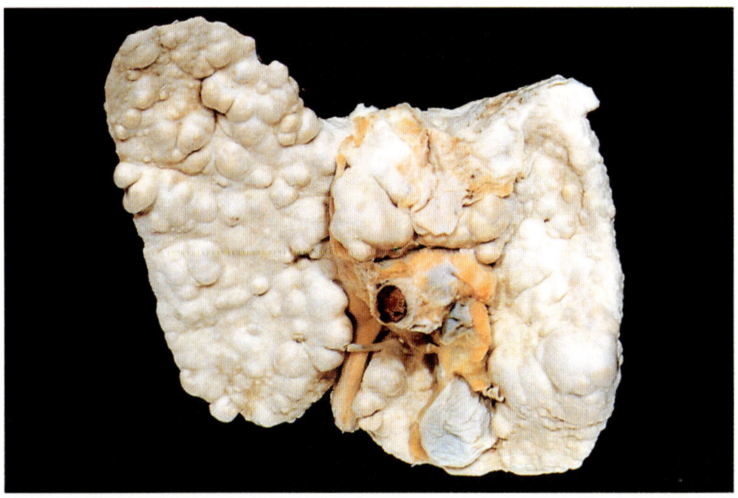

3.217 Liver: Macronodular Cirrhosis with Portal Vein Thrombosis

This is a post-mortem specimen from a 63-year-old woman, known to have cirrhosis for many years, who terminally developed hepatic failure and died following rupture of oesophageal varices.

The liver is markedly shrunken and shows a florid mixed (predominantly macronodular) cirrhosis. The main portal vein, at the porta hepatis, is completely occluded by fairly recent laminated thrombus.

Cirrhosis is the commonest predisposing cause to thrombosis of branches of the portal vein and, particularly in cases of portal hypertension, to occlusion of the main portal vein. This occurrence frequently has little clinical effect since the hepatic arterial blood supply prevents true parenchymal infarction. However, occlusion of smaller portal venous radicles may give rise to pseudoinfarcts (Zahn infarcts), characterised by congestion and atrophy. While some portal venous thromboses remain idiopathic, the majority are associated with a parenchymal lesion, in particular hepatocellular carcinoma invading branches of the portal vein. Other causes include intra-abdominal sepsis and recent abdominal surgery.

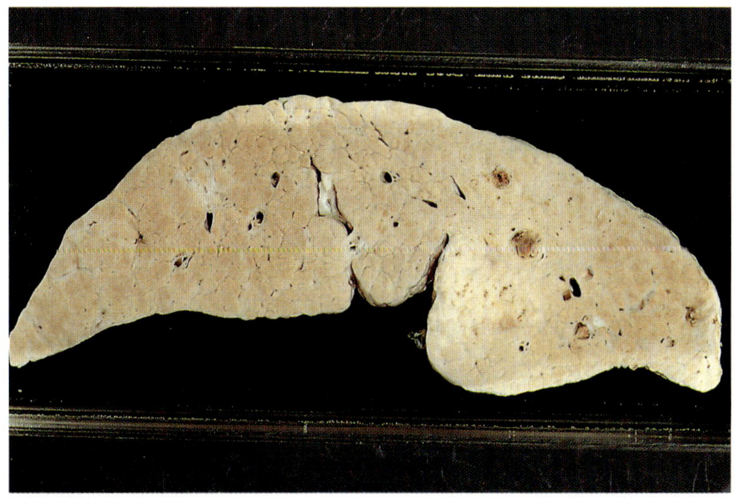

3.218 Liver: Micronodular Cirrhosis with Hepatocellular Carcinoma

This is a post-mortem specimen from an 82-year-old man who died following an episode of bleeding from oesophageal varices. There was a history of viral hepatitis with jaundice 36 years previously.

The cut surface of this liver shows a fine micronodular cirrhosis and is typically rather pale in colour. From beneath the diaphragmatic surface arises an ill-defined, whitish neoplasm which is infiltrating the parenchyma diffusely. Note also the thrombosed vessels.

The development of hepatocellular carcinoma (see Legend 3.25 et seq.) is a well-recognised complication of cirrhosis. The most frequently associated causes of the underlying cirrhosis are viral hepatitis, alcohol abuse and haemochromatosis. It was not possible to establish whether this patient's previous episode of hepatitis was responsible for the development of cirrhosis.

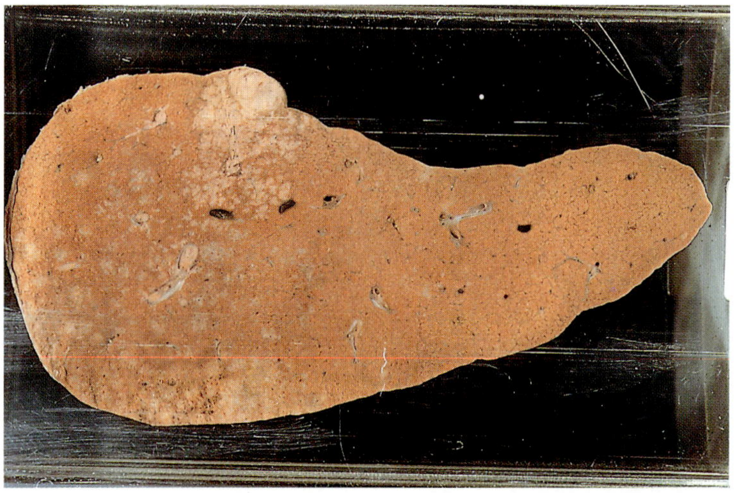

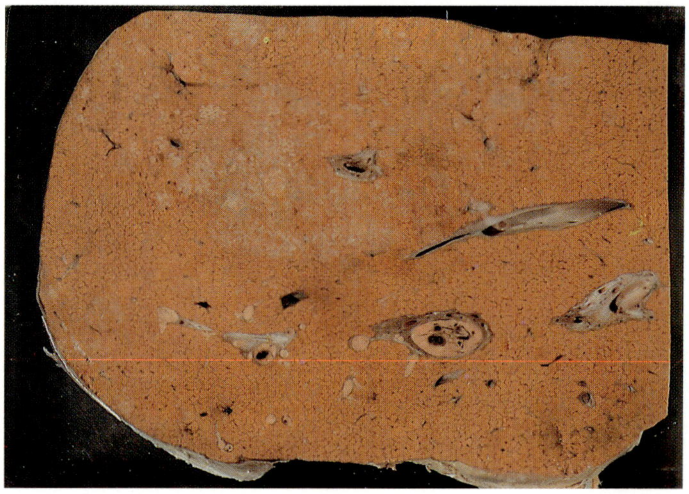

3.219 Liver: Cirrhosis due to Haemochromatosis with Hepatocellular Carcinoma

This is a post-mortem specimen from a 61-year-old man who had been noted to have hepatomegaly for 12 years. Diabetes mellitus and bronze pigmentation of the skin had developed 11 and 9 years ago, respectively. Latterly, he developed ascites and died.

A section through the right lobe of the liver (3.219a) shows a rather ill-defined micronodular cirrhosis, associated with deep brick-red parenchymal pigmentation. Scattered throughout the posterior part are numerous pale nodules of neoplastic tissue, the largest of which projects inferiorly beneath the peritoneal surface. A separate section (3.219b) shows occlusion of the right main portal vein and its branches by similar pale neoplastic tissue.

This is an example of multifocal hepatocellular carcinoma (see Figure and Legend 3.223 et seq.) arising in a case of long-standing haemochromatosis. Haemochromatosis is an uncommon autosomal dominantly inherited condition characterised by the excessive deposition of haemosiderin in a variety of organs throughout the body, especially the liver, pancreas, adrenal glands and skin. The precise underlying defect in iron metabolism is uncertain.

The disease shows a very marked predilection for males but this may reflect, to some extent, the protection conferred upon females by regular menstrual blood (and therefore iron) loss. Deposition of iron in the liver parenchyma leads to extensive fibrosis (hence the cirrhosis) and thereafter up to 20 per cent of patients may develop hepatocellular carcinoma. Similar iron deposition and fibrosis in the pancreas and adrenal glands may give rise to diabetes mellitus and Addison's disease, respectively.

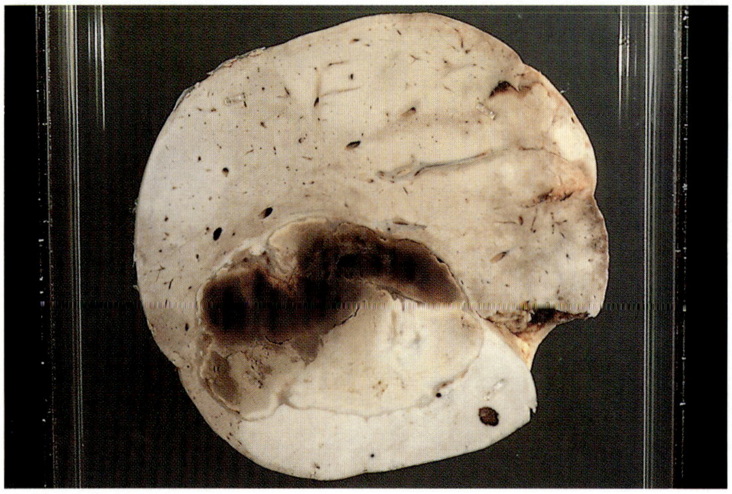

3.220 Liver: Liver-cell Adenoma

This specimen was excised from a 38-year-old woman, who presented with pyrexia and a 5 week history of abdominal pain. The patient had been using an oral contraceptive for several years. At laparotomy, the tumour was found to have given rise to a haemoperitoneum.

Within this segment of hepatic parenchyma is a well-circumscribed, partially encapsulated neoplasm, within which there has been extensive haemorrhage. Several smaller adjacent nodules, which are rather indistinct, also proved histologically to be adenomas.

Hepatic adenomas are rare, benign lesions, which are most often idiopathic but may be associated with the use of oral contraceptives, particularly those high in oestrogen. They are most often solitary, ill-defined lesions. Malignant change is rare. (Courtesy of the Pathology Museum, Royal Free Hospital Medical School)

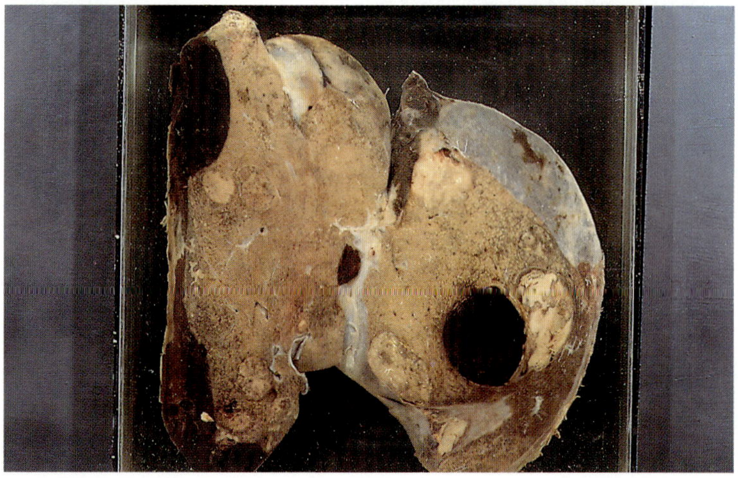

3.221 Liver: Multiple Adenomata

This is a post-mortem specimen from a 29-year-old woman who had been treated with haemodialysis for chronic renal failure for the previous 8 years. She had been taking oral contraceptives to suppress menstruation during this time. Latterly she had presented with a haemoperitoneum due to bleeding from the liver. She died during an operation being undertaken to prevent re-bleeding.

The cut surface of the liver shows multiple well-circumscribed pale lesions, which histologically proved to be liver-cell adenomas. In addition there is a large subcapsular haematoma in the right lobe and a further area of haemorrhage in the left lobe. Note that some of the hepatic vessels are filled with grey barium sulphate, injected at pre-operative angiography.

It is not rare for liver-cell adenomas, of varying size, to be multiple. It is worth noting that about 25 per cent of these lesions present as a result of haemorrhage into the peritoneal cavity, a feature demonstrated by both cases here. (Courtesy of the Gordon Museum, Guy's Hospital School)

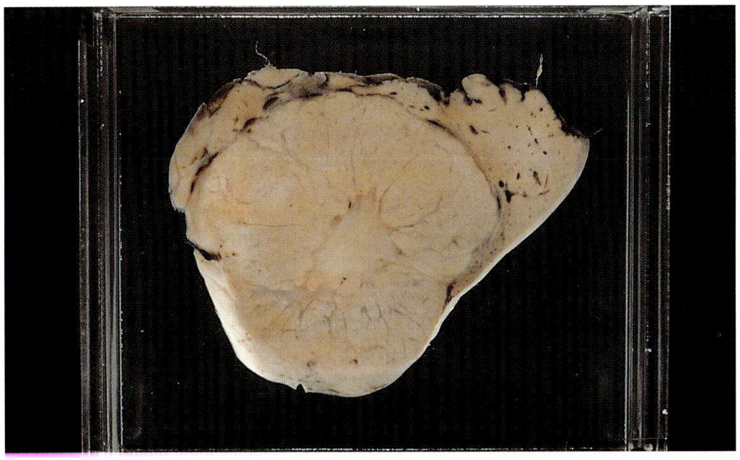

3.222 Liver: Focal Nodular Hyperplasia

This specimen was excised from a 21-year-old woman. No further clinical details are available.

Within the hepatic parenchyma is a well-circumscribed lesion, at the centre of which is a characteristic pale scar. The remainder of the tumour is composed of rather nodular, normally coloured hepatic tissue intersected by delicate fibrous septa, giving an appearance like that of cirrhosis. However, the lesion is focal, rather than diffuse, and the adjacent parenchyma is normal.

Focal nodular hyperplasia is a relatively uncommon benign lesion, which is usually asymptomatic and is typically an incidental finding in an otherwise normal liver, either at laparotomy or post-mortem. It is commonest in young or middle-aged adults and shows a predilection for females. The aetiology is unknown. (Courtesy of the Pathology Museum, Royal Free Hospital Medical School)

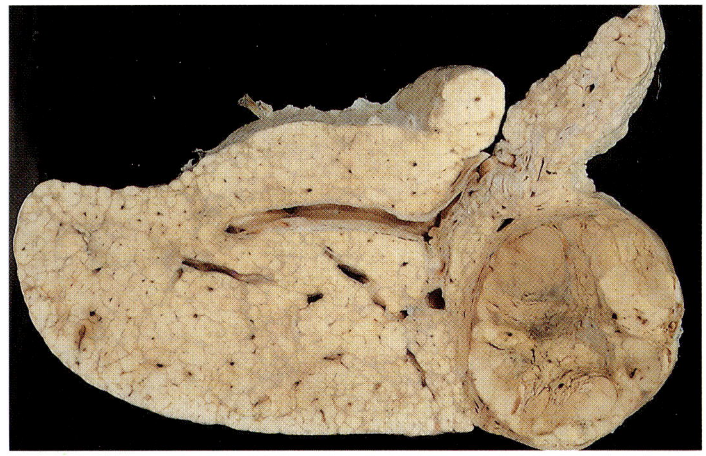

3.223 Liver: Hepatocellular Carcinoma with Micronodular Cirrhosis

This is a post-mortem specimen from a 77-year-old man who collapsed and died while undergoing treatment in a pyschiatric hospital. At autopsy, a hepatic tumour was found to have ruptured through the visceral peritoneum and death resulted from exsanguination with a haemoperitoneum.

The cut surface of this liver shows a fine, uniform, micronodular cirrhosis. A rounded, partly bile-stained tumour, measuring 6.5cm in diameter, arises near the diaphragmatic surface and appears well-circumscribed. A smaller nodule of similar tumour is apparent at the bottom right.

Hepatocellular carcinoma is relatively uncommon in Caucasians but appears to be increasing in incidence. In parts of Africa and Asia, however, it is one of the commonest forms of malignant disease, a difference which is probably attributable to environmental influences (including diet and the increased incidence of hepatitis B). This tumour most often affects adults between the ages of 50 and 70 and, in the majority of Caucasian cases, there is a pre-existing cirrhosis. A well-recognised environmental carcinogen, possibly of importance in African cases, is aflatoxin, derived from the bacterium, *Aspergillus flavus*. In general, the prognosis is very poor with few patients surviving more than 1 year.

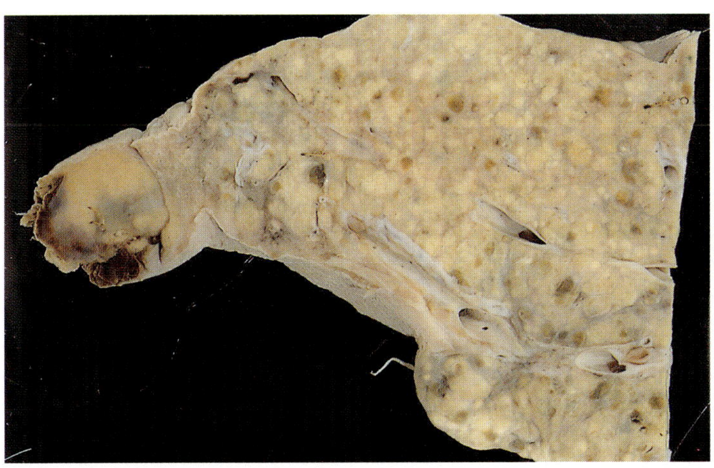

3.224 Liver: Hepatocellular Carcinoma with Micronodular Cirrhosis

This is a post-mortem specimen from a 63-year-old alcoholic male who was admitted to hospital with acute abdominal distension and died rapidly. At autopsy, the carcinoma had ruptured and produced a massive haemoperitoneum.

The cut surface of this liver shows a florid micronodular cirrhosis with a pale, rounded neoplasm, measuring 2.5cm in diameter projecting from the inferior surface. At the site of rupture there is residual blood clot.

Both this and Figure 3.223 represent examples of uninodular primary liver cancer, a macroscopic variant responsible for about 30 per cent of cases. In most cases the tumour adopts a multinodular pattern (see Figure 3.219), often involving almost all of one hepatic lobe while, more rarely, it may show a diffuse pattern, almost indistinguishable from cirrhosis.

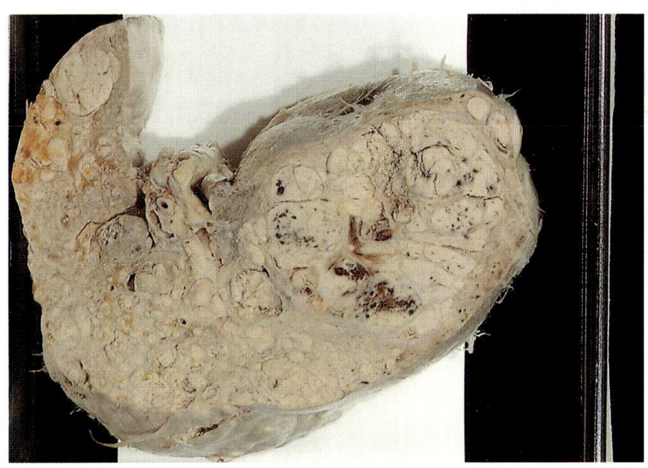

3.225 Liver: Hepatocellular Carcinoma with Micronodular Cirrhosis

This is a post-mortem specimen from an 82-year-old woman who, following investigation for a 2 month history of jaundice with a suspected hepatic mass, died of haemorrhage from oesophageal varices.

Much of the liver parenchyma is replaced by a multinodular pale tumour, the nodules varying in size from 1-10cm in diameter. Note the characteristic foci of haemorrhage and necrosis. The residual liver tissue (bottom right) is bile-stained and shows a micronodular cirrhosis.

This is an example of the most common multinodular variant of hepatocellular carcinoma. It should be noted that, in up to 70 per cent of cases, primary hepatic cancers secrete alpha-fetoprotein, a substance normally produced by the embryonic liver, and this may be of use as a serum tumour marker in both diagnosis and follow-up.

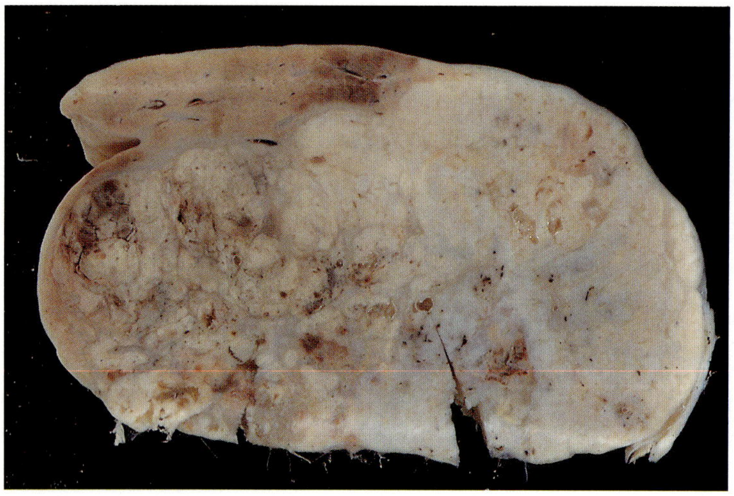

3.226 Liver: Hepatoblastoma

This is a post-mortem specimen from a 2½-year-old boy, who presented with a 2 month history of abdominal swelling and, more recently, diarrhoea. Examination revealed marked hepatomegaly, ascites and a caput medusae. He died 4 days after undergoing an exploratory laparotomy.

The majority of this right hepatic lobe is replaced by a lobulated, pale neoplasm showing foci of necrosis and haemorrhage.

Hepatoblastoma is a rare embryonal malignant neoplasm, comparable to nephroblastoma or neuroblastoma, which typically presents in infancy and shows a predilection for males. It may be associated with a variety of coexistent congenital anomalies. The prognosis is generally extremely poor, with rapid and widespread tumour dissemination. (Courtesy of the Gordon Museum, Guy's Hospital Medical School)

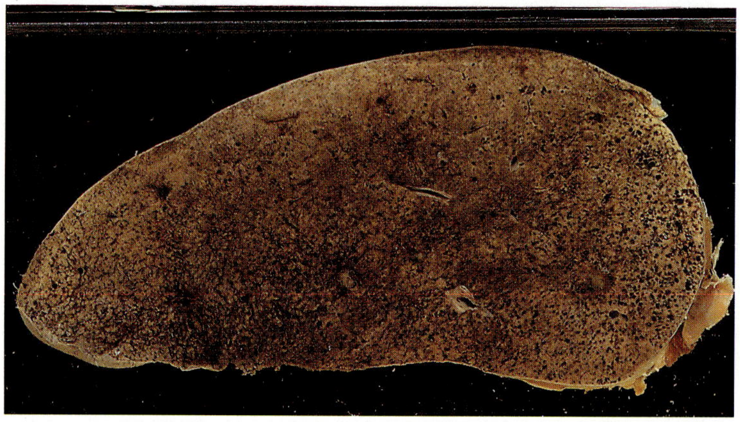

3.227 Liver: Peliosis

This is a post-mortem specimen from a 48-year-old woman who, following radical mastectomy for breast carcinoma, had been treated with radiotherapy, anabolic steroids and Prednisolone for cerebral metastases. She represented with peritonitis and died. At autopsy she was found to have a pelvic abscess due to rupture of an inflamed diverticulum of the sigmoid colon.

The cut surface of the liver shows numerous small blood-filled spaces in the parenchyma, all measuring 0.1cm or less in diameter. There is no evidence of metastatic breast cancer.

Peliosis hepatis is a rare condition, characterised by dilatation of large numbers of sinusoids or small veins in the portal tracts. While many cases remain idiopathic, a proportion are associated with anabolic steroid therapy, use of a high progestogen contraceptive pill or pulmonary tuberculosis. (Courtesy of the Gordon Museum, Guy's Hospital Medical School)

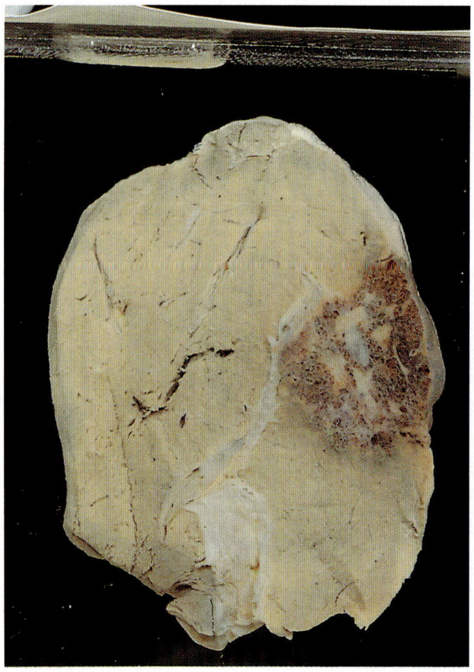

3.228 Liver: Cavernous Haemangioma

This was an incidental finding at post-mortem in an 82-year-old woman who died of a ruptured dissecting aortic aneurysm.

A section through part of the right lobe of the liver shows a reasonably circumscribed angiomatous lesion, measuring 2.5cm in diameter, situated beneath the capsule. Pale areas of fibrosis are located within the tumour.

Cavernous haemangiomas of the liver are relatively common, particularly with advancing age, but are rarely symptomatic. They are hamartomatous developmental lesions, which may be solitary or multiple and are occasionally associated with hereditary haemorrhagic telangieactasia (Osler-Weber-Rendu disease). They are commonly subcapsular and should be distinguished from peliosis hepatis, a diffuse condition characterised by innumerable small, dilated vascular spaces (see Figure 3.227).

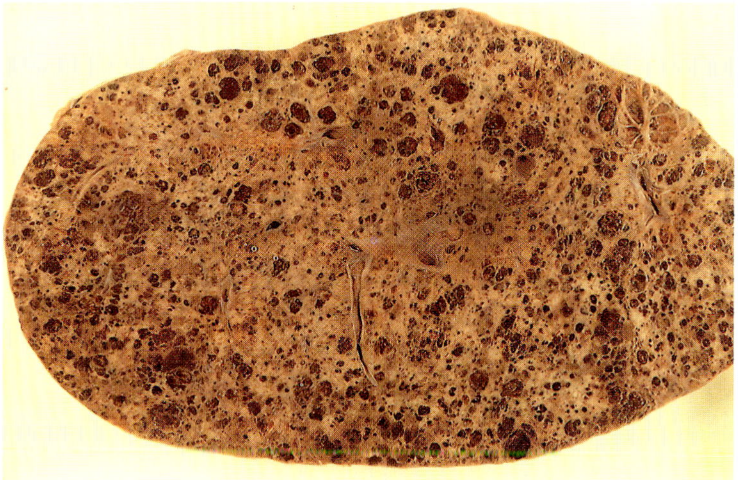

3.229 Liver: Angiosarcoma

This is a post-mortem specimen from a 58-year-old woman who died in hepatic failure. No other clinical details are available. At autopsy, there were metastases in the coeliac lymph nodes and spleen.

The cut surface of the liver shows complete parenchymal replacement by a mass composed of numerous vascular spaces, which show a marked variation in size. Many of the vessels are thrombosed.

Angiosarcoma of the liver is a rare tumour, principally seen in adults, which may be causally related to prior exposure either to Thorotrast (an outdated radiological contrast medium) or to vinyl chloride monomer, used in the plastics manufacturing industry. Chronic arsenical poisoning may be responsible in some cases. Very occasionally, idiopathic cases of a similar tumour are seen in infancy. Characteristically the liver is greatly enlarged by multifocal or diffusely infiltrative tumour. The prognosis is extremely poor. (Courtesy of St. Thomas's Hospital Medical School Museum)

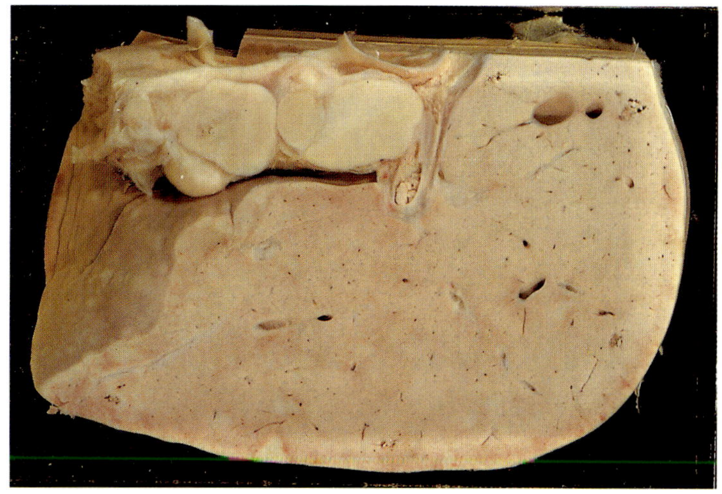

3.230 Liver: Hodgkin's Disease

No clinical details are available.

The cut surface of the hepatic parenchyma is pale and rather greyish, being largely replaced by numerous tiny nodules of lymphomatous tissue. At the porta hepatis are several enlarged, discrete lymph nodes, which are replaced by similar tumour.

The liver is very commonly involved in disseminated Hodgkin's disease but, rarely, may be the primary site of origin; the same applies for non-Hodgkin's lymphoma, particularly the follicular types. (Courtesy of the Gordon Museum, Guy's Hospital Medical School)

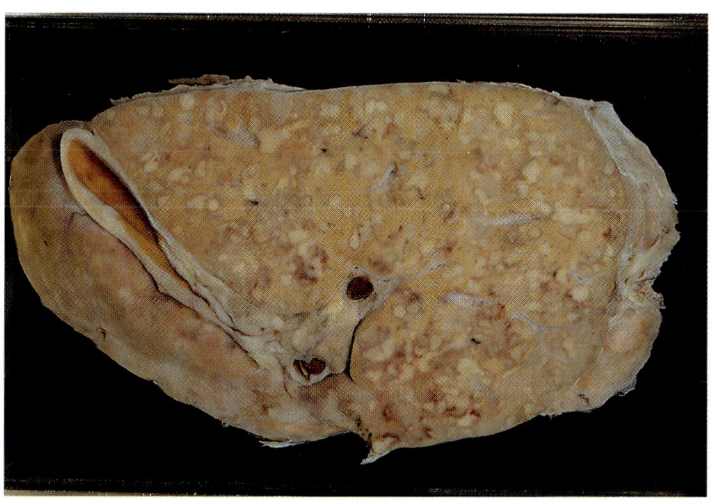

3.231 Liver: Metastatic Breast Carcinoma

This is a post-mortem specimen from a 43-year-old woman who had first noticed a lump in her right breast 3 months previously. She underwent radical mastectomy but rapidly represented with jaundice and ascites and died. Autopsy revealed metastases in the liver, bones, adrenals, pituitary and spleen. The portal and splenic veins were thrombosed.

The cut surface of this liver shows a variegated appearance due to a combination of 3 separate lesions. There are multiple, pale, ill-defined deposits of metastatic tumour, and small yellowish areas of infarction, each having a hyperaemic rim, which have resulted from thrombosis of the portal vein and hepatic artery. The latter is a consequence of extraluminal compression by metastatic carcinoma in lymph nodes at the porta hepatis, which has also occluded the common bile duct, leading to deep bile-staining of the liver parenchyma.

The liver is a particularly common site of metastasis from any disseminated tumour, probably as a consequence of its rich blood supply. Secondary deposits from gastrointestinal carcinomas are especially frequent due to spread within the portal venous system but carcinomas of the breast and bronchus are also often the primary source. It is worth noting that metastases are unusual in a cirrhotic liver, irrespective of the extent of tumour spread, and it is thought that this is a consequence of altered patterns of blood flow, perhaps due to portal hypertension.

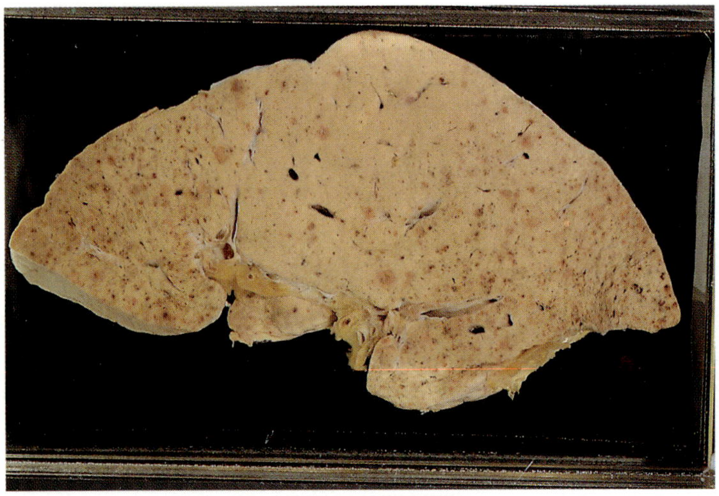

3.232 Liver: Diffuse Metastatic Bronchial Carcinoma

This is a post-mortem specimen from a 93-year-old man who presented with a 3 month history of haemoptysis. A chest X-ray suggested carcinoma of the left lung, but the patient died of bronchopneumonia before any further investigations could be performed. Autopsy revealed an oat cell carcinoma of the left main bronchus with metastases to hilar lymph nodes, the liver and bone.

The cut surface of this liver, which is pale due to fatty change (see Figure and Legend 3.195) shows diffuse parenchymal infiltration by numerous small, ill-defined foci of reddish metastatic tumour.

This appearance, also known as hepatitis carcinomatosa, may be confused with acute hepatitis with multifocal necrosis, particularly since there is smooth, uniform hepatomegaly. It is, in fact, due to massive microscopic infiltration by metastatic tumour, which forms countless small deposits throughout the liver lobules. Jaundice and hepatocellular failure may ensue and, in the majority of cases, the primary source is an oat cell (small cell anaplastic) bronchial carcinoma.

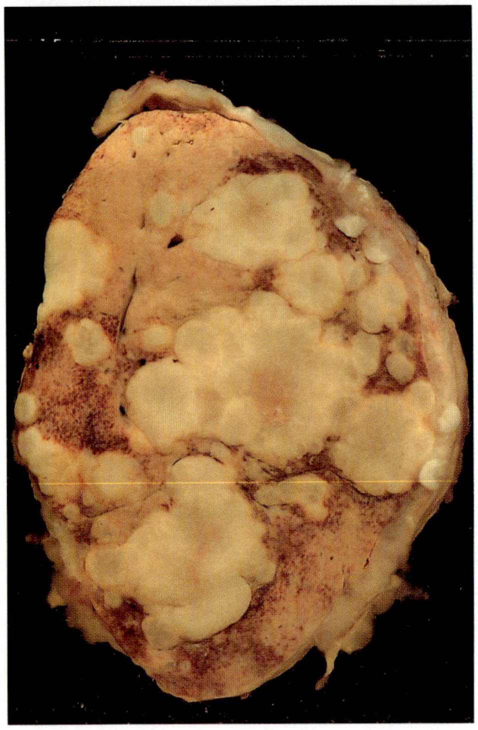

3.233 Liver: Metastatic Ovarian Carcinoma

This is a post-mortem specimen from a 54-year-old woman, who presented with a 2 year history of abdominal distension. She had recently developed dyspnoea and had been vomiting. Examination revealed a very large, hard pelvic mass and she was presumed to have disseminated ovarian cancer; she died rapidly. At autopsy there was a large ovarian mucinous cystadenocarcinoma (see Chapter 5) with metastases throughout the peritoneum, liver and both pleural cavities.

The cut surface of the liver shows replacement of the parenchyma by multiple large, discrete deposits of obviously mucoid neoplastic tissue.

These are the classical appearances of metastatic carcinoma in the liver, the cases described in Legends 3.231 and 3.232 being slightly atypical. Transperitoneal spread is a particularly common feature of ovarian carcinomas. (Courtesy of the Gordon Museum, Guy's Hospital Medical School)

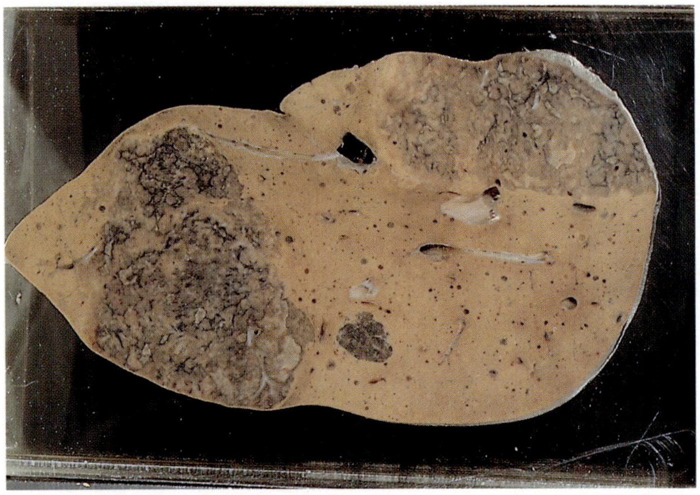

3.234 Liver: Metastatic Cutaneous Malignant Melanoma

This is a post-mortem specimen from a 66-year-old man, who had first noticed enlargement and ulceration of a pigmented 'mole' on the left foot 1 year previously. He had not sought medical treatment and thereafter pigmented nodules had developed in the surrounding skin and in the proximal portion of the leg; he eventually died with widespread metastases.

Within the liver parenchyma are multiple deposits of metastatic melanoma of variable size. Note that the distribution of pigment is very variable, much of the neoplastic tissue being amelanotic.

In almost all cases of disseminated cutaneous malignant melanoma, there is extensive hepatic involvement. It should also be remembered that this tumour shows a marked tendency to spread to unusual or unexpected sites not often involved by other carcinomas. Ocular malignant melanoma shows a similar predilection for spread to the liver; hence, because melanomas may develop metastases after a prolonged latent period (even 20 years or more), the aphorism 'beware the patient with a glass eye and an enlarged liver'.

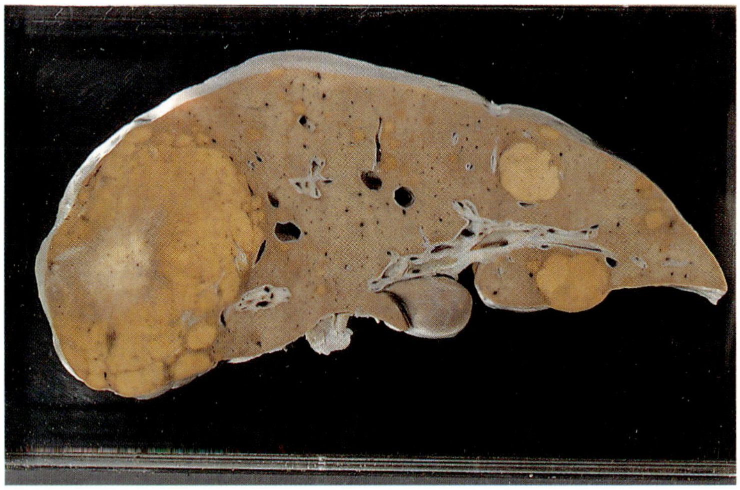

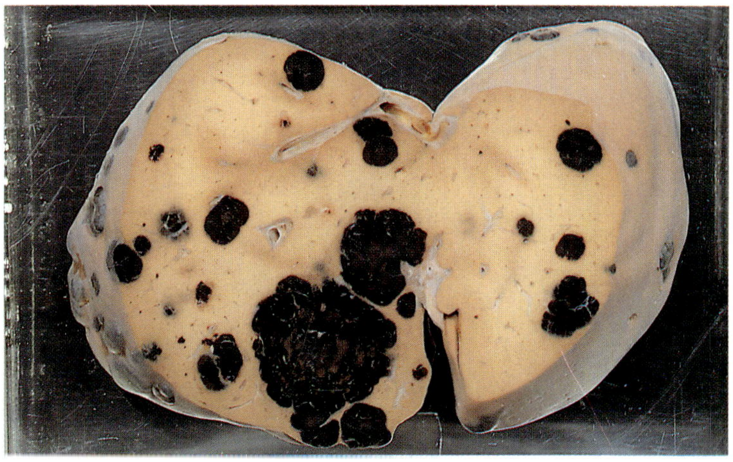

3.235 Liver: Metastatic Carcinoid Tumour

This is a post-mortem specimen from a 66-year-old woman who presented with a 2½ year history of facial flushing, more recently associated with swelling of the hands and feet and desquamation of the skin. On admission to hospital, she was found to have hepatomegaly and large amounts of 5-hydroxyindoleacetic acid in the urine. She rapidly developed signs of tricuspid incompetence, jaundice and ascites and she died shortly afterwards. At autopsy, there were carcinoid tumours in the ileum and within a Meckel's diverticulum and metastases were present in the liver and lungs. There was gross fibrous thickening, (with contraction) of the tricuspid and pulmonary heart valves, associated with marked right atrial dilatation.

Within the liver are several discrete, rounded secondary deposits of typically yellow-brown metastatic tumour. The largest metastasis is undergoing necrosis at its centre.

Gastrointestinal carcinoid tumours (argentaffinomas), whether benign or malignant, typically synthesise significant amounts of 5-hydroxytryptamine (5-HT) (see Small and Large Intestines section), which is usually metabolised in the liver (via the portal venous system) and so does not reach the systemic circulation unless there are hepatic (or more widespread) metastases. Tumour dissemination, hence the carcinoid syndrome, is more often a feature of ileal than appendiceal primary tumours.

3.236 Infantile Liver: Transplacental Metastatic Melanoma

This is a post-mortem specimen from a 10-month-old male infant. His mother had a malignant melanoma of the thigh excised during the first month of her pregnancy and the child had to be delivered by Caesarean section owing to the presence of massive melanomatous metastases in the placenta. The mother died 3 months later with disseminated tumour. The child thrived for the first 8 months of life but was then admitted to hospital with irregular, nodular hepatomegaly. He gradually became cachectic and died; at autopsy, there were deposits of metastatic melanoma in the liver, lymph nodes, pleura and soft tissues. There was no evidence of a primary tumour.

A cross section through this infant's enlarged liver, which weighed 455g, shows multiple, rounded deposits of metastatic melanoma, which are uniformly and heavily pigmented.

Transplacental spread of a maternal malignant tumour to the fetus is a well-described but exceedingly rare occurrence.

Gall Bladder and Bile Ducts

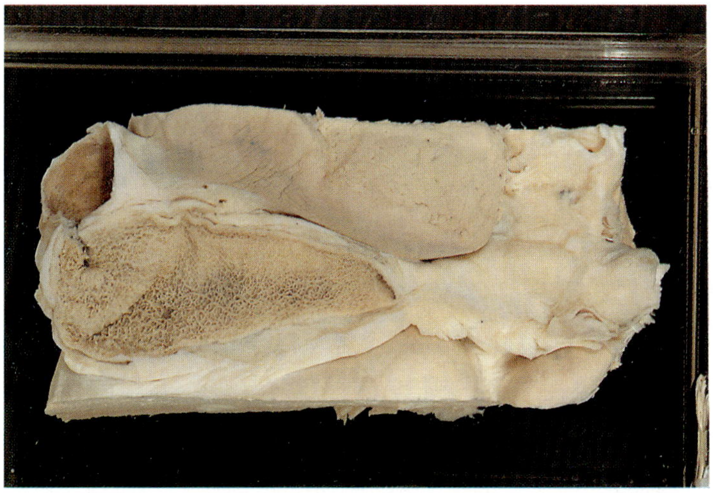

3.237 Gall Bladder: Diverticulum

This was an incidental finding at post-mortem in an 81-year-old man who died of a cerebral thrombosis. There was no past clinical history suggestive of gall bladder disease.

A portion of the liver with the attached, opened gall bladder is shown. In the fundus of the gall bladder there is a small mucosal ostium, leading into a diverticulum which measures 1.5cm in diameter (top left). The gall bladder itself appears normal.

Diverticula of the gall bladder are generally regarded as acquired lesions of mechanical origin. In their commonest form they are only detected microscopically as intramural mucosal outpouchings, known as Rokitansky-Aschoff sinuses, which are very often associated with chronic cholecystitis. Diverticula, which are apparent macroscopically, may be either idiopathic acquired lesions, more frequent with advancing age or, rarely, they may be congenital.

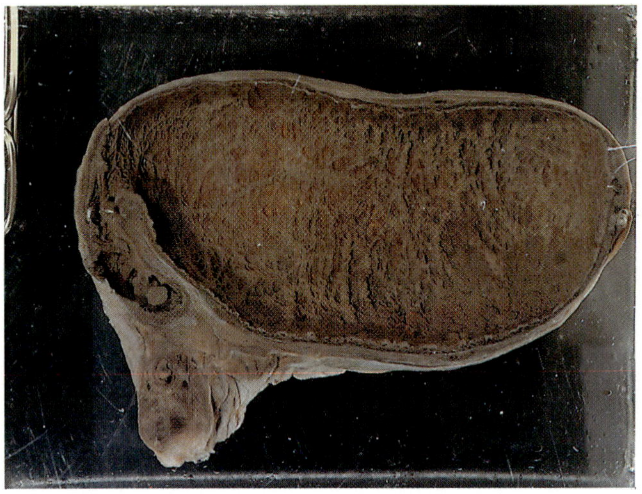

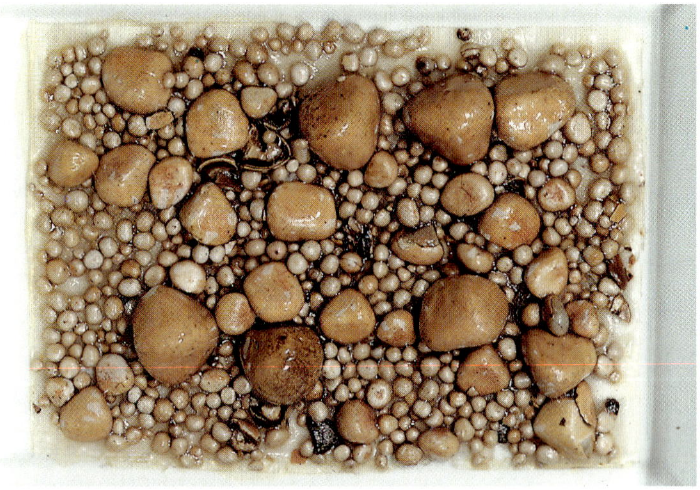

3.238 Gall Bladder: Torsion

This specimen was excised from a 74-year-old woman who presented with acute abdominal pain, severe diarrhoea and a single episode of vomiting during a local epidemic of bacillary dysentery due to *Shigella sonnei*. Examination revealed signs of peritonitis, visible peristalsis and a pyrexia. Laparotomy was performed and a gangrenous, twisted gall bladder was excised. Dense adhesions were noted between the hepatic flexure of the colon and the gall bladder area. Post-operatively the diarrhoea persisted and the patient died the following day.

The gall bladder has been opened to show obvious gangrenous discoloration of the full thickness of the wall, associated with a tight twist in the pedicle containing the cystic duct and main vessels. The cystic vein is thrombosed (top right).

Torsion of the gall bladder is a very unusual event but is most often associated with the presence of a developmentally anomalous short mesentery to which it is attached, instead of being apposed to the undersurface of the liver. In this case it was thought that violent colonic peristalsis (due to the dysentery), in combination with the adhesions described above, had led to torsion of an abnormally mobile gall bladder.

3.239 Gall Bladder: Cholelithiasis

These calculi were removed from the gall bladder of a 71-year-old woman who had undergone cholecystectomy for chronic biliary disease.

The specimen consists of a very large number of yellowish-brown calculi, ranging in diameter from 0.2-2.0cm. Many of the stones have facetted surfaces, a result of their rubbing against one another in the gall bladder.

Cholelithiasis is an extremely common condition, particularly with advancing age, but is often asymptomatic. Females are affected approximately twice as often as males and recognised predisposing factors include obesity, multiparity, diabetes mellitus, previous ileal resection and chronic haemolytic anaemia: there is also an increased familial incidence. There are 3 principal types of gall stone (based on their main constituent) which are cholesterol, bile pigment and mixed, of which the latter is the most common.

The precise pathogenesis of cholelithiasis remains uncertain. The single most important factor seems to be an increased concentration of either cholesterol (perhaps in relation to phospholipids or bile acids) or of bilirubin in excreted bile. Increased bilirubin secretion is typically a feature of the chronic haemolytic anaemias and affected patients classically develop pigment stones. Other proposed initiating mechanisms include local cholestasis within the gall bladder (probably due to incomplete emptying); a qualitative or quantitative alteration in mucosubstances and glycoproteins secreted in the gall bladder which may act as a nidus for stone formation, and biliary infection resulting in bacterial breakdown and precipitation of bile conjugates.

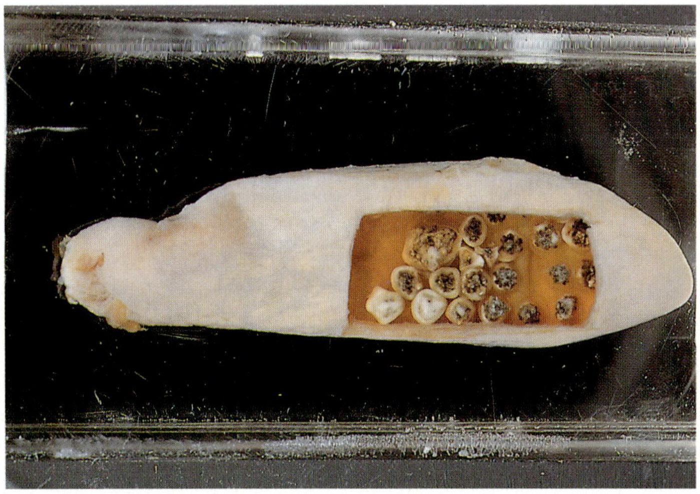

3.240 Gall Bladder: Cholelithiasis

No clinical details are available.

This shrunken gall bladder has been opened to show a number of small mixed stones composed of dark pigment and yellowish cholesterol.

While many such calculi produce no apparent clinical effects, a variety of complications may occur. The commonest of these is cholecystitis (acute or chronic), which most often results from impaction of a stone in the cystic duct or Hartmann's pouch. Many of the other resultant disease processes, such as a mucocele or biliary fistula, should be regarded as complications of cholecystitis. The effects of gall stones within the biliary duct system are dealt with below. However, gall stones *per se*, in the absence of clinically significant inflammation, predispose to the later development of carcinoma of the gall bladder in a very small proportion of cases (see Figure and Legend 3.253 et seq.).

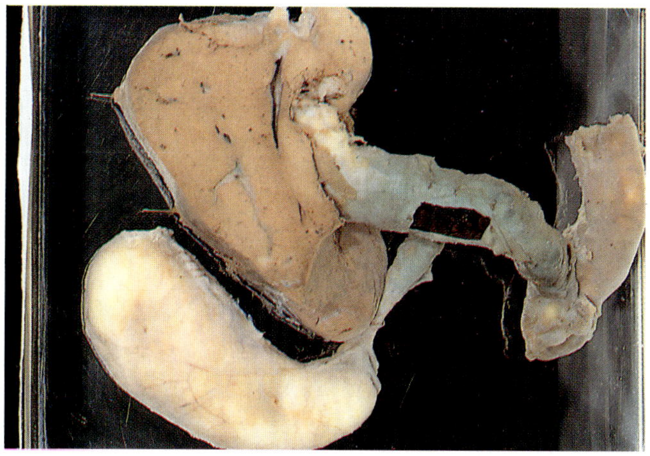

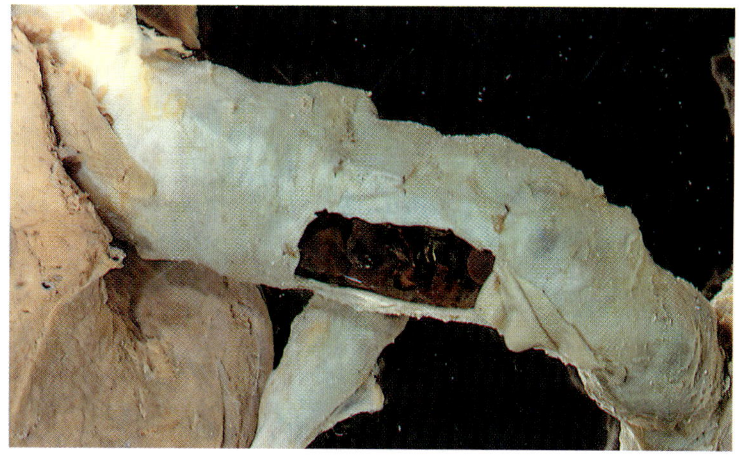

3.241 Common Bile Duct: Cholelithiasis

This is a post-mortem specimen from a 93-year-old woman who for the last 2 months of her life had become mentally confused and had developed a urinary infection. There was no history of abdominal symptoms and she died of bronchopneumonia. Terminally a slight jaundice had been noted.

Part of the liver with the gall bladder, common bile duct and an opened segment of the duodenum are shown (3.241a). The common bile duct is grossly dilated, measuring 3cm in diameter, and the gall bladder is distended but seemingly free from inflammation. A closer view of the opened bile duct (3.241b) shows it to be packed with numerous, dark facetted calculi.

Cholelithiasis of the common bile duct has precisely the same predisposing factors and incidence as that in the gall bladder (see Legends 3.239 and 3.240). Most often such calculi are associated with stones in the gall bladder, whence they are thought to have passed. However, in patients who are prone to the formation of gall stones and who have undergone cholecystectomy, it is not uncommon to find stones developing in the common bile duct at a later date. In this case it would appear that passage of a stone from the gall bladder has resulted in a stricture of the cystic duct (bottom centre), hence the distended gall bladder and the confinement of stones to the bile duct.

Possible effects of calculi in the common bile duct include the development of biliary colic, obstructive jaundice, ascending cholangitis, a biliary stricture and ulceration of a stone through the wall into the gut, leading to a fistula with possible gall stone ileus (see Small and Large Intestines section).

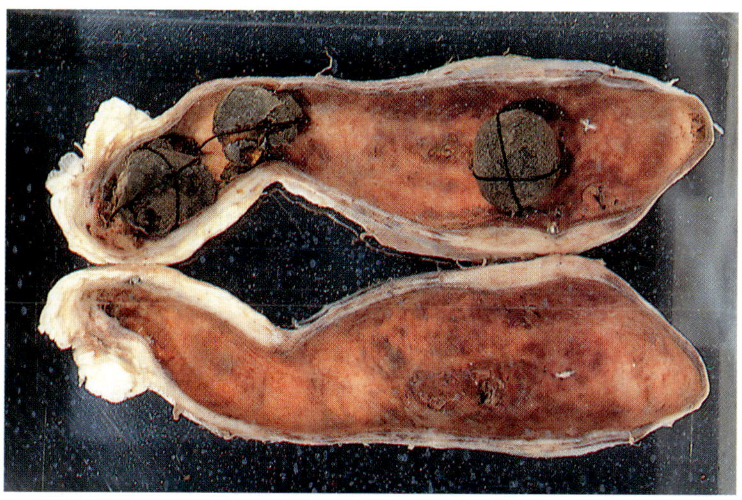

3.242 Gall Bladder: Acute Cholecystitis with Cholelithiasis

No clinical details are available in this case.

This gall bladder is rather distended and has been opened to show florid mucosal and mural congestion, indicative of acute inflammation, associated with three rounded calculi, two of which are impacted in the neck.

Acute cholecystitis is associated with the pre-existence of cholelithiasis in the majority of cases (see above). It is considered likely that in many instances a calculus or calculi become impacted in the neck of the gall bladder or Hartmann's pouch, leading to increased intraluminal pressure, mucosal erosion and a chemical cholecystitis. Whether or not bacteria play a role in the development of this inflammation remains a source of controversy but the weight of evidence would suggest that this is not the case.

Because of the almost invariable association with cholelithiasis, it is predictable that those most often affected tend to be obese, parous females; however, owing to the ubiquity of gall stones, this is by no means invariable. Complications of acute cholecystitis include perforation (with peritonitis) and the development of an empyema (see Figure and Legend 3.247)

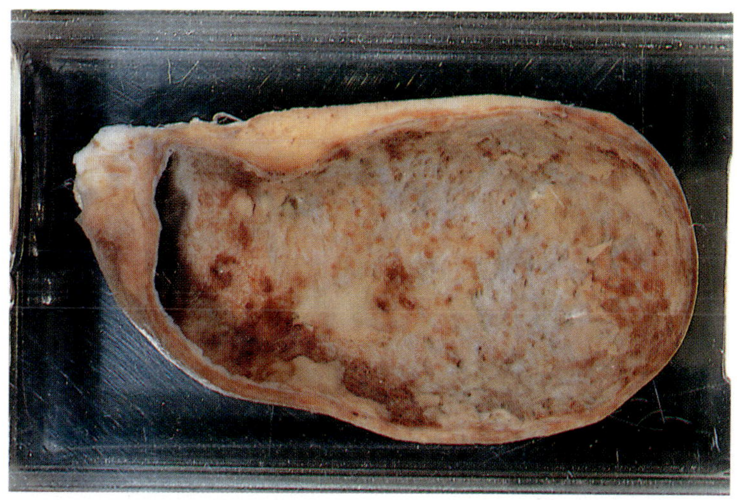

3.243 Gall Bladder: Acute Cholecystitis

This specimen was excised from a 69-year-old woman who, following a long history of non-specific postprandial dyspepsia, presented with acute upper abdominal pain. At operation, no gall stones were found either in the gall bladder or biliary tree.

The gall bladder has been opened to show marked mucosal and transmural congestion and oedema, associated with a multifocal fibrinopurulent exudate.

Acute cholecystitis in the absence of cholelithiasis is uncommon and often idiopathic in origin. However, a variety of causes may be implicated, including kinking of the cystic duct, secretion of an abnormally viscid bile, ischaemia or typhoid infection. This condition may also be seen in post-operative patients who have been starved and in whom the stagnant ('unused') bile may become viscid or hyperconcentrated.

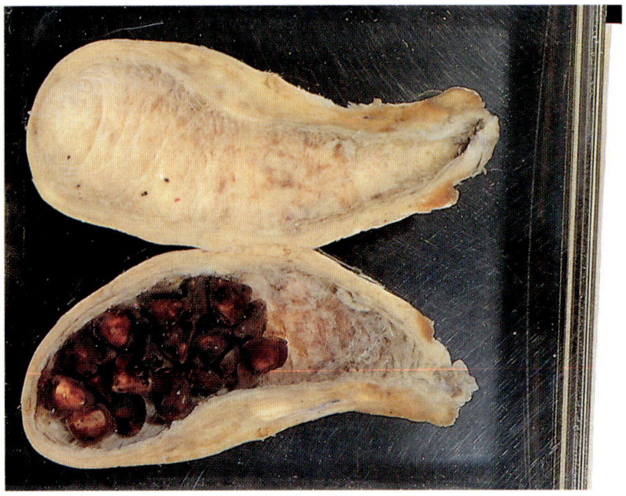

3.244 Gall Bladder: Acute Purulent Cholecystitis

This specimen was excised from a 61-year-old woman who presented with a 4 day history of acute right hypochondrial pain associated with vomiting and a pyrexia. There was marked tenderness and rigidity in the right upper abdomen and laparotomy was performed.

The gall bladder has been opened to show marked congestion associated with florid, yellowish purulent inflammation. Numerous gall stones are present in the fundus and, in the fresh state, these were surrounded by thick pus.

This appearance probably represents a more advanced stage of that seen in Figure 3.242 and reflects the likely development of secondary bacterial infection superimposed upon the initiating chemical cholecystitis.

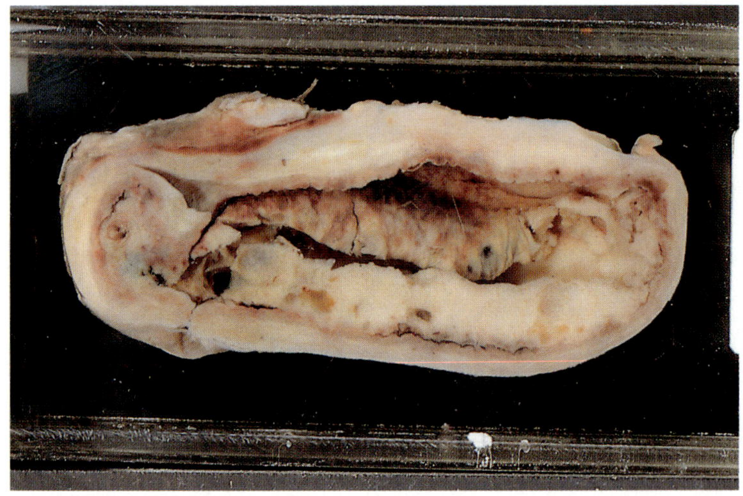

3.245 Gall Bladder: Acute-on-Chronic Cholecystitis

This specimen was excised from a 48-year-old woman who presented with a 2 week history of epigastric pain associated with vomiting. Eight months previously she had suffered similar symptoms and had been jaundiced for 3 weeks on that occasion. Cholecystectomy was performed at which the common bile duct was found to be free from stones.

The gall bladder has been opened to show marked submucosal thickening and fibrosis of the muscle coat. The mucosa is replaced by an expanded layer of pale, focally haemorrhagic, necrotic slough.

This is an example of acute suppurative cholecystitis occurring in a gall bladder that has been the seat of previous chronic inflammation, hence the thickening of the submucosa and muscle coats. Such florid suppuration and mucosal necrosis is infrequently seen in surgical specimens as it is common practice to treat attacks of acute cholecystitis conservatively.

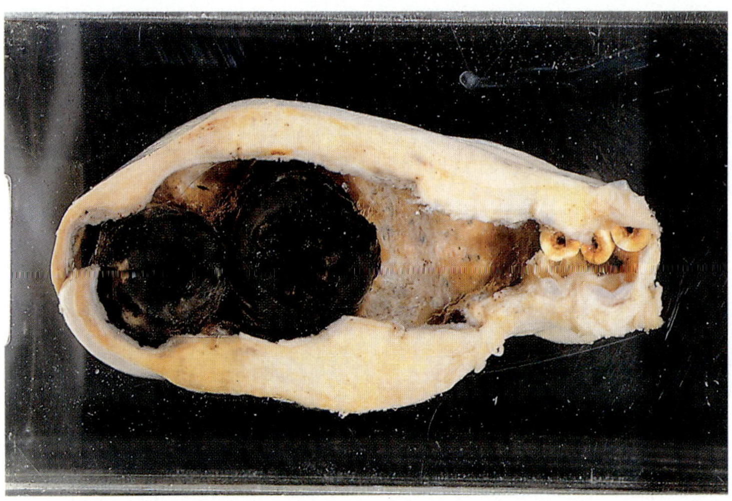

3.246 Gall Bladder: Acute-on-Chronic Cholecystitis

This specimen was excised from a 64-year-old woman who presented with severe right upper quadrant abdominal pain associated with vomiting. She had suffered from bouts of flatulent dyspepsia for several years. Examination revealed signs of peritonitis and a high temperature. Therefore immediate cholecystectomy was performed.

The wall of the gall bladder is grossly thickened, mostly with fibrous tissue, and there is marked mucosal congestion. Two dark pigment stones, each measuring 2cm in diameter, are present in the fundus and three small, paler calculi are impacted in the neck.

Most gall bladders excised for cholecystitis show evidence of previous inflammation with fibrosis and it is often surprising how few biliary symptoms there may have been. Recognised indications for immediate cholecystectomy (which a minority would advocate routinely) are clinical doubt as to the diagnosis, signs of perforation, and the persistence of florid signs or symptoms despite conservative measures.

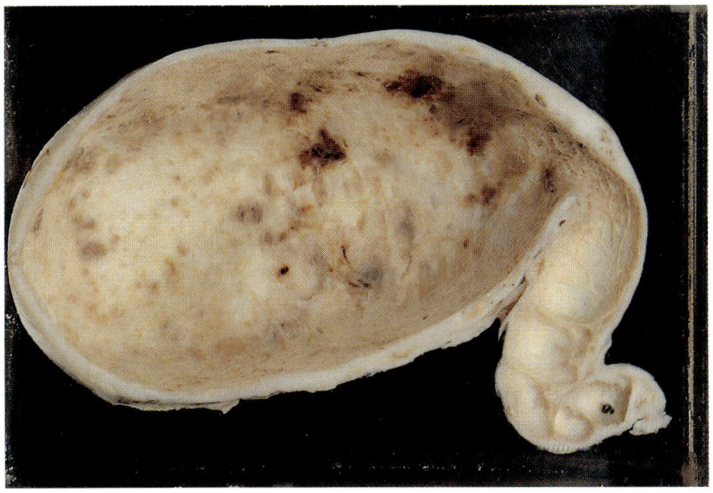

3.247 Gall Bladder: Empyema

This specimen was excised from a 69-year-old man who first presented with indigestion and weight loss. Barium meal suggested a large gastric ulcer but he refused further investigation. Three months later he became jaundiced and, after a further 2 months, he finally presented with severe jaundice and a painless mass beneath the right costal margin. Laparotomy was performed at which a grossly distended gall bladder was excised and 300ml of purulent bile aspirated from the common bile duct. Despite a careful search, no biliary obstruction could be identified and a choledochoduodenostomy was performed empirically.

The gall bladder and cystic duct, which are grossly dilated, have been opened to show intense mucosal congestion with superficial erosions. The wall of the gall bladder is thickened and fibrotic. In the fresh state, the lumen contained a number of small, facetted calculi and copious brown, purulent fluid.

Empyema of the gall bladder is an infrequent complication of acute suppurative cholecystitis and is characterised by the accumulation of copious purulent bile within an obstructed gall bladder. In fact, many cases labelled as 'empyema' are neither truly purulent nor infective and simply represent dilatation of the gall bladder by turbid bile containing inflammatory debris, and precipitated cholesterol and calcium carbonate. The degree of obstruction in this case suggests the possibility of an occult lesion (probably a neoplasm) in the region of the duodenal ampulla or head of the pancreas.

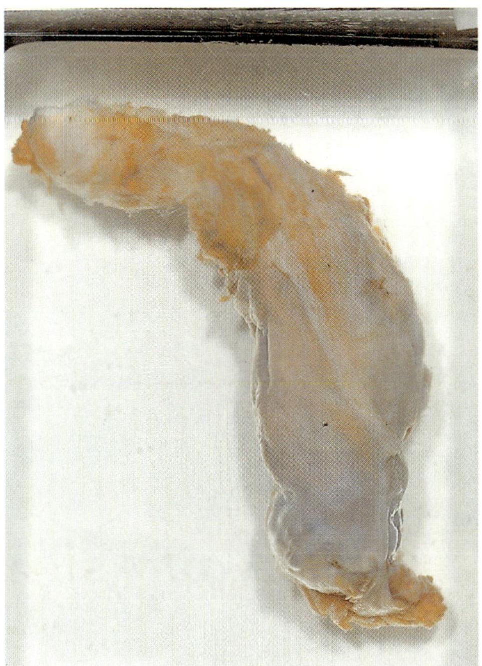

3.248 Gall Bladder: Chronic Cholecystitis

This specimen was excised from a 53-year-old man who had suffered several previous attacks of cholecystitis without jaundice. At operation, the gall bladder was densely adherent to the greater omentum, into which it appeared there had been a small perforation in the past.

The gall bladder (which contains dozens of small calculi not visible in this view) is markedly shrunken and fibrotic, measuring approximately 8 × 2 × 2cm. The omental fat has largely been dissected away but is still adherent over the fundus and around the neck.

Chronic cholecystitis represents the result of either repeated attacks of acute inflammation or of chronic, clinically inapparent low-grade inflammation and, as would be expected (see Legend 3.242) is almost always associated with cholelithiasis. Persistent inflammation leads to fibrous scarring of the gall bladder wall, often associated with mucosal attenuation and the development of intramural 'diverticula' (Rokitansky-Aschoff sinuses).

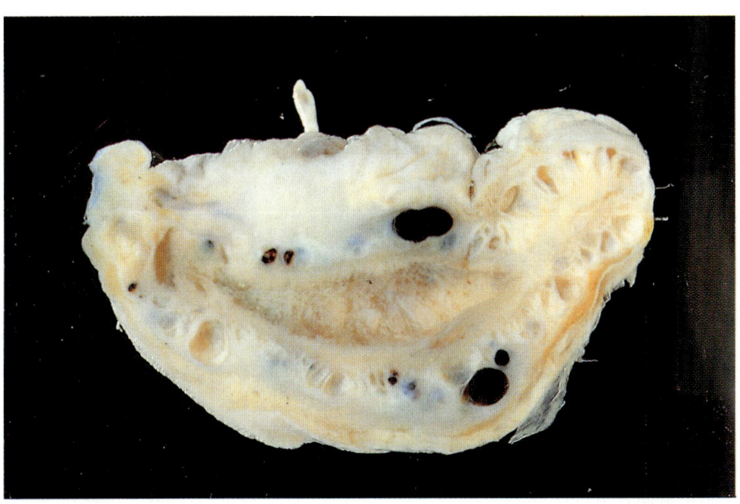

3.249 Gall Bladder: Chronic Cholecystitis

This specimen was excised from a 65-year-old woman who was noted to have a fibrotic gall bladder while undergoing partial gastrectomy for a duodenal ulcer.

This shrunken gall bladder has been sectioned to show gross mural fibrosis with thickening and virtual obliteration of the lumen. Small cystic spaces extend from the lumen into the wall, some of which are filled with pigment concretions. In the fresh state, a cholesterol calculus was impacted in the neck.

In addition to mural fibrous scarring, this case shows obvious (and extreme) development of multiple intramural 'diverticula'. These represent mucosal outpouchings (Rokitansky-Aschoff sinuses) which are characteristic features of chronic cholecystitis, and which have become cystically dilated due to proximal obstruction. This appearance has been known, in the past, as 'cholecystitis glandularis proliferans'.

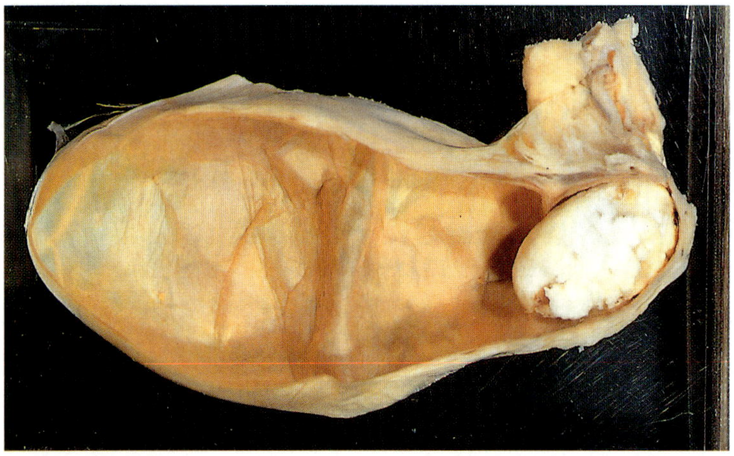

3.250 Gall Bladder: Mucocele

This specimen was excised from a 62-year-old woman who had presented with a history of abdominal pain and repeated vomiting.

The gall bladder is so distended that its wall is almost translucent. Impacted in Hartmann's pouch is a large, ovoid cholesterol stone which has completely obstructed the outlet. In the fresh state, the lumen of the gall bladder contained copious, clear mucoid fluid.

A mucocele of the gall bladder results from persistent complete obstruction of the outflow tract usually by a stone either in the cystic duct, the neck of the gall bladder or in Hartmann's pouch. No further bile can enter the lumen and that which is already present is gradually reabsorbed. The glandular epithelium continues to produce mucinous secretions, which progressively accumulate leading to dilatation. Rupture of such a mucocele may lead to pseudomyxoma peritonei.

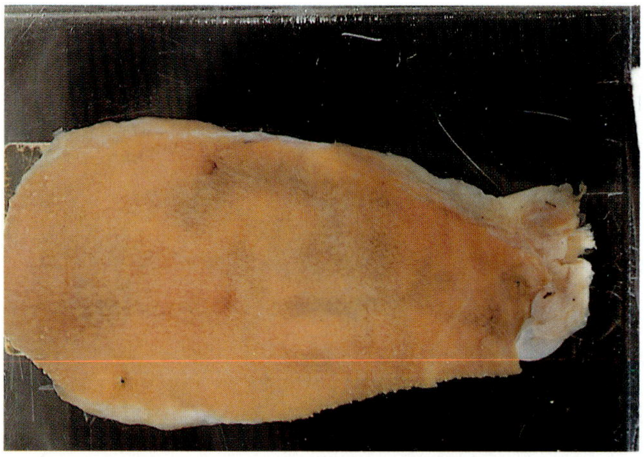

3.251 Gall Bladder: Cholesterolosis

This specimen was excised from a 48-year-old woman who had suffered repeated attacks of biliary colic (without jaundice) for the previous 2½ years. X-rays revealed a single stone in the gall bladder and cholecystectomy was performed.

The gall bladder has been opened to reveal fine yellowish flecks in the superficial mucosal folds.

Cholesterolosis is a common condition of little significance which results from the deposition of cholesterol in the mucosa of the gall bladder. These yellow flecks, when seen in the fresh state against a reddish mucosal surface, have led to the name 'strawberry gall bladder' to describe this condition. The aetiology is unknown but a local abnormality of cholesterol metabolism or absorption is suspected and would account for the frequent coexistence of cholesterol calculi.

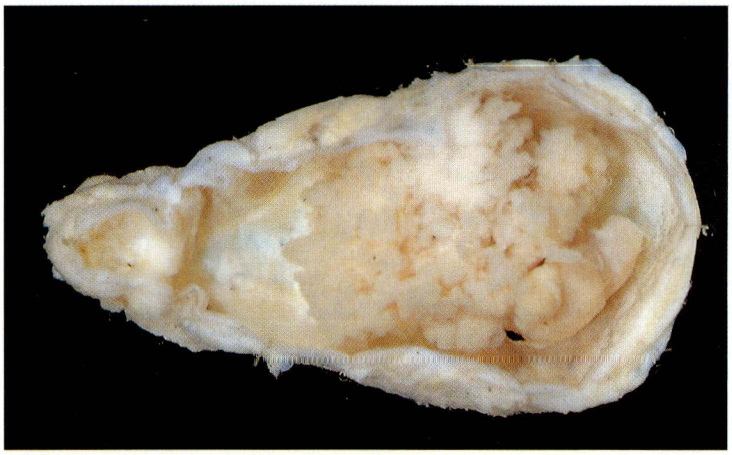

3.252 Gall Bladder: Papillary Adenoma

No clinical details are available.

The gall bladder has been opened to show a papillary, pedunculated lesion arising in the fundus. The gall bladder is otherwise normal and there is no evidence, either macroscopically or histologically, that this tumour has invaded the gall bladder wall.

Adenomata of the gall bladder (i.e. benign epithelial tumours) are extremely rare but may adopt a rounded or papillary appearance. They seem to arise in the elderly and are believed by some to be premalignant lesions (comparable to neoplastic polyps of the large bowel).

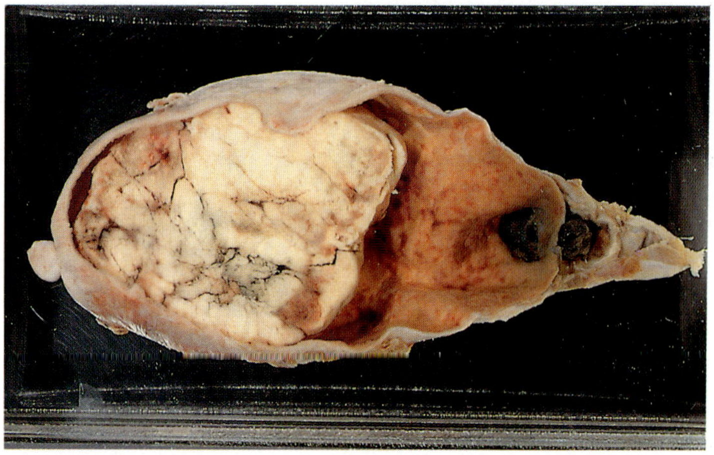

3.253 Gall Bladder: Adenocarcinoma

This specimen was excised from a 71-year-old woman who had suffered from recurrent upper abdominal pain for over 20 years. She finally presented with a severe attack of biliary colic. Examination revealed right hypochondrial tenderness and a cholecystogram showed no concentration of medium in the gall bladder. Cholecystectomy was performed.

This distended gall bladder, measuring 16 × 6 × 6cm, has been opened to show a large (8cm in maximum diameter) pale, partly papillary tumour arising in the fundus. A mixed calculus is impacted in Hartmann's pouch and, in the fresh state, the remainder of the lumen was filled with numerous small gall stones.

Adenocarcinoma of the gall bladder is very uncommon and is seen most often in the elderly with a marked predominance in females. While the precise aetiology is uncertain, this tumour is associated with coexistent gall stones in the majority of cases. The tumour usually adopts a diffuse infiltrative pattern and extensive local invasion (typically with liver involvement) frequently renders the lesion inoperable at presentation. However, polypoid intraluminal growth (as shown here) is also common. These neoplasms also tend to grow directly along the cystic duct and to spread by lymphatics. In general, the prognosis is extremely poor with a 5-year-survival of less than 10 per cent.

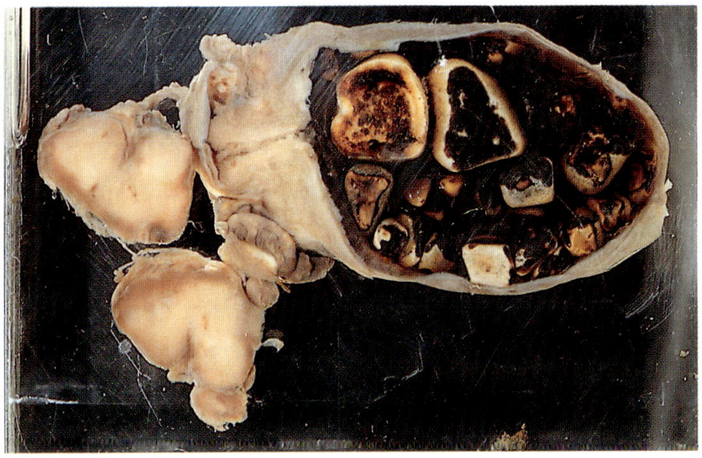

3.254 Gall Bladder: Adenocarcinoma

This specimen was excised from a 46-year-old man, who presented with non-specific upper abdominal discomfort for the past 9 months. On examination the gall bladder was palpable and a laparotomy was performed.

The gall bladder is distended and the lumen contains numerous, facetted mixed calculi. A pale, infiltrative neoplasm has arisen at the neck and spread along the cystic duct, extending to the serosal surface. Lymph nodes (right) located by the portal vein and common bile duct are expanded and infiltrated by tumour, as is the cystic node.

This case demonstrates the propensity of this tumour to spread along the cystic duct and to disseminate via the lymphatic system.

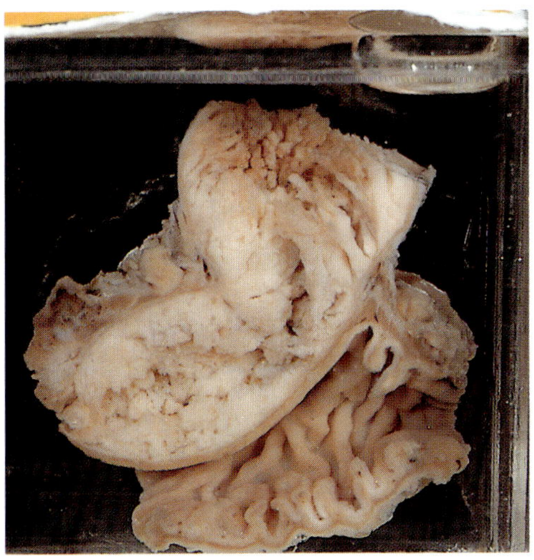

3.255 Common Bile Duct: Adenocarcinoma

No clinical details are available.

A segment of duodenum with the distal portion of the common bile duct (above) is shown; the ampulla of Vater is seen in cross-section at the left hand edge. The bile duct is grossly dilated and its lumen is occluded by an extensive, pale, partly papillary neoplasm.

Carcinoma of the extrahepatic biliary ducts is uncommon and tends to occur in the elderly with an almost equal sex incidence. The two sites most often affected are the periampullary portion of the common bile duct and the junction of the cystic and hepatic ducts. In Western cases the aetiology is uncertain. In the Far East, where this tumour is rather more common, a proportion of cases is associated with biliary infestation by the fluke *Clonorchis sinensis*. Macroscopically, these tumours often adopt a papillary, exophytic configuration (as here) as a result of which biliary obstruction is a common presenting feature. Early lymph node and hepatic metastases are usual and these, combined with the obvious operative difficulties, confer a very poor prognosis.

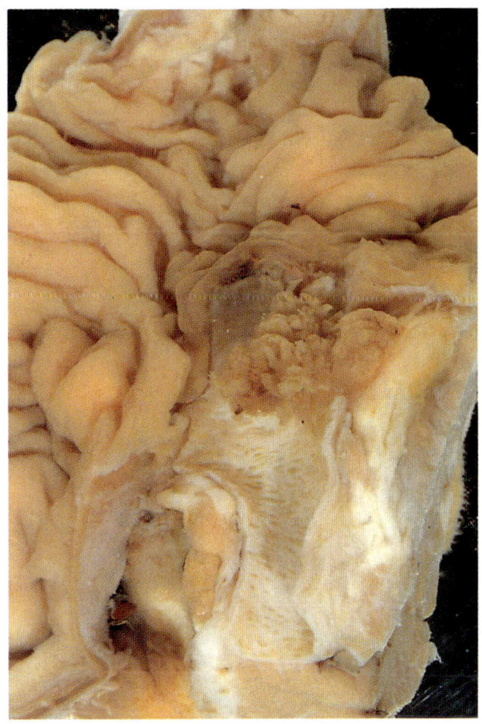

3.256 Common Bile Duct: Papillary Adenocarcinoma

This specimen was excised from a 50-year-old man who presented with obstructive jaundice. An oral cholecystogram revealed only faint opacification of the gall bladder and, at laparotomy, an operative cholangiogram revealed an irregular filling defect near the lower end of the common bile duct. A pancreaticoduodenectomy with cholecystjejunostomy was performed.

A close-up view of the opened duodenum with the distal portion of the common bile duct shows a small papillary neoplasm, measuring 1.5cm in diameter, arising in the bile duct approximately 0.5cm above the ampulla of Vater. Proximally, the bile duct is dilated.

This is a typical example of a papillary carcinoma of the distal common bile duct. In contrast, tumours arising in the more proximal parts of the extrahepatic biliary system usually show a diffuse infiltrative (scirrhous) pattern and may be difficult to distinguish macroscopically from a benign fibrotic process.

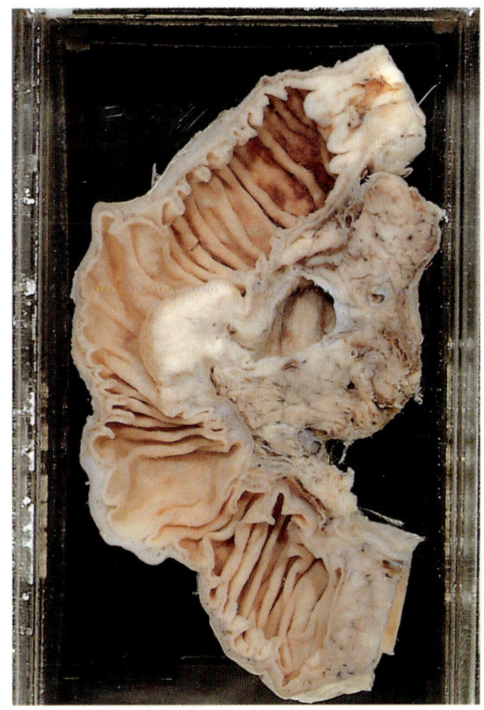

3.257 Ampulla of Vater: Adenocarcinoma

This specimen was excised from a 56-year-old man who presented with a 3 week history of jaundice, itching and a mild pyrexia. Radiological studies were normal but, at laparotomy, the gall bladder and common bile duct were distended owing to distal obstruction. A pancreaticoduodenectomy and cholecystjejunostomy was performed.

The head of the pancreas, duodenum and distal common bile duct have been dissected to reveal a small, nodular, pale neoplasm arising in the ampulla of Vater beneath the duodenal mucosa. The tumour, which measures 1.5cm in diameter, has obstructed the orifice of the ampulla leading to marked dilatation of the common bile duct (middle right).

Ampullary adenocarcinoma usually represents a primary neoplasm of the distal end of the common bile duct rather than a duodenal lesion; some would regard this site as the commonest of all extrahepatic biliary carcinomas. Tumours located in the ampulla tend to cause obstructive jaundice early in the course of the disease and this fact may account for the comparatively good prognosis that adenocarcinoma at this location carries.

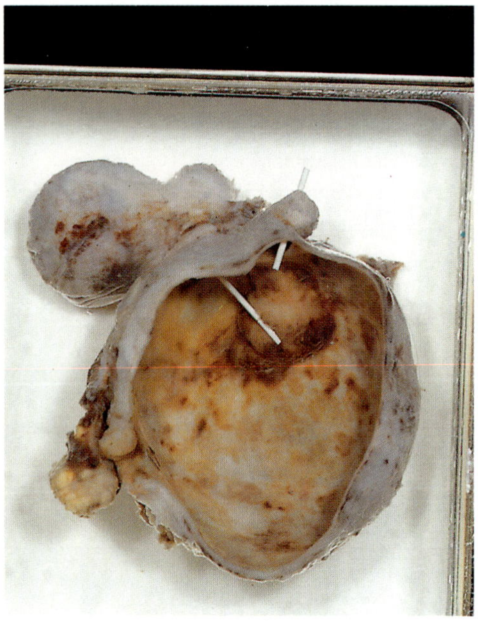

3.258 Common Bile Duct: Choledochus Cyst with Adenocarcinoma

This specimen was excised from a 50-year-old woman, who presented with a 4 year history of recurrent right upper abdominal pain. A tender cystic mass was palpable in the right upper quadrant and a cholecystogram suggested the diagnosis of a mucocele. Laparotomy revealed the mass to be a choledochus cyst within which a small tumour was present. Resection with hepaticojejunostomy and a bypassing entero-enterostomy was performed.

The specimen consists of an enormously cystically dilated portion of the common bile duct, measuring 7cm in diameter, with attached gall bladder (top left), and into which the dilated common hepatic duct drains (upper probe). The point at which the cystic duct enters the lesion is marked by the lower probe. In the upper part of the posterior wall of the cyst is a rounded, rather flattened tumour which, at operation, had visibly infiltrated adjacent soft tissues.

This is another example of an adenocarcinoma arising at the confluence of the cystic and common bile ducts. Its precise relationship to the choledochus cyst (which is simply a dilated segment of the common bile duct) is uncertain. True choledochus cysts are usually congenital lesions which represent incomplete canalisation of the developing bile duct with partial obstruction and typically present in childhood with obstructive jaundice. It is impossible to determine whether this lesion has developed secondarily to obstruction by the tumour with herniation of a 'pseudocyst' through a congenital weakness in the bile duct wall. However, congenital lesions of the biliary tree, including choledochus cyst, are prone to malignant change.

Pancreas

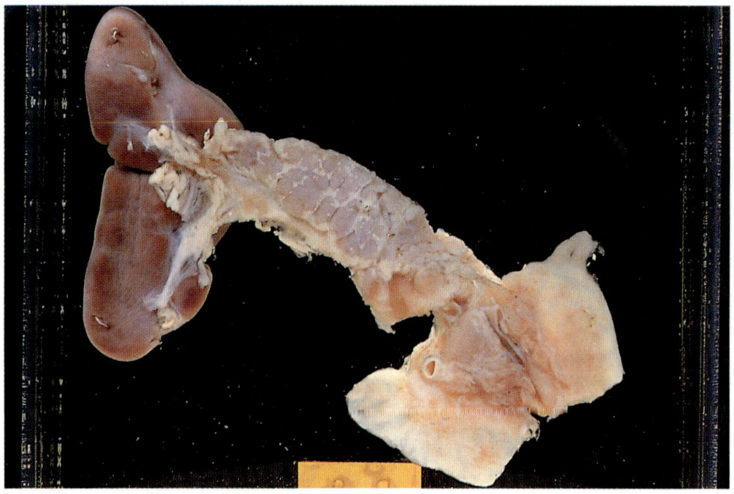

3.259 Pancreas: Cystic Fibrosis

This is a post-mortem specimen from a 21-month-old girl who had been noted to have pale, offensive stools and who died of respiratory infection.

The spleen, pancreas and duodenum are viewed from behind. The surface of the pancreas shows very marked lobulation (reflecting underlying scarring), but otherwise appears relatively normal.

Cystic fibrosis (synonym: mucoviscidosis) is an autosomal recessively inherited condition which affects up to 1 in 2500 live-born Caucasian infants, but is much rarer in Asians and Africans. The disease is characterised by abnormal exocrine secretory function, leading to excessively viscid secretions containing a high concentration of electrolytes. The sweat glands, salivary glands and respiratory mucous glands are affected as well as the pancreas. Clinical features may include meconium ileus (see Small and Large Intestines section), malabsorption, pancreatic insufficiency and repeated respiratory infections leading to bronchiectasis. Patients surviving into adolescence may develop secondary biliary cirrhosis, usually associated with involvement of the common bile duct by the disease process. Treatment remains purely palliative and only a small proportion of affected individuals survive into their 3rd decade. (Courtesy of the Gordon Museum, Guy's Hospital Medical School)

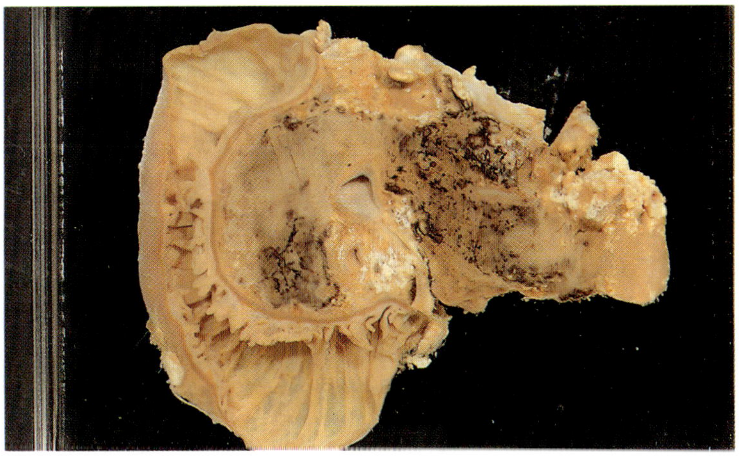

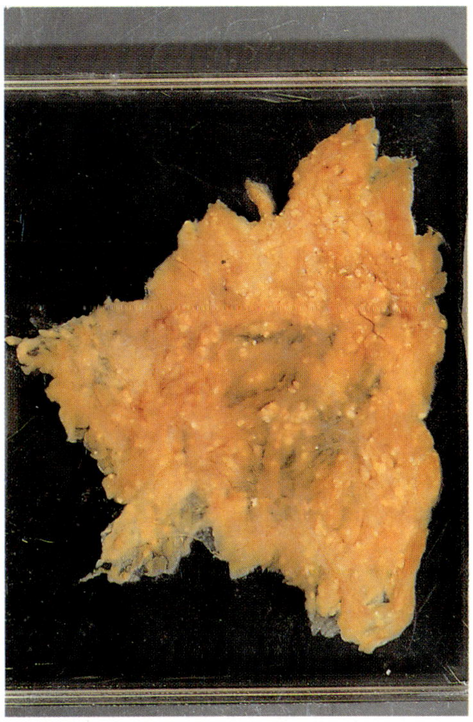

3.260 Pancreas: Acute Haemorrhagic Pancreatitis

No clinical details are available.

The pancreas and part of the duodenum are shown in coronal section (3.260a). The pancreas is markedly swollen and shows extensive haemorrhagic necrosis, particularly in the body. Small fragments of adjacent adipose tissue show multiple foci of bright yellow necrosis, which can be seen more clearly in the portion of greater omentum mounted separately (3.260b).

Acute pancreatitis is very common, accounting for approximately 1 in 500 hospital admissions in the Western world, and results from the sudden onset of enzymatic autodigestion of the pancreatic parenchyma and adjacent tissues. It largely affects adults in the 4th and 5th decades and is rather more common in males. Several theories for its development are postulated, the suggestion of reflux of duodenal contents into the pancreatic duct being the most favoured. While some cases are idiopathic, the commonest known predisposing causes are alcohol abuse (particularly in males) and the pre-existence of biliary tract disease, especially gall stones (particularly in females). There are many other recognised causes including upper gastrointestinal or hepatobiliary surgery or instrumentation, any adjacent inflammatory process, bacterial or viral infection, ischaemia, hypothermia, various drugs, hypercalcaemia, and hyperlipoproteinaemia.

Activation of proteases, elastases and lipases leads to the destruction of pancreatic tissue, blood vessel walls (hence the haemorrhage) and adjacent adipose tissue. This extensive tissue damage, associated with loss of blood and body fluids, may lead to the development of shock and renal failure. Other immediate complications include the development of secondary infection, disseminated intravascular coagulation, 'shock lung', and death in up to 10 per cent of cases. Possible delayed complications are the development of a pancreatic pseudocyst, exocrine or endocrine pancreatic insufficiency and a tendency to further attacks of inflammation.

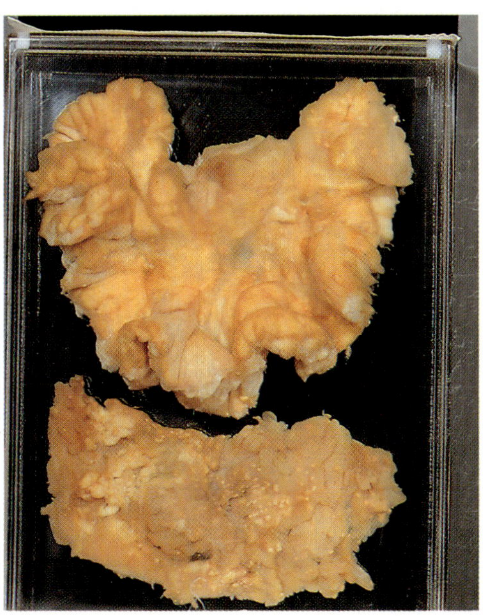

3.261 Mesentery and Omentum: Fat Necrosis due to Acute Pancreatitis

These are post-mortem specimens from a 53-year-old man who died one week after the onset of acute pancreatitis. At autopsy there was extensive fat necrosis throughout the peritoneal cavity.

Both the mesentery (above) and greater omentum (below) show numerous foci of yellowish fat necrosis, many of which have undergone dystrophic calcification.

Release of lipases from the damaged pancreas leads to this characteristic feature of acute pancreatitis. Digestion of adipose tissue causes release of triglycerides and fatty acids and the latter then undergo saponification which, in turn, predisposes to the deposition of calcium salts. Sequestration of calcium to necrotic fat may be so marked as to give rise to hypocalcaemia in patients with acute pancreatitis, and tetany may develop.

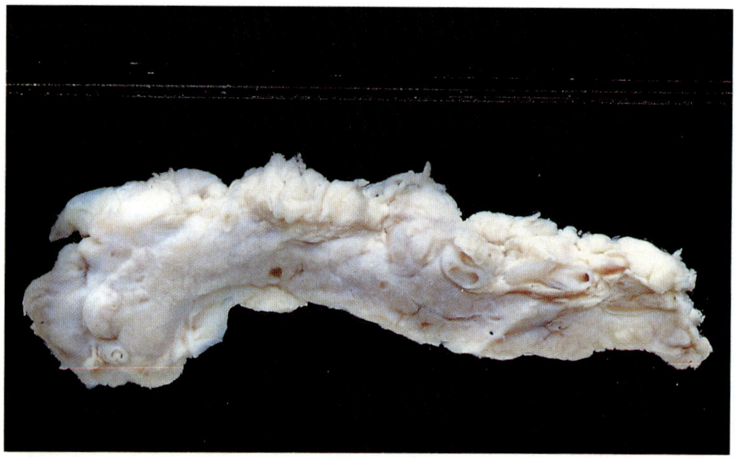

3.262 Pancreas: Chronic Pancreatitis

This is a post-mortem specimen from a 46-year-old man who died of a myocardial infarct. At the age of 25 he had undergone partial gastrectomy for a duodenal ulcer and, 3 years previously, a cholecystenterostomy had been performed following repeated attacks of pancreatitis.

The entire pancreas is pale and has a rather irregular surface, being largely replaced by fibrous tissue.

Chronic pancreatitis may present *de novo* following prolonged low-grade inflammation or may be the end result of repeated symptomatic attacks of acute inflammation. It is commonest in males, often being related to alcohol abuse, although there may be coexistent pancreatic duct obstruction or dysfunction. Complications include calcification, stone formation in the pancreatic ducts, liver disease, pancreatic exocrine hypofunction and occasionally, diabetes mellitus. At laparotomy, the hard fibrotic nature of the pancreas is easily mistaken for infiltration by a carcinoma. (Courtesy of the Gordon Museum, Guy's Hospital Medical School)

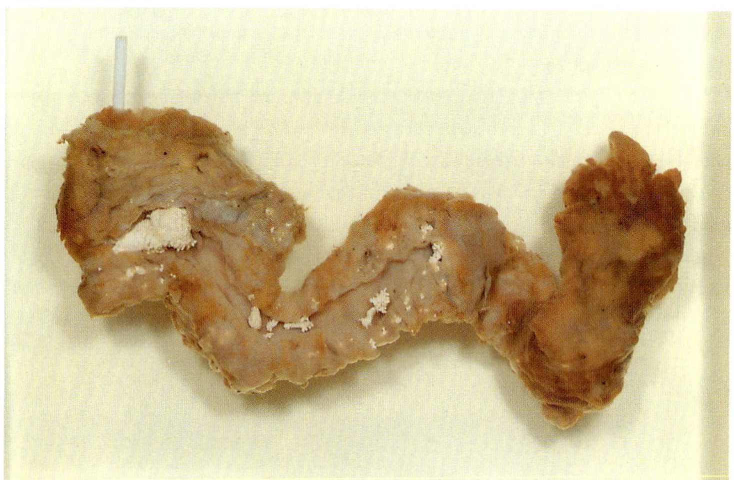

3.263 Pancreas: Calculi with Duct Obstruction

This is a post-mortem specimen from a 72-year-old man who died of acute myocardial infarction. The pancreatic pathology was an incidental finding and the remainder of the abdominal organs were normal.

The pancreas has been dissected to show the main pancreatic duct within which are located numerous pale calculi of varying size. The largest of these is impacted at the opening of the duct. Numerous small branches of the pancreatic duct, seen in cross-section, also contain small calculi and the pancreatic parenchyma is irregularly scarred and fibrotic.

The development of pancreatic calculi is often associated with duct obstruction and chronic pancreatitis but it is uncertain whether the stones are the initiating factor or a secondary phenomenon. An underlying abnormality of exocrine secretory drainage may possibly predispose to both lesions. Frequently such calculi are an incidental finding in the elderly, either at post-mortem or on a plain abdominal X-ray, suggesting that they develop independently in the absence of clinically significant inflammation. Any cause of hypercalcaemia may be a predisposing factor.

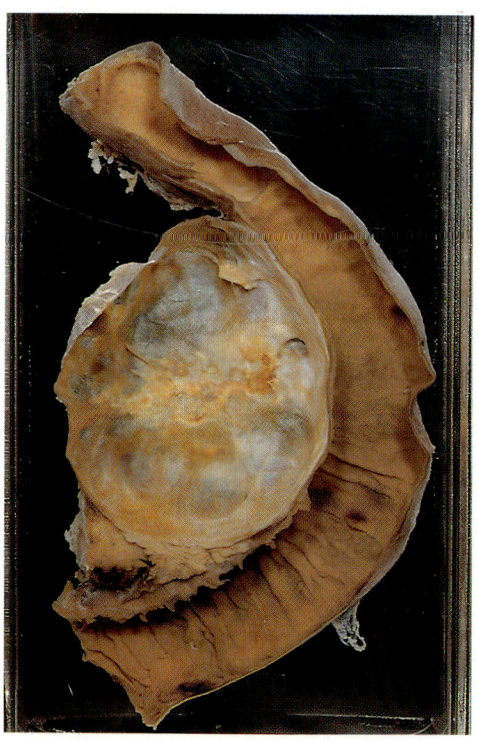

3.264 Pancreas: Cyst

This specimen was excised from a 47-year-old woman who presented with a symptomless mass in the upper abdomen. X-rays revealed a rounded lesion with focal calcification in the region of the head of the pancreas and, following discovery of the cyst at laparotomy, a pancreaticoduodenectomy was performed.

The head of the pancreas adjacent to the duodenum is replaced by a large unilocular cyst, measuring 8cm in diameter. The wall of the cyst shows pale mucinous areas and foci of dystrophic calcification. In the fresh state it contained clear gelatinous fluid. The body and tail of the pancreas, which were not excised, appeared completely normal.

The precise nature of this cystic lesion is uncertain; histologically, it is a true cyst lined by mucin-secreting columnar epithelium. True pancreatic cysts may be divided into 3 principal types – congenital, retention and neoplastic – which should be distinguished from the pseudocyst of acute pancreatitis, which simply represents a walled-off area of necrotic tissue.

Congenital pancreatic cysts are most often associated with renal or hepatic polycystic disease and there may be a coexistent cerebellar haemangioblastoma (von Hippel-Lindau disease). Retention cysts follow pancreatic duct obstruction and are therefore usually seen in chronic pancreatitis or cystic fibrosis (mucoviscidosis). Neoplastic cysts most often represent either a cystadenoma (see Figure and Legend 3.265) or a cystadenocarcinoma.

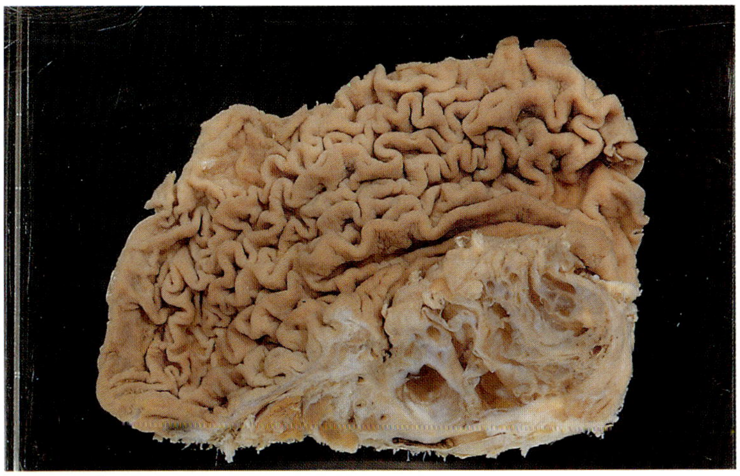

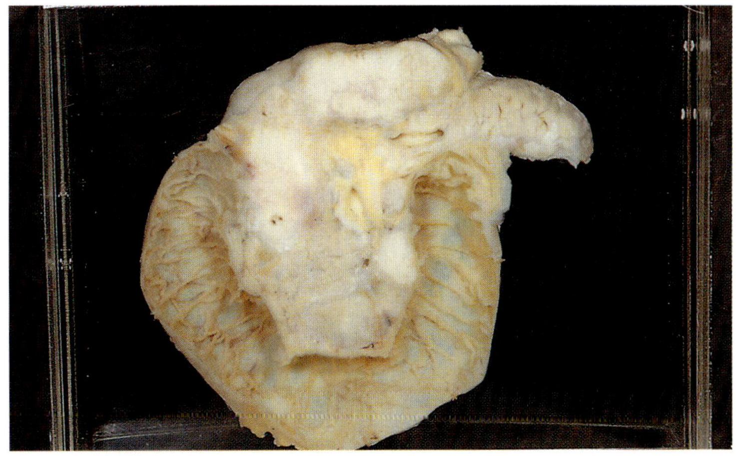

3.265 Pancreas: Cystadenoma

This specimen was excised from a 35-year-old woman who had suffered periodic attacks of epigastric pain and vomiting for 6½ years. More recently she had developed haematemesis and melaena. A barium meal suggested a tumour on the greater curvature of the stomach and laparotomy revealed a mass in the body of the pancreas, compressing the stomach, over which the gastric mucosa had ulcerated.

Part of the gastric greater curvature and a portion of the body of the pancreas have been dissected to show a reasonably circumscribed pancreatic tumour, measuring 5cm in diameter. The lesion is partly solid and partly cystic and, in the fresh state, the multilocular cystic areas contained pale, mucoid fluid. The gastric mucosa over the tumour is attenuated and ulcerated. Histologically there is no evidence of malignancy.

Pancreatic cystadenomas are fairly rare benign lesions which tend to present in the 4th and 5th decades, the majority of cases being seen in females. They are typically multilocular lesions, usually located in the body or tail of the pancreas, which tend only to produce symptoms when they exceed about 5cm in diameter. Whether they may predispose to the development of cystadenocarcinoma or whether the latter is malignant from the outset is difficult to determine.

3.266 Pancreas: Adenocarcinoma

This is a post-mortem specimen from a 67-year-old woman who presented with colicky abdominal pain and vomiting. She had been known to have diabetes mellitus for some years. On examination there was tenderness in the right hypochondrium with pyrexia; cholecystitis was suspected but her condition deteriorated rapidly and she died. At autopsy there was a pancreatic tumour with metastases in the liver and right adrenal gland.

The pancreas and distal half of the duodenum are shown. Arising in the head of the pancreas is an infiltrative, pale neoplasm and there are separate tumour nodules close to the serosal surface of the duodenum (middle right).

Adenocarcinoma of the pancreas, which arises from exocrine ductal epithelium in 99 per cent of cases, accounts for approximately 5 per cent of malignant neoplasms in the Western world; the incidence appears to be increasing. Patients in the 6th and 7th decades are most often affected and up to 65 per cent of cases arise in males. The aetiology is uncertain but there is an increased incidence in cigarette smokers. At least two-thirds of such tumours arise in the head of the pancreas, the tail being the least common primary site. They tend to be diffusely infiltrative lesions which lead to obstruction of the common bile duct at an early stage, hence the frequent coexistence of a dilated gall bladder. Patients may present with an associated migratory thrombophlebitis (Trousseau's sign). While lymphatic and blood-borne metastases eventually occur, the majority of patients die of hepatobiliary dysfunction beforehand. The prognosis is abysmal, 5-year-survival being less than 5 per cent. Complications of this neoplasm, other than obstructive jaundice and gastrointestinal haemorrhage due to direct invasion, include the development of chronic obstructive pancreatitis, diabetes mellitus (the reasons for which are unclear), and non-bacterial thrombotic endocarditis.

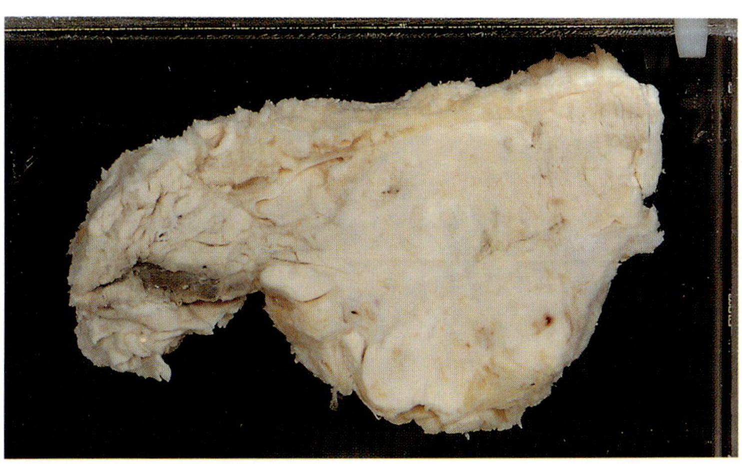

3.267 Pancreas: Adenocarcinoma

This is a post-mortem specimen from a 63-year-old man, who presented to an orthopaedic department complaining of very severe low back pain. He was cachectic and was found to have gross, irregular hepatomegaly and a bone scan revealed multiple metastases. Following admission he developed a right hemiparesis and a pathological fracture of the right femur and, shortly thereafter, died.

A coronal section through the pancreas shows a large, pale neoplasm virtually replacing the body and invading the neck. The head of the organ and common bile duct (lower left) are spared.

Up to 25 per cent of pancreatic carcinomas develop in the body of the organ. These tumours, along with those in the tail, tend not to produce biliary obstruction and very commonly present with metastases (as here) since any preceding symptoms may be nonspecific or entirely absent.

4. URINARY SYSTEM

KIDNEY

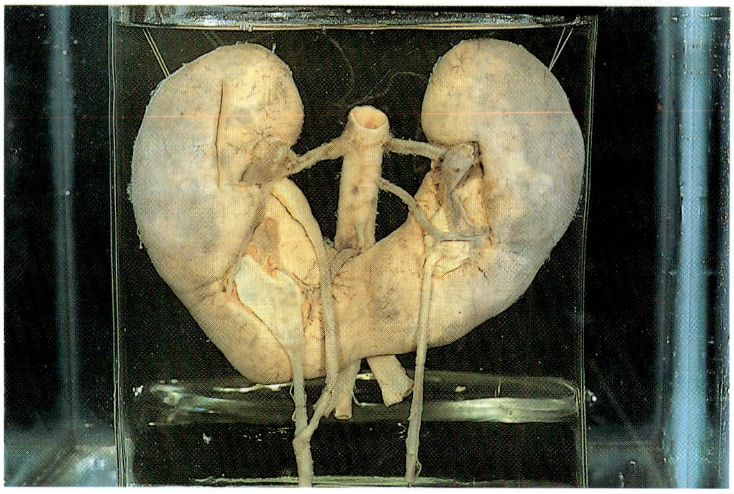

4.1 Horseshoe Deformity

This was an incidental post-mortem finding in a 34-year-old soldier, dying as a result of gunshot wounds sustained during the First World War.

Both kidneys with the aorta, renal arteries and ureters are shown. The kidneys are enlarged and united at their lower poles by an isthmus of renal tissue which lies over the aortic bifurcation. Due to a failure of rotation, both renal hila lie anteriorly.

The left kidney has a single ureter but two main renal arteries are present. On the right side, the ureter has a double origin and the upper and lower poles of the kidney are supplied by two arteries with widely separated origins from the aorta.

Renal fusion is not a very rare abnormality, being found in about 1 in 250 autopsies. It probably results from an embryological failure of ascent of nephrogenic tissue. Associated abnormalities of the vascular supply and ureters are common and it is as a result of these that horseshoe kidneys are prone to hydronephrosis, infection and stone formation. This deformity is more common in males than females and may be associated with other congenital abnormalities.

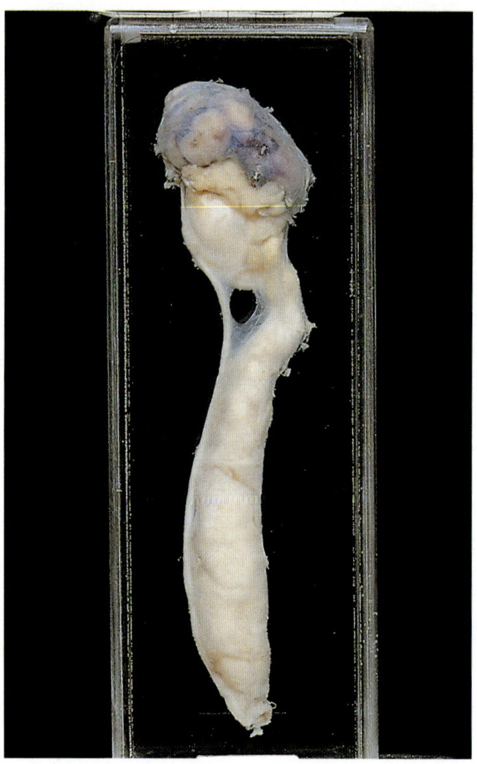

4.2 Hypoplasia with Congenital Hydronephrosis

This specimen was excised from a 3½-year-old girl who complained of left-sided abdominal pain and was found to have a urinary tract infection associated with a left-sided hydronephrosis and hydroureter.

A small kidney is seen, forming a cap over the grossly distended pelvis which is continuous with a dilated, tortuous ureter. The pale, thin, cordlike structure attached to the posterior surface of the ureter (left) is a second rudimentary ureter.

True renal hypoplasia is extremely rare and is defined as a small kidney, with 5 or less calyces, but which is otherwise normal. Most often the condition is unilateral and prognosis is largely dependent upon the contralateral renal function. The hydronephrosis is a consequence of abnormal ureteric drainage and serves to reiterate the frequency with which more than one congenital abnormality may be found in an anomalous urinary system.

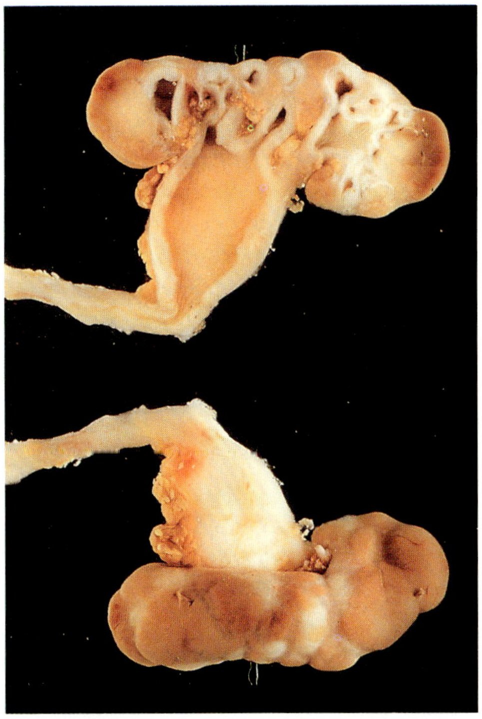

4.3 Dysplasia with Urinary Obstruction

This is a nephro-ureterectomy specimen from a 7-year-old boy who suffered recurrent urinary tract infections. Investigation revealed a very small left kidney and bilateral vesicoureteric reflux. At operation, right ureteric advancement reimplantation was also carried out.

The kidney is small and has an abnormal architecture. Histologically, areas are composed only of primitive metanephric tissue. There is moderate dilatation of the pelvicalyceal system and ureter (left). The cortical surface (right) shows marked fetal lobulation.

This is an example of segmental renal dysplasia, rather than hypoplasia, since parts of the kidney are histologically maldeveloped. Associated anomalies of the urinary tract are common, particularly vesicoureteric reflux which some would say is a causative factor of the abnormal renal development.

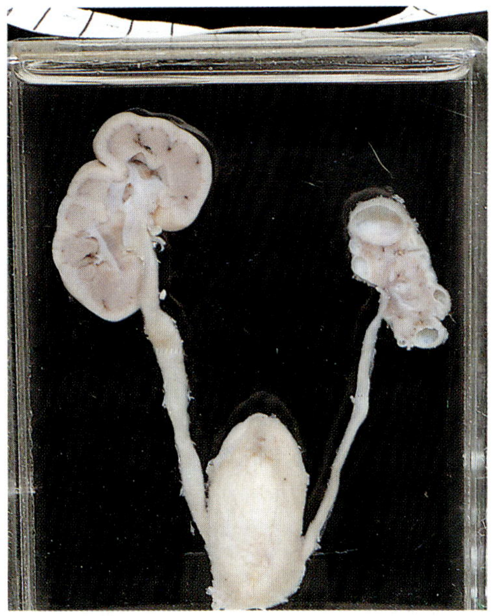

4.4 Dysplasia with Contralateral Hypertrophy

This was a post-mortem finding in a female neonate who died of pneumonia.

The left kidney and ureter are small and the renal parenchyma is largely composed of smooth-walled cysts. The right kidney shows compensatory enlargement.

This is an example of unilateral total renal dysplasia since no normal renal tissue is present on the left side. This is the commonest renal cystic abnormality in neonates and may be associated with congenital abnormalities of the heart or oesophagus.

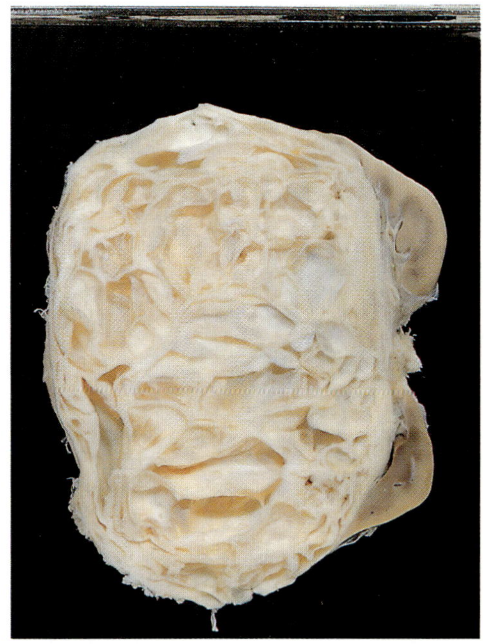

4.5 Multicystic Nephroma

This specimen was removed from a 19-month-old child.

The enlarged right kidney has been bisected to show virtual replacement of the renal parenchyma by a well-demarcated mass composed of multiple smooth-walled cysts. The remaining normal renal tissue (right) is attenuated.

Multicystic nephroma (synonyms: multilocular cyst, differentiated nephroblastoma) is a rare developmental malformation which most often presents in childhood. It is a sporadic condition, rather than inherited, and is usually unilateral. Pre-operatively it may be indistinguishable from a nephroblastoma, but its behaviour is entirely benign.

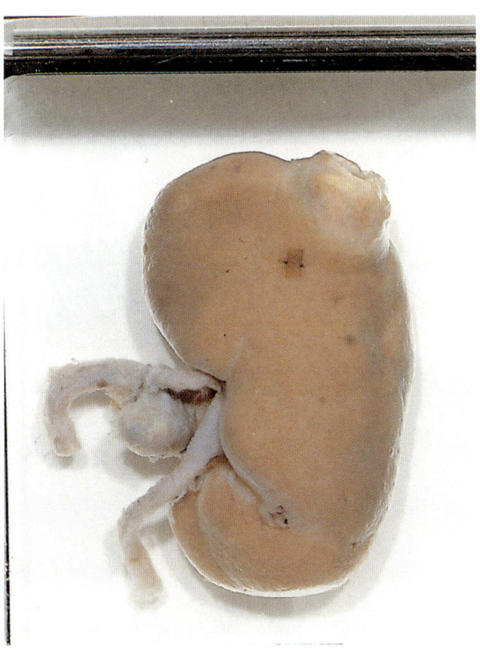

4.6 Aberrant Renal Artery with Aneurysm

This specimen was excised from a 66-year-old man who presented with a ureteric calculus but was also found to have an aneurysm of the renal artery.

The posterior surface of the right kidney, bearing a simple subcapsular cyst, is shown. In the region of the hilum, the renal artery divides into two branches and a yellowish aneurysmal sac, measuring 1.5 × 1cm, arises from the upper branch.

Anomalies of the renal arterial system are common and the development of an aneurysm is probably coincidental. The possible importance of aberrant renal vessels is that their path is thought occasionally to distort the pelviureteric junction, resulting in urinary obstruction.

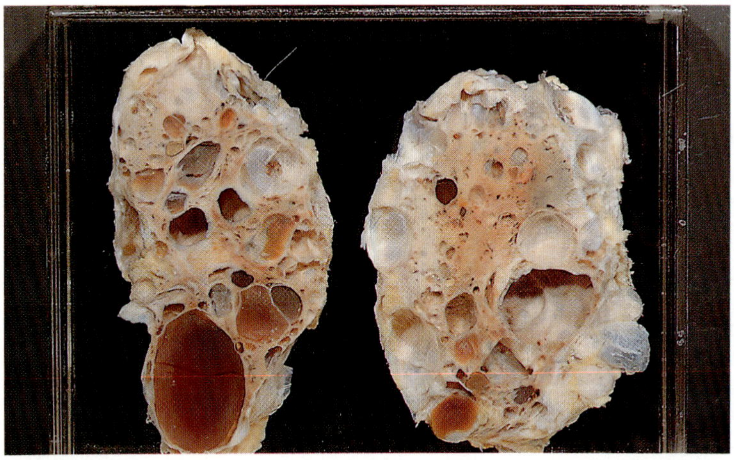

4.7 Adult Polycystic Disease

These are post-mortem specimens from a 53-year-old hypertensive woman who died of bronchopneumonia. At autopsy, hepatic cysts were also present.

Both kidneys are enlarged and show virtual replacement by multiple cysts of varying size. The cysts are smooth-walled and some contain gelatinous material.

Adult polycystic disease is a common condition which has an autosomal dominant inheritance. Patients most often present in middle age, either with hypertension, pyelonephritis or haematuria. Associated hepatic or pancreatic cysts are a common finding as are cerebral berry aneurysms. Survival from the time of presentation varies from 10-20 years and those affected usually succumb to the complications of chronic renal failure, hypertension or cerebral haemorrhage.

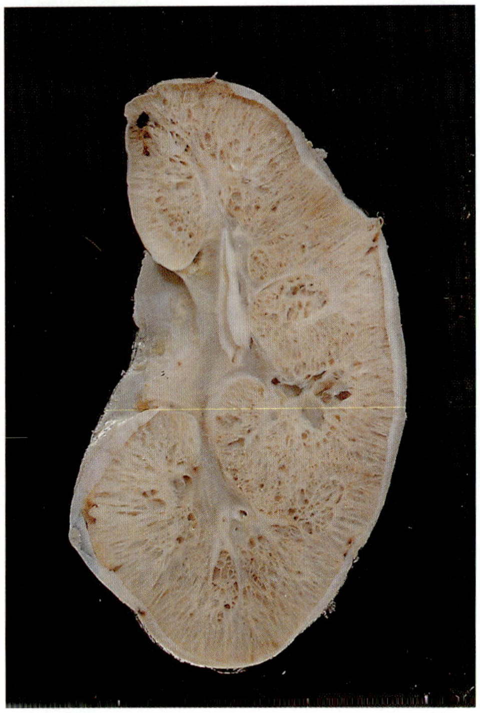

4.8 Infantile Polycystic Disease

No clinical details are available concerning this infant's kidney.

The kidney is greatly enlarged and the parenchyma is replaced by a mass of small, narrow, radially-arranged cysts. The normal shape of the kidney is retained.

Infantile polycystic disease is an inherited autosomal recessive condition which is much rarer than its adult counterpart. All those affected have associated congenital hepatic abnormalities and death commonly ensues from chronic renal failure by early childhood.

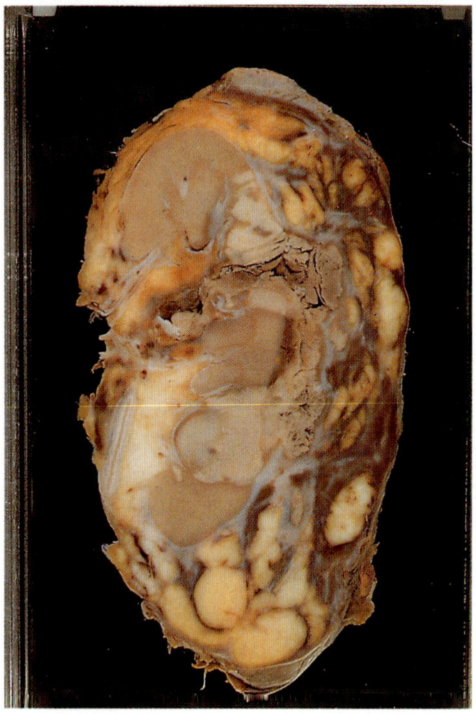

4.9 Rupture

This specimen was excised from a 33-year-old man who complained of loin pain and haematuria after falling from a bicycle. Haematuria persisted for 2 weeks and a nephrectomy was performed.

A section through the left kidney shows a transverse tear which has separated the upper pole. There is haemorrhage both around the tear and extending into the perirenal fat. Note the widespread infarction which is apparent as pale, wedge-shaped areas in both portions of the ruptured kidney.

Renal trauma is not uncommon, particularly with loin injuries. While conservative management is often adequate, it is clearly important to examine the contralateral kidney before more radical treatment is undertaken.

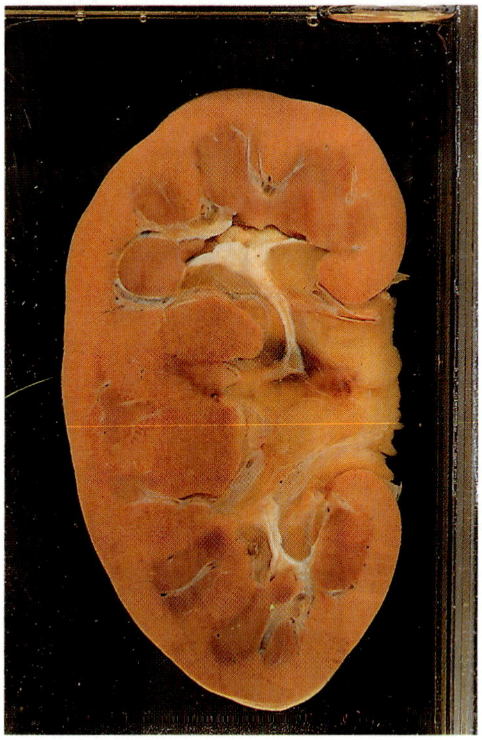

4.10 Venous Congestion

This is a post-mortem specimen from a 55-year-old man who died in cardiogenic shock, 12 days after a massive myocardial infarction.

The kidney is mildly enlarged and shows red engorgement which is most marked in the medulla. Passive congestion is manifest in the cortex by red radial streaks.

Passive venous congestion of the kidney may result in mild haematuria or proteinuria but significant renal damage does not ensue.

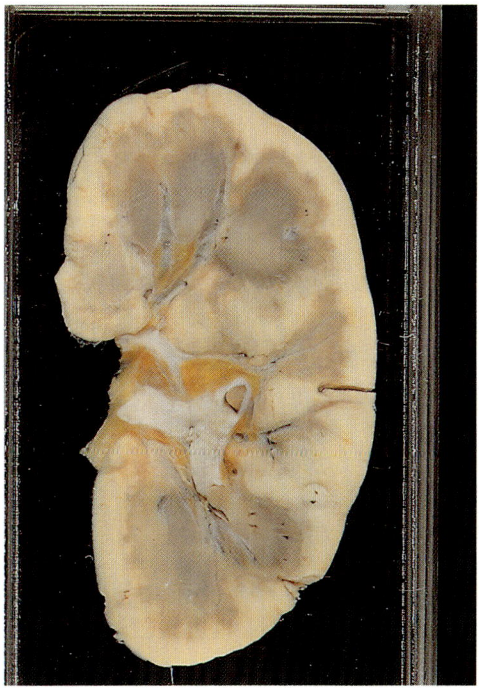

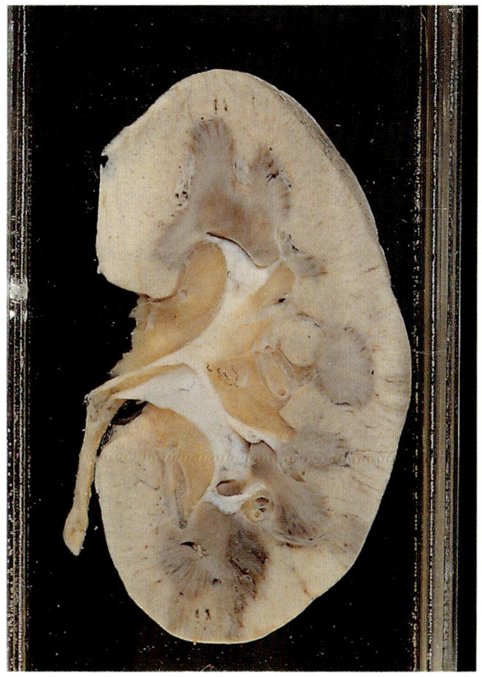

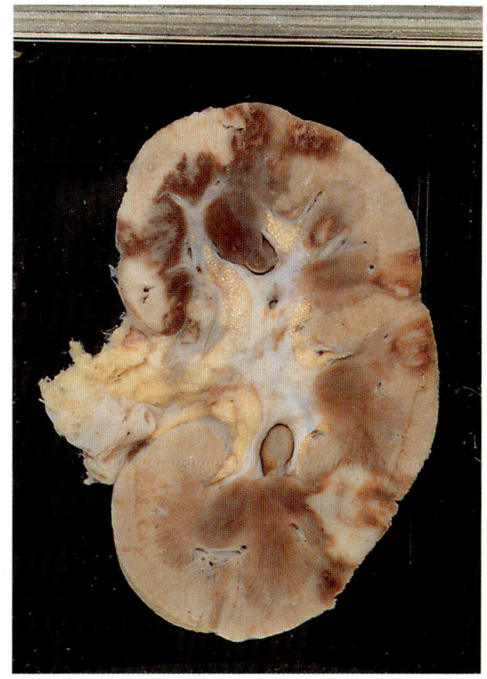

4.11 Cortical Necrosis

This is a post-mortem specimen from a 22-year-old woman who developed pre-eclampsia in her second pregnancy and delivered a still-born infant after suffering placental abruption. Postnatally she went into acute renal failure and died.

The kidney has been sectioned to show almost complete necrosis of the cortex, standing in marked contrast to the congested medulla. Very small areas of viable cortex remain beneath the capsule and at the corticomedullary junction.

Renal cortical necrosis is a rare cause of acute renal failure but is most often associated with complications of pregnancy, in particular *abruptio placentae*. It is thought to be a consequence of disseminated intravascular coagulation and, in pregnancy, may be associated with similar lesions in the pituitary and adrenal. The prognosis is very poor, although haemodialysis may be of value.

4.12 Pale Infarct

This is a post-mortem specimen from a 68-year-old man who died of a myocardial infarction. At autopsy, there was extensive atheroma with adherent mural thrombus in the abdominal aorta.

The kidney has been sectioned to show a pale, wedge-shaped infarct in the lower pole. The infarcted area shows no shrinkage and is still level with the surrounding tissue, indicating its recent origin. The typically congested and haemorrhagic margins of the infarct are well seen and extend into the adjacent medulla.

This is the classical appearance of a pale renal infarct which, in this case, was due to thrombosis of an arteriole at the apex of the lesion.

4.13 Multiple Infarction

This is a post-mortem specimen from a 65-year-old woman who died of subacute bacterial endocarditis; blood cultures were positive. At autopsy, in addition to the cardiac lesions, there were infarcts in the brain, liver, spleen and kidneys.

The kidney has been sectioned to show several recent infarcts with adjacent haemorrhage.

Systemic emboli, originating from vegetations on the valve cusps are a common complication of bacterial endocarditis. Organisms within these emboli may produce septic infarcts. The other important renal complication of infective endocarditis is the development of glomerulonephritis.

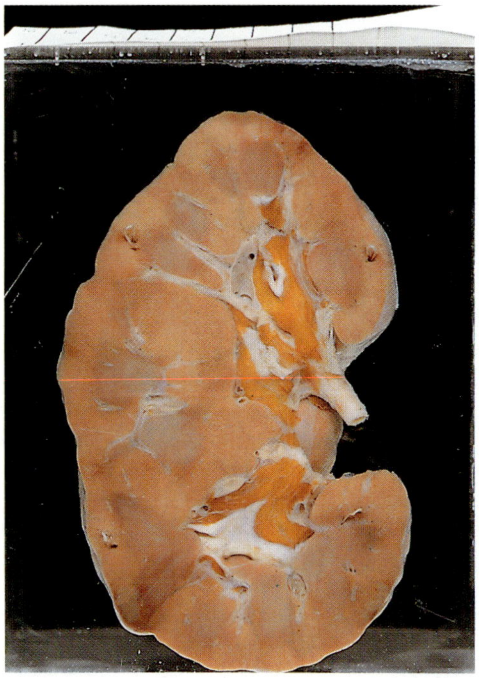

4.14 Benign Essential Hypertension

This is a post-mortem specimen from a 55-year-old man with long-standing hypertension who died of a myocardial infarction.

The kidney has been sectioned to show irregular capsular scarring, attenuation of the cortex and passive venous congestion. Three small subcapsular infarcts are also present, two in the region of the lower pole and one at the apex of the upper pole.

Essential hypertension, by promoting the development of atheroma and causing hyaline thickening of smaller renal vessels, results in relative renal ischaemia. This leads to fine cortical scarring and mild cortical atrophy but generally there is little, if any, impairment of renal function. The venous congestion and infarcts seen here are complications of this patient's terminal illness.

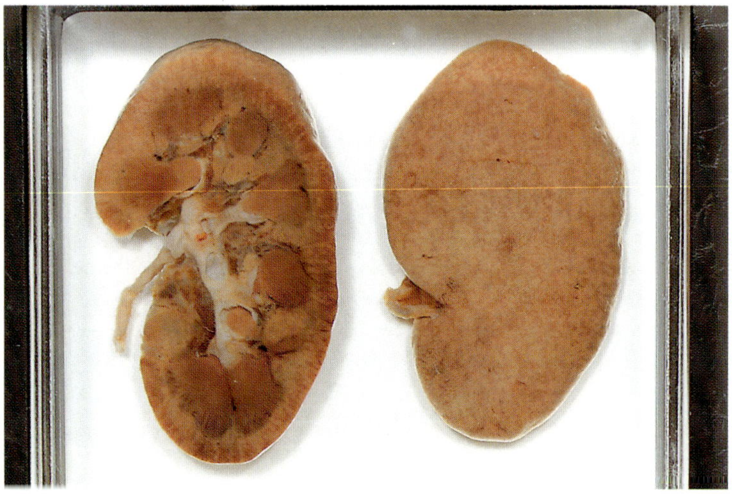

4.15 Progressive Systemic Sclerosis

This is a post-mortem specimen from a 31-year-old woman who had proven systemic sclerosis for some years. Terminally she developed hypertension and heart failure.

The kidney has been bisected: on the left, the cortex is attenuated and the medulla is engorged; on the right, the capsular surface is congested and shows fine granular scarring.

Progressive systemic sclerosis is one of the collagen diseases and is probably auto-immune in origin. It affects both sexes equally, usually between the 3rd and 5th decades. Features of the disease include skin atrophy, pulmonary, cardiac and gastrointestinal fibrosis and intimal thickening with fibrosis of small arteries and arterioles. This latter component is responsible for the renal lesion which is very similar to that seen in hypertension.

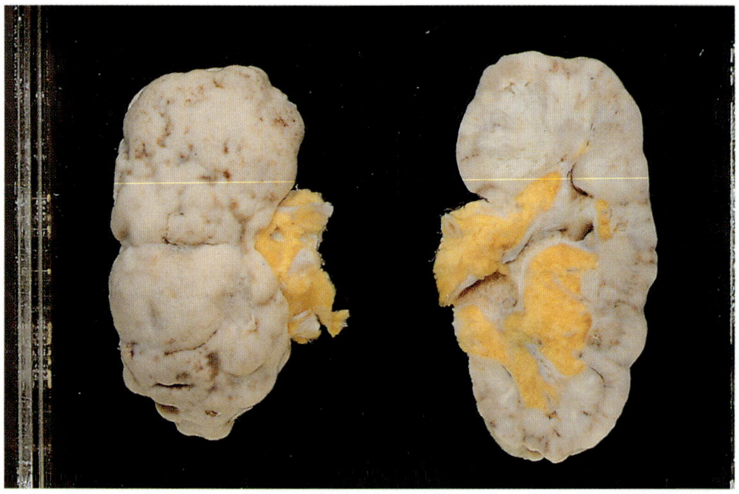

4.16 Active Chronic Pyelonephritis

These are post-mortem specimens from a 66-year-old man who died with widely disseminated carcinoma of the prostate.

Both kidneys are shown, one of which has been bisected. Both are shrunken and, on the left, coarse, irregular scarring and pitting of the capsular surface is apparent. The cut surface (right) shows relatively normal areas of renal parenchyma separated by contracted fibrotic segments. The pelvis is thickened and inflamed, and multiple, small, linear abscesses are present in the medulla, particularly in the upper pole.

Chronic pyelonephritis is defined as chronic inflammation not only of the renal parenchyma but also of the pelvicalyceal system and as such is almost always due to infection. The commonest predisposing causes are chronic urinary obstruction (e.g. due to prostatic enlargement or urolithiasis) or vesicoureteric reflux. A very small proportion of cases are idiopathic. Irregular, asymmetrical renal scarring is characteristic. A large proportion of cases develop hypertension but only late in the course of the disease do a small number show evidence of renal failure.

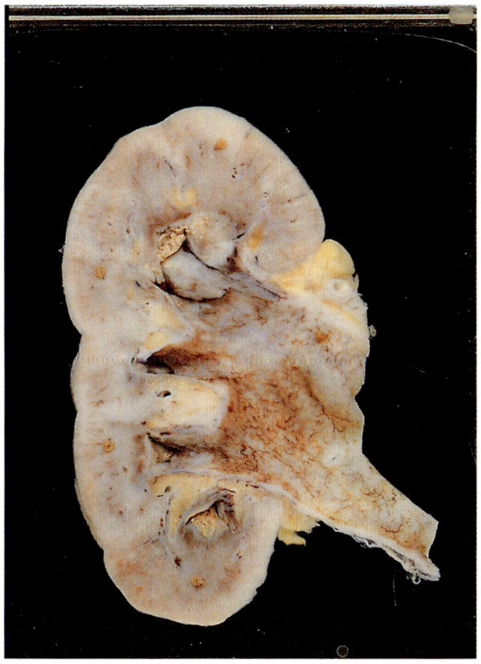

4.17 Pyelonephritis with Papillary Necrosis

This is a post-mortem specimen from a 77-year-old man who had symptoms of prostatic enlargement for years and died in chronic renal failure.

A section through the kidney shows dilatation and acute inflammation of the pelvis. The renal papillae are blunted, necrotic and show adjacent haemorrhage. The cortex is irregularly contracted and contains several small abscesses. The subcapsular surface is irregularly scarred.

The features seen here are those of acute or chronic pyelonephritis, complicated by renal papillary necrosis. Papillary necrosis is most often associated with either diabetes mellitus or analgesic nephropathy but urinary obstruction with superadded infection is a well recognised cause; very rarely, haematological disorders, particularly sickle cell disease, may be responsible.

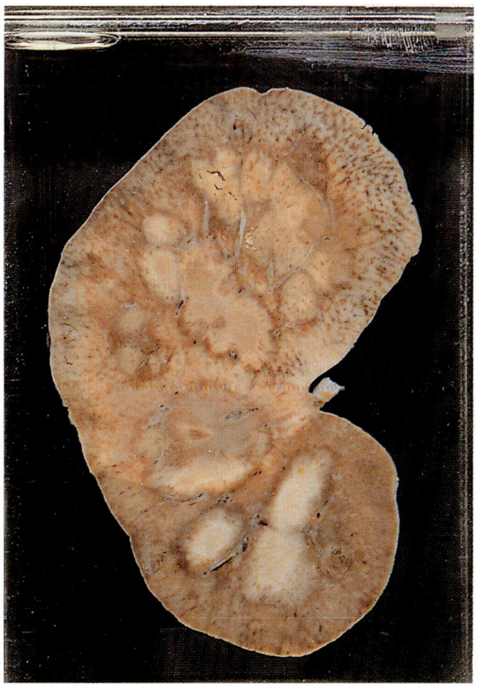

4.18 Acute Pyelonephritis with Papillary Necrosis

This is a post-mortem specimen from a 69-year-old woman who had ischaemic heart disease and congestive cardiac failure. Terminally, she was admitted with a cerebrovascular accident; she developed acute renal failure and purulent bronchitis and died.

The kidney has been sectioned away from the renal pelvis to show generalised parenchymal oedema. The medullary papillae are strikingly yellow and necrotic, each being bounded by a zone of haemorrhage.

There was no apparent history of either diabetes or analgesic abuse in this case and the aetiology of the papillary necrosis remains uncertain.

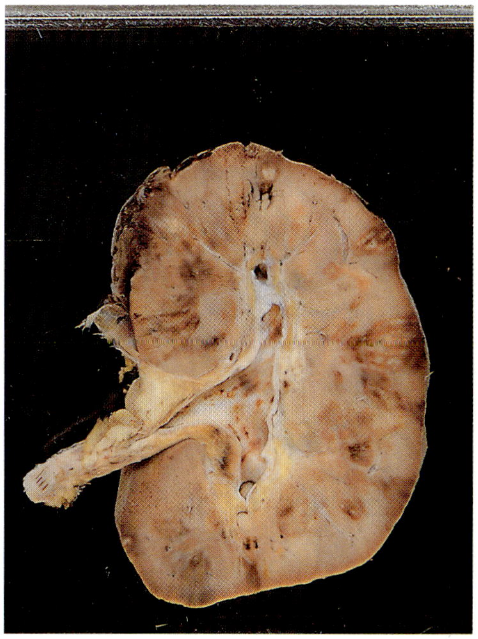

4.19 Acute Suppurative Pyelonephritis

This specimen was excised from a young woman who was acutely ill with *Escherichia coli* septicaemia. Because of severe pain in the left loin, ureteric catheter specimens of urine were examined and only that on the left was infected. Nephrectomy was performed and the patient made a rapid recovery.

The kidney has been sectioned to show numerous abscesses, principally in the cortex, surrounded by zones of hyperaemia. Note that the pelvis is neither dilated nor thickened, although it is clearly inflamed.

Acute pyelonephritis is due to Gram-negative bacilli (particularly *E. coli* and *Proteus spp.*) in the vast majority of cases. Infection is most commonly ascending in origin, although a small proportion of cases develop due to a florid septicaemic illness. In young adults females are most often affected, while in older adults males predominate. Common predisposing causes include urinary obstruction, intrumentation of the urinary tract, pregnancy, vesicoureteric reflux, diabetes mellitus or pre-existent renal disease. Females of all ages are more prone to urinary infection than males and up to 5 per cent may have asymptomatic bacteruria. This is most probably due to vulval contamination by faecal organisms. Modern antibiotic therapy had led to greatly improved treatment of acute pyelonephritis and, nowadays, nephrectomy is very rarely necessary.

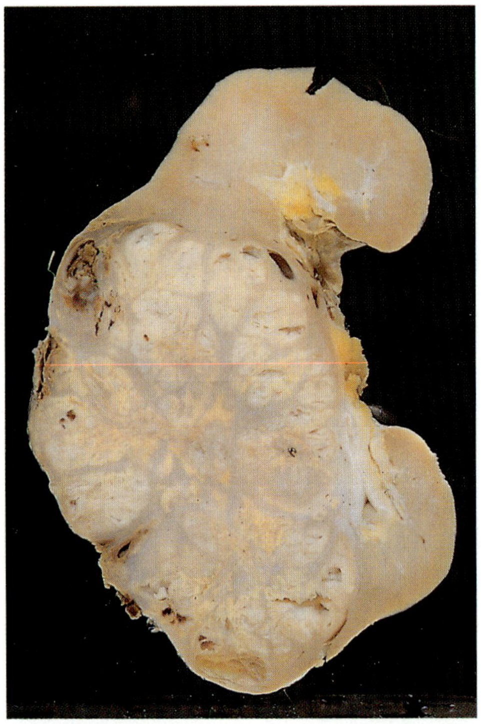

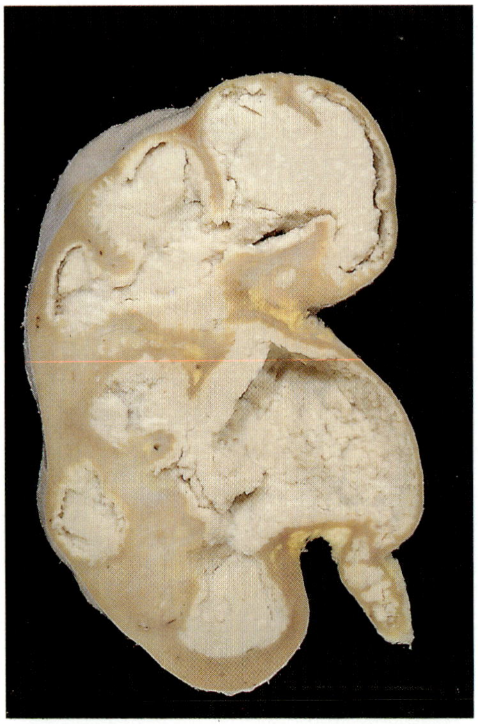

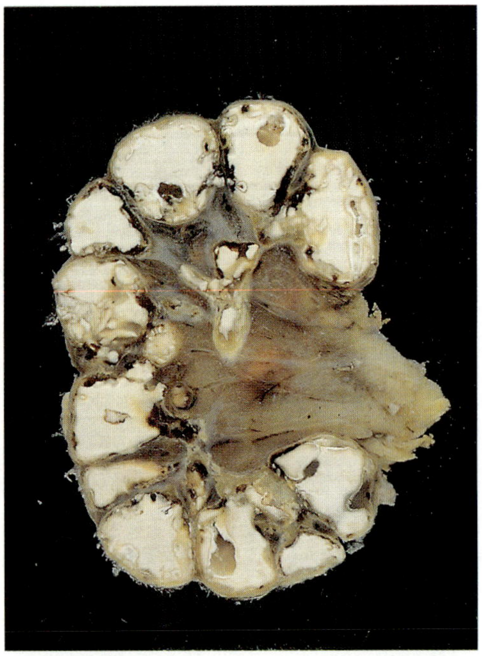

4.20 Localized Abscess ('Carbuncle')

This specimen was excised from a 33-year-old man who presented with loin pain and a swinging fever. A palpable mass developed in the left flank and exploration revealed a small perinephric abscess from which *Staphylococcus aureus* was cultured. A week later, nephrectomy was performed and the fever abated.

The kidney has been bisected to show a large loculated abscess, measuring 8 × 4cm, which is composed of yellowish foci of suppuration intersected and surrounded by dense fibrous septa.

Formation of a renal carbuncle in the absence of pelvicalyceal infection is uncommon and most probably arises as a consequence of an undetected bacteraemic or septicaemic illness. Such lesions are commonest in patients with diabetes mellitus or those who are immunosuppressed.

4.21 Caseous Tuberculosis

This specimen was excised from a 42-year-old woman who presented with urinary frequency, haematuria and a mass in the loin.

The kidney has been sectioned to show an advanced stage of tuberculosis. The pelvicalyceal system is greatly distended by pale, caseous material, which is extending down the ureter and causing obstruction. A thin layer of unaffected renal cortex remains.

Renal tuberculosis, while still endemic in underdeveloped countries, has become uncommon in Caucasians. Adult males are most often affected. The disease may arise either by haematogenous spread from a focus of infection in the lungs or female reproductive tract, or by direct spread from a male genital infection. This spread may become manifest fairly rapidly, but the infection can remain latent for years such that no primary source can be identified by the time of presentation. Bilateral renal involvement is usual. Involvement of the ureter can lead to stricture formation, which may require surgical treatment if the renal infection is cured conservatively.

4.22 Healed Tuberculosis

This was an incidental finding at post-mortem in an 87-year-old man who died of myocardial infarction. No other tuberculous lesions were found and he had no clinical history of known infection.

The kidney is shrunken and shows extensive calcification of the previously necrotic parenchyma. Each pyramidal system is sharply outlined and projects from the capsular surface to give a lobulated appearance.

These are the typical appearances of burnt-out tuberculosis which has healed by scarring; dystrophic calcification is common. A kidney such as this is readily identifiable on a plain abdominal X-ray.

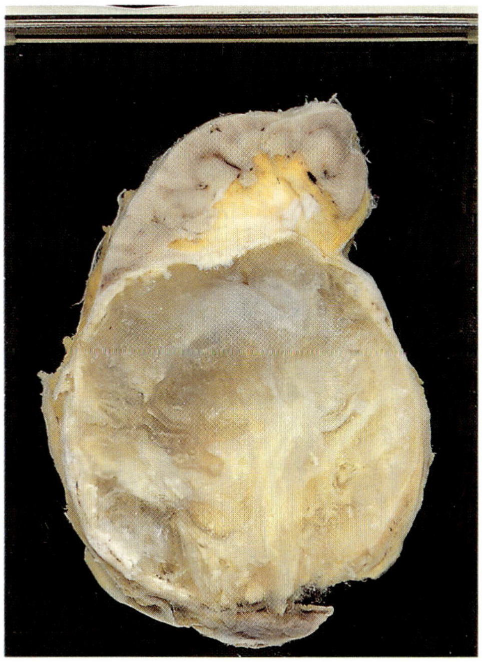

4.23 Hydatid Cyst

This was an incidental post-mortem finding in a 64-year-old man who died of a cerebrovascular accident.

The kidney has been sectioned to show a cyst, measuring 8cm in diameter, in the lower pole. The wall of the cyst is extensively calcified and the cavity contains folded hydatid membranes and debris.

Hydatid disease is due to infestation by the tapeworm, *Echinococcus granulosus*, and is most often seen in sheep-farming communities. The cysts are typically multilocular, containing numerous daughter cysts within which the brood capsules are formed. The cyst shown here appears to be 'burnt-out', there being little evidence of disease activity. Hydatid cysts of the kidney are rare but the diagnosis may be made by demonstration of cutaneous hypersensitivity to hydatid antigen, the Casoni intradermal test.

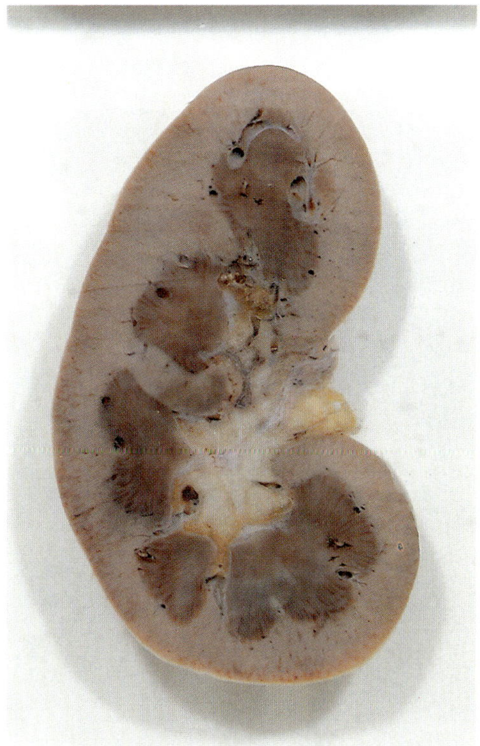

4.24 Acute Glomerulonephritis

This is a post-mortem specimen from a 30-year-old man who developed haematuria and proteinuria 3 days after an upper respiratory tract infection. He developed dyspnoea and haemoptysis and died.

A section through the kidney shows cortical swelling and marked medullary engorgement. The subcapsular surface is smooth.

Glomerulonephritis is an immense subject, too complex to be covered properly here. However, those cases presenting with the nephrotic syndrome most commonly have either acute, post-streptococcal, proliferative glomerulonephritis (seen particularly in children) or rapidly progressive glomerulonephritis, which may be either idiopathic, post-infective or a manifestation of Goodpasture's syndrome. The pulmonary involvement and the rapidly fatal clinical course in the case described here suggests that the preceeding upper respiratory tract infection may have been coincidental, and that this patient probably had Goodpasture's syndrome.

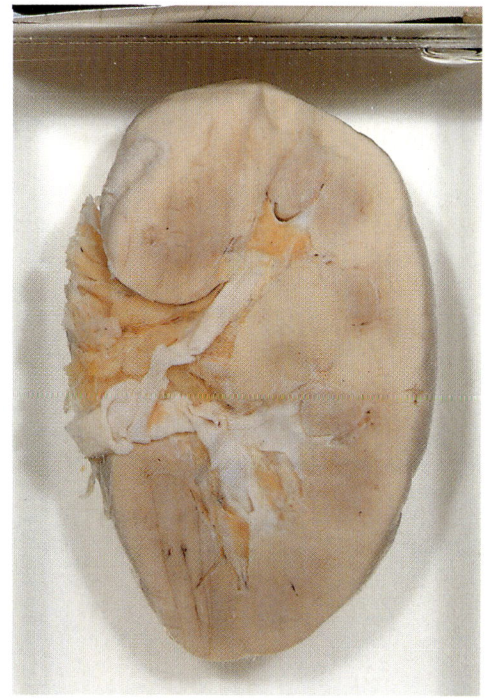

4.25 Membranous Glomerulonephritis

This is a post-mortem specimen from a 67-year-old man, who presented with malaise, oedema and proteinuria. Despite treatment with steroids, the patient developed chronic renal failure and died 11 months later.

A section through the kidney shows the swollen, pale cortex with blurring of the corticomedullary junction.

Membranous glomerulonephritis is largely a disease of adults and affects males more than females. It is thought to be due to the deposition of circulating immune complexes in the glomeruli but, with a few exceptions, the source of these complexes is unknown. Up to 70 per cent of patients show progressive deterioration in renal function and many die in chronic renal failure, although it should be noted that the time course of this disease is extremely variable.

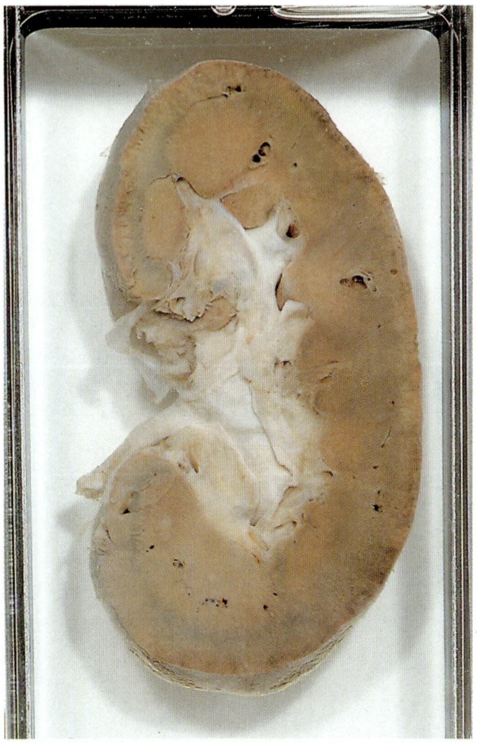

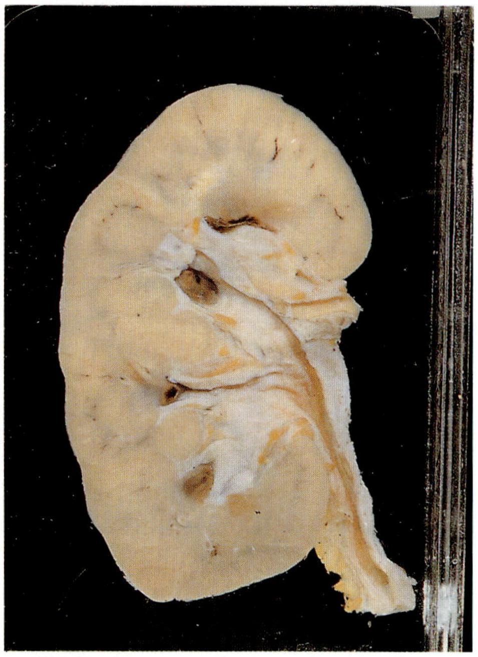

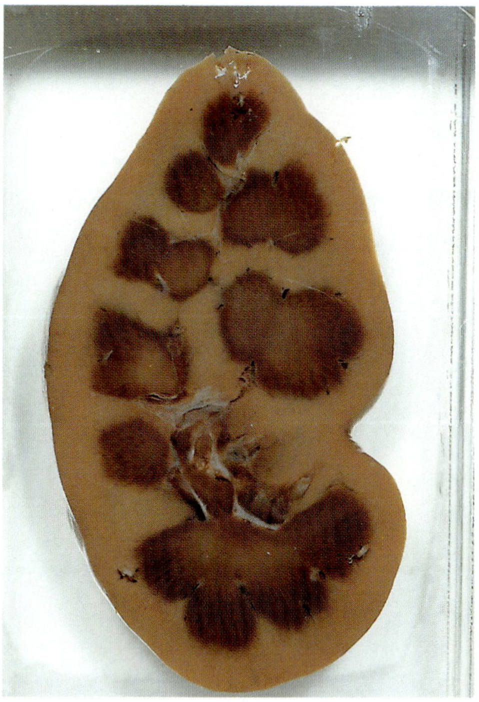

4.26 Microscopical Polyarteritis

This is a post-mortem specimen from a 52-year-old man who died in acute left ventricular failure with hypertension.

A section through this enlarged kidney shows swelling of the cortex, parenchymal congestion and blurring of the corticomedullary junction.

Renal involvement by polyarteritis may take two forms. In the classical form, there is loin pain, haematuria associated with fibrinoid necrosis of medium-sized arteries and the formation of small saccular aneurysms. In the microscopical form, fibrinoid necrosis affects mainly the glomeruli and the course is similar to that of rapidly progressive glomerulonephritis.

4.27 Analgesic Nephropathy

This is a post-mortem specimen from a 32-year-old man who had suffered unexplained gastrointestinal haemorrhage in the past and presented terminally in chronic renal failure. It was subsequently discovered that the patient had been consuming very large amounts of analgesic tablets containing aspirin, phenacetin and codeine.

The kidney is slightly small and shows pallor and atrophy of the cortex. The renal papillae are reddish-brown in colour due to necrosis.

Excessive consumption of analgesics, in particular aspirin or phenacetin derivatives, results in the development of renal papillary necrosis and chronic interstitial nephritis. Females are most often affected and the condition may be complicated by tubular acidosis, urolithiasis, urinary tract infection and ureteric obstruction by papillary slough. There is an increased risk of transitional cell carcinoma of the renal pelvis.

4.28 Acute Tubular Necrosis

This is a post-mortem specimen from a woman who committed suicide by taking 42.5g of paracetamol.

The kidney shows pallor and swelling of the cortex and intense congestion of the medulla.

Acute tubular necrosis is an important cause of acute renal failure. It most often results from severe renal ischaemia as seen in hypotensive shock of whatever cause, or it may be nephrotoxic in origin, for example after ingestion of heavy metals, organic solvents or certain antibiotics. Up to 90 per cent of cases may be reversible.

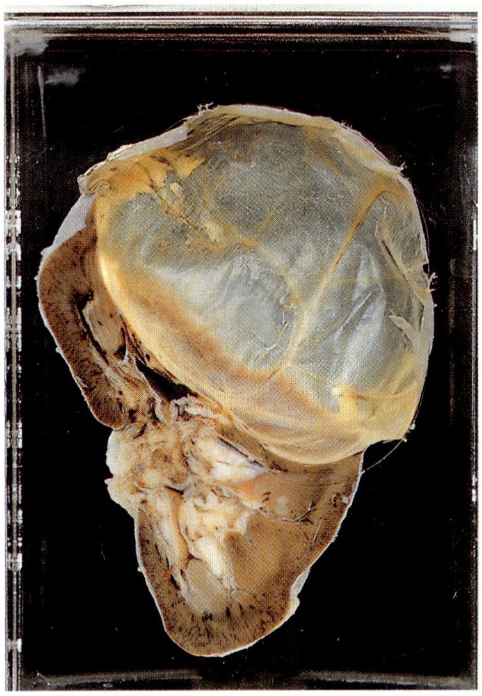

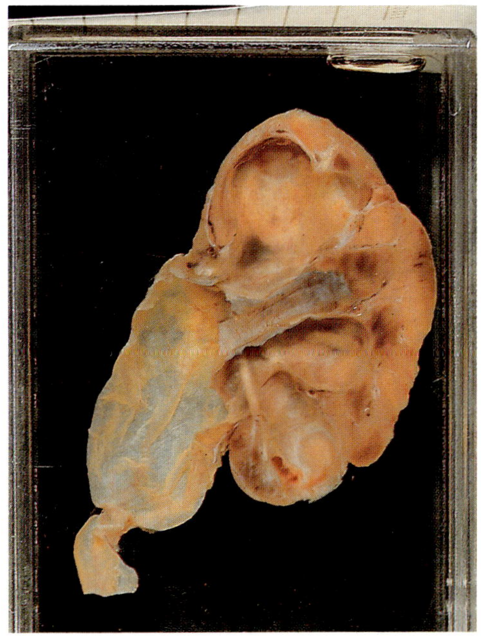

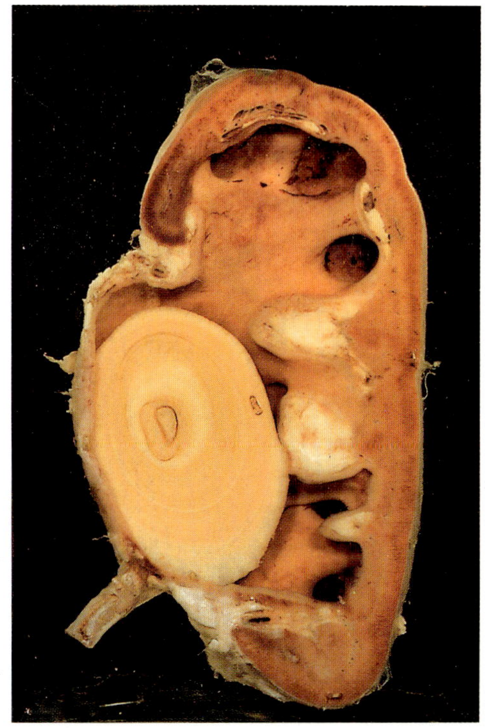

4.29 Simple Cortical Cyst

No clinical details are available.

A section through the kidney shows a single, thin-walled cyst, measuring 7cm in diameter, which has arisen in the upper pole and projects from its convex border.

Simple renal cysts are an extremely common incidental finding at post-mortem. They are most often solitary and arise in the cortex. They have no clinical significance and are thought to arise as a consequence of previous local obstruction or ischaemia.

4.30 Hydronephrosis

This is a nephrectomy specimen from a 25-year-old woman who suffered recurrent urinary tract infections and loin pain for 3 years. Micturating cystography showed gross vesicoureteric reflux on the affected side.

The kidney has been sectioned to show gross dilatation of the pelvis and calyces with severe attenuation of the remaining parenchyma. The kidney is shrunken and shows coarse scarring. There is also a stricture at the pelviureteric junction.

Hydronephrosis occurs as a complication of outflow obstruction; dilatation of the urinary drainage system leads to progressive renal atrophy. There are very many causes, dependent upon the level of obstruction, including prostatic hypertrophy, pelvic tumours, a ureteric stricture or stone, retroperitoneal fibrosis or kinking of the pelviureteric junction. Some cases may arise as a result of an idiopathic functional disorder of pelviureteric coordination and it is also important to remember that hydronephrosis may complicate such neurological disorders as multiple sclerosis or spina bifida. The most common complication is urinary tract infection but, unless the obstruction is bilateral, significant impairment of renal function is uncommon.

4.31 Hydronephrosis with a Pelvic Calculus

This is a nephrectomy specimen from a 40-year-old man who presented with renal colic and haematuria. X-rays revealed a large renal calculus.

The hydronephrotic kidney shows a rounded, laminated calculus, measuring 5 × 4cm, which is distending and obstructing the renal pelvis. The calyces are grossly distended and the remaining parenchymal tissue is markedly attenuated.

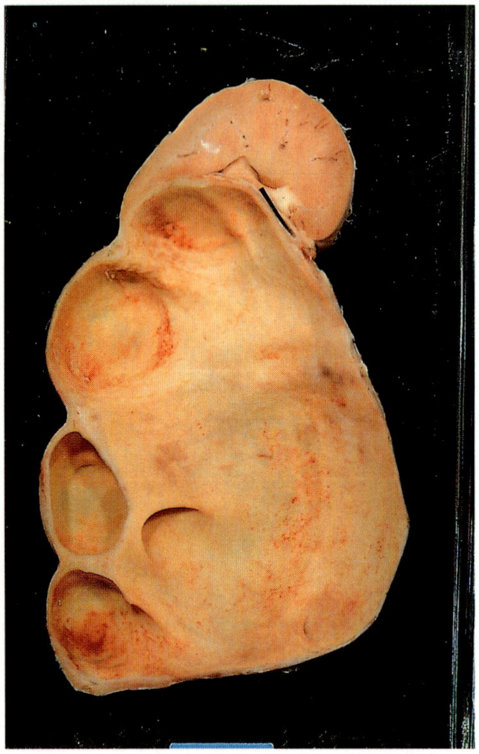

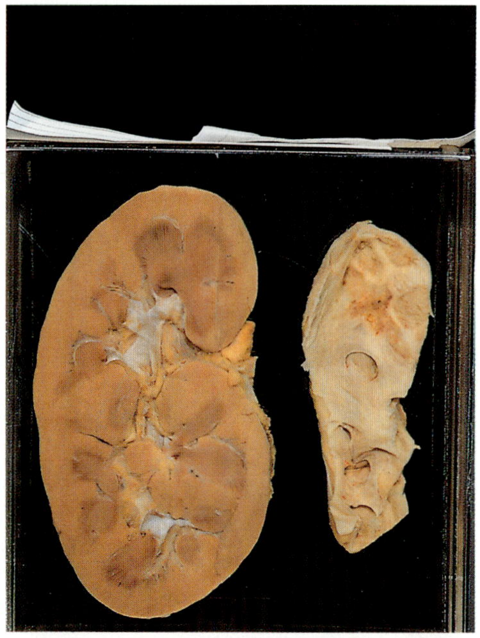

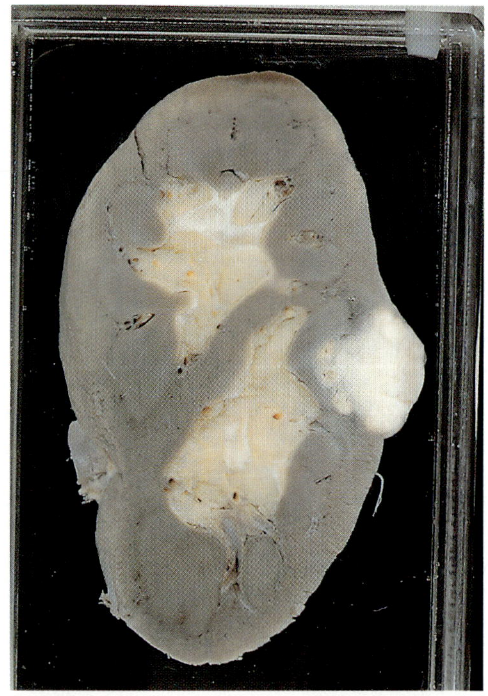

4.32 Pyonephrosis

This is a nephrectomy specimen from a 39-year-old woman who presented with dysuria, frequency and loin pain. Investigation revealed bilateral duplex ureters, one of which was not functioning on the affected side.

The kidney has been sectioned to show that its lower half, which was drained by the non-functioning ureter, is distended to form a thin-walled, loculated sac in which no recognisable renal tissue remains. This cavity contained copious purulent urine at operation.

Pyonephrosis signifies infection of the stagnant urine in a hydronephrotic kidney, and as such is not an uncommon condition.

4.33 Compensatory Hypertrophy associated with Contralateral Hydronephrosis

These are post-mortem specimens from a 68-year-old man who died of bronchopneumonia, associated with an episode of acute renal failure shortly before death.

The kidney on the left, greatly enlarged, weighs 475g (normal adult male kidney circa 150g). The parenchyma is congested with blurring of the corticomedullary junction, comparable with acute renal failure. The kidney on the right is grossly hydronephrotic and consists solely of a dilated pelvis.

It is well recognised that if function of one kidney is impaired or non-existent then the contralateral kidney undergoes hypertrophy.

4.34 Cortical Adenoma

This was an incidental post-mortem finding in a 78-year-old woman who died of cardiac failure.

The kidney has been sectioned to show a pale, clearly demarcated tumour, measuring 2cm in diameter, protruding from the cortex of the convex border.

Renal adenomas are very common and usually asymptomatic. They most often arise in the cortex and are frequently multiple or bilateral. They rarely exceed 1-2cm in diameter. Their incidence increases with age and very occasionally these lesions may undergo malignant change.

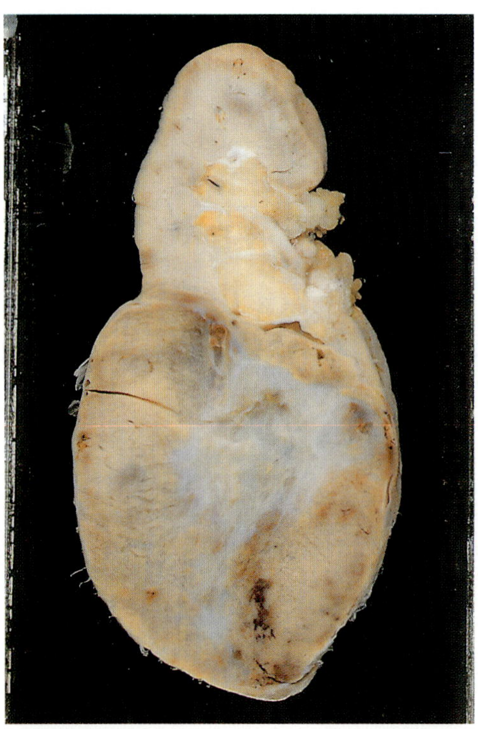

4.35 Oncocytoma

This is a nephrectomy specimen from a 78-year-old man who was found to have a palpable tumour in the left loin on routine examination.

The kidney has been sectioned to show a rounded, well-circumscribed tumour, measuring 8cm in diameter, in the lower pole. The tumour has a yellowish-brown appearance with a central area of pale scarring. Note the absence of necrosis or haemorrhage.

These are the typical appearances of a renal oncocytoma, defined as a tumour composed solely of bland, monomorphic, granular eosinophilic cells. This entity has only been recognised in recent years, formerly being classified as a variant of renal adenocarcinoma, largely because of its propensity to attain a considerable size (cf. renal adenoma). Typically it is found incidentally, in the absence of symptoms, in the 6th or 7th decades. The sex incidence appears equal. Its behaviour is entirely benign, thereby warranting separation from adenocarcinoma, and many now believe that this entity is a variant of a renal adenoma, showing oncocytic change.

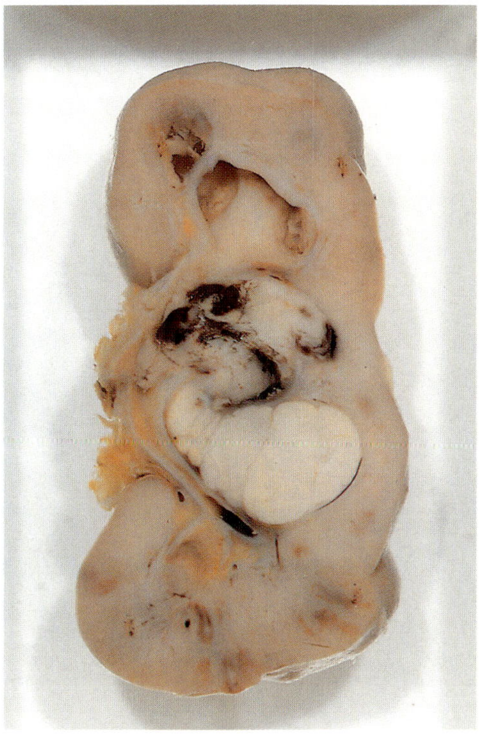

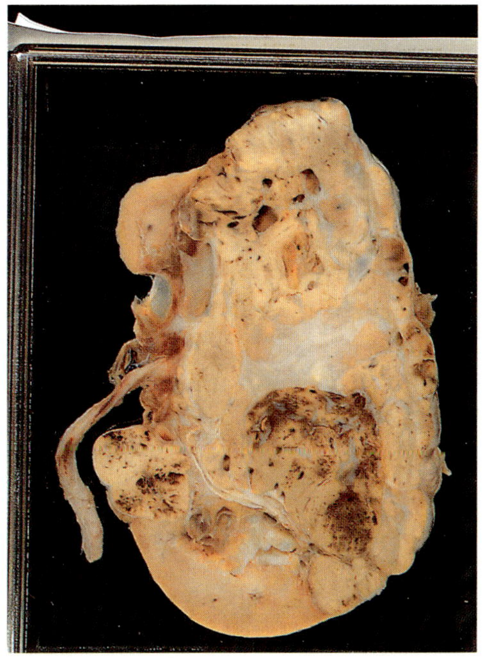

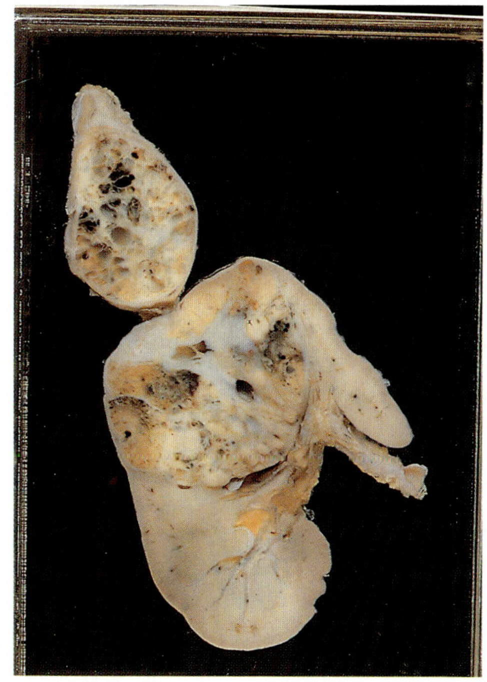

4.36 Adenoma causing Pyelonephritis

This is a nephrectomy specimen from a 34-year-old woman who presented with recurrent urinary tract infection. Intravenous pyelography showed minimal function on the affected side.

A section through the kidney shows a rounded, well-circumscribed yellowish tumour, measuring 3cm in diameter, which is distorting the renal pelvis. The upper and lower calyces are dilated and pyelonephritic scarring is apparent.

In causing urinary obstruction, this adenoma has given rise to symptoms by predisposing to infection of the stagnant urine. Occasionally tumours similarly situated may cause hydronephrosis.

4.37 Adenocarcinoma

This is a nephrectomy specimen from a 65-year-old woman who had suffered intermittent haematuria for 7 years.

A section through the kidney shows virtual replacement of the parenchyma by a tumour measuring 13 × 10cm It has the characteristic variegated appearance of a renal carcinoma, being predominantly golden-yellow in colour, interspersed by foci of haemorrhage, fibrosis and cyst formation. The adjacent renal pelvis is compressed.

Adenocarcinoma of the kidney (synonyms: clear cell carcinoma, hypernephroma, Grawitz tumour) is the commonest primary renal malignant tumour and predominantly occurs in older adults, affecting males more than females. These tumours are derived from renal tubular epithelium and usually arise in the cortex. Associated systemic manifestations are common and include fevers, amyloidosis, hypercalcaemia and polycythaemia — the latter two being due to tumour production of parathormone and erythropoietin respectively. These tumours tend to invade and grow along the renal vein, giving rise to early, blood-borne metastases. Up to 30 per cent of patients have detectable metastatic tumour at presentation, as a consequence of which the 5-year-survival is only of the order of 40 per cent.

4.38 Adenocarcinoma with Adrenal Metastasis

No clinical details are available.

The kidney and ipsilateral adrenal gland have been sectioned. In the upper half of the kidney there is a rounded tumour measuring 4cm in diameter, which has the characteristic appearance of a renal carcinoma. In the medullary zone of the adrenal, there is a deposit of similar tumour which is rather more cystic.

Metastases, from any tumour, are more commonly located in the medulla of the adrenal than the cortex. While renal carcinomas have no particular tendency to spread to the adrenal, the commonest primary tumours to metastasise to this gland are carcinomas of the bronchus and breast and malignant melanoma.

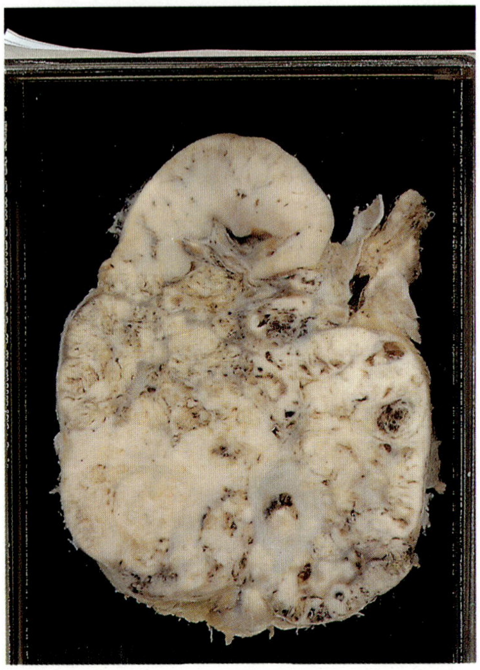

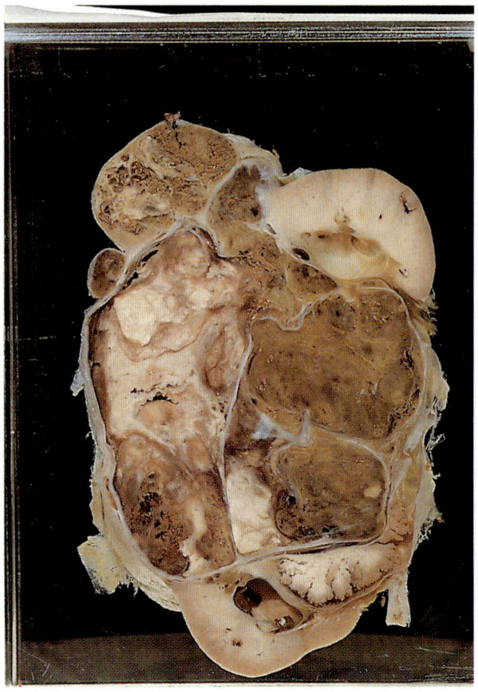

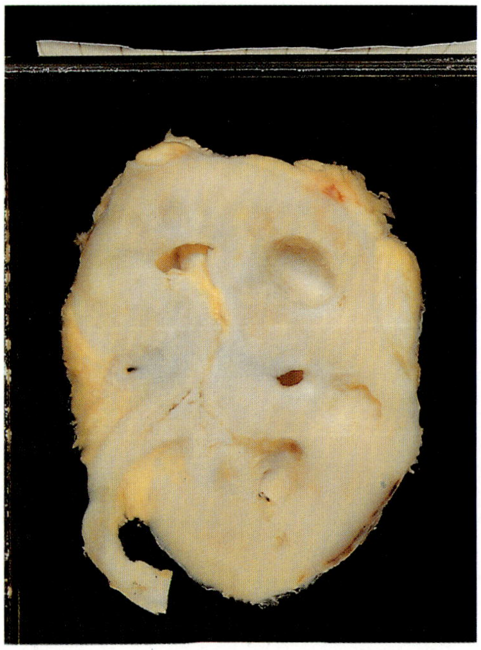

4.39 Adenocarcinoma invading Renal Vein

This is a post-mortem specimen from an 80-year-old woman who died of pneumonia, following a pathological hip fracture through a metastasis from the kidney.

The kidney has been sectioned to show replacement of its lower ⅔ by a tumour with the typical appearances of a renal carcinoma. A finger-like process of the tumour can be seen extending along the lumen of the displaced renal vein.

As already mentioned (see Legend 4.37), invasion of the renal vein is typical of these tumours. Indeed they may extend to involve the inferior vena cava and give rise to venous obstruction.

4.40 Adenocarcinoma and Transitional Cell Carcinoma of the Pelvis

This is a nephrectomy specimen from a 63-year-old man who presented with two episodes of painless haematuria.

The kidney has been sectioned to show a lobulated tumour, measuring 9cm in diameter, replacing the middle segment and extending through the renal capsule on the convex border. The upper and lower poles with their dilated calyces remain uninvolved. The pelvis is stretched over this tumour and in its lower portion there is a separate papillary growth projecting from the urothelium.

The coexistence of these tumours is very rare and probably coincidental. Transitional cell carcinoma of the renal pelvis is discussed below (see Legend 4.41 et seq.).

4.41 Papillary Transitional Cell Carcinoma

This is a nephrectomy specimen from a 45-year-old man who complained of haematuria. The kidney was palpable.

The kidney has been sectioned to show a bulky papillary tumour, which is filling and distending the renal pelvis. Surprisingly, there is no associated calyceal dilatation.

Transitional cell carcinoma of the renal pelvis is not uncommon and may be associated with similar tumours in the ureter and bladder. It most often presents in the 6th or 7th decades and affects males more than females. Individuals with a known predisposition include workers in the aniline dye and rubber industries, and cigarette smokers show an increased incidence of these tumours throughout the urinary tract. Patients with analgesic nephropathy or endemic Balkan nephropathy are also at increased risk. The majority of these tumours have a papillary pattern but the term transitional cell papilloma is only applied to the very rare tumours, which are small, well differentiated and follow a benign course. It has been recognised that many lesions labelled as papillomas in the past will eventually invade and metastasise. The clinical course is variable but 5-year-survival is only of the order of 40 per cent.

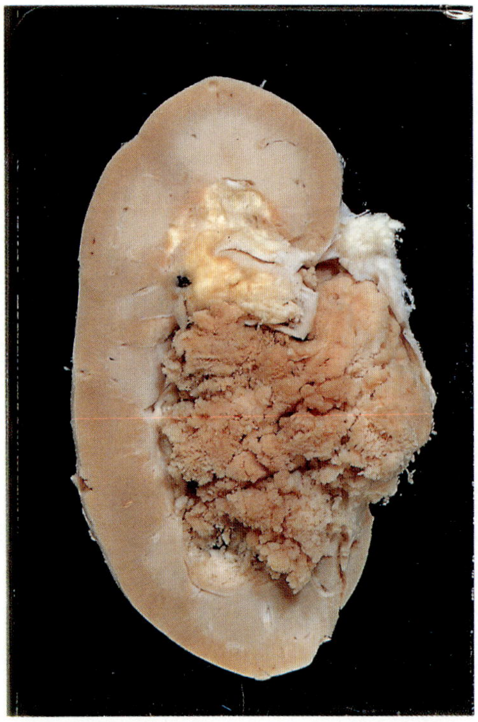

4.42 Solid Transitional Cell Carcinoma

This is a nephrectomy specimen from a 33-year-old man who presented with haematuria. He died 4 months postoperatively with pulmonary metastases.

The kidney has been sectioned to show almost total replacement by a diffuse pale tumour. A small area of uninvolved renal parenchyma is visible in the upper pole. The calyces are dilated and distorted and appear focally ulcerated. Histology revealed widespread squamous metaplasia in this neoplasm.

This is the solid variant of transitional cell carcinoma which carries a worse prognosis than the more common papillary type, with very few cases surviving even two years. Similarly squamous metaplasia in these tumours is associated with a reduced survival.

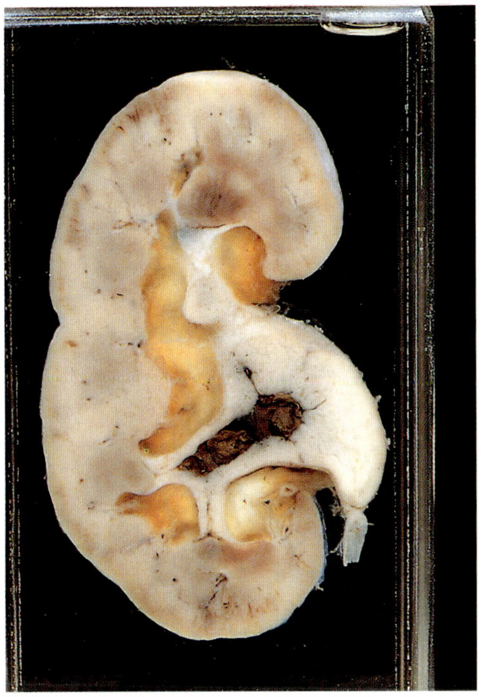

4.43 Transitional Cell Carcinoma of Pelvis

This is a nephrectomy specimen from a 74-year-old man who complained of painless haematuria for several weeks.

A section through the kidney shows a solid mass arising from the walls of the renal pelvis. The remaining cavity is filled with blood clot. There is mild associated calyceal dilatation.

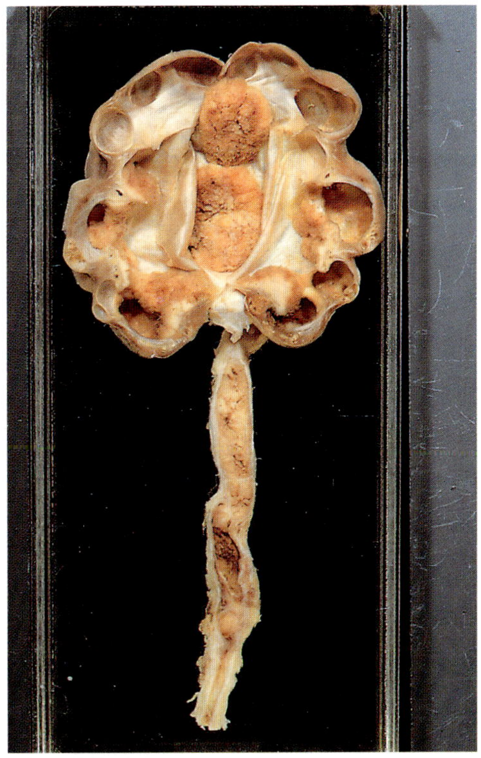

4.44 Multifocal Transitional Cell Carcinoma

This is a nephroureterectomy specimen from a 56-year-old man with a 13 year history of intermittent painless haematuria and abdominal pain. He had undergone several previous cytoscopic resections of papillary tumour in the lower ureter.

A hydronephrotic kidney and grossly dilated and thickened ureter are shown. The pelvis and calyces contain many nodules of papillary tumour and little recognisable renal tissue remains. Tumour is also seen filling the upper ureter and further discrete nodules are visible in the middle third.

Multiple transitional cell carcinomas in the urinary tract are common and represent either a 'field change' effect in response to an unknown carcinogenic stimulus, or metastatic seeding down the urinary tract.

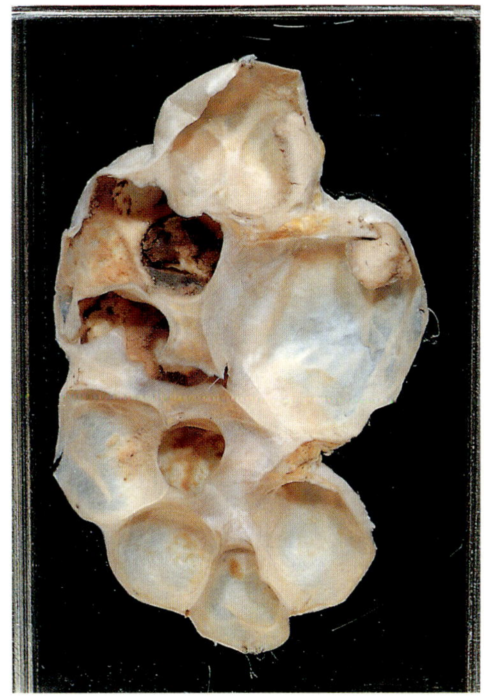

4.45 Transitional Cell Carcinoma causing Hydronephrosis

This is a nephrectomy specimen from a 69-year-old woman who complained of intermittent haematuria for 12 years. Investigation revealed a non-functioning right kidney with complete obstruction at the pelviureteric junction.

The right kidney has been opened to show a tumour, measuring 1cm in diameter, at the pelviureteric junction and a second nodule in the adjacent calyx. The kidney is grossly hydronephrotic and no recognisable renal tissue remains.

Hydronephrosis is a well-recognised, although uncommon, complication of transitional cell tumours arising in the pelvis or ureter. Similarly, transitional cell carcinoma may occasionally occur in a hydronephrotic kidney. In the absence of any other cause of obstruction in the case here, it would seem that the former statement applied.

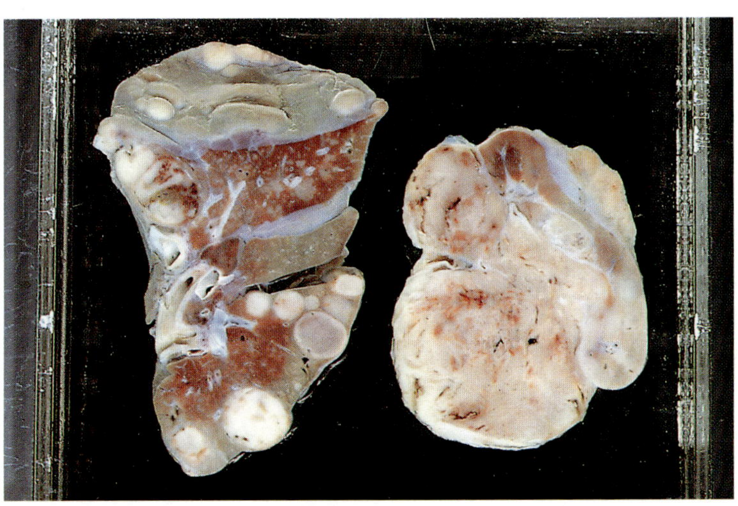

4.46 Nephroblastoma with Pulmonary Metastases

No clinical details are available.

Sections of the kidney and lung of a child are shown. The hilum of the kidney is replaced by a solid, lobulated tumour, measuring 5cm in diameter; the remaining renal parenchyma is stretched over the tumour's outer surface. The lung contains multiple, discrete metastatic deposits of similar tumour.

Nephroblastoma (synonym: Wilms' tumour) is the most common malignant tumour of infancy and early childhood. At least half of these tumours present before the age of 3 years and males are more often affected than females. Up to 10 per cent of cases may be bilateral. There may be a positive family history and other clinical associations include aniridia and hemihypertrophy. These tumours arise from embryonic renal tissue (the metanephric blastema) and therefore may contain any mesodermal elements. With modern multimodal treatment, the majority of these tumours are cured but poor prognostic features include older age and the extent of spread at presentation. The lungs are one of the commonest sites for metastases.

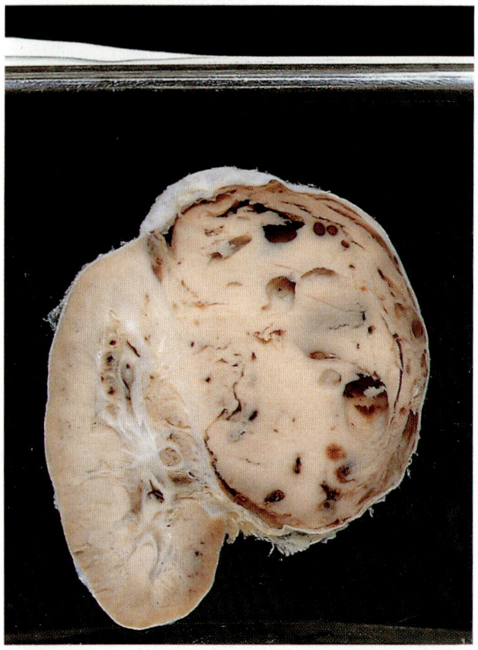

4.47 Nephroblastoma

This is a nephrectomy specimen from a 20-month-old boy who presented with haematuria and a large mass in the loin. He died 2 months after operation with disseminated metastases.

The kidney has been sectioned to show a rounded, pseudo-encapsulated tumour projecting from the hilum. The tumour is largely homogeneous with focal cystic and haemorrhagic spaces.

These are the typical appearances of a nephroblastoma.

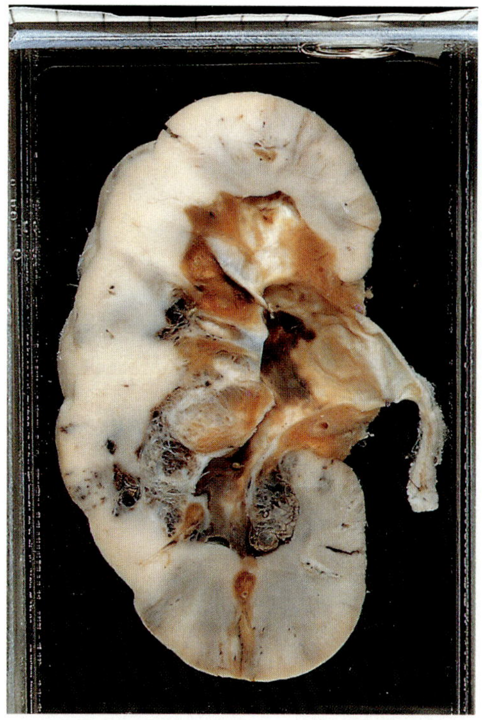

4.48 Cavernous Haemangioma

This is a nephrectomy specimen from a 61-year-old woman who complained of intermittent haematuria, occasionally associated with renal colic, for over 40 years. Renal function was normal.

A section through the kidney shows numerous blood-filled spaces concentrated around the lower pole calyx. There is a blood clot in the renal pelvis.

Renal haemangiomas are rare and show no predilection for any age or sex. Their principal importance lies in their ability to cause profuse haematuria, which may lead to the mistaken pre-operative diagnosis of adenocarcinoma. Occasionally they may be associated with haemangiomas elsewhere, for example, on the face and meninges as in the Sturge-Weber syndrome.

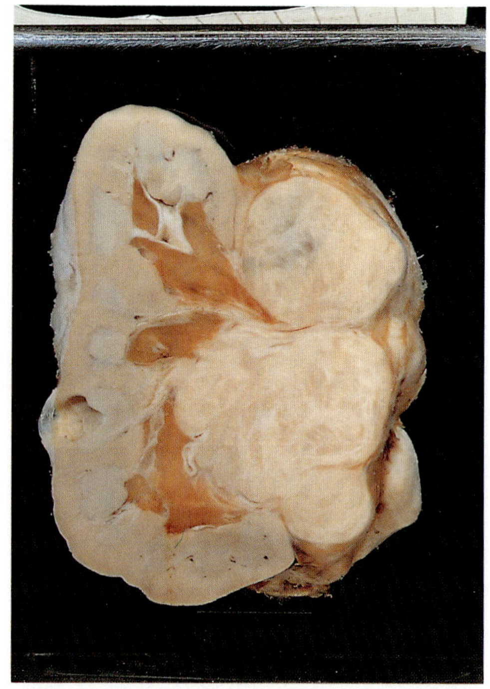

4.49 Leiomyoma

This is a nephrectomy specimen from a 77-year-old woman who had suffered abdominal pain for 2 years. A mobile mass was palpable in the loin and an intravenous pyelogram showed calyceal distortion.

A section through the kidney shows an ovoid, well-circumscribed mass, measuring 8cm in maximum diameter, arising from the hilum. The cut surface has a whorled appearance with foci of haemorrhage and cystic degeneration.

Benign leiomyomas of the kidney are not uncommon and are most often an incidental finding. When situated in the renal cortex, they are usually very small but, as seen here, hilar lesions may attain a considerable size and give rise to symptoms.

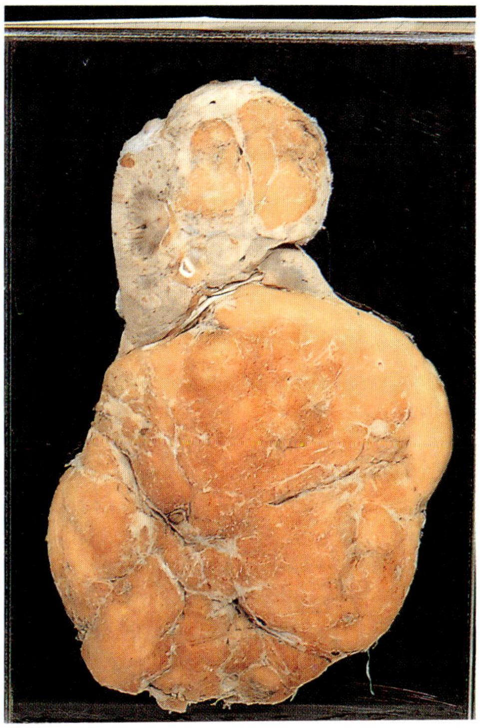

4.50 Angiomyolipoma

This was a post-mortem finding in an 18-year-old girl with known tuberous sclerosis who died of a pulmonary embolism. At autopsy there were multiple adenomata sebaceum of the skin, lipomas in the heart and liver, a lymphoid hamartoma in the spleen and typical cortical and ependymal nodules in the brain.

A section through the kidney shows a large, lobulated tumour, measuring 16cm in maximum diameter, situated in the lower pole. There are several similar, although smaller, lesions in the upper part of the organ. The tumours are solid and yellowish.

Angiomyolipoma is a rare hamartomatous lesion of the kidney, composed of mature adipose tissue, large blood vessels and smooth muscle. In approximately one third of cases there may be bilateral tumours and up to 30 per cent of patients, usually with multiple tumours, have tuberous sclerosis. Macroscopically the typical yellow colour may give rise to confusion with an adenocarcinoma.

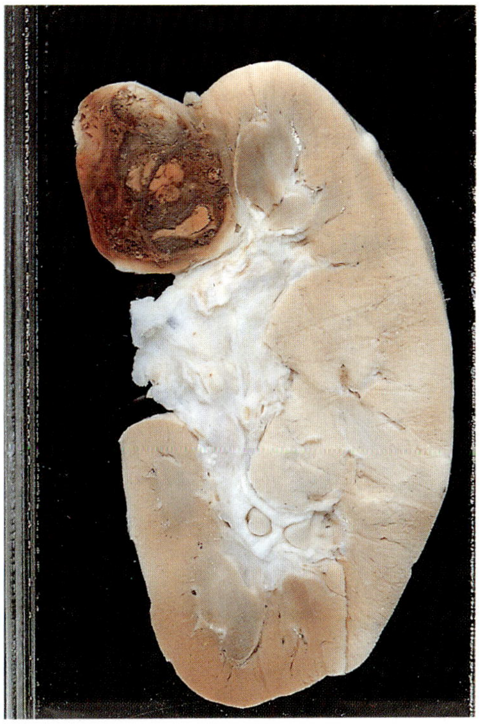

4.51 Secondary Carcinoma

This specimen is from a 31-year-old woman who died with disseminated anaplastic carcinoma of unidentified primary origin.

In the upper pole of the kidney there is a solitary, well-circumscribed deposit of haemorrhagic tumour, measuring 3 × 2 × 1cm.

Metastatic involvement of the kidney by malignant tumours is not uncommon but is rarely symptomatic. The most frequent primary site is carcinoma of the bronchus.

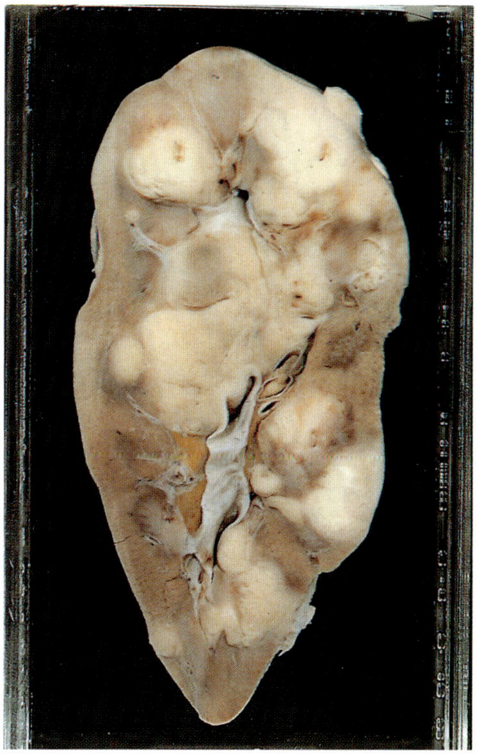

4.52 Involvement by Lymphoma

This was a post-mortem finding in a 46-year-old woman who died with disseminated non-Hodgkin's lymphoma 3 months after presentation.

A section through the kidney shows multiple, irregular deposits of pale tumour throughout the renal parenchyma and involving the capsule.

Renal involvement by lymphoma is not uncommon but most frequently occurs in Burkitt's lymphoma.

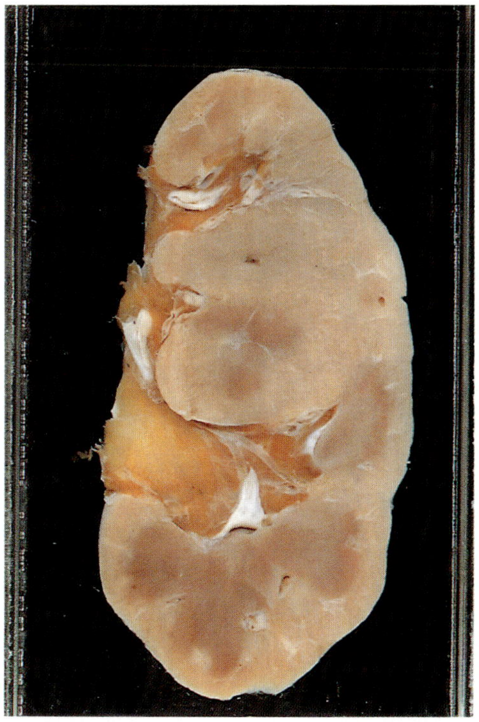

4.53 Amyloidosis

This is a post-mortem specimen from a 73-year-old woman who developed chronic renal failure and died of myocardial infarction. An incidental finding at autopsy was an anaplastic carcinoma of the bronchus.

The kidney has been sectioned to show the pale, waxy appearance and blurring of the cortico-medullary junction typical of amyloidosis.

Involvement of the kidney is commoner in secondary amyloidosis than in primary. Amyloid is a fibrillary protein, arranged in ß-pleated sheets; it is derived from immunoglobulin light chains in primary or myeloma-associated disease and from a naturally occurring serum amyloid A protein in secondary disease. Common causes of secondary amyloidosis include tuberculosis, bronchiectasis, rheumatoid arthritis and almost any chronic inflammatory disease. Rarely tumours may give rise to generalised amyloidosis – renal adenocarcinoma and Hodgkin's disease being the commonest culprits. It was not possible to determine whether amyloidosis was primary or secondary in the case shown here.

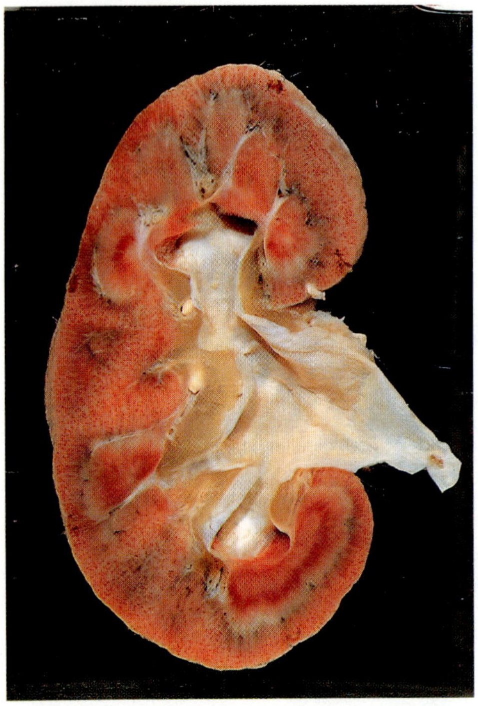

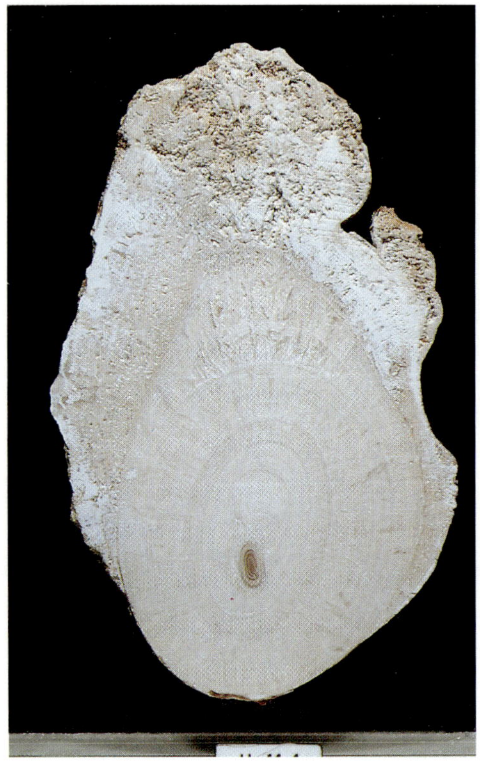

4.54 Secondary Amyloidosis

This is a post-mortem specimen from a 31-year-old woman who died in renal failure. She had been treated for unremitting pulmonary tuberculosis for the past 15 years.

The kidney has been stained with Congo red to show the extensive deposition of amyloid throughout the renal parenchyma. Amyloid may also be demonstrated in gross specimens by the application of Lugol's iodine which gives a brown colour.

4.55 Calculus

This specimen was removed from a 64-year-old man who was asymptomatic but was found to have a mass in the loin.

This large renal calculus has been sectioned to show the typical laminated appearance around the original nidus, the origin of which is not clear. Note the irregular calcification at the edge of the specimen.

Stones in the urinary tract are most common in the kidney and are usually unilateral. They most often present in adults, males being affected more than females. Their true incidence is impossible to ascertain but it is estimated that up to 5 per cent of the population may have urolithiasis. The majority of stones are composed of calcium in combination with oxalate or phosphate and many of the patients with such stones show an idiopathic increase in urinary calcium concentration. About 15 per cent of stones are of 'triple' phosphate type, the formation of which is usually triggered by urinary tract infections by urea-splitting organisms such as *Proteus spp.* While an increased urinary concentration of the relevant stone's constituents is the best recognised aetiological factor, there is no clear predisposing cause in very many cases. It is thought that alterations either of urinary mucoproteins or of crystal-forming inhibitors in the urine may be pathogenetically important. Complications of urolithiasis include obstruction of the affected portion of the urinary tract, a predisposition to infection and haematuria (see Urinary Calculi section).

URETER

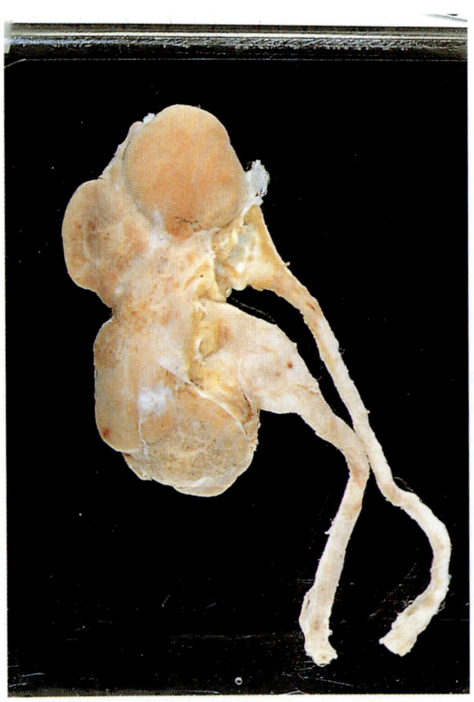

4.56 Reduplication of Pelvis and Ureter

This specimen was excised from a 45-year-old woman who had suffered intermittent attacks of right-sided renal colic for the previous 3 years. An intravenous pyelogram showed a small, scarred duplex kidney and renal function on that side was assessed to be minimal. A right nephrectomy was performed at which time a segmental blood supply, consisting of three renal arteries and veins, was also found.

The kidney is irregularly shrunken and scarred and has two pelves and ureters. Both pelves are slightly dilated. The ureters entered the bladder separately, the one draining the upper pole being abnormally situated as is often the case.

Congenital anomalies of the ureter are comparatively common and are said to account for between 5 and 10 per cent of patients attending urological clinics. There may be associated abnormalities of the genitalia. It is more common for the ureter to bifurcate along its upward path and to retain a single opening into the bladder than to be totally duplicated as seen here. Complete duplication is probably due to the separate development of two ureteric buds on the same side. Infective or obstructive complications are to be expected in any abnormality of urinary drainage.

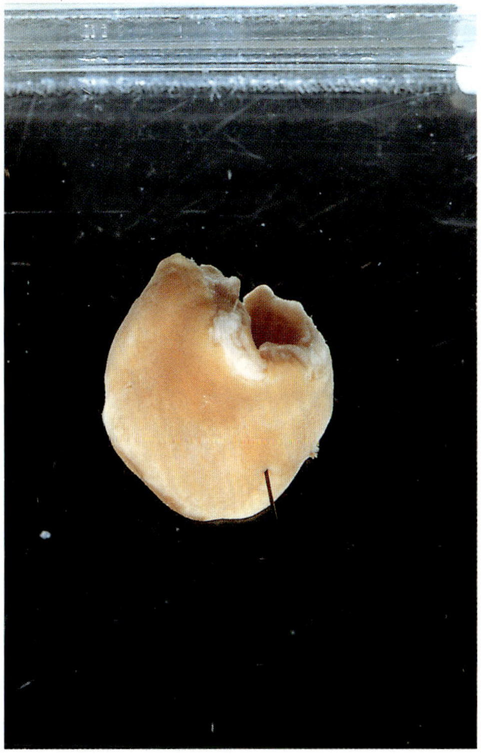

4.57 Ureterocele

No clinical details are available.

The specimen consists of a cystic swelling excised from the bladder wall, measuring 1cm in diameter. A portion of the wall has been removed to demonstrate the cystic cavity. At the bottom of the picture a fine bristle has been used to demonstrate the ureteric orifice.

A ureterocele represents a cystic dilatation of the lower end of the ureter. It is commoner in females and may be bilateral. It is thought to arise as a consequence of stenosis of the ureteric orifice, whether congenital or acquired, and it may be complicated either by infection or the development of a stone within the cavity.

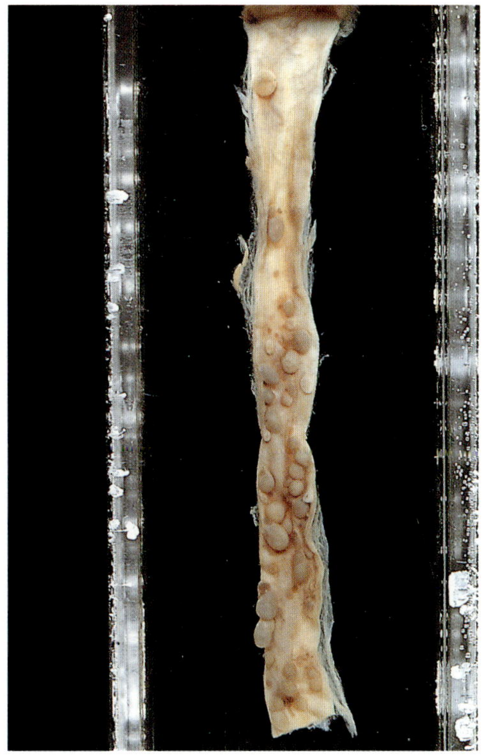

4.58 Ureteritis Cystica

This was an incidental post-mortem finding in a woman who died of disseminated breast carcinoma. There was no history of renal disease.

A portion of the upper end of the ureter has been opened to show a number of smooth, rounded cysts projecting from the urothelial surface.

Ureteritis cystica represents a response to non-specific chronic inflammation, similar to that seen in the bladder, in which small cysts are formed within von Brunn's nests. Development of such lesions within the ureter may give rise to ureteric obstruction. The pathogenesis is variable but urinary tract infection is the most common cause. The condition is recognised by a 'cobblestone' appearance on an ureterogram.

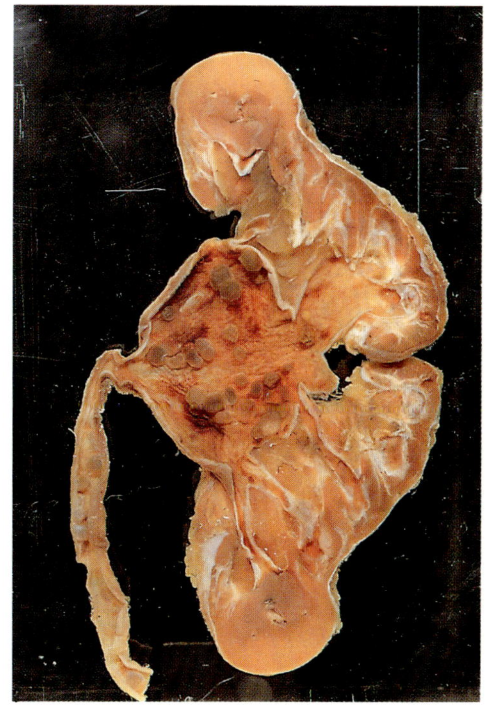

4.59 Pyelo-ureteritis Cystica

This is a nephro-ureterectomy specimen from a 60-year-old women who had suffered recurrent urinary tract infections for 15 years. Cystoscopy also revealed gross cystitis cystica with bladder neck obstruction.

There is moderate extrarenal and intrarenal hydronephrosis with attenuation of the renal parenchyma. Numerous confluent spherical cysts can be seen in the pelvis and ureter which have led to partial ureteric obstruction.

This is a more extensive example of cystic change resulting from long-standing infection.

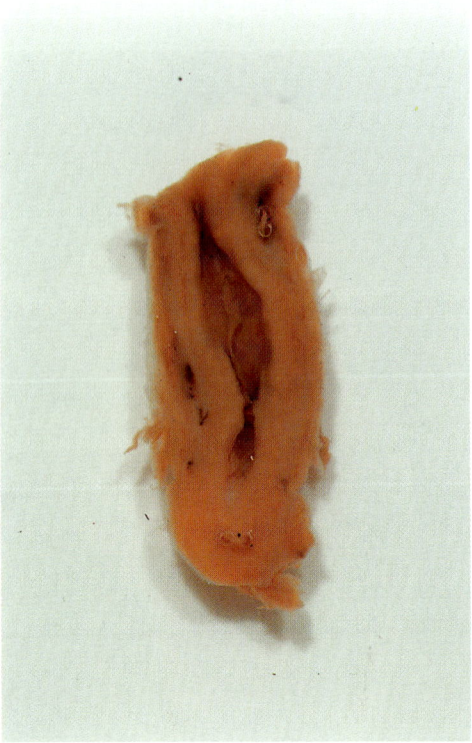

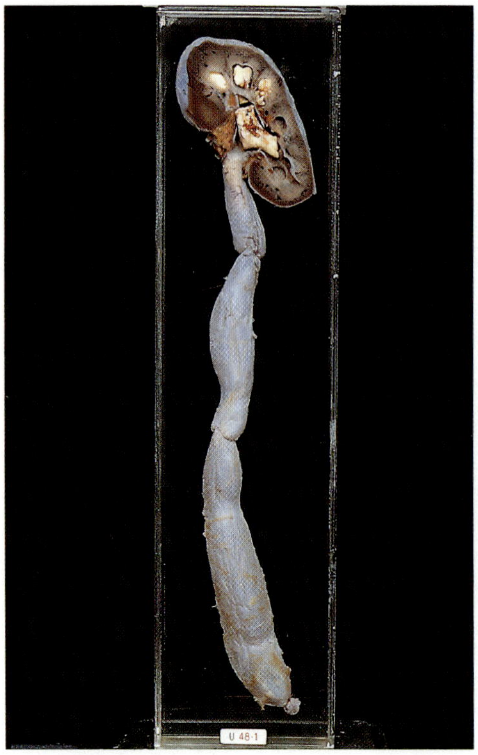

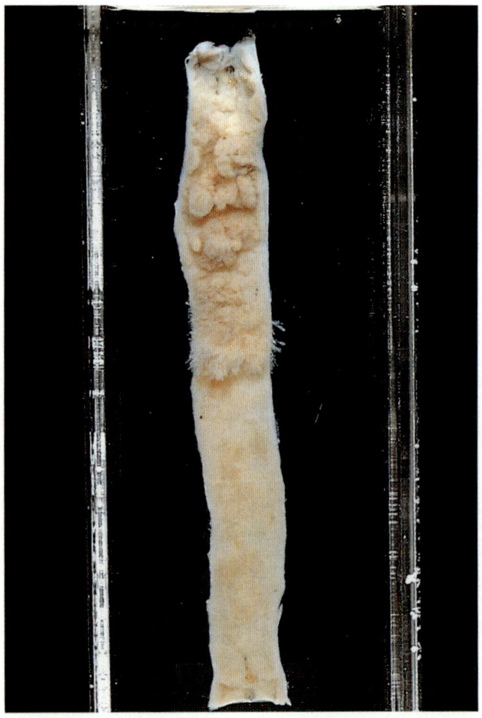

4.60 Schistosomiasis

This is a partial ureterectomy specimen from a 15-year-old boy who presented with renal colic. He was found to have florid schistosomiasis of the lower urinary tract and, despite drug treatment, renal colic due to ureteric obstruction persisted.

The lower segment of the ureter has been obliquely bisected to show gross thickening of the wall, due to fibrosis, with obvious stenosis. There is ulceration of the urothelium.

Schistosomiasis of the urinary tract most often affects the bladder and lower ureters and is almost always due to infection by the trematode, *Schistosoma haematobium*. It is commonly referred to as Bilharzia and is endemic in certain countries, particularly Egypt. The intermediate host is a species of water snail. Marked fibrosis, with the development of ureteric obstruction, is common. Dystrophic calcification of dead ova may facilitate a pre-operative radiological diagnosis. Schistosomiasis predisposes to the development of squamous or transitional cell carcinoma of the bladder and ureter.

4.61 Hydroureter and Calculous Hydronephrosis

This is a nephro-ureterectomy specimen from a 17-year-old boy who complained of transient haematuria. He was found to have a urinary tract infection and radiography revealed a calculus in the right kidney with hydronephrosis and hydroureter and moderate dilatation of the left ureter with no renal abnormality.

The kidney has been sectioned to show a large branched calculus occupying the somewhat dilated pelvicalyceal system. The ureter is grossly and irregularly dilated, particularly towards the distal end where it measures 3cm in diameter.

The clinical history and radiological findings suggest that this boy suffered from a congenital anomaly resulting in urinary obstruction. Possibilities include neuromuscular incoordination (megaureter), abnormal sites of ureteric implantation in the bladder or urethral valves, although the latter is unlikely in view of the degree of asymmetrical ureteric dilatation. Distal ureteric obstruction predisposes to infection and stone formation in the upper urinary tract and this is the probable source of the calculus seen here.

4.62 Papillary Transitional Cell Carcinoma

This is a partial ureterectomy specimen from a 72-year-old woman who complained of haematuria. She had undergone nephrectomy and excision of the upper ureter for a transitional cell carcinoma of the renal pelvis 1 year previously.

The lower end of the ureter has been opened to show several papillary lesions at the proximal end. Elsewhere the urothelium is inflamed and thickened.

The pathology of transitional cell carcinoma of the urinary tract and its tendency to multifocality have already been described (see Legend 4.41 et seq.). The ureter is far less often affected than either the bladder or kidney, but ureteric neoplasms may be prone to invasion of adjacent tissues owing to the thinness of the ureteric wall.

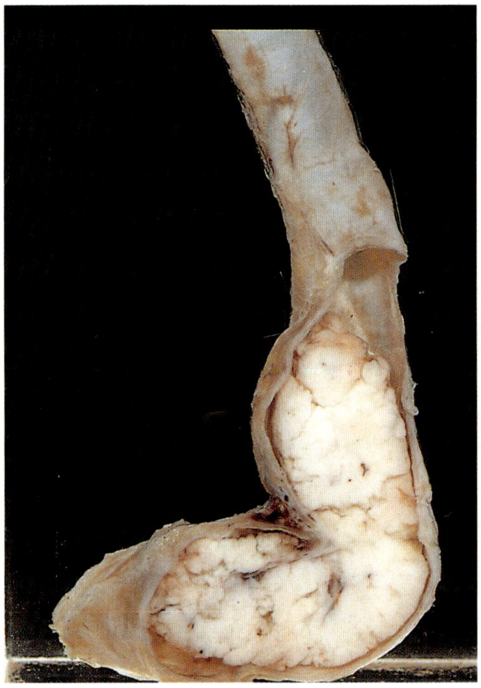

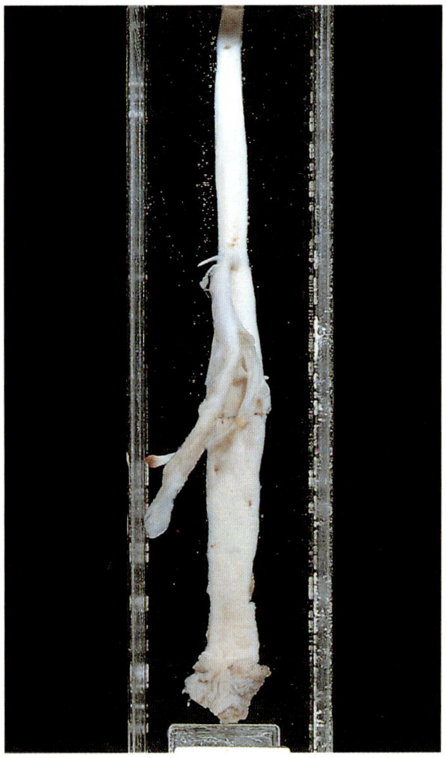

4.64 Fibro-epithelial Polyp

This is part of a nephro-ureterectomy specimen from a 63-year-old man who presented with haematuria. X-rays revealed a filling defect in the lower ureter with proximal dilatation.

The ureter has been opened to display an elongated polyp, measuring 7.5cm in length, arising 10cm proximal to the lower end of the ureter. The lesion is pedunculated and several smaller filamentous polyps protrude from its surface.

Fibro-epithelial polyps of the ureter are comparatively rare and usually present in adulthood. They are benign lesions but may give rise to haematuria or urinary obstruction.

4.63 Solid Transitional Cell Carcinoma

This is part of a nephro-ureterectomy specimen from a 70-year-old man who complained of painless haematuria. He was found to have a filling defect in the lower ureter with an associated hydronephrosis and hydroureter.

The lower end of the ureter is totally occluded by a bulky, solid polypoid tumour. Proximal ureteric dilatation is clearly seen.

As already stated (Legend 4.42), the solid variant of transitional cell carcinoma carries a worse prognosis than its more common papillary counterpart.

BLADDER

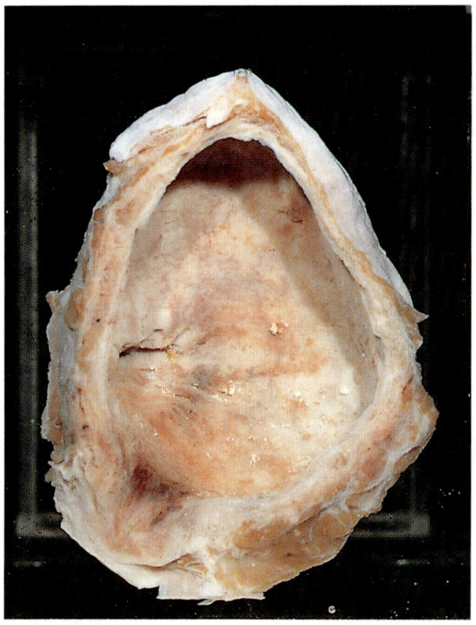

4.65 Cystitis

This is a post-mortem specimen from a 70-year-old woman who suffered from a cerebrovascular accident and developed rapidly progressive Parkinson's disease. For the last few weeks of her life, her urine was foul-smelling and *Proteus spp.* was cultured.

The bladder has been opened to show intense congestion of the posterior wall. On the left, the ostium of a small diverticulum is visible just above the ureteric orifice and on the right there are small flecks of calcific material adherent to the urothelium.

Acute infection of the urinary tract is most often due to *E. coli*, *Proteus spp.* or other enterobacteriaceae. Predisposing factors to urinary infection have already been mentioned (see Legend 4.19). In this case, both the diverticulum and the small stone could have been contributory.

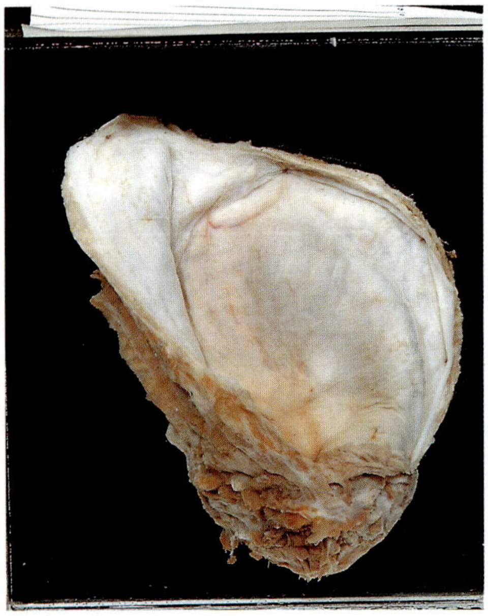

4.66 Schistosomiasis

This is a post-mortem specimen from a 42-year-old man who had been treated for some months for schistosomiasis contracted in South Africa. He was also receiving psychiatric treatment and committed suicide.

The urothelial surface of the bladder is studded with very small yellow nodules, similar in appearance to miliary tubercles. These are aggregated into areas, known as 'sandy patches', on the lower right and upper left of the specimen.

Urinary schistosomal infection has already been mentioned (see Legend 4.61). Degenerate ova deep in the bladder wall may undergo dystrophic calcification, giving rise to an unusual radiological appearance. It should be reiterated that schistosomiasis predisposes to squamous carcinoma and, less often, transitional cell carcinoma of the bladder. Squamous carcinoma arises in areas of squamous metaplasia brought about by chronic inflammation.

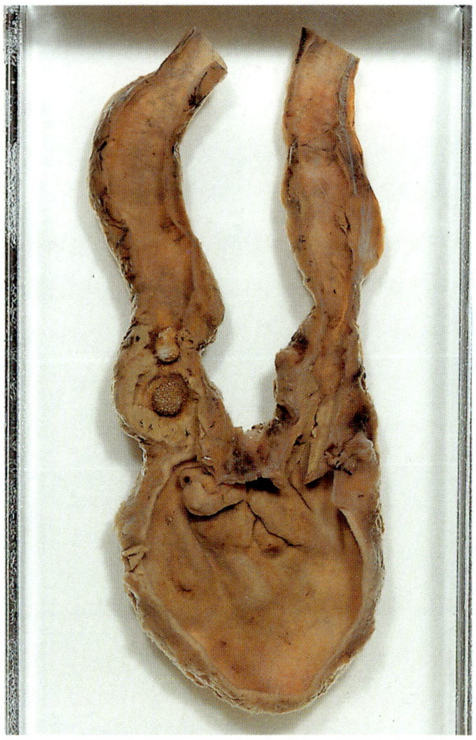

4.67 Schistosomiasis

This is a surgical specimen from a 26-year-old Saudi Arabian man who had advanced schistosomiasis. X-rays revealed calcification of the bladder wall and ureters up to the level of the third lumbar vertebra and there were multiple ureteric stones. He underwent cystectomy and reimplantation of the upper ureters into the ileum.

The bladder is grossly contracted with thickened walls and a granular, puckered lining. There is bilateral stenosis at the lower end of the ureters, the walls of which are also fibrotic. Proximally the ureters are dilated and two stones are visible in the ureteric lumen on the left of the specimen.

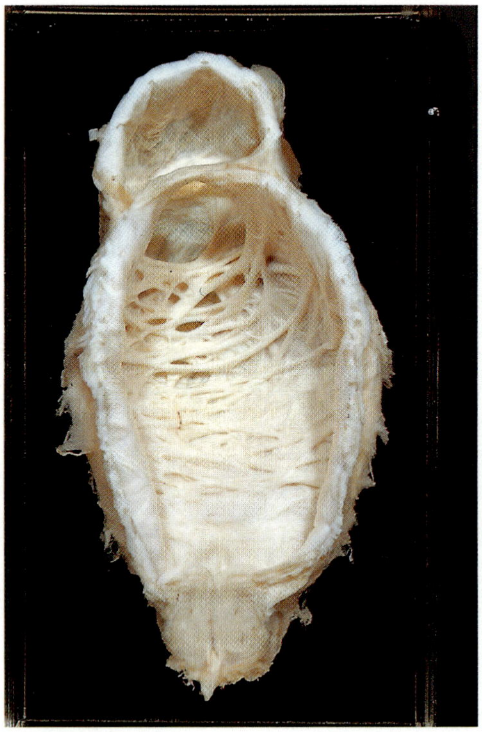

4.68 Diverticulum

No clinical details are available.

The bladder has been opened to show marked dilatation and trabeculation of the muscle due to obstruction of the outflow tract by a hypertrophied prostate. In the fundus, a large thin-walled diverticular sac is present.

Bladder diverticula are found predominantly in males, usually in the 6th and 7th decades. They are a result of long-standing outflow obstruction, the commonest cause of which is benign prostatic hypertrophy. They are not uncommonly multiple. Clearly their development will lead to incomplete emptying of the bladder during micturition and the remaining stagnant urine predisposes both to infection and the development of stones. As a probable result of chronic irritation and inflammation of the diverticular urothelium, there is an increased risk of transitional cell and squamous carcinoma in diverticula.

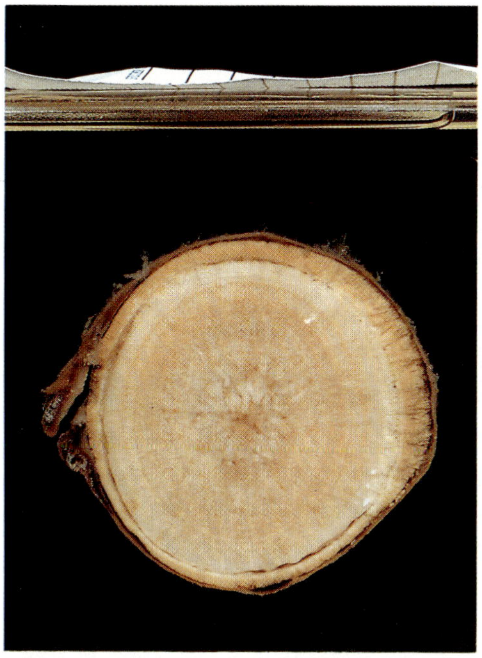

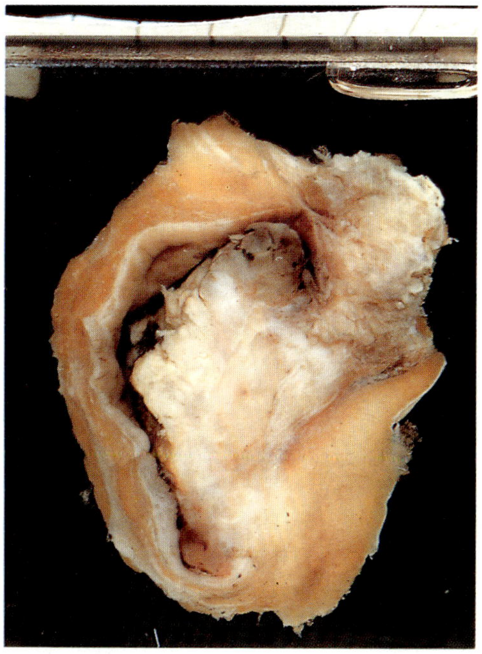

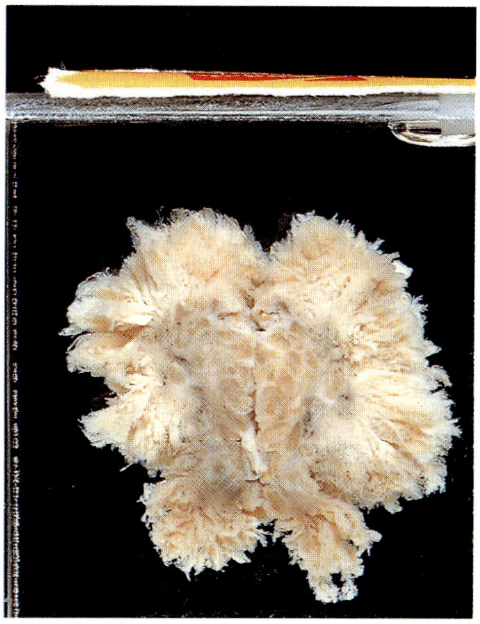

4.69 Diverticulum Containing Calculus

This diverticulum was excised from a 29-year-old man who complained of dysuria and haematuria.

A thin-walled diverticulum, measuring 5cm in diameter, is shown completely filled by a laminated stone. The communication with the bladder cavity is visible on the left of the specimen.

Diverticula are rare in children and young adults but may occur in association with either congenital urinary obstruction (of whatever cause) or an abnormally weak area of the bladder wall. Clearly the complications in such individuals are the same as in the more common elderly patients.

4.70 Anaplastic Carcinoma in a Diverticulum

This diverticulum was excised from a 51-year-old woman who had long-standing recurrent cystitis. More recently she had complained of haematuria.

The diverticulum with perivesical tissue has been sectioned to show that its cavity is completely filled with pale tumour which, in places, has invaded through the full thickness of the diverticular wall.

4.71 Papillary Transitional Cell Carcinoma

No clinical details are available.

This papillary tumour, measuring 2cm in diameter, has been excised from the bladder. It has been bisected to show the typical long, branching villous processes. At the core is a small fragment of muscle from the bladder wall which shows superficial invasion by tumour.

Transitional cell carcinoma of the urinary tract has already been described (see Legend 4.41 et seq. and 4.62 et seq.). The bladder is by far the commonest site and particular predisposing factors include bladder diverticula, schistosomal infection and exstrophy. While these tumours tend to be multiple, the trigone is the single most common site. The various systems of grading and staging correlate well with prognosis. Death may eventually result in up to 50 per cent of patients, either from the complications of urinary tract obstruction and infection or from metastases in those cases which have benefited from improved methods of repeated local treatment.

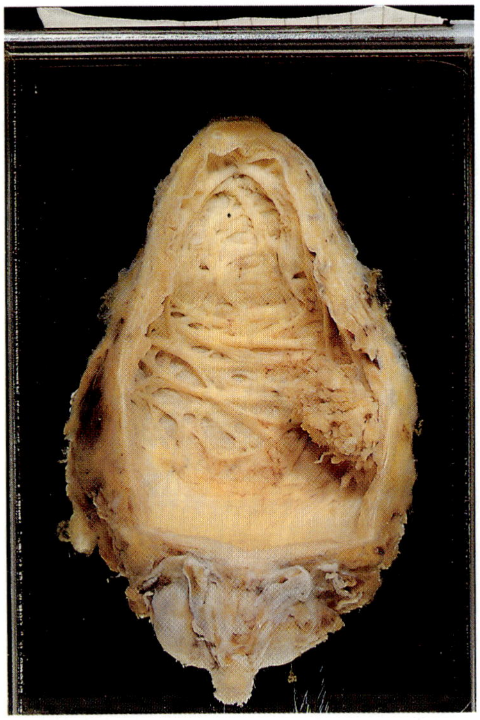

4.72 Papillary Transitional Cell Carcinoma

This is a cystectomy specimen from a 67-year-old man who complained of frequency and haematuria.

The bladder, with the prostate, has been sectioned to show a papillary tumour, measuring 2cm in diameter, arising from a narrow base in the lateral wall.

It should be restressed that the term bladder papilloma, so often used in the past to denote an apparently benign tumour is now only very rarely applied. Lesions showing a normal thickness epithelium with no multilayering and no atypia whatever are extremely uncommon and are the only transitional cell neoplasms thought not to invade or metastasise.

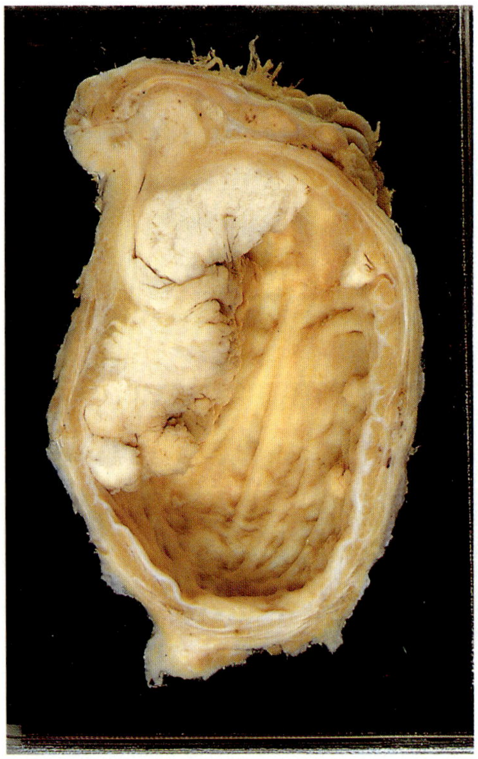

4.73 Solid Transitional Cell Carcinoma

This is a post-mortem specimen from a 68-year-old man who had a 9-month history of frequency and haematuria.

The bladder has been opened to show a largely solid tumour, measuring 6cm in diameter, with a focally papillary surface arising from the base. The tumour has invaded the muscle coat at several points. Separate tumour nodules are visible on the opposite wall of the bladder.

As already stated, solid transitional cell carcinomas carry a worse prognosis than their more common papillary counterparts.

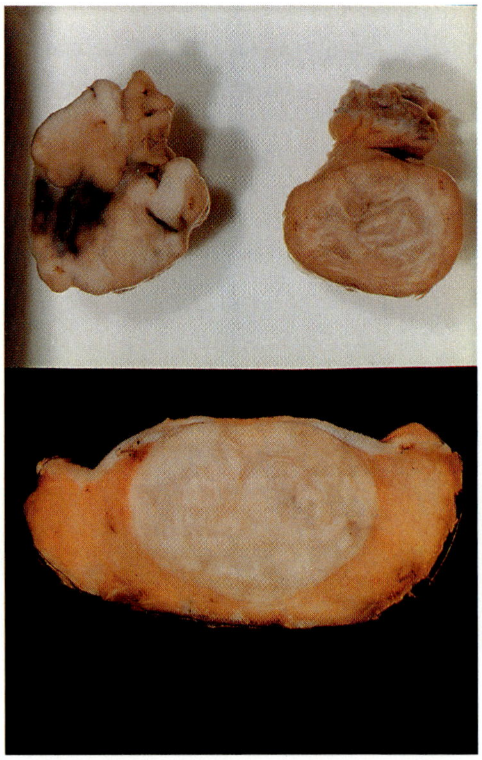

4.74 Leiomyosarcoma

These specimens were excised from a 43-year-old woman who had complained of haematuria and dysuria for 3 months. Cytoscopy revealed a smooth, rounded and pedunculated bladder tumour which was removed with a wide cuff of normal urothelium. Seven years later, a recurrent lesion in the bladder was similarly excised and 5 years after that a further deposit was removed from the abdominal wall.

On the left, the primary neoplasm, mounted below the intravesical recurrence, is a firm, rounded tumour, measuring 3cm in diameter. It has a short pedicle and is covered by attenuated and focally ulcerated urothelium. The cut surface shows the characteristic whorled appearance. The first recurrence (above) has a coarsely lobulated appearance and shows foci of haemorrhage and necrosis. On the right, a portion of the abdominal wall has been sectioned to show a circumscribed, ovoid deposit of tumour, measuring 3cm in diameter. The surface again shows a whorled appearance.

Sarcomas of the bladder are extremely rare, but leiomyosarcoma is the least uncommon. It most often presents in late adulthood and clinical behaviour is directly related to the degree of histological differentiation. The protracted course of the case here is typical of well differentiated leiomyosarcoma, of which this tumour is an example.

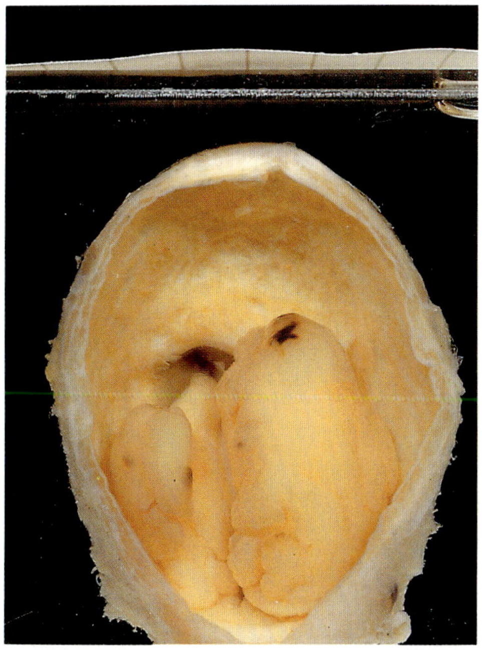

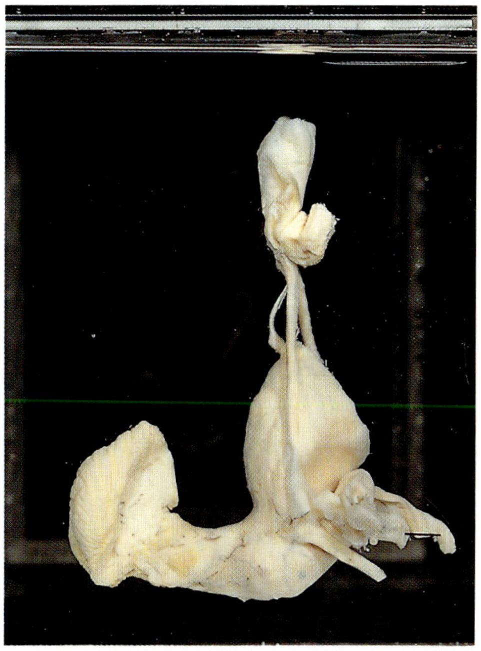

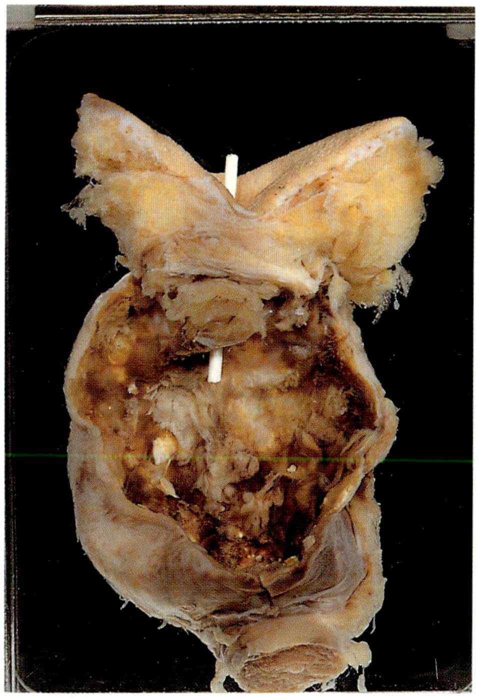

4.75 Embryonal Rhabdomyosarcoma

This is a cystectomy specimen from a 12-month-old boy who presented with a 3 day history of haematuria. The bladder was distended and a polypoid tumour was found arising from the left side of the base. This was locally excised but recurrence 2 months later prompted a cystectomy and partial prostatectomy.

The bladder has been opened to show a soft, lobulated polypoid tumour arising adjacent to the trigone and obstructing both the ureteric orifices and the urethra. The bladder is dilated and hypertrophied and a saccular diverticulum is visible in the posterior wall.

The tumour, while histologically a typical embryonal rhabdomyosarcoma, may be described macroscopically as sarcoma botryoides. This describes the grape-like polypoid appearance that occurs when such tumours arise beneath an epithelial surface. These neoplasms are rare in the bladder but most often affect infants of less than 2 years of age, predominantly of the male sex. They usually originate close to the trigone, and give rise to urinary obstruction. Embryonal rhabdomyosarcoma is a highly malignant tumour but, with radical multimodal treatment, there are now hopes of long-term survival.

4.76 Persistent Urachus

No clinical details are available.

The bladder, uterus and vagina of a female neonate have been dissected to show the partly patent urachus passing from the bladder to the umbilical cord.

The urachus is derived embryologically from the ventral portion of the cloaca and forms the apex of the vesicourethral canal. *In utero* it connects the bladder lumen with the umbilical arteries in the allantois. Normally, as the bladder is drawn downwards, the connection is obliterated, leaving only the umbilical ligament. However, if the urachus persists, a sinus tract or complete vesicoumbilical fistula may develop. It should be remembered that the urachal remnant, even if normally situated, may be the site of origin of carcinomas in adulthood.

4.77 Urachal Cyst

This specimen was excised from 50-year-old man who had noticed minor umbilical swelling, associated with an intermittent purulent discharge from the umbilicus, for 2 years. Clinically the swelling was considered to be a retro-umbilical hernia but at operation a cyst was found which was connected to the dome of the bladder by a pedicle containing an epithelium-lined tract.

An ellipse of periumbilical skin with underlying subcutaneous tissue is shown. In the soft tissues is a cyst, measuring 5cm in diameter, which has been opened to show its irregular lining with foci of myxoid change, haemorrhage, calcification and lipid deposition. A very thin pale pedicle with a central duct is visible at the bottom of the specimen. A white probe has been used to demonstrate the fistula between the umbilicus and the urachal cyst.

Cystic dilatations of a persistent urachus occur most often at the inferior aspect of the median umbilical ligament and are extraperitoneal. They may be single or multiple and, if associated with an umbilical fistula, are particularly prone to infection.

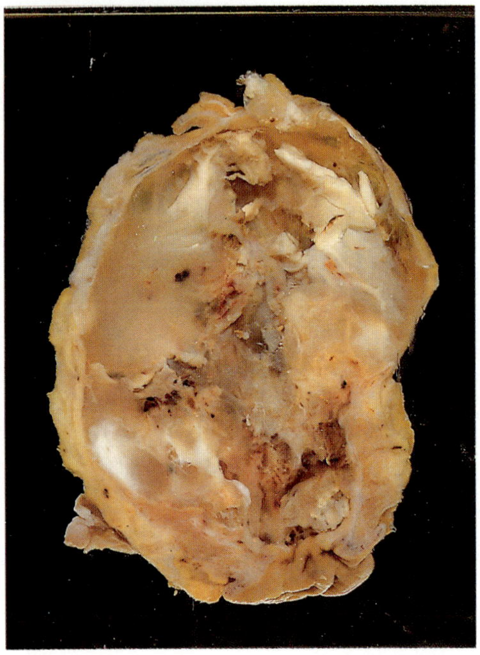

4.78 Adenocarcinoma in Urachal Remnant

This is a partial cystectomy specimen from a 75-year-old woman who presented with frequency and haematuria. At operation a large, gelatinous tumour was found arising adjacent to the dome of the bladder.

The specimen consists of a large saccular structure, measuring 10 × 9 × 5cm, which has been sectioned and is continuous with a small fragment of urothelium from the bladder dome, seen at the bottom of the picture. Within the cavity, there is a mass of neoplastic tissue which is focally mucoid, necrotic and haemorrhagic. Histologically, the sac is lined entirely by glandular epithelium.

Urachal epithelium often undergoes metaplasia to either mucus-secreting glandular epithelium or squamous epithelium. The development of adenocarcinomas in the urachal remnant is well-recognised and is thought to account for at least 35 per cent of adenocarcinomas of the bladder. It is usually possible to identify the site of origin of such tumours outside the bladder lining, thus distinguishing them from adenocarcinomas arising in foci of metaplasia due to chronic cystitis.

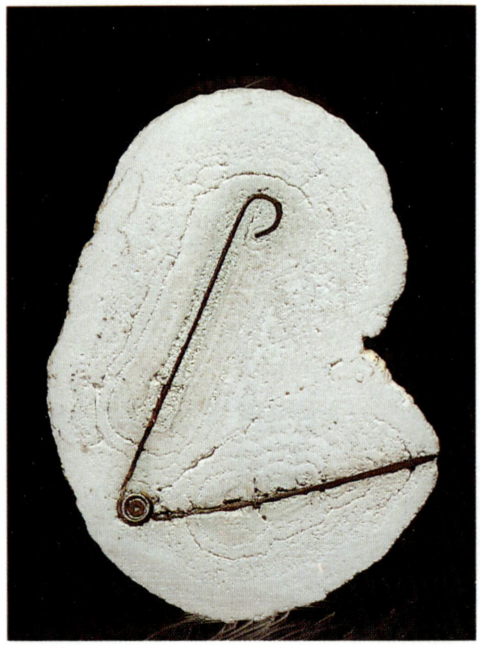

4.79 Calculus containing Tie-Pin

This specimen was removed suprapubically from the bladder of a 29-year-old man who was severely mentally retarded. He had been noted to suffer frequency and dysuria, and urine culture grew *E. coli*.

This laminated calculus is reniform in shape, measuring 6cm in maximum diameter, and has been sectioned to show a brass tie-pin embedded in the centre.

The vast majority of vesical calculi occur in males and may originate either in stagnant infected urine, for example in a diverticulum, or else around a nidus, such as a stone that has descended from higher in the urinary tract or a foreign body. These calculi are almost all of mixed type and the same predisposing factors apply as in the kidney stones (see Legend 4.55). Frequently multiple stones are found (see Urinary Calculi section).

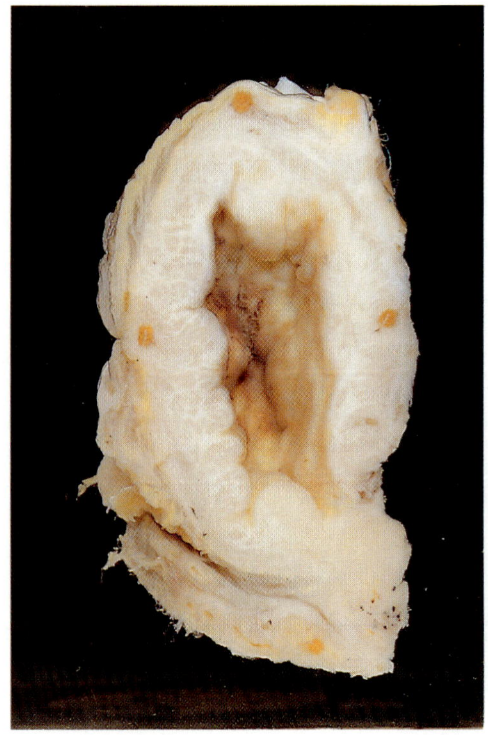

4.80 Irradiation Damage

This is a cystectomy specimen from a 53-year-old man who had undergone radiotherapy for an ulcerated bladder carcinoma 4 years previously. Recurrence of the tumour prompted removal of the bladder.

The bladder is contracted and has been sectioned to show marked fibrous thickening of the wall with atrophy of the muscular layers. The urothelium is congested and focally ulcerated. The recurrent tumour is not present in this portion of the bladder.

Radiation cystitis and fibrosis are common complications of radiotherapy to any pelvic tumour, although each patient's response to treatment is very variable. Vascular ectasia may predispose to haematuria while ulceration and necrosis may give rise to infection or urinary obstruction. Shrinkage of the bladder often causes distressing frequency.

URETHRA

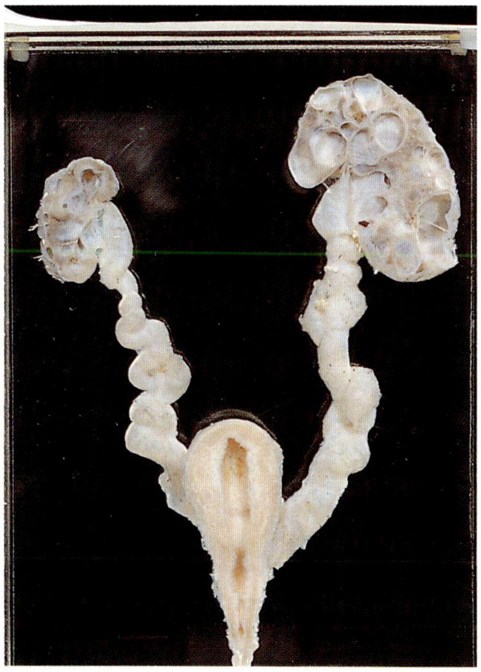

4.81 Congenital Obstruction

This is a post-mortem specimen from a still-born male infant.

The urinary tract of this infant has been dissected to show that the vesicourethral orifice and proximal prostatic urethra are dilated so as to form a single cavity with the bladder. The bladder is hypertrophied and dilated and there is a bilateral hydroureter and hydronephrosis. This obstructive picture has arisen as a consequence of narrowing in the posterior urethra. In addition, the kidneys also show infantile polycystic disease.

Congenital urethral obstruction is virtually confined to male infants and may arise as a result of either urethral valves (abnormal flaps of urothelium near the verumontanum), congenital stenosis or atresia of the urethra or defective neuromuscular coordination. Note again the frequency with which more than one congenital anomaly may be found in the urinary tract.

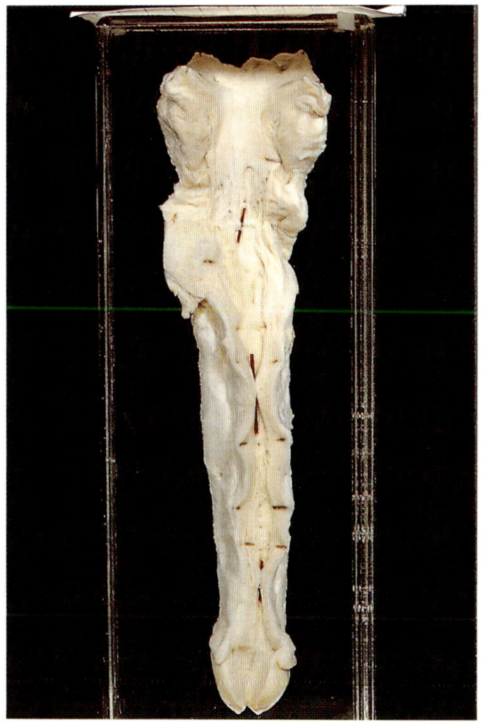

4.82 Acquired Strictures

This specimen was removed at post-mortem from a 36-year-old man, known to have a long-standing stricture, who died after an attack of 'ague' in 1841.

The penis and prostate are shown with the urethra laid open. There are two very narrow strictures, 3cm and 8cm from the external urinary meatus. Proximally the urethra is dilated with flattening of the verumontanum and, on the left of the membranous urethra, a closed cavity, which represents an abscess in Cowper's gland, is present.

Acquired urethral strictures usually occur as a result of trauma or inflammation. Traumatic causes include direct external injury or instrumentation of the lower urinary tract. Multiple strictures are usually inflammatory in origin, most particularly post-infective. The common infective causes are gonorrhoea, syphilis and tuberculosis. In the presence of a bulbourethral gland abscess in the case here, it would appear that this patient's problems were gonococcal in origin.

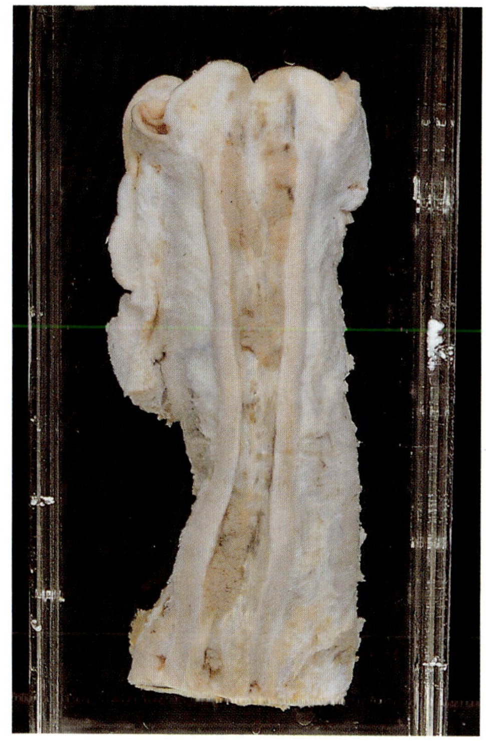

4.83 Transitional Cell Carcinoma

This specimen was excised from a 67-year-old man who had proven papillary carcinoma of the bladder for some years.

A portion of the penis with the urethra has been laid open to show numerous small papillomatous tumours arising from the urethral epithelium.

Transitional cell carcinoma of the urethra most often occurs in association with a coexistent bladder tumour and, as already mentioned, represents either a separate tumour arising as a 'field-change' effect or a seedling metastasis down the urinary tract. Primary carcinoma of the urethra, in the absence of any other tumour, is rare and occurs in the elderly, usually with a previous history of recurrent inflammation. The prognosis is poor.

URINARY CALCULI

Urinary calculi are said to affect up to 5 per cent of the population at some time in their life, although many will remain asymptomatic. Most calculi arise in the kidney and tend to be unilateral; the majority present in adulthood, males predominating over females.

General predisposing factors, applicable to all types of stone, are as follows:

1) An elevated urinary concentration of the relevant constituent, due either to increased excretion or decreased urinary volume.
2) Alterations in urinary pH which promote precipitation of the relevant constituent.
3) Urinary obstruction.

Frequently, no clear predisposition can be demonstrated and it is thought that many stones arise as a consequence of either a deficiency of inhibitors of crystal formation (e.g. citrate, pyrophosphate) or an alteration in urinary mucoproteins, which form the matrix or core of most calculi (see table on page 179).

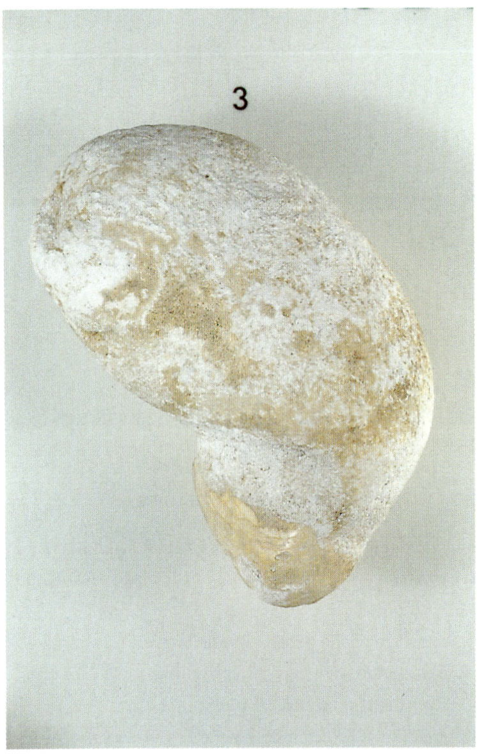

4.84 Calcium Phosphate Stone from Renal Pelvis

This specimen was removed from a 41-year-old woman who had suffered increasing loin discomfort and intermittent haematuria for some years. Sixteen years previously she had an episode of urinary tract infection. IVP showed a non-functioning left kidney containing many small stones and the right kidney showed limited function, but the pelvicalyceal system contained a large branched stone.

This irregularly ovoid, white phosphate stone measured 10 × 6 × 4.5cm and weighed 341g. It has the shape of a dilated renal pelvis and the surface is largely smooth.

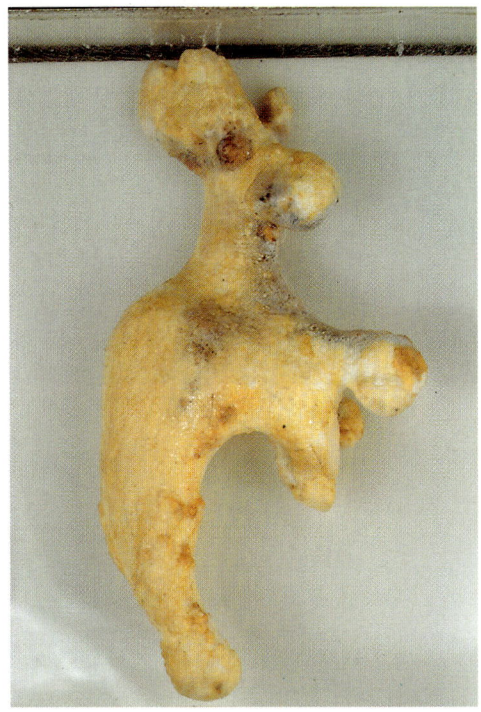

4.85 Staghorn Phosphate Stone from Renal Pelvis

No clinical details are available.

This stone has a complex, branched appearance which forms an accurate cast of the pelvicalyceal system and upper ureter; the resemblance to the horns of a stag is obvious.

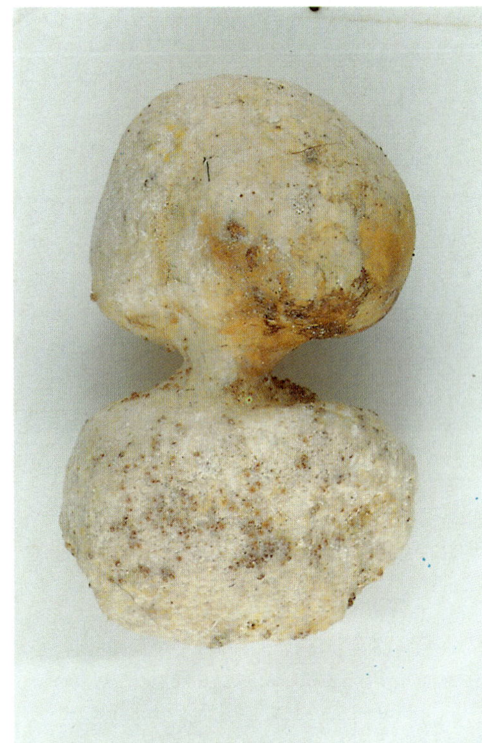

4.86 Dumbell Phosphate Stone

This stone was found partly within, and partly protruding from, a bladder diverticulum.

This smooth, white phosphate stone measured 6 × 4 × 4cm in maximum dimensions and resembles a dumbell.

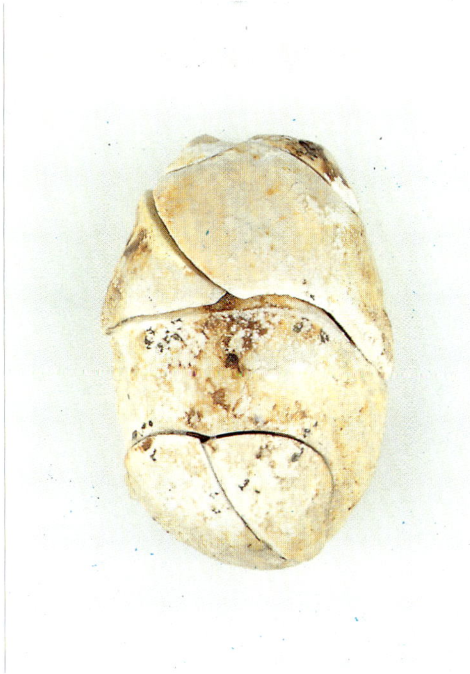

4.87 Articulating Phosphate Stones

This specimen was removed from the urethra of a 50-year-old woman.

A pale, smooth stone, measuring 3.5 × 2.5 × 1.5cm, is seen to consist of 5 separate pieces which fit together closely so as to form a single composite unit.

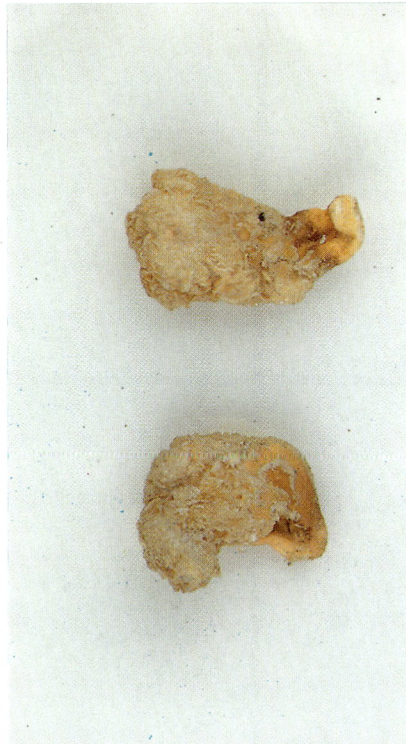

4.88 Mixed Calcium Phosphate and Oxalate Stone

These stones were removed from a 42-year-old woman who had suffered dysuria and frequency since having a colporrhaphy two years previously. It appeared that these stones had formed in the bladder adjacent to the ligatures remaining from her operation.

These two irregular, pale brown stones, each measuring approximately 1.5cm in length, have granular areas typical of oxalate stones but there are also smooth areas of phosphate origin.

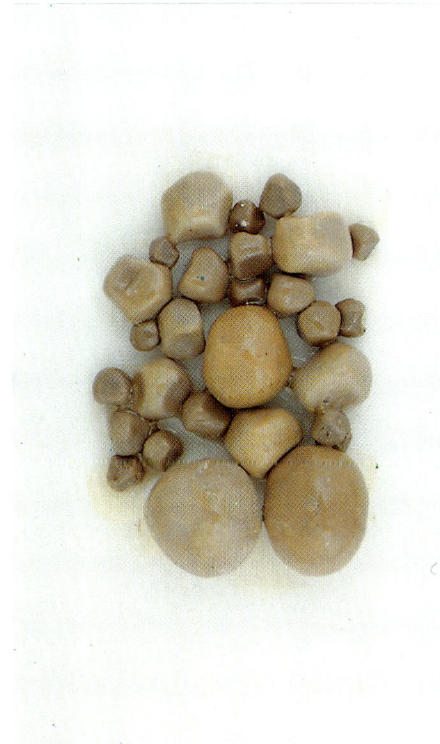

4.89 Mixed Faceted Phosphate and Oxalate Stones

These stones were removed from an upper pole calyx in the kidney.

This collection of small stones show a smooth, faceted appearance and are greyish-brown in colour.

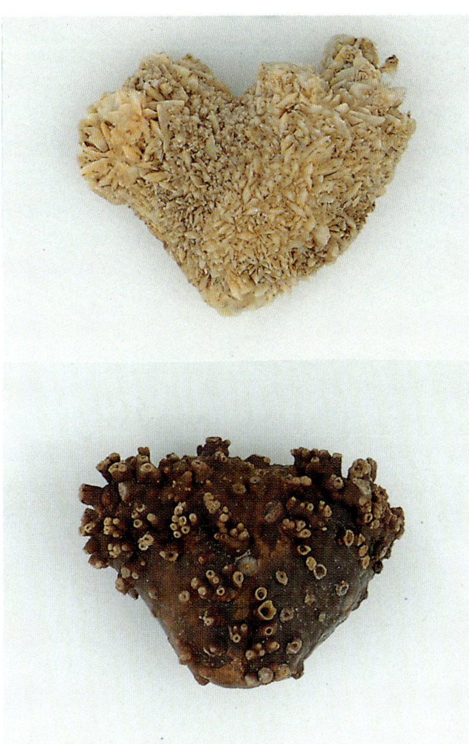

4.90 Oxalate Stones from Renal Pelvis

The specimen on the left was removed from the kidney of a 25-year-old soldier who presented with a 12 year history of intermittent painless haematuria. Plain abdominal X-ray showed a large stone occupying the left renal pelvis. No clinical details are available for the specimen on the right.

Both stones have formed a cast of the renal pelvis and are covered with small, sharp crystalline projections. While the one on the left is pale, the right-hand stone is dark brown in colour. This is due to deposition of blood pigments from pelvicalycaeal haemorrhage due to abrasion by the rough edges of the stone.

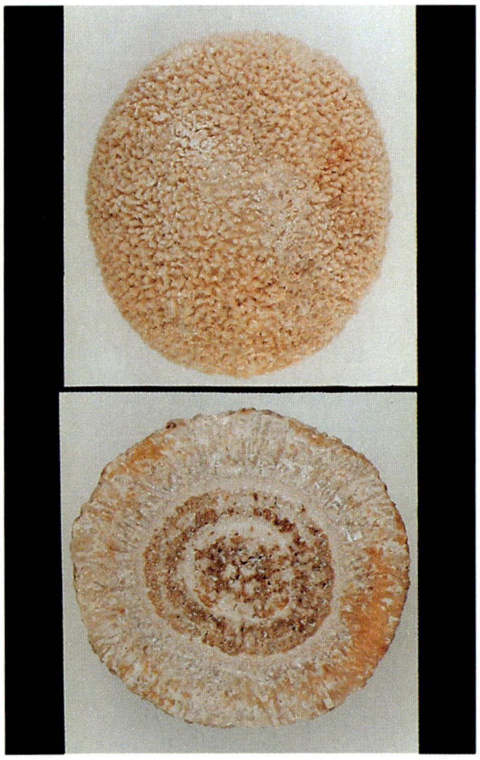

4.91 Pale Oxalate Stones from the Bladder

The specimen on the left was removed from the bladder of an airman who complained of increasing dysuria, frequency and difficulty in defaecation. The one on the right was passed spontaneously by a multiparous woman who presented with abdominal swelling and a pelvic mass, and was thought to be pregnant. However, closer examination revealed the abdominal swelling to be a distended bladder and the pelvic mass to be a stone at the neck of the bladder. The patient attempted to exonerate the doctor of his erroneous diagnosis by stating that, during the passage of the stone, she 'felt as though she was giving birth to a hedgehog'.

Both stones are rounded and measure approximately 4.5cm in diameter. Each has a rough, granular surface and the one on the right has been bisected to demonstrate the laminated structure, seen in many stones, which represents the consecutive laying down of material around a central nidus. Note that, in mixed stones, the outer laminations may conceal a central core of the pathogenetic urinary salt. Careful sampling and biochemical estimations may be required to identify an underlying metabolic defect.

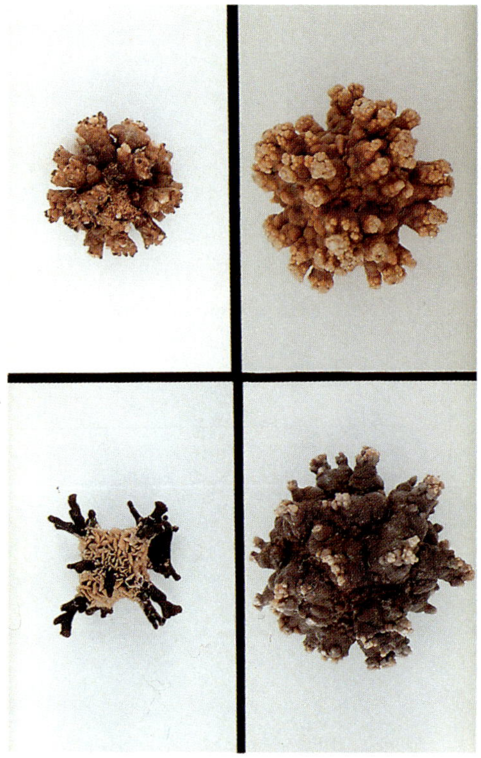

4.92 Stellate Vesical Oxalate Stones

These specimens were all removed from the bladder, three of them being found in elderly men with benign prostatic hypertrophy.

Each of these stones has the irregular crystalline projections typical of oxalate stones. The two on the left show the characteristic 'mulberry' colour due to deposition of blood pigments. It is easy to appreciate that the bladder epithelium might he abraded and bleed when stones such as these are present.

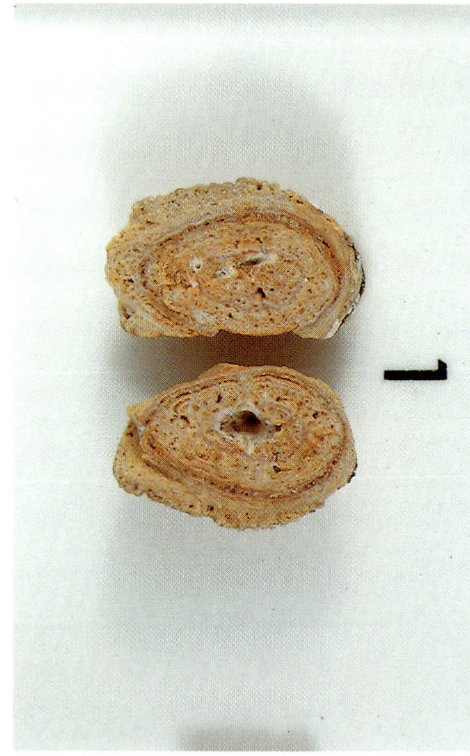

4.93 Urate Stone from Kidney

This specimen was removed from the kidney of a 40-year-old Middle European woman.

This rounded brown stone, measuring 1.3cm in maximum dimension, has been bisected to demonstrate the concentric lamination which may be a feature of any urinary calculus. It should be noted that the original nidus at the core of these laminae is often not identifiable.

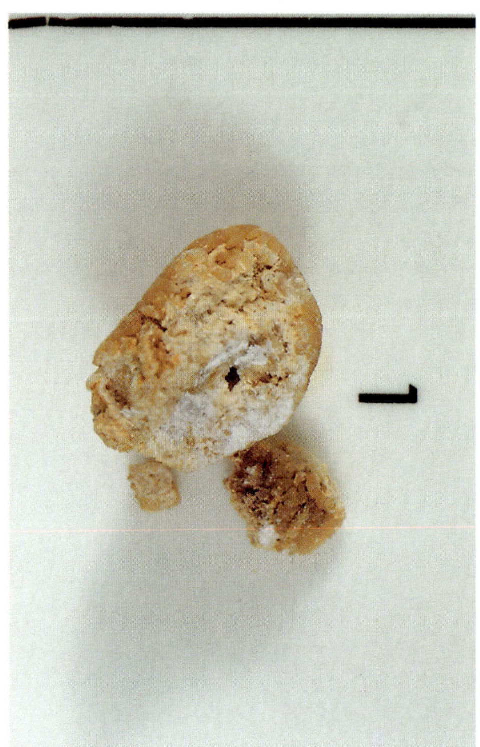

4.94 Cystine Stone from Kidney

This specimen was removed from the kidney of a man whose age was unstated.

These are three fragments of one irregular, yellow-brown stone; the surface is largely smooth but some small areas have an irregular crystalline appearance. Cystine stones commonly turn a greenish-blue in colour if left exposed to the air for a long period.

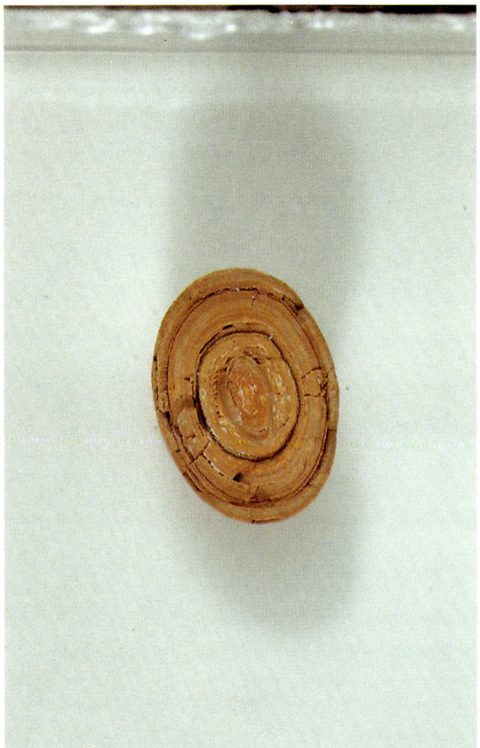

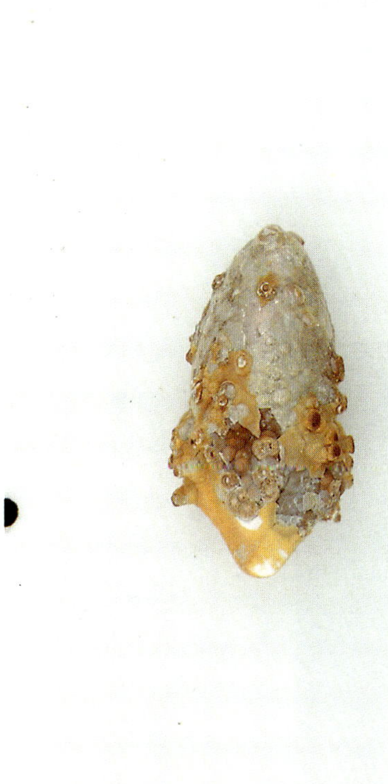

4.96 Mixed Urate/Oxalate/'Triple' Phosphate Stone

This specimen was removed from the ureter of a patient with unilateral pyonephrosis.

The stone is ovoid with blunt ends, measuring 3cm in length, and conforms in shape to a dilated ureter. The lower pole, which is smooth and greyish, is composed largely of urate while the brown irregular projections above are oxalate. The yellowish 'cap' at the upper pole is composed of 'triple' phosphate and was thought to be the consequence of *Proteus spp.* infection prior to surgery.

This stone simply serves to show that the pathogenesis of urinary calculi is inconsistent, often not being attributable to a single predisposing cause, so that mixed or complex calculi are not uncommon.

4.95 Xanthine Stone from Bladder

This specimen was removed from the bladder of a 10-year-old Indian boy.

This stone has the typical reddish-brown colour of xanthine stones and measures 1.4 × 1 × 0.7cm. It has a smooth surface and has been bisected to show its concentric lamination.

URINARY CALCULI

TYPE OF STONE	FREQUENCY (% all stones)	TYPICAL APPEARANCES	KNOWN PREDISPOSING FACTORS	FAVOURABLE URINARY pH
Calcium Phosphate		White; smooth/faceted, may form staghorn	Hypercalciuria ± Hypercalcaemia	
Calcium Oxalate	65-75	White/red/black/'mulberry'; irregular/sharp	Hyperoxaluria - primary - secondary	Alkaline
Mixed Calcium Phosphate + Oxalate		Variable		
Calcium Ammonium Magnesium Phosphate (triple phosphate)	15	Pale; soft, may form staghorn	Urinary tract infection with urea-splitting organisms, such as *Proteus spp.*	Aklaline
Urate	6	Yellow-brown; hard/smooth	Hyperuricaemia - primary - secondary	Acid
Cystine	2-3	Yellow to green/blue; soft, may form staghorn	Primary Cystinuria	Acid
Xanthine	1-2	Red-brown; smooth	Primary Xanthinuria	Acid

Extremely rarely, urinary calculi may also be composed of lysine, ornithine, arginine and indican.

It is important to re-stress that, in very many cases, no clear predisposing cause for the development of a calculus can be identified.

5. REPRODUCTIVE SYSTEM

FEMALE GENITAL SYSTEM

Ovary and Fallopian Tube

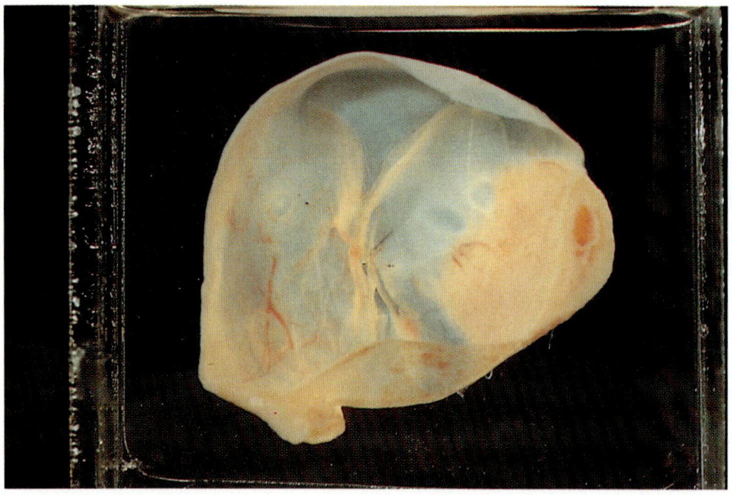

5.1 Ovary: Torsion

This specimen was excised from a multiparous 49-year-old woman who presented with acute abdominal pain. A uterine myomectomy had been performed 10 years previously.

The left ovary, fallopian tube and uterus are shown. The ovary is swollen, dark-red and engorged due to torsion of its pedicle. Note also the multiple leiomyomata in the uterine wall (see Figure 5.37 et seq.).

Ovarian torsion occurs when the ovary twists either on the ovarian ligament or the mesovarium: this occurs more often when ovarian cysts or tumours are present. Acute cases may progress rapidly to gangrene or peritonitis. A chronic torsion may lead to the condition of massive ovarian oedema, which can simulate an ovarian tumour.

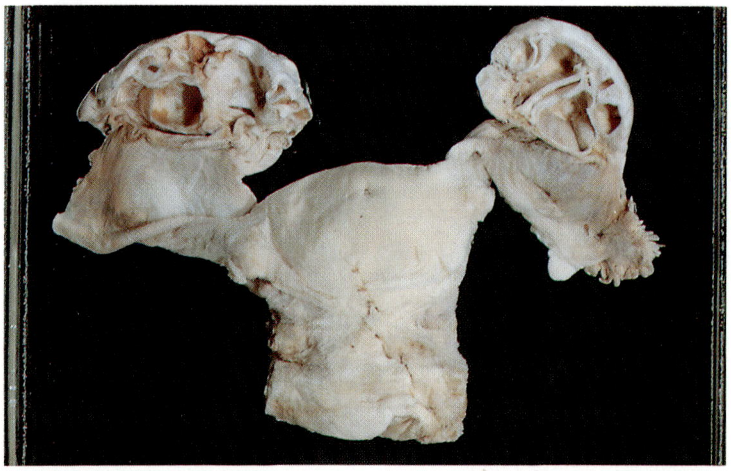

5.2 Ovaries: Multiple Follicular Cysts

These were an incidental finding at post-mortem in a 79-year-old woman who died after a road traffic accident.

The uterus, fallopian tubes and ovaries are shown. The ovaries are enlarged and have been bisected to show virtual replacement by multiple, smooth-walled cysts of varying size.

Follicular cysts are common, usually small and arise most often in perimenopausal women in whom failing ovarian function leads to the partial maturation of many germinal follicles which then become atretic and undergo cystic change. Occasionally the granulosa and theca cell layers remain active, thereby secreting excess oestrogen which gives rise to endometrial hyperplasia. In the Stein-Leventhal syndrome, each ovary contains very many follicular cysts.

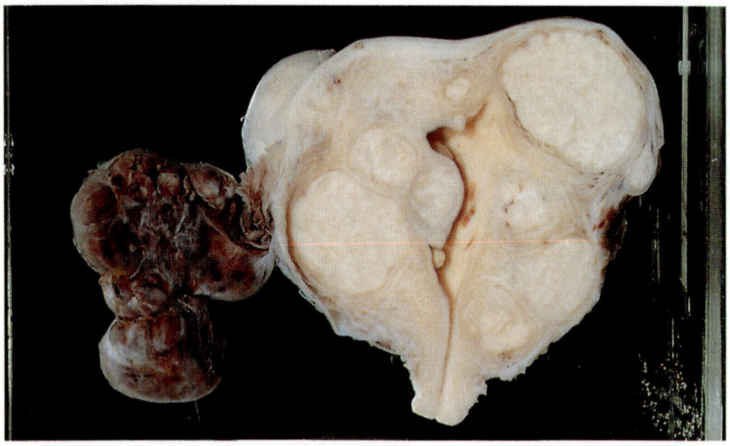

5.3 Ovary: Luteal Cyst

This specimen was an incidental finding at laparotomy in a 34-year-old multiparous woman. The cyst had been entirely asymptomatic.

This is a thin-walled cyst containing clear material, which measures approximately 3cm in diameter. On the left, a solid yellowish portion of the corpus luteum remains.

Corpus luteum cysts are common and they most often develop after excessive haemorrhage into a normal corpus luteum or after organisation of an involuting corpus luteum of pregnancy. Although corpus luteum cysts are usually of no clinical significance, they may sometimes rupture and cause intraperitoneal bleeding, thus occasionally presenting as an acute abdomen. (Courtesy of the Royal College of Obstetricians and Gynaecologists)

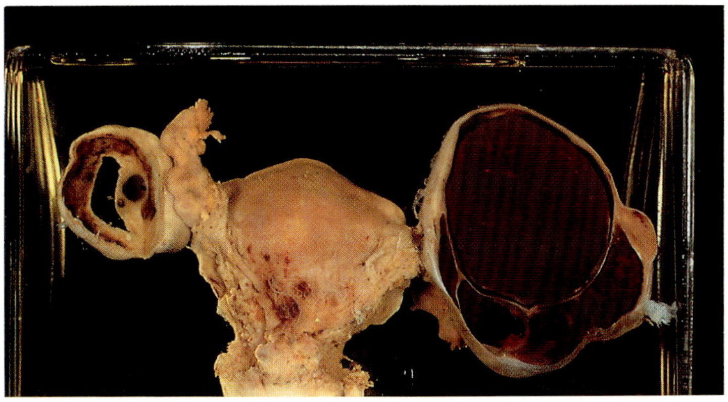

5.4 Ovaries: Bilateral 'Chocolate' Cysts

This specimen was excised from a 43-year-old woman who had a one year history of dysmenorrhoea. At operation, in addition to the ovarian lesions, several leiomyomata were present in the uterus.

The uterus with both tubes and ovaries are shown. Both ovaries contain cystic lesions within which there is organised blood clot. In the ovary on the left there is also a solid, reddish area which represents an endometriotic focus.

Endometriosis is defined as the presence of ectopic endometrial tissue outside the uterus. The commonest sites are the ovary, broad ligament, pouch of Douglas and pelvic peritoneum. Other sites include the bowel, hernial sacs, umbilicus and bladder. Very rare cases have been identified at almost any site in the body. The pathogenesis is uncertain; the following hypotheses have been put forward to explain the sites involved: retrograde menstruation down the fallopian tube; endometrial metaplasia in peritoneal tissue, and blood-borne or lymphatic dissemination of endometrial tissue. Ovarian endometriosis may be first recognised as small reddish nodules but, with repeated cyclical stimulation, cysts most commonly develop into which menstrual bleeding occurs. It is this blood which becomes organised giving rise to the 'chocolate' cysts seen here. (Courtesy of the Royal College of Obstetricians and Gynaecologists)

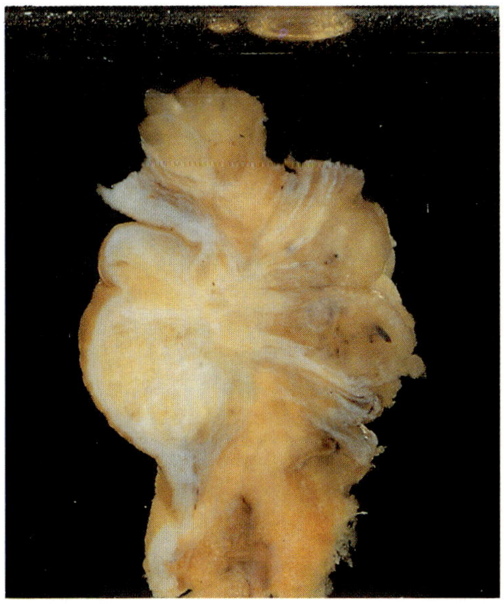

5.5 Umbilicus: Endometriosis

This specimen was excised from a 39-year-old woman who had noticed a pigmented nodule at the umbilicus for 3 years. The nodule steadily increased in size and bled at the menstrual periods. There was no evidence of endometriosis elsewhere.

The umbilicus has been sectioned to show a smooth, rounded, fibrous nodule projecting from the surface. Numerous tiny cysts and foci of brown discolouration are barely visible within the lesion.

Endometriosis only causes symptoms during the reproductive years and this is due to the normal cyclical changes that the ectopic tissue undergoes. Some patients with endometriosis present with infertility but, interestingly, others are often cured by undergoing a normal pregnancy. Very occasionally, endometriotic foci may develop hyperplasia or even carcinoma.

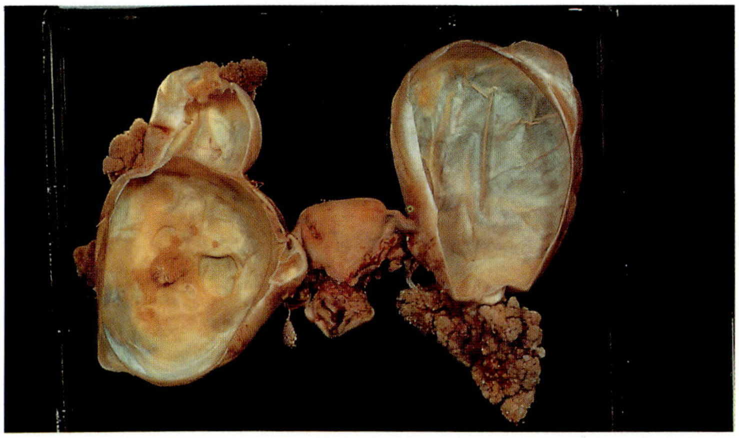

5.6 Ovaries: Bilateral Serous Cystadenoma

This specimen was excised from a 50-year-old, postmenopausal woman who presented with a one year history of right iliac fossa pain associated with abdominal swelling. A total abdominal hysterectomy with bilateral salpingo-oöphorectomy was performed.

On the right, there is a large unilocular, thin-walled cyst replacing the ovary, from the surface of which numerous sessile papillae project. On the left there is a similar bilocular cyst which also shows several surface papillomata.

Serous cystadenoma is a common benign epithelial ovarian tumour, which probably accounts for about 25 per cent of all ovarian tumours. The tumour is, like most epithelial ovarian neoplasms, derived from the surface epithelium of the ovary; cells in this epithelium retain a potentiality to differentiate into various Müllerian structures, and differentiation into tubal type epithelium gives rise to a serous neoplasm. Such tumours are commonly thin-walled, unilocular and rarely exceed 20cm in diameter. Papillary projections from either the internal or external surface are frequently found. Bilaterality occurs in up to 30 per cent of cases. (Courtesy of the Royal College of Obstetricians and Gynaecologists)

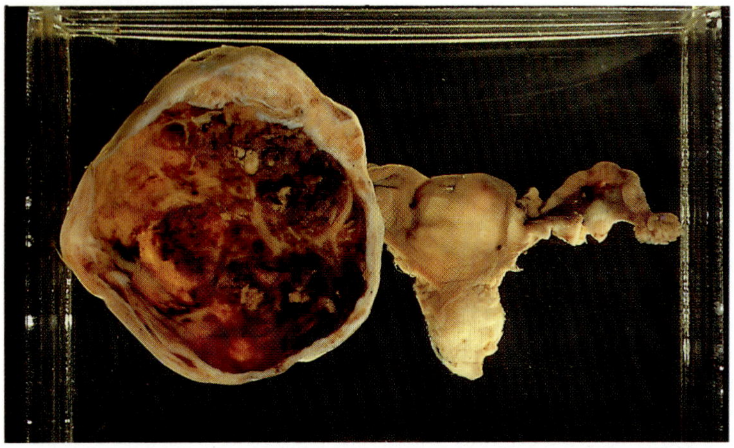

5.7 Ovary: Serous Cystadenocarcinoma

This specimen was excised from a 70-year-old woman who complained of intermittent left lower abdominal pain and had recently noticed swelling of the abdomen.

The left ovary is replaced by a cystic tumour, measuring 11cm in maximum diameter. The wall of the cyst is focally thickened and there are numerous irregular, solid intraluminal masses of haemorrhagic tumour. Note also the uterine leiomyomata.

Distinction between benign and malignant serous ovarian tumours is largely dependent upon histological examination. However, a serous cystadenocarcinoma tends to be larger than its benign counterpart and often shows extensive haemorrhage or necrosis. It is the commonest primary ovarian malignant tumour and arises bilaterally in up to 40 per cent of cases. Women in the 6th and 7th decades are predominantly affected, as is the case for all ovarian epithelial malignancies. Prognosis is closely related to tumour staging but the overall 5-year-survival is only of the order of 20-25 per cent. (Courtesy of the Royal College of Obstetricians and Gynaecologists)

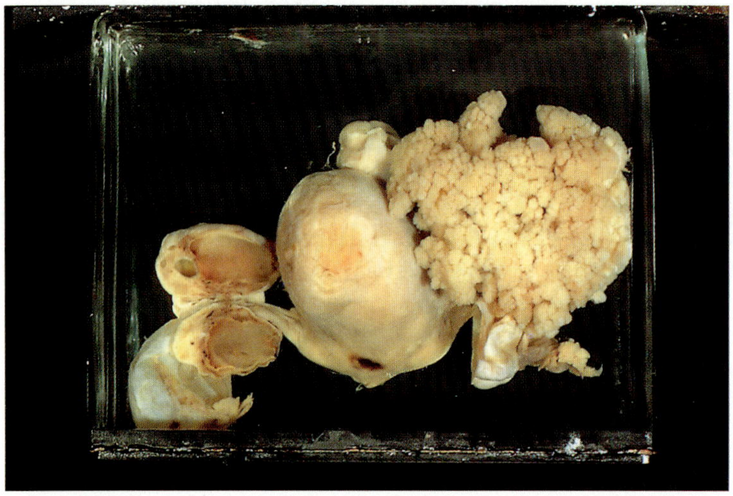

5.8 Ovary: Papillary Serous Tumour of Borderline Malignancy

This specimen was excised from a 29-year-old woman who presented with menorrhagia.

The uterus with both tubes and ovaries are shown. The left ovary is largely replaced by a tumour covered in sessile papillae. At its upper pole, note also a small mature (benign) teratoma. The uterus is distorted by leiomyomata and the right ovary contains a follicular cyst and corpus luteum cyst.

Both serous and mucinous tumours of borderline malignancy are now well defined histologically, and clearly recognised clinically; both are relatively common and are macroscopically very similar to their benign counterparts. Histologically, however, there is cellular proliferation and atypia, together with multilayering and mitotic activity; stromal invasion is absent and this is the definitive feature of a neoplasm of borderline malignancy. The majority of these neoplasms behave in a benign fashion and 5-year-survival is in the region of 95 per cent. The long-term prognosis, though generally believed to be good, is not clearly defined, however. A small proportion of cases will behave in a malignant fashion though the progress of the disease is usually indolent. There are currently no pathological criteria for distinguishing those tumours which will progress from those that will not. The case shown here is remarkable for the variety of gynaecological pathology it displays. (Courtesy of the Royal College of Obstetricians and Gynaecologists)

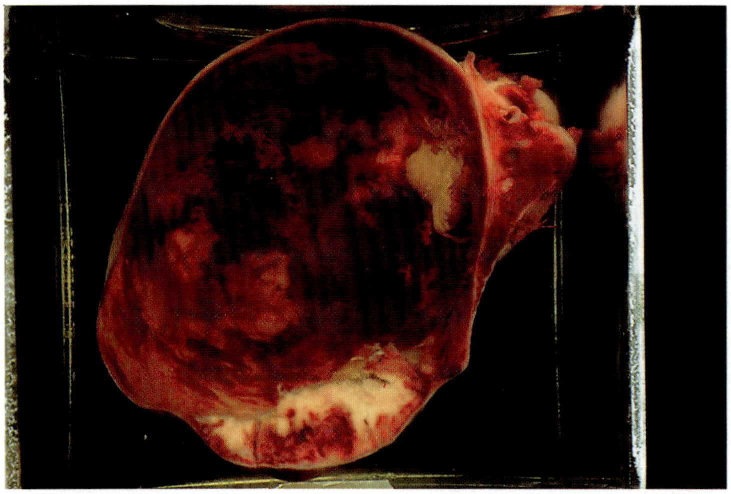

5.9 Ovary: Torsion of Serous Cystadenocarcinoma

This specimen was excised from a 37-year-old woman who had noticed an increase in her abdominal girth for the previous 6 weeks. She presented as an emergency with sudden onset of lower abdominal pain and vomiting.

A large, unilocular ovarian cyst with solid tumour masses on the internal surface is shown. The cyst is intensely congested and focally necrotic as a result of torsion.

Torsion of any ovarian tumour of significant size is common and results from twisting of the ovary on its pedicle. Sudden abdominal pain is characteristic and such cases should be treated as a surgical emergency. (Courtesy of the Royal College of Obstetricians and Gynaecologists)

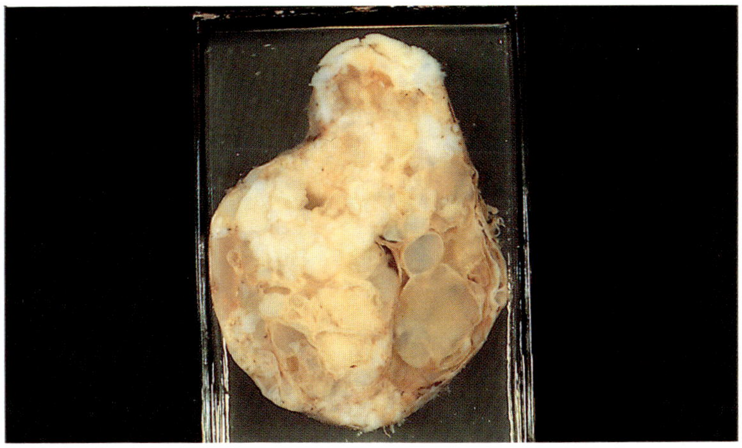

5.10 Ovary: Mucinous Cystadenoma

No clinical details are available.

This is a well-circumscribed multilocular tumour, some areas of which are solid. Many of the locules contain thick, viscid mucinous material while others are more translucent.

Mucinous cystadenomas are common, representing approximately 20 per cent of benign ovarian neoplasms. They are again derived from the ovarian surface epithelium but, in contrast to serous tumours, differentiate along an endocervical-type Müllerian pathway. They are classically multilocular and are usually much larger than their serous counterparts, often attaining an enormous size: tumours weighing up to 35kg have been recorded. These tumours arise most often during the reproductive years and may be bilateral in up to 10 per cent of cases. An important complication of mucinous tumours is that rupture or leakage may lead to the development of pseudomyxoma peritonei, typified by bulky gelatinous masses throughout the peritoneal cavity. (Courtesy of the Royal College of Obstetricians and Gynaecologists)

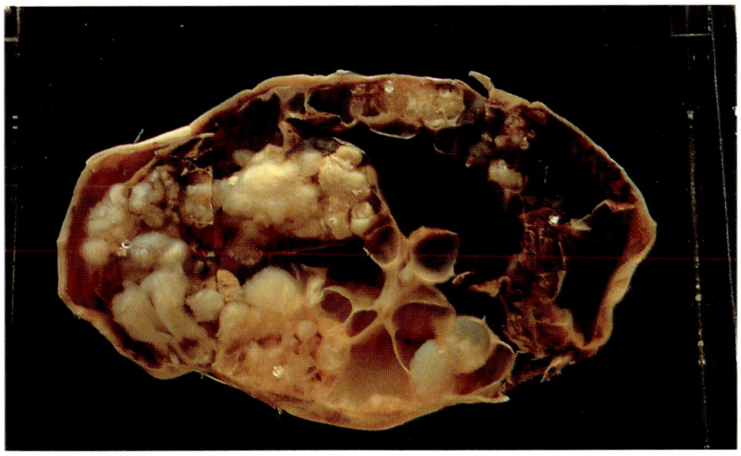

5.11 Ovary: Mucinous Cystadenocarcinoma

This specimen was excised from a young woman who complained of intermittent abdominal pain for 2 years and had recently noticed an increase in her abdominal girth.

This ovoid ovarian cyst is multilocular and many of the smaller loculi contain viscid grey fluid. However, in areas, the wall of the cyst is composed of pale, friable solid tissue. It was in these areas that foci of frank malignancy were detected.

As in serous tumours, distinction between benign and malignant mucinous ovarian neoplasms is often only possible by careful histological examination. The presence of solid nodular areas on either the internal or external surface should be regarded with suspicion. Mucinous cystadenocarcinoma accounts for about 15 per cent of primary ovarian malignancies and, like its serous equivalent, is commonest in middle-aged or elderly females; the case here in which the tumour presented in a young woman is unusual. The 5-year-survival is of the order of 40-50 per cent which is rather better than that for serous tumours; the reasons for this are unknown though it may possibly reflect a different degree of inherent biological malignancy in this type of neoplasm. As already stated (see Legend 5.10), rupture of a mucinous tumour, or slow leakage of its contents from a small perforation, may be complicated by pseudomyxoma peritonei. (Courtesy of the Royal College of Obstetricians and Gynaecologists)

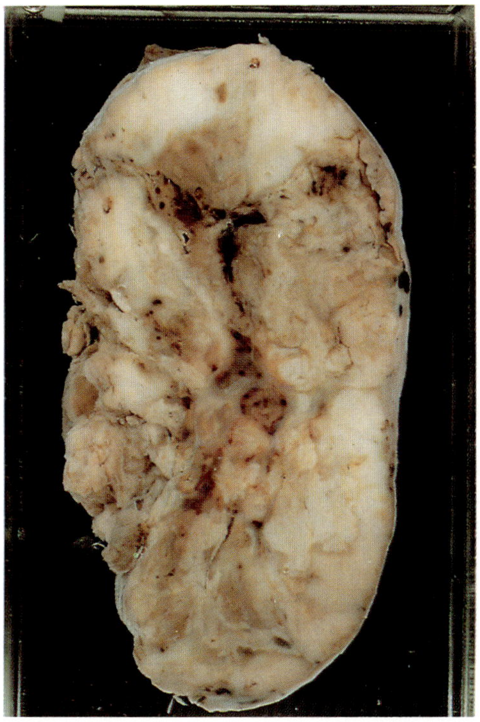

5.12 Ovary: Mesonephroid (Clear Cell) Adenocarcinoma

This specimen was excised from a 48-year-old woman who presented with weight loss and menorrhagia for 3 months. Examination revealed a mass in the right iliac fossa which was adherent to the uterus and pelvic wall.

This large ovarian tumour, measuring 12 x 6 x 6cm, has been bisected to show total replacement of the ovarian tissue by a pale neoplasm showing focal cystic change and widespread necrosis.

Mesonephroid adenocarcinoma accounts for only about 4 per cent of ovarian carcinomas. The term 'mesonephroid' reflects a mistaken historical belief that these tumours were derived from the mesonephric (Wolffian) duct and were similar in nature to a renal (clear cell) adenocarcinoma. It is now thought that these tumours arise from the ovarian surface epithelium and are undoubtedly of Müllerian origin; they appear to be related to, and can be considered a variant of, the endometrioid carcinoma of the ovary. The clinical features are much the same as for other ovarian adenocarcinomas (see Legends 5.7 and 5.11) and 5-year-survival is of the order of 25-35 per cent. Benign mesonephroid, or clear cell, tumours are rare, and usually take the form of an adenofibroma.

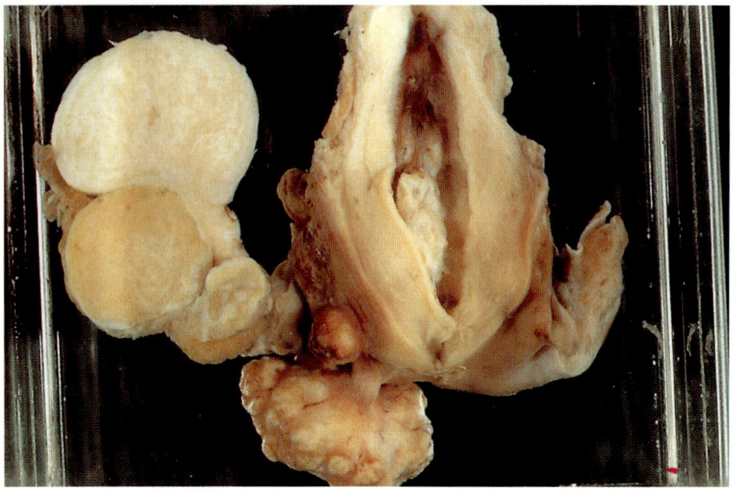

5.13 Ovary: Brenner Tumour

This specimen was excised from a 79-year-old woman who presented with a 3 month history of lower abdominal pain. On examination there was a palpable mass in the left iliac fossa and a laparotomy was performed.

The uterus, both fallopian tubes and the left ovary, are shown. The ovary is replaced by a bilobular, well circumscribed tumour, measuring 6cm in maximum dimension. The cut surface of the tumour is yellowish-white and the lower moiety has a whorled, fibrous appearance. The uterus shows several subserosal leiomyomata and there is a large endometrial polyp.

Brenner tumours are relatively uncommon neoplasms and are thought to arise from ovarian surface epithelium. They are formed of uroepithelium (transitional type epithelium) and thus represent a tumour showing Wolffian, rather than Müllerian, differentiation. The old belief that they arose from Walthard nests is no longer valid. Brenner tumours occur at any age and are usually small, often microscopic only, the example shown here being larger than average. They are occasionally bilateral and the majority are entirely benign. Malignant Brenner tumours are thought to be rare. Brenner tumours may also be found in association with mucinous cystadenomas or mature teratomas.

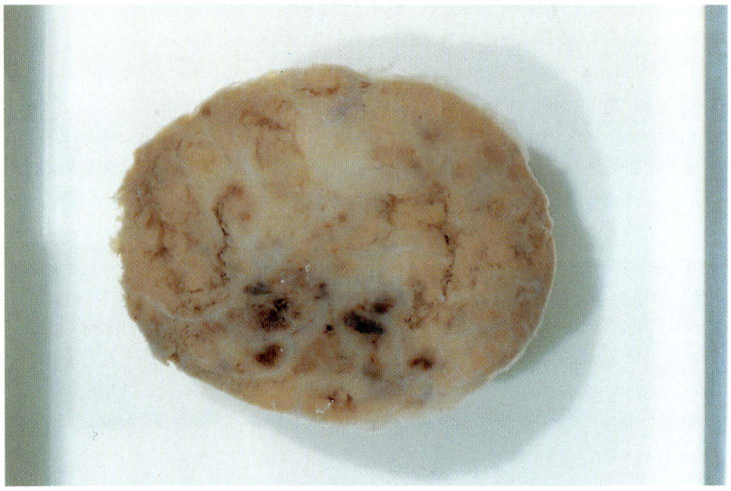

5.14 Ovary: Granulosa Cell Tumour

This specimen was excised from a 46-year-old woman. At the age of 36 she had undergone left salpingo-oöphorectomy after 4 years of amenorrhoea but details of the findings at that time are not available. For the following 5 years she had regular periods but then developed metrorrhagia and more recently suffered a further 18 months of amenorrhoea.

The tumour is well circumscribed, measuring 4cm in diameter, yellow in colour and largely solid. Small foci of ill-defined cystic change are also visible.

These are the typical appearances of a granulosa cell tumour, classified as a sex-cord stromal tumour, the latter group accounting for about 12 per cent of ovarian tumours. These lesions can occur at any age, including childhood, but present most commonly in the perimenopausal years; this is thought to be related to increased gonadotrophin production at this time. Granulosa cell tumours frequently secrete excessive amounts of oestrogen leading to menstrual irregularity or postmenopausal bleeding; a further consequence may be the development of endometrial hyperplasia or adenocarcinoma. All granulosa cell tumours should be regarded as malignant, despite the lack of well-defined histological criteria, but it should be stressed that the clinical course is often indolent.

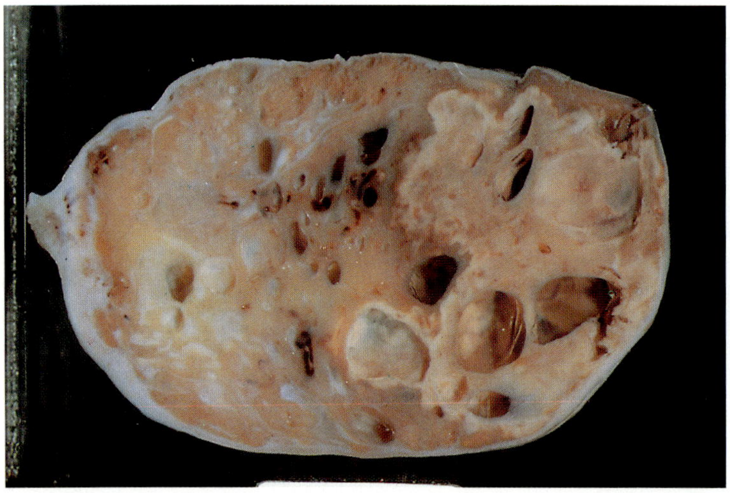

5.15 Ovary: Juvenile Granulosa Cell Tumour

This specimen was excised from a 3½-year-old girl who presented with a short history of abdominal pain. Examination revealed a large mass in the right iliac fossa, coarse pubic hair and well-developed external genitalia.

This ovarian tumour, which weighed 480g, has been bisected to show that it is pale and largely solid but with cystic areas, some of which show evidence of previous haemorrhage.

About 4 per cent of granulosa cell tumours occur in young girls, not uncommonly before the menarche. The term 'juvenile granulosa cell tumour' is a diagnosis based on a specific pattern of histological findings. About 90 per cent of granulosa cell tumours occurring in young girls are of the juvenile variety, but such neoplasms may occur at any age up to and including the 4th decade. Granulosa cell tumours, of whatever type, occurring in pre-menarchial girls usually cause precocious iso-sexual pseudopuberty. Most juvenile granulosa cell tumours are benign but about 5 per cent behave in a malignant fashion, and, unlike the adult form, pursue a rapidly malignant course, usually being fatal within 2 years.

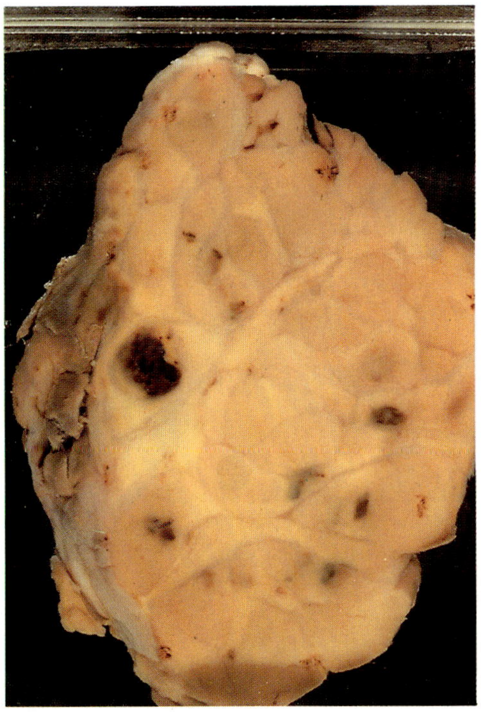

5.16 Ovary: Thecoma

This specimen was excised from a 44-year-old woman who presented with a 6 week history of an abdominal mass and dysuria.

The tumour measures 12 x 10 x 6cm and has been bisected to show that the cut surface is multinodular, greyish-yellow in colour and shows several small foci of haemorrhage.

Thecomas are also sex-cord stromal tumours and are more common than granulosa cell tumours. They can occur at any age but are most frequent, again, in the perimenopausal period. They commonly secrete excessive amounts of oestrogen and may be associated with endometrial adenocarcinoma. The vast majority are entirely benign.

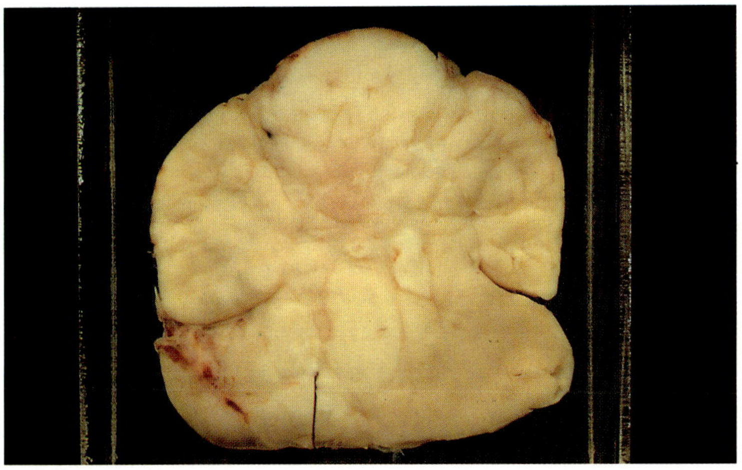

5.17 Ovary: Dysgerminoma

This specimen was excised from a 23-year-old woman who presented with an 8 month history of lower abdominal pain. On examination, there was a firm pelvic mass extending into the lower abdomen. At laparotomy the tumour was adherent to the sigmoid colon and had locally invaded the perimetrium.

This ovarian tumour has been bisected to show that it is solid, lobulated and has a uniform, pale cut surface, reminiscent of a potato. The capsular surface is smooth and there is a small area of haemorrhage in the lower left quadrant.

Dysgerminoma is a tumour of germ cell origin which shows no evidence of differentiation into either embryonic or extra-embryonic elements and it is therefore directly comparable to a seminoma of the male testis. It comprises about one per cent of ovarian tumours, may occasionally be bilateral and is commonest in the 2nd and 3rd decades. In very young patients, a dysgerminoma may occasionally give rise to precocious pseudopuberty. Typically, these tumours do not exceed 15-20cm in diameter and the uniform, potato-like cut surface is characteristic. All dysgerminomas should be regarded as malignant, since they show a clear tendency to local invasion and early lymphatic spread. They are, however, extremely radiosensitive and, in the absence of any identifiable spread, 5-year-survival approaches 90 per cent. (Courtesy of the Royal College of Obstetricians and Gynaecologists)

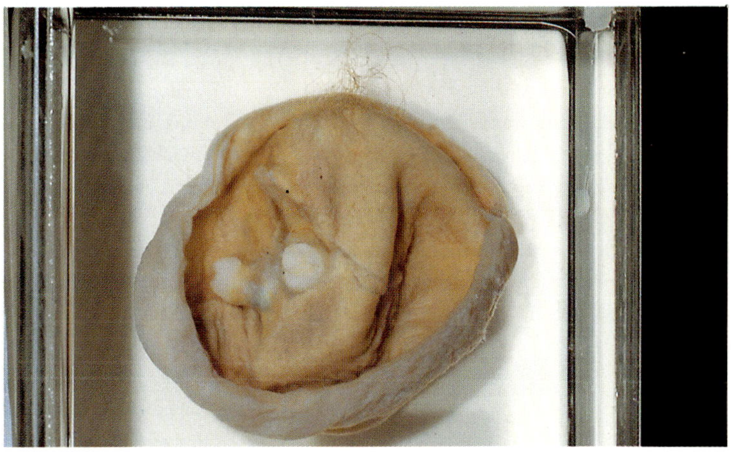

5.18 Ovary: Mature (Benign) Cystic Teratoma

This specimen was excised from a 32-year-old woman who presented with acute pain in the right iliac fossa. Plain abdominal X-ray revealed an ovarian cyst containing several teeth.

The lesion is a rounded cyst measuring 4cm in diameter, the lining of which is largely smooth but there is a central ridge from which project teeth and a tuft of hair.

Mature (benign) cystic teratomas, known by many as ovarian dermoids, constitute about 15 per cent of all ovarian tumours and are approximately 30 times more common than their malignant counterparts. Teratomas are germ cell tumours which show variable differentiation into each of the three germ layers. They occur most often in the 2nd to 4th decades and may be bilateral in up to 10 per cent of cases. Typically they are pedunculated, as a consequence of which these tumours frequently undergo torsion and present acutely as in the case here. The benign nature of the lesion is verified by the presence of mature or full differentiation in all the elements present.

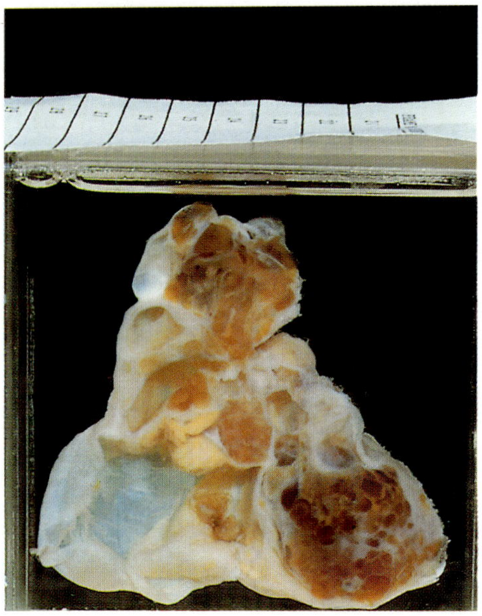

5.19 Ovary: Struma Ovarii

This specimen was excised from a 41-year-old woman who had noticed an enlarging abdominal mass for 3 months.

The tumour is partly solid and partly cystic but shows 2 well-defined nodules of apparently normal thyroid tissue with prominent colloid follicles. The cyst on the lower left shows protrusions, covered with hair, that are typical of benign teratomas.

Struma ovarii refers to a mature (benign) teratoma in which thyroid tissue is predominant. Such tumours are rare, most often unilateral and may be associated with ascites. The thyroid tissue is physiologically normal and, on occasion, may give rise to thyrotoxicosis or carcinoma.

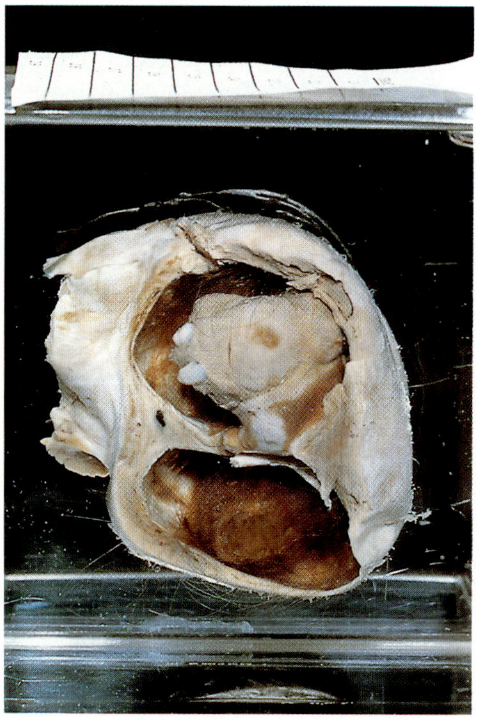

5.20 Ovary: Strangulated Cystic Teratoma

This specimen was excised from a 24-year-old woman who presented in the 7th month of pregnancy with a painful swelling in the right side of the abdomen. Plain abdominal X-ray revealed an intra-uterine anencephalic fetus and teeth in the region of the swelling, suggesting a teratoma. Labour was induced and post-partum the ovarian tumour became much more apparent but the pain subsided. At laparotomy, one month later, the tumour was found to have twisted 4 times on its pedicle.

This cystic teratoma has been sectioned to show a felted mass of hair (below) and a fleshy protuberance bearing 2 well-formed teeth. Features of acute infarction are no longer apparent but there is some organised fibrous thickening of the cyst wall.

Torsion of cystic teratomas is their commonest complication and may occur in up to 10 per cent of cases: the size or weight of the lesion is probably contributory. Infrequently, torted tumours may rupture, leading to a granulomatous peritonitis, or gangrene may supervene.

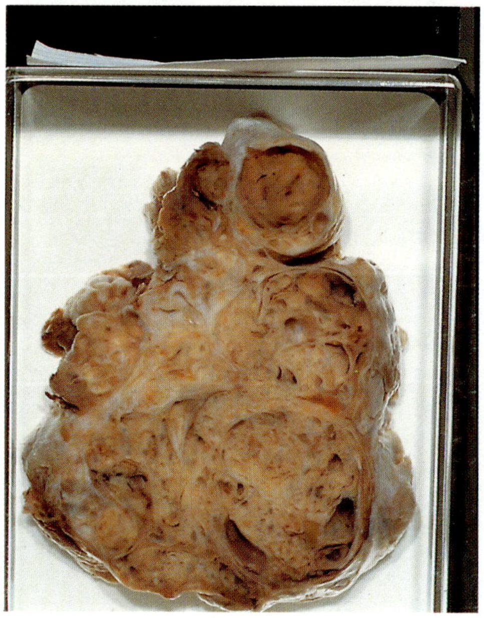

5.21 Ovary: Immature Solid Teratoma

This specimen was excised from a 24-year-old woman who was admitted for investigation of primary infertility, abdominal pain and an abdominal mass. At laparotomy both ovaries contained solid teratomas but no histologically immature areas were identified. However, 5 months later, a large pelvic recurrence and multiple peritoneal and omental metastases were found.

The ovary is greatly enlarged and is largely replaced by solid, pinkish tissue showing small foci of cystic degeneration.

Immature solid teratomas are rare malignant tumours which arise most often in the second decade. They are typically large and multinodular and histology reveals an admixture of mature and immature (embryonal) tissues. The prognosis is dependent upon the proportion of immature tissue present but modern multimodal therapy has led to a greatly improved survival rate in what was regarded to be a high grade tumour. The case here demonstrates well the importance of adequate tissue sampling for a pathological diagnosis: in a large tumour such as this it is easy to miss the immature elements.

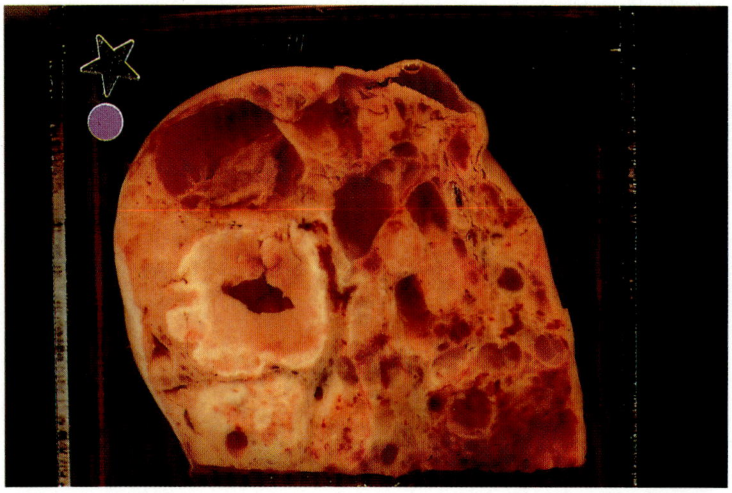

5.22 Ovary: Yolk Sac (Endodermal Sinus) Tumour

This specimen was excised from a 23-year-old woman who complained of gradual abdominal swelling for 3 months. The patient died with disseminated tumour 7 months post-operatively.

The tumour has been bisected to show the typical cut surface, which has a variegated appearance: there are solid yellowish and cystic areas associated with foci of haemorrhage and necrosis.

Yolk sac tumours are of germ cell origin but differentiate into extra-embryonic tissues which bear a close resemblance to the yolk sac in the rat. hence the original name. These tumours are uncommon but usually arise in the second decade. They are extremely malignant, being uniformly and rapidly fatal in the past, but recent chemotherapeutic advances have led to prolonged survival in a small number of cases. A useful tumour marker, alphafetoprotein, is typically produced by these tumours and serial serum estimations are useful in the follow-up of affected patients. (Courtesy of the Royal College of Obstetricians and Gynaecologists)

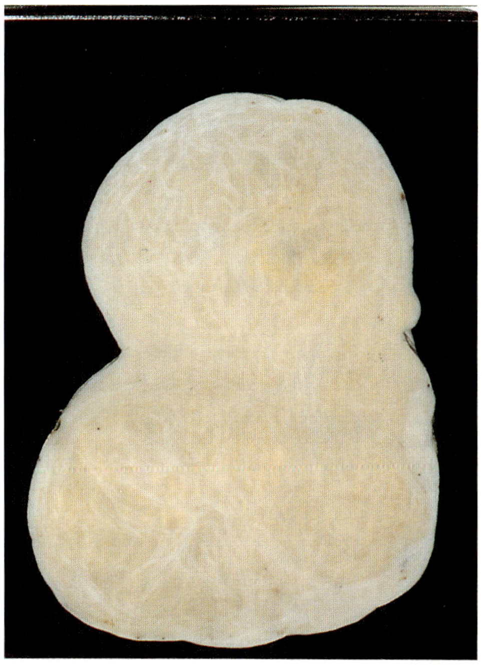

5.23 Ovary: Fibroma

This specimen was excised from a 65-year-old woman who had developed ascites associated with recurrent attacks of abdominal pain over the previous 6 months. Her recovery was uncomplicated and the ascites did not recur.

The tumour, measuring 12cm in maximum diameter, is firm, smooth and well circumscribed. It has a pale, whorled appearance typical of a fibroma. No recognisable ovarian tissue remains.

Fibromas constitute about 5 per cent of ovarian tumours and are derived from stromal mesenchyme. They arise most often in the 5th and 6th decades and larger tumours may be associated with the development of ascites and/or pleural effusions (Meigs's syndrome), the cause of which is unknown. Only extremely rarely do these lesions undergo malignant change.

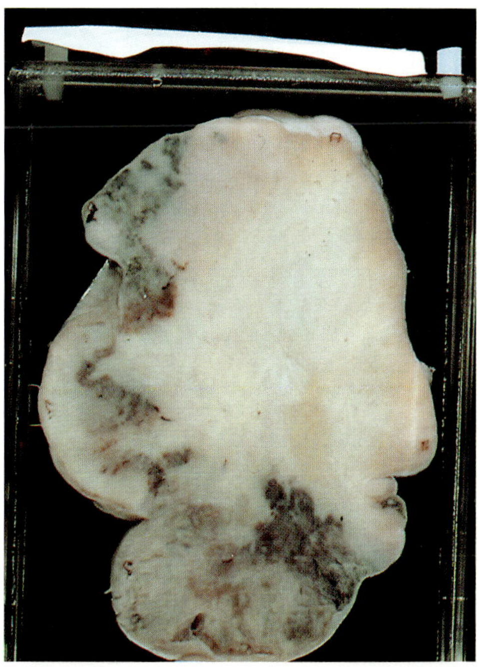

5.24 Ovary: Krukenberg Tumour

This specimen was found at post-mortem in an elderly woman who died of carcinomatosis from a primary adenocarcinoma of the stomach. Both ovaries were diffusely infiltrated by tumour, but only the right was enlarged.

The right ovary is enlarged by a coarsely nodular mass, measuring 12cm in maximum dimension. The cut surface shows almost complete replacement of the ovarian tissue by a pale neoplasm showing foci of necrosis and haemorrhage.

The term Krukenberg tumour is applied to metastatic adenocarcinoma in the ovary which has a specific histological pattern, characterised by the presence of signet ring mucus-containing cells and a pseudosarcomatous reaction of the stroma. The term should not be applied to metastatic adenocarcinomas not showing this specific histological picture. Most often these tumours are bilateral and occasionally may be misconstrued as primary ovarian adenocarcinomas in the absence of symptoms from elsewhere. The majority of Krukenberg tumours arise from primary neoplasms in the stomach, colon or breast.

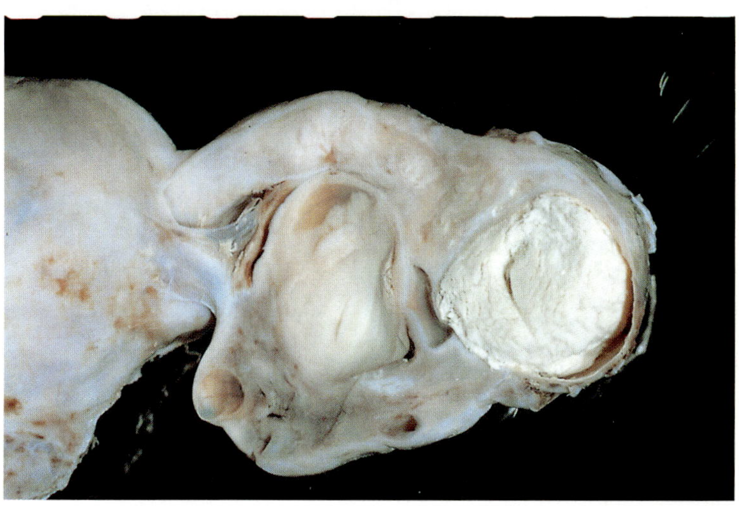

5.25 Fallopian Tube: Pyosalpinx

This specimen was excised from a 34-year-old woman who presented with infertility and dysmenorrhoea. A uterosalpingogram showed no filling of either tube. A bilateral salpingo-oöphorectomy and hysterectomy were performed. At operation both fallopian tubes were dilated and had thickened walls.

The right fallopian tube, attached to the uterus, and ovary are shown. There are dense adhesions, the wall of the fallopian tube is thickened and fibrotic, and there are a series of abscesses within the tube, the largest of which has been bisected (right). Histologically, there was no evidence of tuberculosis.

Pyosalpinx is usually bilateral and represents the result of prolonged or particularly severe bacterial salpingitis. By the time this chronic state is reached, it is uncommon to isolate the organism responsible but the most frequent bacteria giving rise to the primary infection are chlamydia, mycoplasma and anaerobic organisms; commonly the infection is polymicrobial and the gonococcus, previously thought to be an important cause, is now held only to be an initiating factor, incapable of giving rise to an established salpingitis. Predisposing factors include surgical instrumentation, abortion, parturition and the use of an intrauterine contraceptive device, but nevertheless, most cases are sexually transmitted.

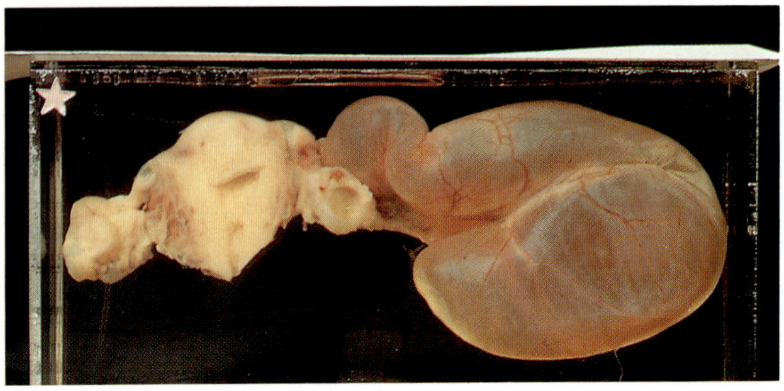

5.26 Fallopian Tube: Hydrosalpinx

This specimen was excised from a 47-year-old woman who presented with backache and a vaginal discharge, from which *Trichomonas vaginalis* was isolated.

A portion of the uterine corpus, with both fallopian tubes and ovaries, is shown. On the right, the fallopian tube is grossly dilated and filled with clear fluid. The wall of the fallopian tube is markedly attenuated.

A hydrosalpinx is thought to represent the end-stage of low-grade chronic tubal inflammation of whatever cause. It should be noted that, while the fimbrial end of the tube is typically occluded, the uterine opening is patent, suggesting that altered tubal motility, rather than obstruction, gives rise to the dilatation. The source and nature of the inflammation in most cases are probably similar to those in a pyosalpinx (see Legend 5.25) but some cases of hydrosalpinx occur in the presence of idiopathic pelvic inflammatory disease. (Courtesy of the Royal College of Obstetricians and Gynaecologists)

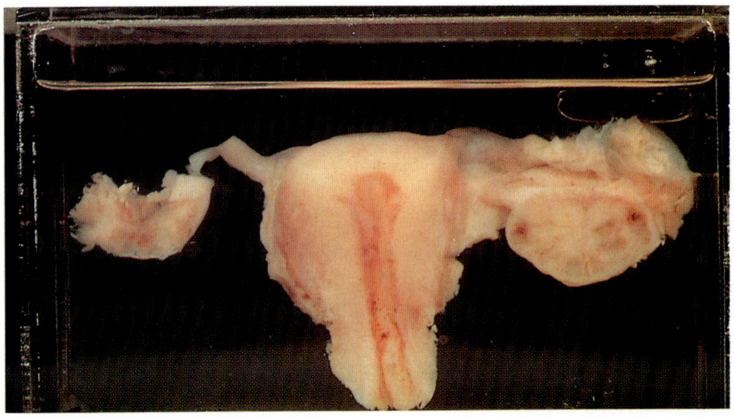

5.27 Fallopian Tube: Tuberculosis

This specimen was excised from a 30-year-old woman, with a long-standing history of infertility, who had recently complained of intermittent right iliac fossa pain and menorrhagia.

The uterus, with both fallopian tubes and the right ovary, is shown. The tube on the right is markedly dilated and there is obvious caseous material both in its wall and lumen. The ampullary portion of the tube on the left is also dilated and its serosal surface is covered in fibrinous adhesions.

Tuberculous salpingitis is now uncommon in Caucasians and is invariably associated with infection by *Mycobacterium tuberculosis* elsewhere in the body. Young women are predominantly affected and bilateral tubal involvement is usual. The associated inflammation and fibrosis, which is often prolonged prior to detection, almost invariably leads to tubal adhesions, occlusion and as here, infertility. Histologically, there is often very marked tubal epithelial hyperplasia in tuberculosis and it is very easy for the unwary to make a mistaken diagnosis of adenocarcinoma. (Courtesy of the Royal College of Obstetricians and Gynaecologists)

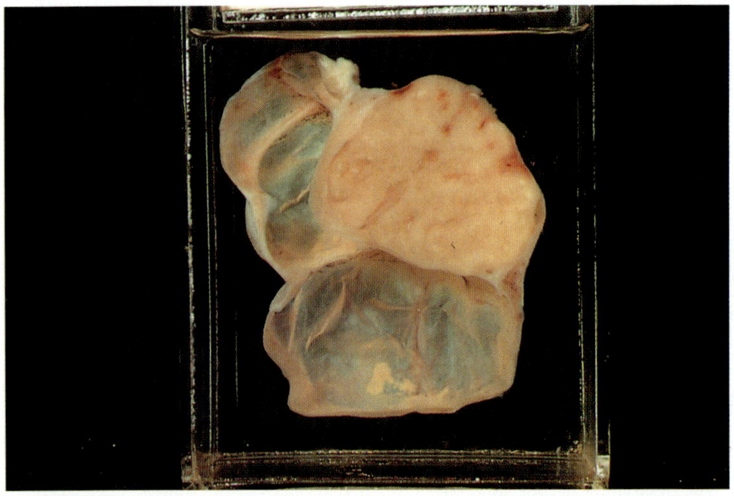

5.28 Fallopian Tube: Tuberculous Hydrosalpinx

This specimen was excised from a 42-year-old woman who presented with a 6 week history of dysuria and pyuria. She also had a 16 year history of infertility and menorrhagia. Cystoscopy revealed a fistulous orifice in the trigone and a tender mass was palpable to the left of the uterus. A left tubo-ovarian mass was excised.

A portion of the left fallopian tube, which is densely adherent to the ovary, is shown. The tube is grossly dilated and attenuated and there are small areas of calcification in the wall. The cut surface of the ovary shows multiple small foci of caseous necrosis.

Tuberculous salpingitis commonly leads to adhesions between the affected tube and other pelvic organs, and tissue necrosis often gives rise to fistula formation. Involvement of the ovary by adjacent tuberculous infection is uncommon but may occur in advanced cases, such as the one here: spread to the endometrium is, however, common. The development of a thin-walled hydrosalpinx is unusual since extensive fibrosis in the tubal wall is to be expected. (Courtesy of the Royal College of Obstetricians and Gynaecologists)

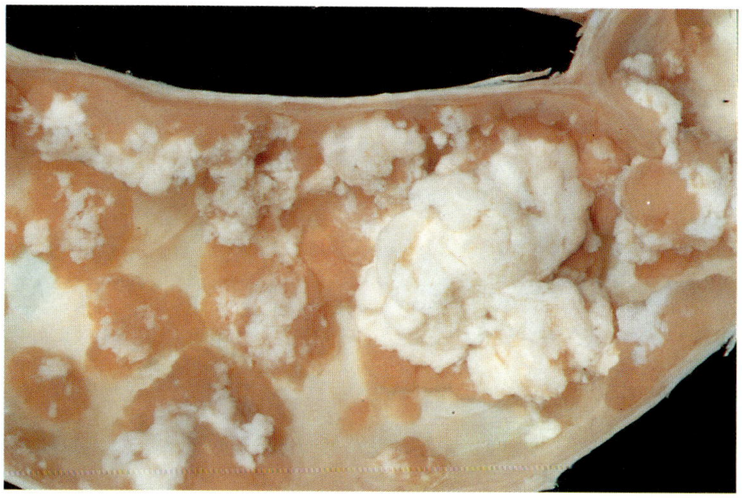

5.29 Fallopian Tube: Adenocarcinoma

This specimen was excised from a 44-year-old woman who complained of intermittent abdominal pain, dysmenorrhoea and menorrhagia.

The fallopian tube has been opened to show the epithelial surface studded with pale papillomatous tumour. Note also the marked luminal dilatation, the tube measuring up to 3cm in diameter.

Primary adenocarcinoma of the fallopian tube is extremely rare but may occasionally be associated with long-standing salpingitis. It is not uncommonly bilateral and spread to the serosal surface of the tube prior to presentation means that 5-year-survival is less than 50 per cent.

Uterus

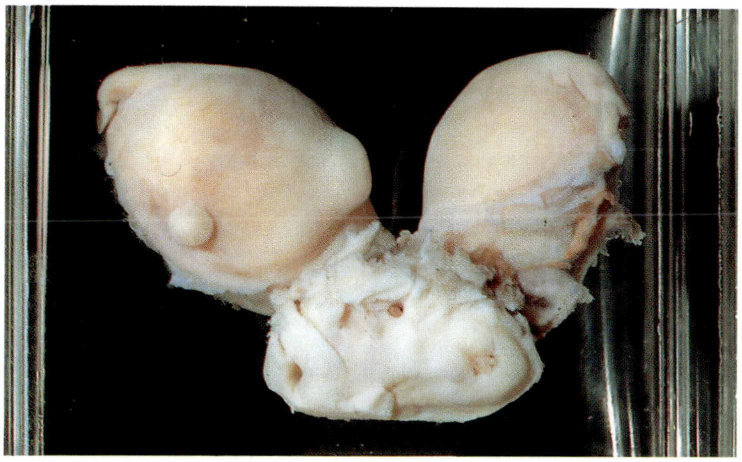

5.30 Uterus: Bicornis Bicollis

This specimen was excised from a 50-year-old woman who presented with premenstrual discomfort and menorrhagia.

Two uteri with 2 distinctly separate cervices are seen. The uterus on the left is distorted by fibroids.

This congenital malformation in which 2 uteri and cervices, but only one vagina, are present represents a partial failure of fusion of the 2 Müllerian ducts. The incidence of developmental anomalies of the female genital tract is about 1 in 500 women: the commonest presentations are menstrual irregularity, a poor obstetric history, infertility or dyspareunia.

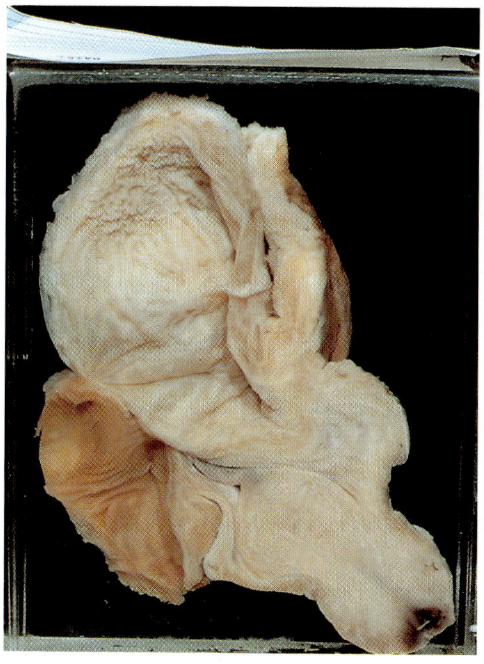

5.31 Uterus: Complete Prolapse

This was an incidental finding at post-mortem in a 62-year-old woman who died of coronary thrombosis. She was multiparous and the prolapse had been present for over 20 years.

This is a sagittal mid-line section through the bladder, rectum, uterus and vagina. There is complete prolapse of the uterus and vagina so that they project outwards from the vulva. The neck of the bladder has been drawn down behind the prolapsed mass.

Uterine prolapse is common and is usually associated with partial descent of the vagina. Prolapse is effectively a form of hernia and is classified by the degree of downward movement that has occurred. Aetiological factors include damage to the musculature of the pelvic floor during childbirth, raised intra-abdominal pressure or congenital weakness of the pelvic floor. The condition is most often seen in postmenopausal women in whom it is assumed that general atrophy of genital tissues plays a contributory role. Allied lesions, without actual uterine prolapse include cystocele and rectocele. Complete prolapse (synonym: procidentia) may be complicated by ulceration or irreducibility.

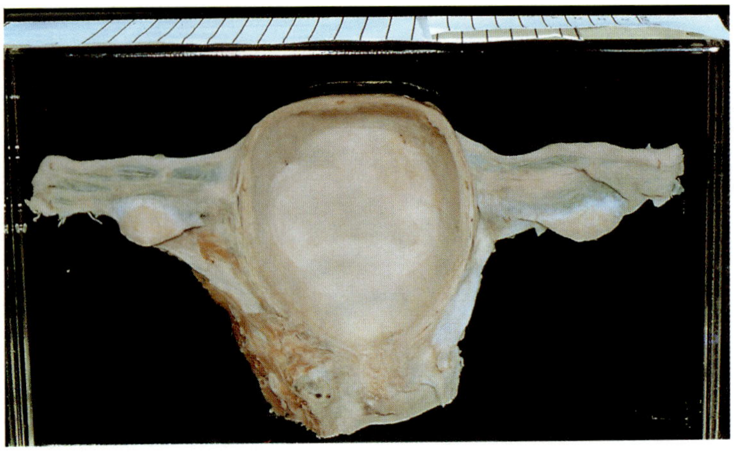

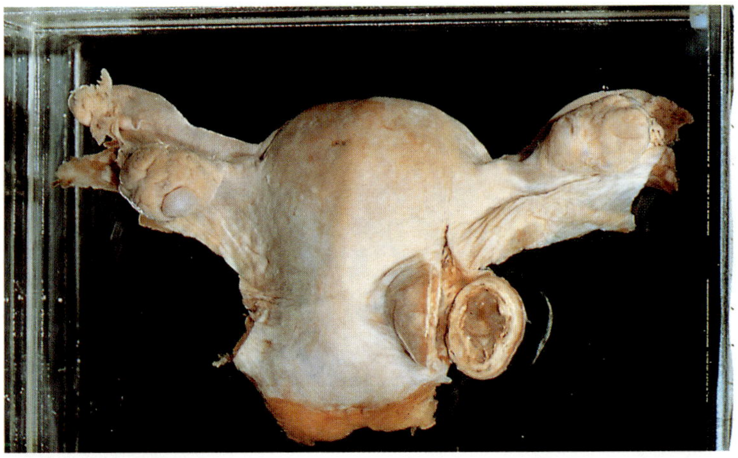

5.32 Uterus: Chronic Pyometria

This was an incidental finding at post-mortem in an 85-year-old woman who died of myocardial failure. She had no past history of ill-health.

The uterus has been bisected in the coronal plane. It is enlarged and globular and the endometrial cavity is distended, measuring up to 7cm in diameter. A quantity of pus has been removed to show the smooth, flattened endometrial lining.

A chronic pyometria is most often seen in postmenopausal women. It results from stenosis of the cervical canal which, in conjunction with atrophy of the uterine muscle, prevents expulsion of inflammatory exudate from the uterine cavity. Most often no organism can be isolated. The condition is sometimes associated with a squamous cell carcinoma of the endometrium.

5.33 Uterus: Hydatid Cyst

This was an incidental finding at post-mortem in a 47-year-old Australian woman who died of unrelated causes. Cysts were also found in the omentum and liver.

The uterus with the tubes and ovaries are shown: there is an ovoid cyst, measuring 2cm in maximum diameter, projecting from the postero-lateral aspect of the uterus at the level of the internal os. The cyst has been bisected to show the compressed hydatid membrane encased in a fibrotic, partly calcified capsule.

Hydatid disease is due to infestation by the tapeworm *Echinococcus granulosus*, and is most often seen in sheep-farming communities. The cysts are typically multilocular, containing numerous daughter cysts within which the brood capsules are formed. The diagnosis may be made by demonstration of cutaneous hypersensitivity to hydatid antigen, the Casoni test. Involvement of the uterus is extremely rare and the cyst shown here appears to a large extent to be 'burnt out', there being little evidence of disease activity.

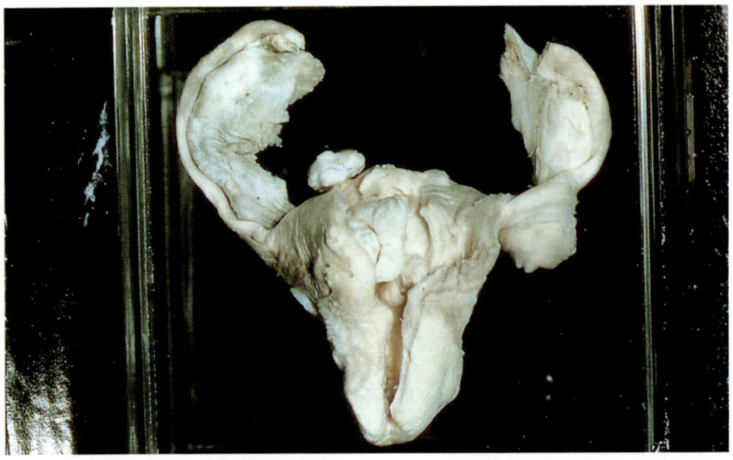

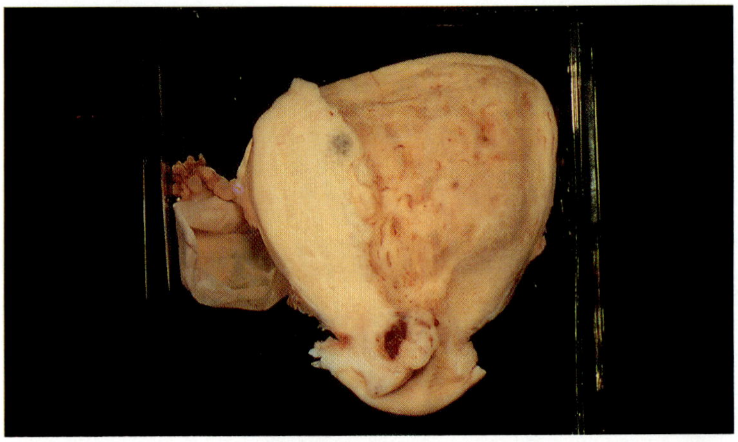

5.34 Uterus: Endometrial Polyps

These were an incidental finding at post-mortem in a 72-year-old woman who died of ischaemic heart disease.

This atrophic postmenopausal uterus has been opened from the front to show a number of large endometrial polyps projecting into the cavity of the fundus. Note also a small, pedunculated, subserosal leiomyoma at the top left.

Endometrial polyps are common and arise most often in the perimenopausal years, usually presenting with menorrhagia. Their exact nature is unclear: they may represent the effect of a localised increased sensitivity to oestrogens or they may be true benign neoplasms. Multiplicity is common and a small percentage are associated with adjacent endometrial adenocarcinoma: malignant change within a polyp is, however, extremely rare.

5.35 Uterus: Adenomyosis

This specimen was excised from a 34-year-old woman who presented with a 2 year history of dysmenorrhoea and menorrhagia. The uterus was found to be uniformly enlarged.

The uterus and cervix have been sectioned in the sagittal plane and the right ovary, containing a follicular cyst, is visible posteriorly. The uterine wall is diffusely hypertrophied and the endometrial cavity has a trabeculated appearance. In the posterior wall, irregular portions of endometrial tissue can be seen penetrating up to 1cm into the muscle coat. The depressed areas in the endometrial cavity correspond to similar foci of adenomyosis, viewed *en face*. Note also a more clearly defined, haemorrhagic focus of the same process just above the internal cervical os.

Adenomyosis is defined as the presence of endometrial tissue deep in the myometrium. Adenomyosis is a common condition which occurs predominantly in women who have borne children, but are now approaching the menopause. It represents downward extension of the basal endometrium into the myometrium and may be diffuse, as in the case here, or localised (see Figure 5.36). It is unusual for adenomyotic tissue to undergo cyclical menstrual changes, probably because of the unresponsive basal nature of the endometrial tissue. The aetiology is unclear but excessive oestrogenic stimulation is the most widely held hypothesis. (Courtesy of the Royal College of Obstetricians and Gynaecologists)

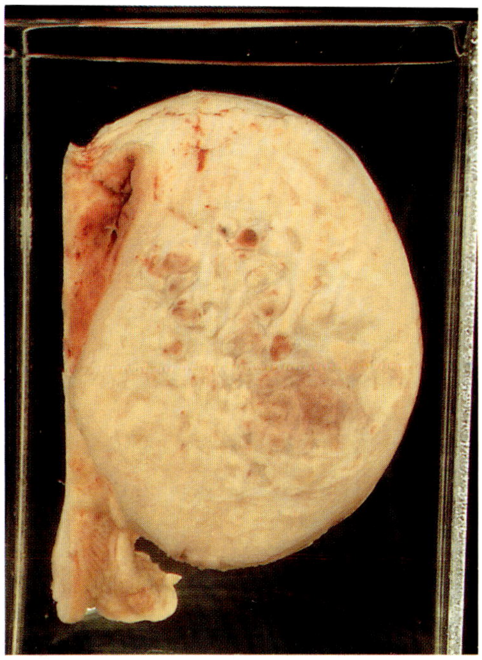

5.36 Uterus: Localised Adenomyosis (Adenomyoma)

This specimen was excised from a 23-year-old woman who complained of menorrhagia.

A sagittal section through the uterus shows a relatively well-circumscribed mass in the anterior wall. The mass has a whorled appearance and shows irregular yellowish and haemorrhagic foci.

This is an example of localised, tumour-like adenomyosis, also known as an adenomyoma. It is again typified by deep nodules of endometrium associated with myometrial hypertrophy and is not pre-malignant. The patient in the case here was unusually young to develop adenomyosis. (Courtesy of the Royal College of Obstetricians and Gynaecologists)

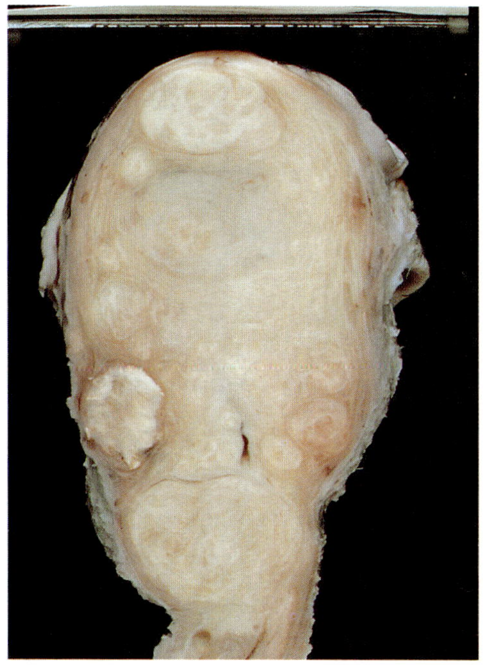

5.37 Uterus: Leiomyoma

This specimen was excised from a 47-year-old woman who presented with a 3 year history of dysmenorrhoea and metrorrhagia. Most recently she had noticed an abdominal mass and she developed intermittent constipation and urinary frequency.

This grossly enlarged and distorted uterus has been sectioned to show multiple, well-circumscribed intramural and submucosal tumours which have displaced and compressed the uterine cavity. The lesions all have a typical whorled appearance except one on the left which has undergone degeneration and dystrophic calcification.

Leiomyomas, known by many as 'fibroids', are very common benign neoplasms of uterine smooth muscle which arise only during the reproductive years. They are most often multiple and are thought to result from oestrogenic stimulation: enlargement is common during pregnancy or with the use of oral contraceptives and they tend to atrophy after the menopause. Various forms of degenerative change are common and are thought to occur when the tumour outgrows its blood supply: calcified lesions, as seen here, are often referred to as womb stones. Malignant change in a leiomyoma is very rare.

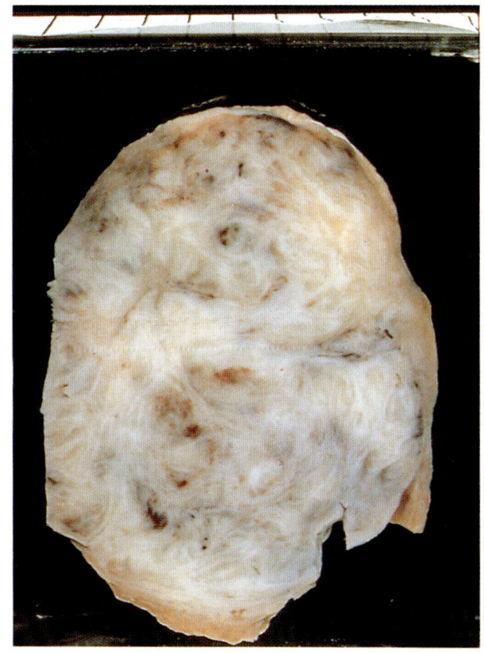

5.38 Uterine Leiomyoma: Red Degeneration

This specimen was removed from the wall of a pregnant uterus.

The tumour, measuring 5cm in maximum diameter, has been sectioned to show irregular foci of haemorrhagic degeneration.

Red degeneration in a leiomyoma occurs most often during pregnancy or in the puerperium and results from haemorrhagic infarction and necrosis, usually within a particularly hyalinised lesion. Ischaemia is the most probable cause and this occurrence may give rise to pain or a fever.

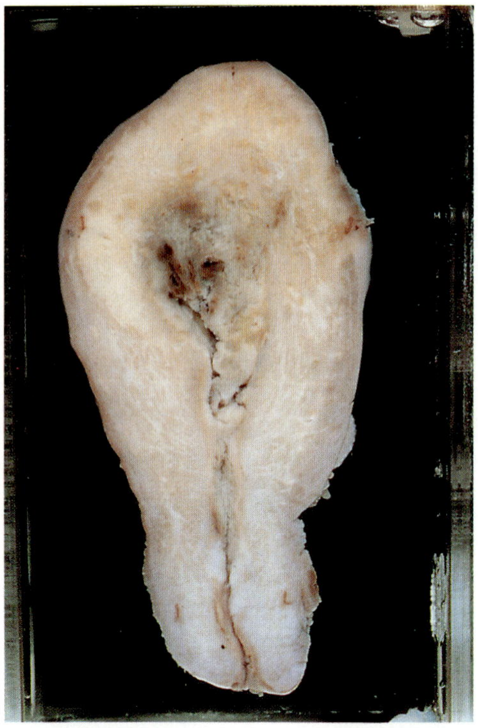

5.39 Uterus: Endometrial Adenocarcinoma

This specimen was excised from a nulliparous 58-year-old woman in whom the menopause had occurred 9 years previously and who presented with postmenopausal bleeding. Pre-operatively she was treated with intra-uterine radium.

The uterus has been sectioned in the sagittal plane to show a pale neoplasm arising in the fundus and projecting into the uterine cavity, widely infiltrating the muscle coat. The uninvolved endometrium also appears necrotic and this is probably a consequence of the irradiation.

Endometrial carcinoma accounts for about 10 per cent of malignant disease in women. The majority of cases arise postmenopausally and known associations include infertility, nulliparity, obesity and possibly hypertension and diabetes mellitus. The underlying pathogenetic origin appears to be prolonged unopposed oestrogenic stimulation of the endometrium. Prognosis is dependent upon tumour grade, depth of myometrial invasion and clinical stage, but the overall 5-year-survival is of the order of 70 per cent. The less common adenosquamous, clear cell and papillary serous variants carry a significantly worse outlook.

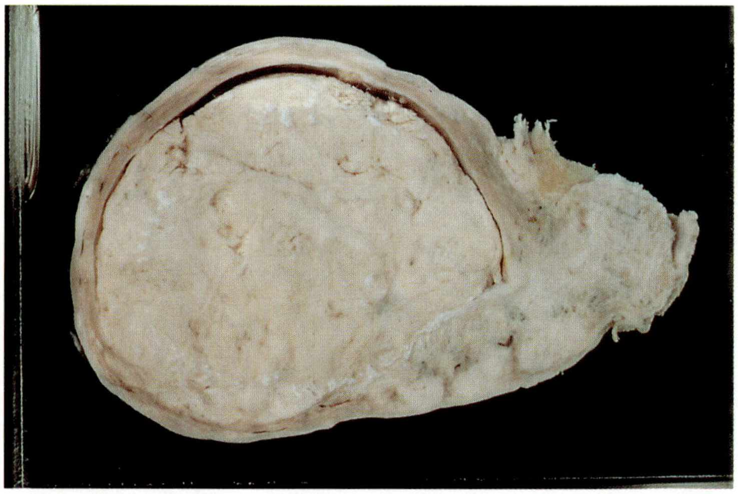

5.40 Uterus: Anaplastic (Grade III) Endometrial Carcinoma

This was an unexpected post-mortem finding in a 72-year-old woman who died following a hip fracture. In addition there were widespread metastases in the liver, omentum and mesentery.

A sagittal section through the uterus shows a large polypoid mass of pale tumour which has distended the endometrial cavity and is infiltrating the lower part of the uterine wall.

Anaplastic (Grade III) carcinomas of the endometrium are rare and carry a poor prognosis; these tumours tend to invade the myometrium deeply and show early spread to lymph nodes.

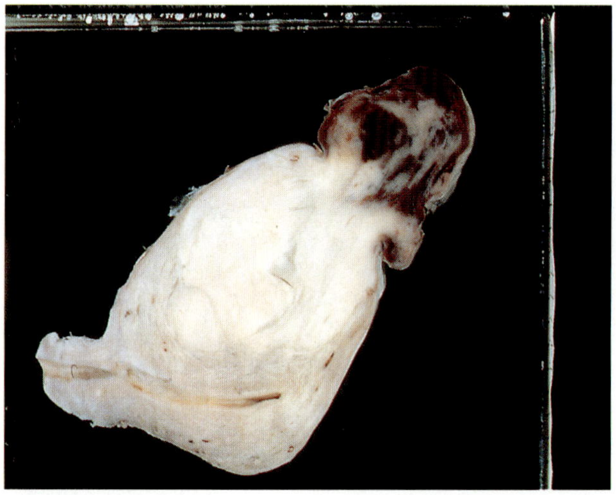

5.41 Uterus: Leiomyosarcoma

This specimen was excised from a 34-year-old woman who had noticed a painless abdominal swelling for the past 2 months. She had undergone simple myomectomy 5 years previously. On examination and at operation there was no evidence of metastases.

A sagittal section through the uterus shows a large, rounded tumour, measuring 7cm in diameter, in the anterior wall. The tumour is not well circumscribed and there is no clear whorling (cf. benign leiomyoma). A portion of the tumour, projecting subserosally, appears to have undergone haemorrhagic infarction.

Uterine leiomyosarcoma is rare and most often presents between the ages of 40 and 60 years. Not infrequently there is a history of nulliparity. Macroscopically, the malignant nature of the lesion may not be apparent since some cases closely mimic a benign leiomyoma. The histological diagnosis of malignancy rests upon the number of mitotic figures seen which, unfortunately, has led to the recognition of a borderline group of lesions. In truly malignant neoplasms, spread is blood-borne and 5-year-survival is only of the order of 30 per cent. It should be noted that the vast majority of leiomyosarcomas appear to arise *de novo* and not from pre-existing leiomyomas.

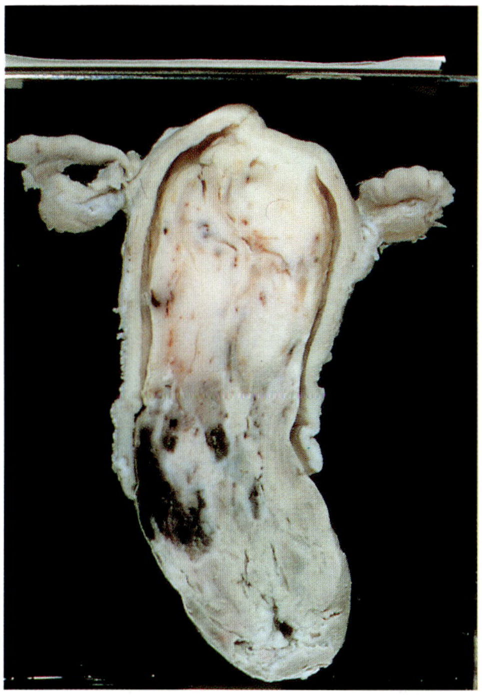

5.42 Uterus: Mixed Müllerian Tumour of High Grade Malignancy

This specimen was excised from a 69-year-old woman who presented after 2 episodes of recent vaginal bleeding. Examination revealed an enlarged uterus with a necrotic tumour protruding through the cervical canal.

A caudal section through the uterus shows a soft, polypoid tumour, measuring 13cm in length, arising from the fundus by a narrow pedicle. The lower 5cm of the tumour projects through the markedly dilated cervix and shows extensive haemorrhage and necrosis.

Mixed Müllerian tumours are derived from undifferentiated mesenchyme of the Müllerian duct and therefore contain both epithelial and connective tissue elements to a varying degree. In some tumours, both components are benign (Müllerian adenofibroma), in others only one component is malignant. In malignant mixed tumours, both derivatives are histologically malignant. This latter group arises most often in elderly women, the clinical features in the case here being typical. These tumours behave in an aggressive fashion with rapid lymphatic and blood-borne spread and survival for any length of time is very uncommon.

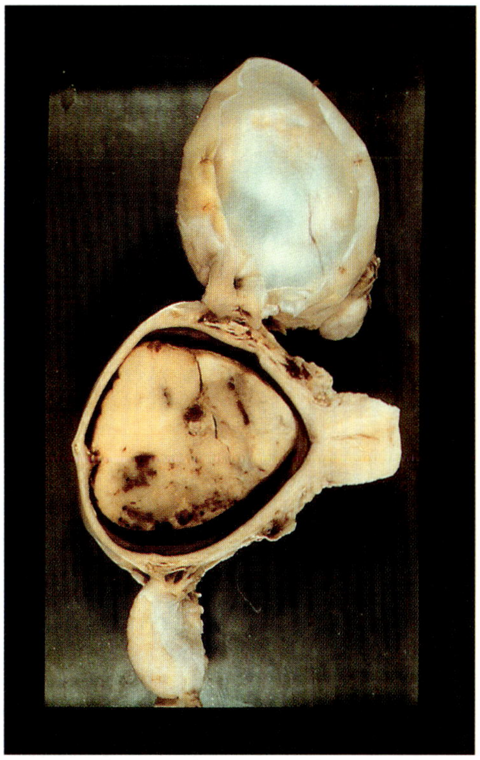

5.43 Uterus: Müllerian Adenosarcoma

This specimen was excised from a 63-year-old woman who presented with postmenopausal bleeding and a blood-stained vaginal discharge. Post-operatively she remained well for 3 years, before developing ascites and disseminated metastases.

The uterus, with the fallopian tubes and ovaries, is shown. Arising in the fundus of the uterus is a large, rounded polypoid tumour, measuring 5cm in diameter. The tumour shows foci of haemorrhage and necrosis and has markedly distended the uterine cavity. The endometrium is smooth and atrophic. In the left ovary is a large follicular cyst, measuring 6cm in diameter.

This is the variant of mixed Müllerian tumour in which the epithelial component is benign and the stromal element is malignant. The clinical features are much the same as those of the malignant mixed Müllerian tumours (see Figure 5.42), although more cases are identified in younger women. The example here is unusual in showing haemorrhage and necrosis; Müllerian adenosarcoma is commonly more papillary and cystic. Adenosarcomas are of low grade malignancy but about 50 per cent of cases show long-term local recurrence; metastasis, as has occurred in this case, is unusual. When the tumour does recur it tends to do so in a rather indolent manner.

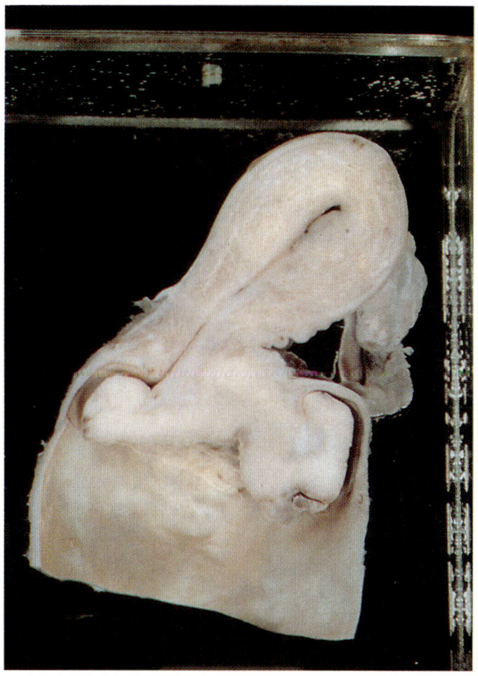

5.44 Uterus: Squamous Carcinoma of Cervix

This specimen was excised from a 49-year-old multiparous woman who had noticed irregular vaginal bleeding for the last 3 months. At operation there was no apparent involvement of either the parametrium or adjacent lymph nodes.

A sagittal section through the uterus and upper vagina shows a bulky, polypoid tumour arising from the external cervical os and extending into the vaginal vault. The surface of the tumour is extensively ulcerated.

Carcinoma of the cervix is common and despite screening procedures, the incidence seems to be increasing, particularly in younger women. It occurs most often in the 5th and 6th decades and the majority are squamous in type, largely arising in pre-existing areas of intra-epithelial neoplasia which may have been present for 10-20 years. The single most important risk factor is early age at first coitus, of which promiscuity, early marriage or pregnancy, multiparity and lower social class are co-variables. It is thought that the carcinogenic agent responsible is transmitted sexually when the cervix is undergoing squamous metaplasia in adolescence. The two most likely culprits appear to be *Herpes simplex* virus Type II and human papillomavirus. The prognosis is largely dependent upon staging: 5-year-survival for tumours confined to the cervix is about 85 per cent while, for pelvic involvement, the figure falls to 50 per cent. Death is commonly due to uraemia caused by local invasion obstructing the ureters.

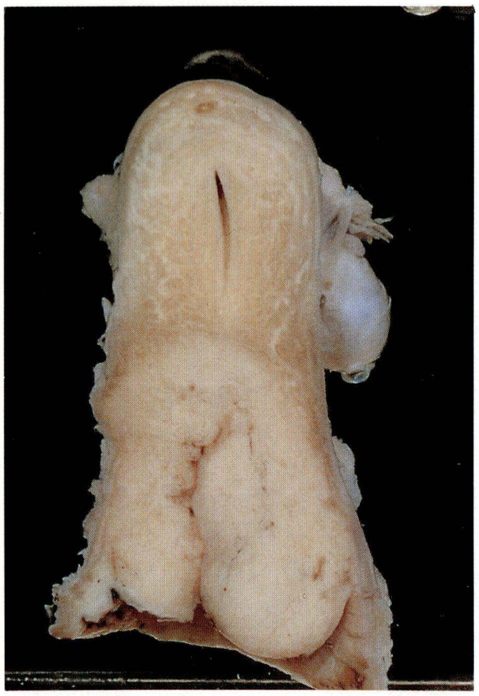

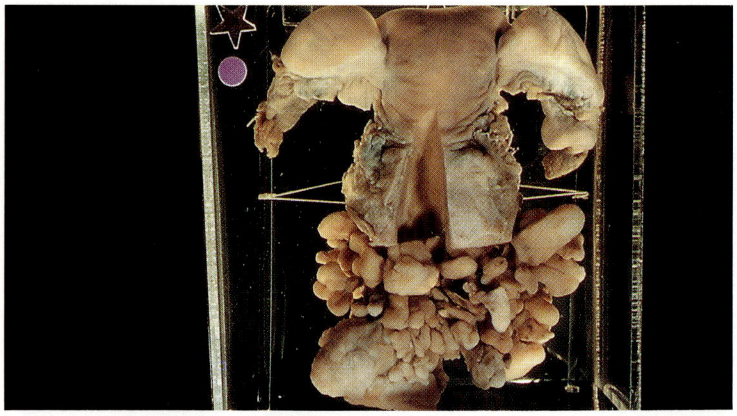

5.45 Uterus: Squamous Carcinoma of Cervix

No clinical details are available.

A sagittal section through the uterus and upper vagina reveals a fungating carcinoma of the cervix which has infiltrated the full thickness of the cervix and invaded the body of the uterus.

This is a more advanced example than Legend 5.44 and would be regarded as Stage II.

5.46 Uterus: Embryonal Rhabdomyosarcoma of the Cervix

This specimen was excised from a 20-year-old woman who presented with a polypoid vaginal mass, protruding from the vaginal orifice. She was treated with radiotherapy prior to a Wertheim's hysterectomy. Fourteen months later she developed a large vaginal recurrence.

The uterus with both fallopian tubes and ovaries, is shown. Arising from the ectocervix is a large mass composed of multiple, rather oedematous polyps which bear a resemblance to a bunch of grapes.

Embryonal rhabdomyosarcoma of the female genital tract is rare but most often arises in the vagina. Primary involvement of the cervix is even more uncommon. Irrespective of site, these tumours typically arise in female infants less than 5 years of age and probably develop from primitive skeletal muscle in the Müllerian tubercle. The grape-like masses occur as a consequence of sub-epithelial proliferation of tumour and it is this feature which has led to the use of the purely descriptive term, sarcoma botryoides. Extensive local invasion is common and involvement of other pelvic structures may be fatal before there is extensive blood-borne spread. While, in the past, these tumours were uniformly fatal, improved survival is being reported in a minority of cases using modern multimodal therapy. Note that the patient here is very unusual by virtue of her age. (Courtesy of the Royal College of Obstetricians and Gynaecologists)

Vagina and Vulva

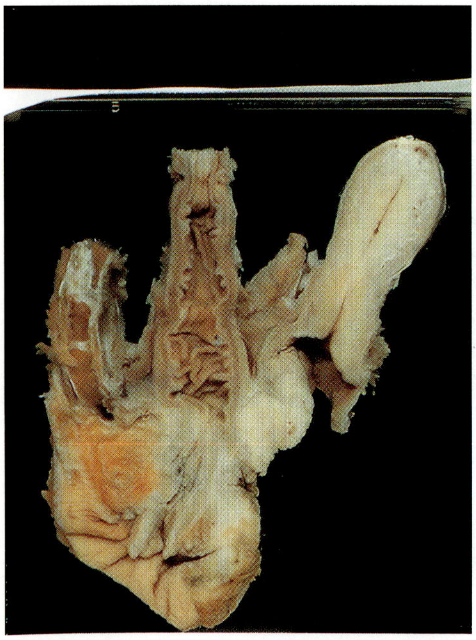

5.47 Vagina: Squamous Carcinoma

No clinical details are available.

The uterus, posterior vaginal wall, rectum, anus and lower coccyx have been sagittally sectioned to show a large, pale fungating neoplasm arising from the upper end of the posterior vaginal wall. The tumour shows extensive local invasion and has infiltrated the rectal wall to produce an annular stricture, approximately 2cm in length, within which the hypertrophied rectal muscle is prominent.

Primary malignant tumours of the vagina are rare, most cases representing spread from either the vulva or the cervix. However, squamous carcinoma is the most common and usually presents in the 6th or 7th decades. It is suggested that similar aetiological agents to carcinoma of the cervix (see Legend 5.44) are important but this is unproven. Prognosis is largely dependent upon clinical stage; tumours confined to the vaginal wall having a 90 per cent 5-year-survival. In the case here, which would be classified as Stage III, survival would be reduced to about 30 per cent.

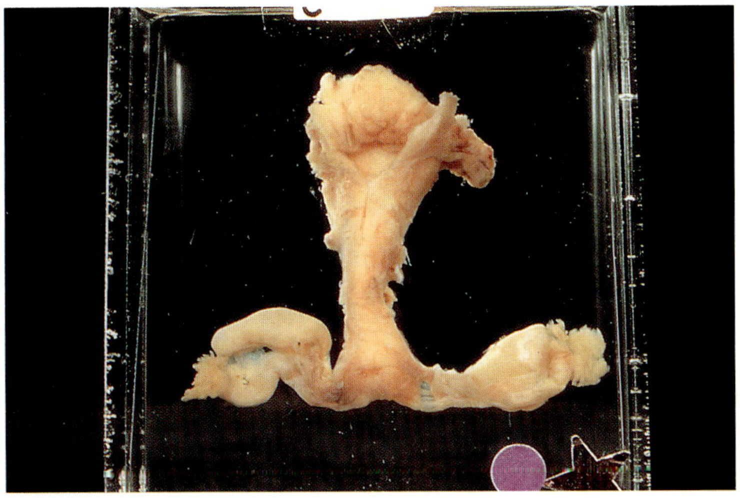

5.48 Vagina: Adenocarcinoma

This specimen was excised from an 18-month-old female infant who was noted to have vaginal bleeding for the preceding 3 weeks.

Both ovaries, fallopian tubes, the uterus and vagina are shown. Arising in the posterior wall of the vagina is a rounded, rather polypoid tumour.

Vaginal adenocarcinoma is very uncommon but has shown a recent increase in incidence. This has been explained by the fact that most females who develop this tumour have been exposed to diethylstilboestrol, a synthetic oestrogen, *in utero*, usually prior to 18 weeks gestation. Approximately 1 in 1000 females whose mothers were treated with this drug develop vaginal adenocarcinoma, most often during the 2nd decade of life. It is probable that this neoplastic change occurs in foci of vaginal adenosis which represents sequestration of Müllerian remnants in the vaginal epithelium, an event caused by the same drug. The prognosis is closely related to tumour staging but the survival rate is up to 80 per cent in localised cases. (Courtesy of the Royal College of Obstetricians and Gynaecologists)

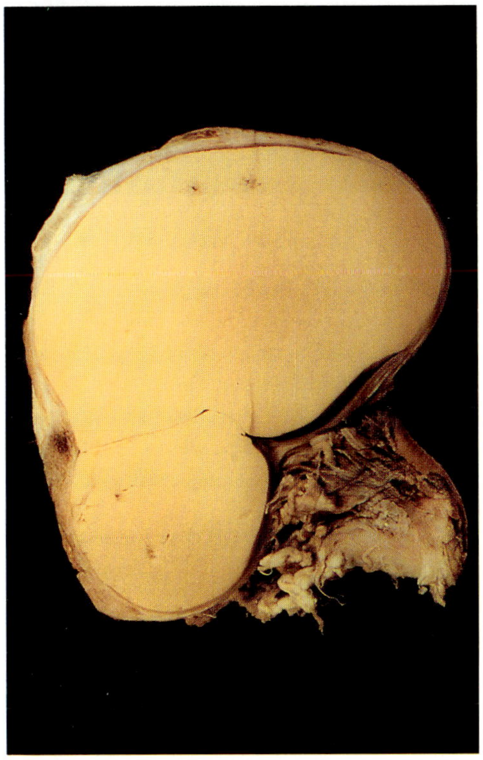

5.49 Vulva: Bartholin's Cyst

This specimen was excised from a 52-year-old woman who had noticed a swelling on the left side of her vulva for the previous 27 years. This had slowly increased in size but was not painful. Arising beneath the attenuated skin of the labium majus is a very large bilocular cystic lesion, containing inspissated yellow material. In the fresh state, the cyst measured 15cm in maximum diameter. A Bartholin's cyst simply represents the end-stage of low-grade chronic inflammation or an abscess in Bartholin's glands. Acute inflammation in Bartholin's glands is common and is most often due to *Staphylococcus aureus* or faecal contaminants. Other causative organisms include the gonococcus, *Mycoplasma hominis* and, very occasionally, *Mycobacterium tuberculosis*. (Courtesy of the Royal College of Obstetricians and Gynaecologists)

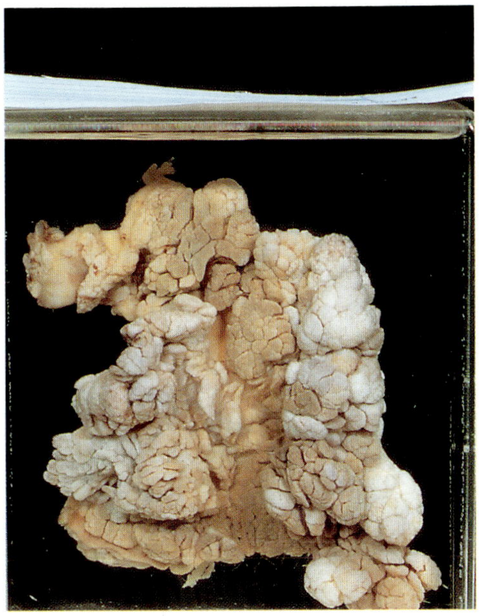

5.50 Vulva: Condylomata Acuminata

This specimen was excised from a 63-year-old woman who complained of 'warty' lesions of the vulva which had been present for 34 years. She had undergone local excisions in the past.

The anatomical features of this partial vulvectomy specimen have been obscured by multiple pale, sessile papillomatous lesions.

Condylomata acuminata are sexually-transmitted genital warts caused by human papillomavirus infection. They are usually multiple, focally confluent and arise most frequently on the labia minora. Malignant change is extremely rare and it is thought that the verrucous variant of squamous carcinoma, which is similar in appearance to a large wart, probably arises *de novo* and goes unrecognised as a condyloma, leading to the mistaken belief that a benign viral lesion has become malignant.

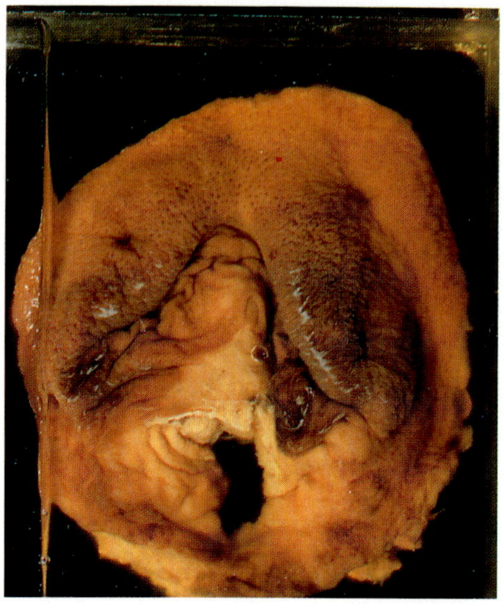

5.51 Vulva: Intra-epithelial Carcinoma

This specimen was excised from a 56-year-old woman who presented with vulval soreness for 2 years. A small reddish area was excised but a few months later a separate scaly plaque appeared elsewhere on the vulva. A simple vulvectomy was performed.

This vulvectomy specimen shows several raised, reddish areas around the introitus. In places the affected skin is white and rather scaly.

Intra-epithelial carcinoma (synonym: carcinoma-*in situ*, Bowen's disease, erythroplasia of Queyrat) represents the presence of atypical ('dysplastic') cells occupying the full thickness of the vulval epithelium and as such is the most severe form of intra-epithelial neoplasia. This change is not uncommon and, although the incidence increases with age, it is being seen with increasing frequency in young women below the age of 30. It may be associated with similar changes in the cervix and the current most likely hypothesis regarding aetiology is that of viral infection, perhaps affecting much of the lower genital tract as a 'field-change' effect. *Herpes simplex* Type II or human papillomavirus are the most likely culprits. It is probable that progression to invasive squamous carcinoma is very uncommon, but this tends to occur particularly in elderly women or those who are immunosuppressed. (Courtesy of the Royal College of Obstetricians and Gynaecologists)

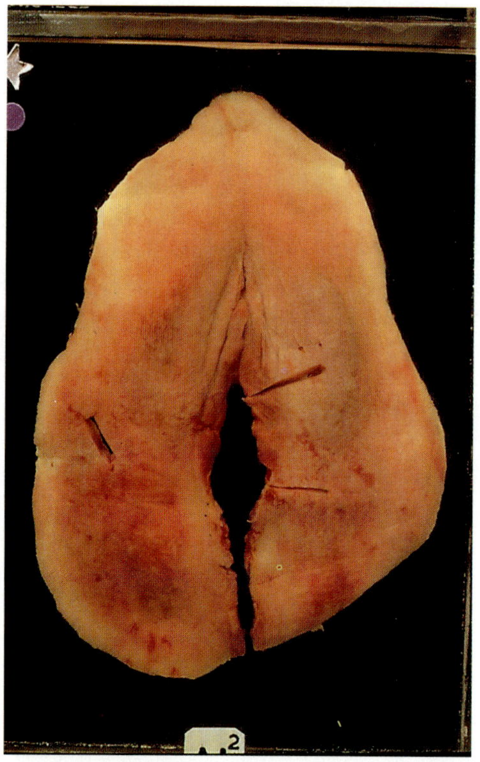

5.52 Vulva: Paget's Disease

This specimen was excised from a 60-year-old woman who presented with a 10 month history of unrelieved pruritis vulvae.

This is a simple vulvectomy specimen and shows that much of the skin is raised, reddish and focally excoriated. On the right, one area has assumed a whitish appearance.

Paget's disease of the vulva is uncommon and affects predominantly post-menopausal women. It is typically a multifocal and ill-demarcated lesion. The pathogenesis of extra-mammary Paget's disease is varied: at least 50 per cent of cases represent epidermal spread of an underlying adnexal tumour; others may indicate similar spread of a subcutaneous metastatic adenocarcinoma and occasional cases arise by epidermotropic spread of a distant adenocarcinoma, particularly cervical, endometrial or colonic. While some examples are genuinely idiopathic, all patients with extra-mammary Paget's disease should be thoroughly examined for a primary tumour. The principle that Paget's disease of the nipple is *always* associated with an underlying breast carcinoma does not hold true in the vulva. Clearly the prognosis in vulval disease is dependent upon any associated pathology. (Courtesy of the Royal College of Obstetricians and Gynaecologists)

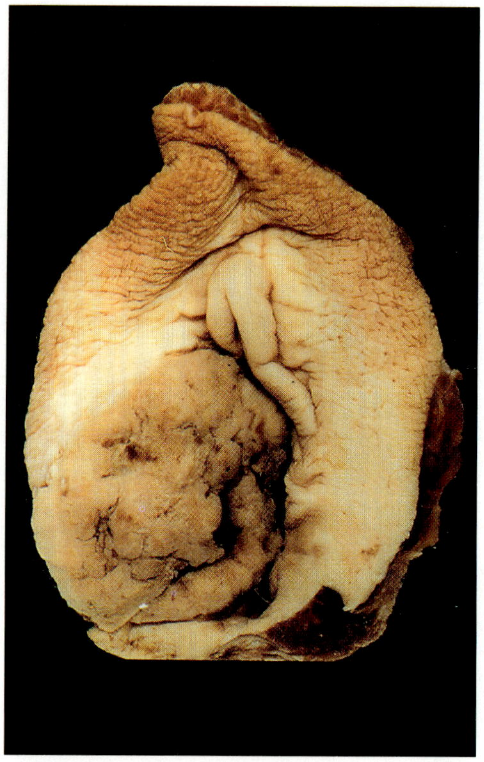

5.53 Vulva: Squamous Carcinoma

This specimen was excised from a 79-year-old woman who had noticed a lesion on the left labia.

This is a simple vulvectomy specimen and shows a large, irregular, flattened tumour, measuring 4cm in maximum diameter, which has arisen on the left labium majus. Note also the white area, which clinically would be called leukoplakia, at the muco-cutaneous junction above.

Carcinoma of the vulva accounts for about 5 per cent of female genital malignancies and is almost always squamous in type. It presents most often in elderly women in the 7th and 8th decades and commonly arises in cases of pre- existing vulval intra-epithelial neoplasia or chronic inflammation. The most frequent site is the labia, with fewer cases originating around the clitoris or mons. Survival is dependent upon histological grading and staging but the overall 5-year-survival is about 70 per cent. A rare variant, verrucous carcinoma, usually appears similar to a genital wart both clinically and microscopically. These latter lesions rarely metastasise to lymph nodes, but are aggressively locally invasive; radiotherapy is contraindicated in their treatment as this may lead to a deterioration in clinical behaviour.

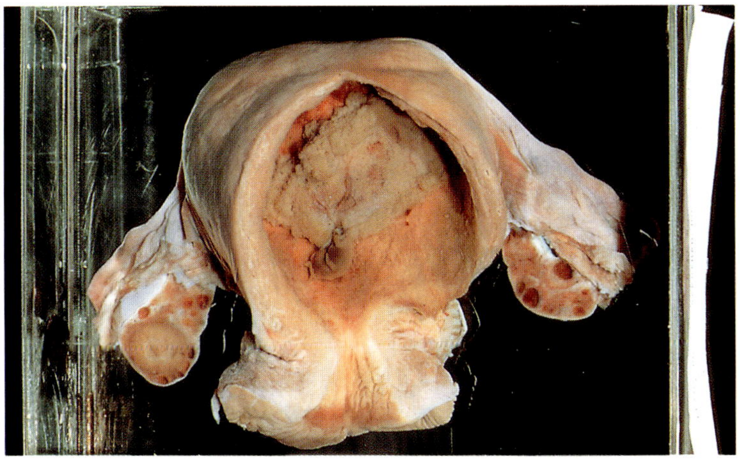

5.54 Uterus: Early Pregnancy

This is a post-mortem specimen from a 26-year-old multiparous woman who died of a pulmonary embolism during the 2nd month of pregnancy.

The uterus has been opened to show an enlarged endometrial cavity, measuring 7 x 7 x 3cm, compatible with this patient's multiparity. Attached to the fundus is a small placenta with umbilical cord and a fetus, measuring 1.5cm in length. The fallopian tubes and ovaries are normal; note the presence of a corpus luteum of pregnancy in the right ovary. The size of the fetus suggests about 6 weeks gestation.

Pregnancy itself, predisposes to deep venous thrombosis although this more usually occurs in the 2nd or 3rd trimesters. It is possible that a high circulating level of oestrogen may have been contributory in the case here.

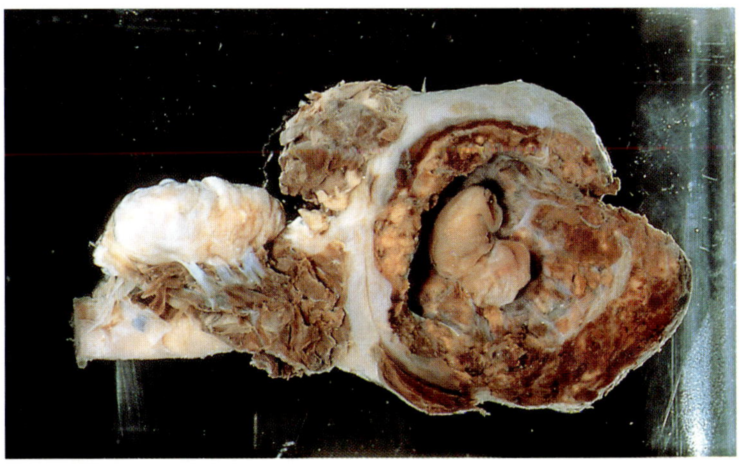

5.55 Fallopian Tube: Ectopic Pregnancy

No clinical details are available.

The left fallopian tube and ovary have been dissected to show a small fetus, within its amniotic sac, implanted in the ampullary portion of the tube. There is gross luminal dilatation, with widespread haemorrhage and blood clot, extending to involve the fimbrial end of the tube.

Ectopic implantation of a fertilised ovum is increasing in incidence and occurs in approximately 1 in 100 pregnancies, the vast majority involving the fallopian tube. Postulated aetiological factors in tubal ectopic pregnancy include chronic salpingitis or fibrosis, impaired tubal motility or over-ripeness of the ovum. In about 80 per cent of cases, implantation occurs in the ampullary portion of the tube and it is extremely rare for tubal pregnancies to remain viable for more than about 12 weeks. Inadequate decidualisation and the thinness of the tubal wall lead either to resorption of the conceptus, separation of the placenta with local haemorrhage (as in the case here), tubal rupture or abortion into the peritoneum. About 15 per cent of tubal pregnancies occur in the isthmus. The wall of the fallopian tube at this site is comparatively thick, so that these cases often present with haemorrhage or rupture rather later than ampullary pregnancies.

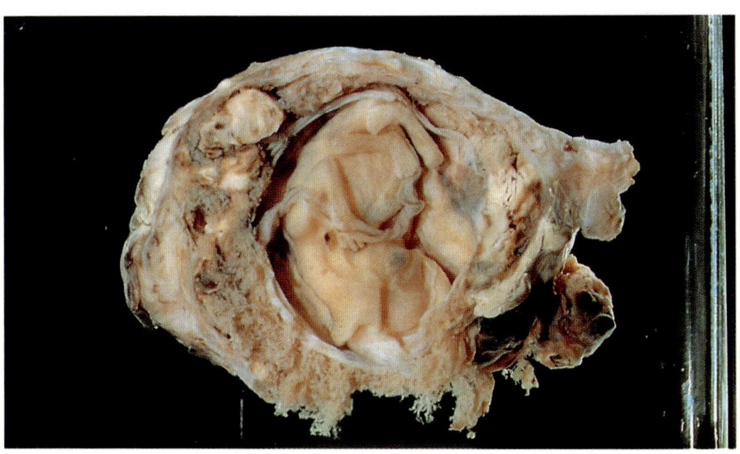

5.56 Fallopian Tube: Ruptured Ectopic Pregnancy

No clinical details are available.

The fallopian tube is grossly distended, measuring up to 4cm in diameter, and has been sectioned to show a fetus of about 14 weeks gestation within its lumen. The peritoneal surface of the tube is covered with blood clot and there is a rupture along the lower border, through which chorionic villi protrude.

Tubal rupture complicates up to 60 per cent of tubal ectopic pregnancies. Very occasionally, re-implantation of the placenta may occur in the broad ligament or peritoneal cavity but the principal importance of tubal rupture is that the rapid and profuse haemorrhage which commonly occurs constitutes an acute surgical emergency.

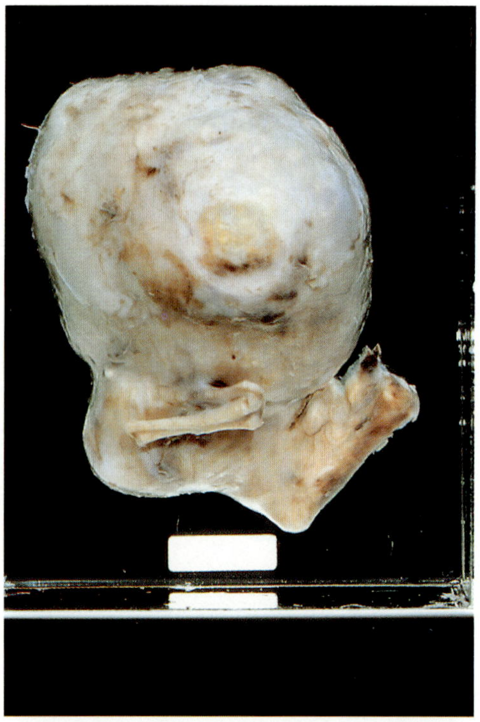

5.57 Fallopian Tube: Lithopaedion

This specimen was excised from a 34-year-old Jamaican woman who had 2 normal pregnancies, 5 years and one year previously. She presented with a 2 month history of abdominal pain and was found to have an abdominal mass which was interpreted as uterine leiomyomata. At operation the mass was found to involve the left fallopian tube and was adherent to the omentum.

The mass, measuring 10cm in maximum diameter, has been bisected to show a compressed, inspissated fetus and placenta.

A lithopaedion represents mummification of an undetected fetus, most often implanted at an ectopic site. In the case here, since the patient could not recall anything suggestive of either an ectopic pregnancy or a suspected pregnancy, which came to nothing, it is possible that this lithopaedion may have been a twin associated with either of the 2 preceding pregnancies.

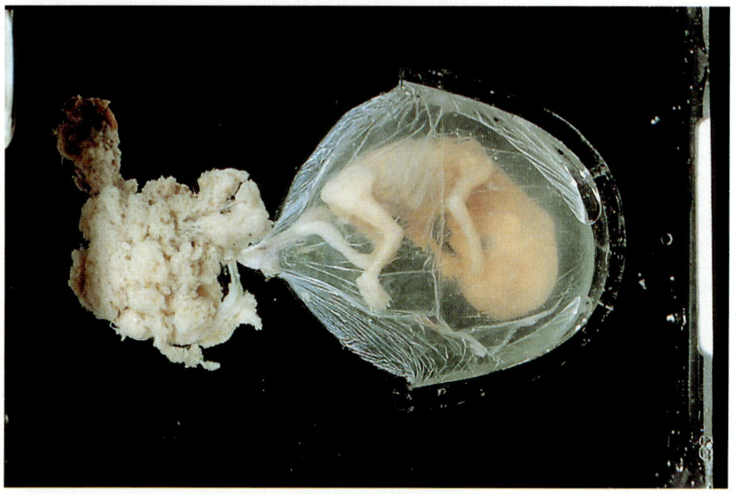

5.58 Pelvic Haematocele: Ectopic Pregnancy

This specimen was found within a pelvic haematocele in a patient diagnosed as having an ectopic pregnancy.

A fetus, measuring 4cm in length, can be seen enclosed in an amniotic sac and attached by an umbilical cord to a mass of placental tissue.

Primary peritoneal implantation of the conceptus is rare and it is probable that most of these cases in fact represent tubal or ovarian pregnancies which have been dislodged and reimplanted. Very occasionally intra-abdominal pregnancies progress successfully to term, reflecting the ability of ectopic sites to show at least a partial response to hormonal stimulation.

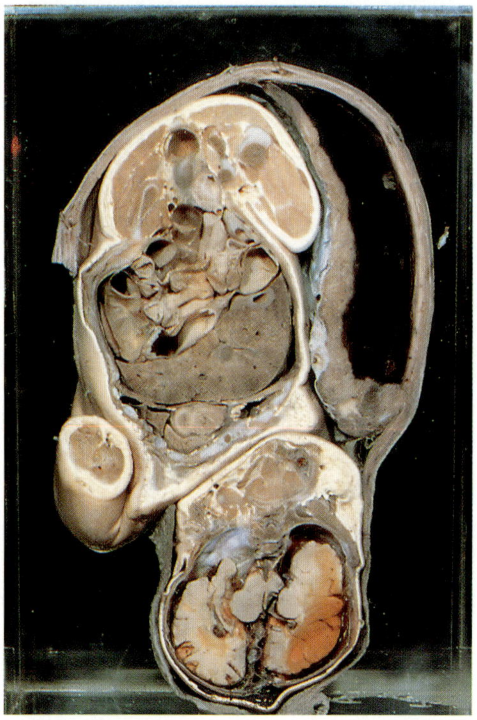

5.59 Uterus: Retroplacental Haemorrhage

This is a post-mortem specimen from a woman who died after placental abruption close to term.

A sagittal section through the gravid uterus with fetus shows a mass of blood clot between the placenta, situated anteriorly, and the uterine wall. Except for a very small area in the lower segment, the placenta has been completely separated from the endometrium.

Placental abruption of varying degree, is one of the commonest causes of antepartum haemorrhage in the 3rd trimester. In principle, the degree of placental separation determines the amount of bleeding but, without uterine contractions, bleeding becomes uncontrollable and unless appropriate action is taken haemorrhage may be profuse. The aetiology is unclear, but up to 50 per cent of cases may be associated with pre-eclampsia. Well recognised complications include disseminated intravascular coagulation and Sheehan's syndrome.

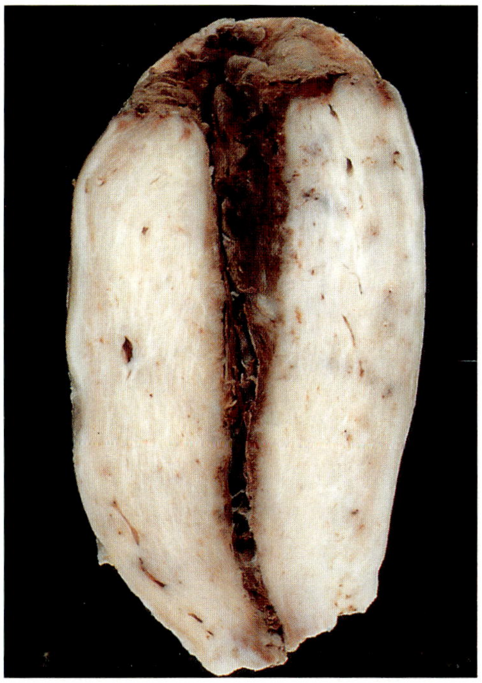

5.60 Uterus: Rupture during Pregnancy

This specimen was excised from a 30-year-old woman who presented with severe abdominal pain and shock during the 35th week of pregnancy. Her previous pregnancy had been terminated by curettage owing to severe pulmonary tuberculosis. Laparotomy revealed the uterine rupture and an intact fetus in the abdominal cavity.

A coronal section through the uterus shows a rupture in the fundus with adjacent haemorrhage and the remnants of thin fibrous scar tissue. In the fresh state, the tear was 10cm in length and extended in the antero-posterior plane.

Uterine rupture is very uncommon, particularly if the patient avails herself of regular obstetric care. However, predisposing causes include prolonged obstruction of labour and fibrous scarring of the uterine wall from previous Caesarean section or incautious curettage. Rupture may also occur as a complication of placenta accreta. Clearly the condition represents a surgical emergency for there may be torrential haemorrhage.

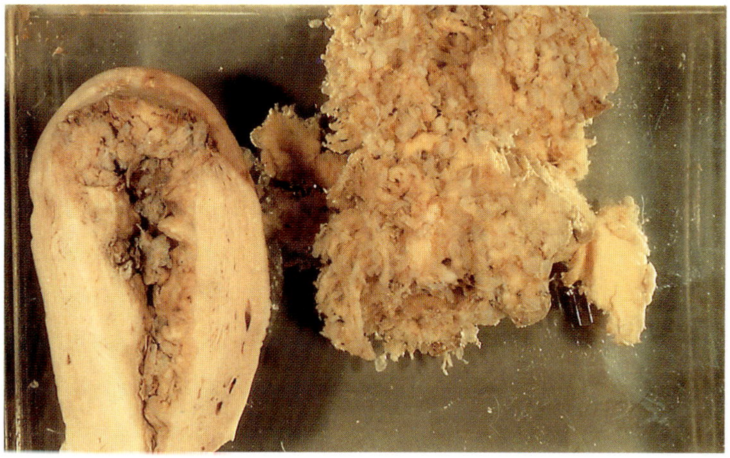

5.61 Uterus: Complete Hydatidiform Mole

This specimen was excised from a 46-year-old woman who presented in the 5th month of pregnancy with vaginal bleeding. A subtotal hysterectomy was performed and she remained well when seen 2½ years later.

On the left, a coronal section through the uterus shows a ragged layer of cystic chorionic tissue lining the endometrium. At the site of implantation in the fundus, the invasive nature of the chorion is well demonstrated. On the right, the uterine contents are shown. There is no trace of a fetus but, instead, there is a mass of cystic and vesicular chorionic villi, bearing some resemblance to a bunch of grapes.

The incidence of complete hydatidiform mole in Britain is about 1 in 1500 pregnancies but this lesion is seen much more often in parts of the Far East and Africa. Females at the extremes of reproductive life are most often affected. Pathogenetically, moles are thought to arise primarily from an abnormal proliferation of the villous trophoblast and, interestingly, 85 per cent of complete moles show XX sex chromosomes, both chromosomes being paternal in origin. It is thought that this is due to penetration of an 'empty' ovum by a single sperm which then replicates. Fifteen per cent of complete moles have an XY sex chromosomal complement, again both of paternal origin. It is thought that these moles are due to 2 spermatozoa entering an 'empty' ovum and then combining and replicating. In Caucasians, up to 3 per cent of affected patients will go on to develop choriocarcinoma (see Figure and Legend 5.63) but unfortunately there are, as yet, no reliable means of predicting this complication. By contrast, incomplete or partial moles, which are probably more common, show a proportion of normal placental tissue and often a fetus, either apparently normal or malformed, is also present. It is not clear whether the latter group have any malignant potential. All moles, whether complete or incomplete, should be followed up by serial human chorionic gonadotrophin estimations. (Courtesy of the Royal College of Obstetricians and Gynaecologists)

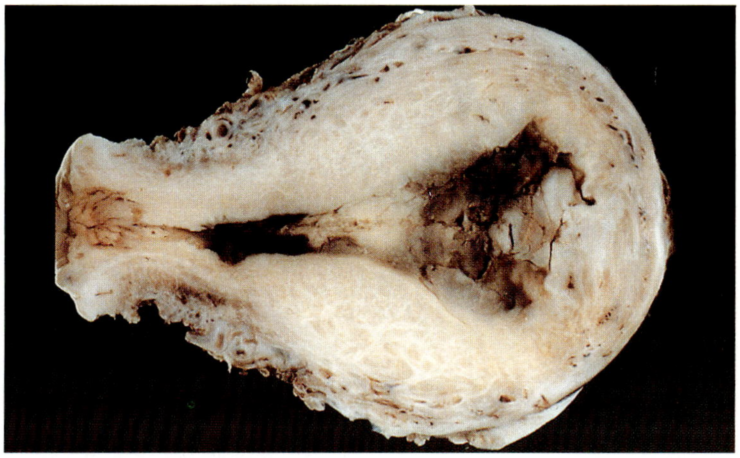

5.62 Uterus: Invasive Complete Hydatidiform Mole

This specimen was excised from a 31-year-old woman who was admitted in the 11th week of pregnancy with hyperemesis. She had also noticed a persistent blood-stained vaginal discharge and intermittent haemoptysis. Examination revealed the uterus to be enlarged to a size compatible with 18 weeks gestation. A hysterotomy with removal of the mole was performed but, due to continuing symptoms, she underwent hysterectomy 2 weeks later. Thereafter recovery was uneventful.

This coronal section of the uterus shows necrotic and haemorrhagic material in the endometrial cavity. Rather pale, hydropic tissue is visible penetrating the myometrium in the fundus. The excised mole was not submitted to the museum.

Invasive hydatidiform mole is defined as a lesion in which hydropic villi and trophoblast extend deeply into the myometrium and invade blood vessels. The presence of recognisable villi allows differentiation from choriocarcinoma. To some extent this invasion simply represents an exaggeration of the normal physiological process of implantation. Similarly the pulmonary symptoms, as seen in this patient, probably reflect increased vascular dissemination of trophoblastic tissue, which occurs to a minor degree in every normal pregnancy. It is, therefore, important to realise that an invasive mole is not a malignant lesion and in fact, surprisingly, it shows a reduced tendency to progress to choriocarcinoma than non-invasive hydatidiform mole.

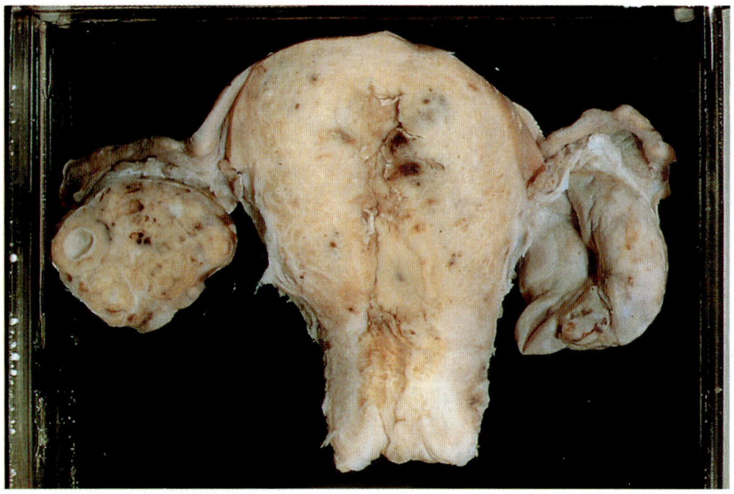

5.63 Uterus: Choriocarcinoma

This specimen was excised from a 23-year-old woman who was admitted to hospital with a threatened abortion. Examination revealed that the uterus was much more enlarged than expected for her stated 16 weeks amenorrhoea. Shortly afterwards, she spontaneously passed a large vesicular mole but, 3 weeks later, the uterus remained enlarged and the pregnancy test was still strongly positive.

The uterus, with both tubes and ovaries, is shown. The uterus is markedly enlarged and has been sectioned coronally to show numerous small foci of haemorrhagic tissue extending deeply into the myometrium. Both ovaries contain multiple follicular cysts and the larger cystic structure in the right ovary is a corpus luteum cyst.

Choriocarcinoma is a malignant trophoblastic tumour and is, therefore, of fetal origin. In Britain this lesion is rare, complicating about 1 in 50,000 pregnancies, but in the Far East, and parts of Africa it is much more common. Females in the 3rd decade are most often affected; 50 per cent of cases follow a hydatidiform mole, 30 per cent develop after spontaneous abortion and 20 per cent arise after an apparently normal pregnancy. These tumours are classically multinodular and haemorrhagic and show a marked predilection for vascular invasion. While in the past the outcome was invariably fatal, the use of modern chemotherapy and careful follow-up, using serum estimations of ß-human chorionic gonadotrophin, results in up to 90 per cent of patients being cured.

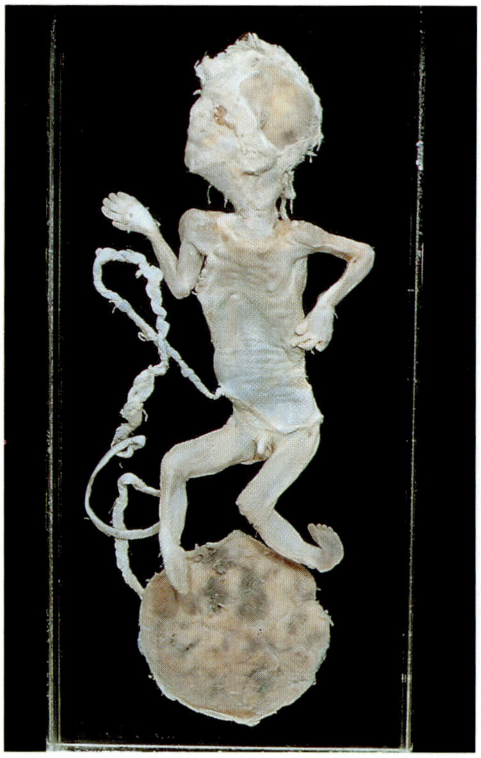

5.64 Umbilical Cord: Torsion leading to Fetus Papyraceus

This specimen was delivered spontaneously by a 28-year-old woman in her first pregnancy. She was known to have a twin pregnancy and was delivered of a normal female infant, which was followed 2 minutes later by this papyraceous fetus.

The fetus is dehydrated, compressed and partly mummified. A radiological skeletal survey suggested development had progressed to between 24-28 weeks. The umbilical cord shows multiple tight twists and the placenta is rather pale.

Fetus papyraceous may develop for a variety of reasons, the commonest of which are missed abortion or concealed intra-uterine death. In a twin pregnancy it is not uncommon for one fetus to gradually monopolise the placental blood supply, leading to progressive ischaemia and death of the other one. Similarly, genuine rather than delivery-induced twists or knots in the umbilical cord may cause fetal ischaemia, death and subsequent mummification. Torsion of the cord is predisposed to by excessive fetal movement, cord stricture and an excessively long cord. Care has to be taken to distinguish between post-mortem twisting of the cord and true ante-mortem torsion.

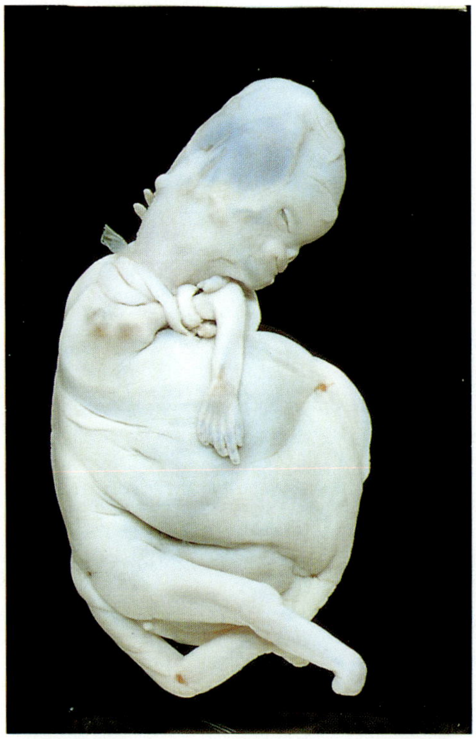

5.65 Fetus: Strangulation by Umbilical Cord

This specimen was delivered from a 25-year-old primiparous woman who suffered an intra-uterine fetal death at about 16 weeks of gestation.

The fetus is rather compressed and the umbilical cord is wound very tightly around the neck and right arm. The abdomen is grossly distended and this is probably due to post-mortem autolysis.

True fetal strangulation by the umbilical cord is rare. It is thought that, as the fetus becomes progressively hypoxic, its subsequent agitation unfortunately leads to the cord being pulled even tighter.

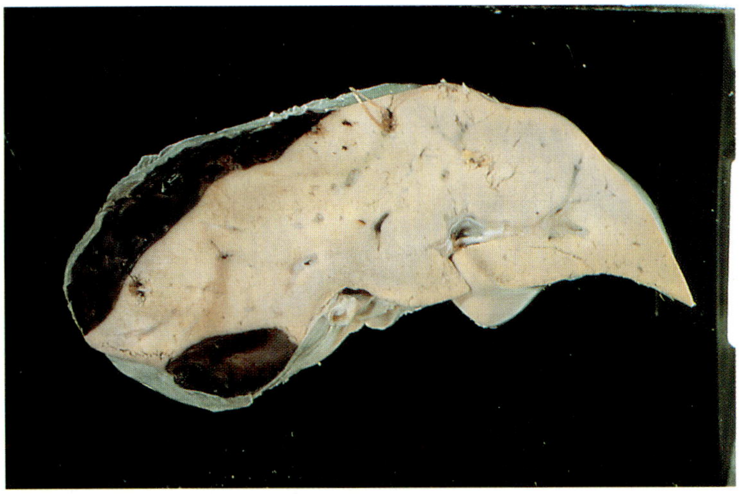

5.66 Fetal Liver: Subcapsular Haemorrhage

This is a post-mortem specimen from a 3-day-old infant who died following breech extraction. A tentorial tear, with intracerebral haemorrhage, was also noted at autopsy.

The liver has been sectioned to show a mass of recent blood clot beneath the capsule.

A subcapsular hepatic haemorrhage is a well-recognised complication of birth trauma, whether due to instrumentation (e.g. forceps) or breech delivery. Other possible consequences include cephalhaematoma, cerebral haemorrhage, fractures either of the skull or limbs and rupture of the spleen.

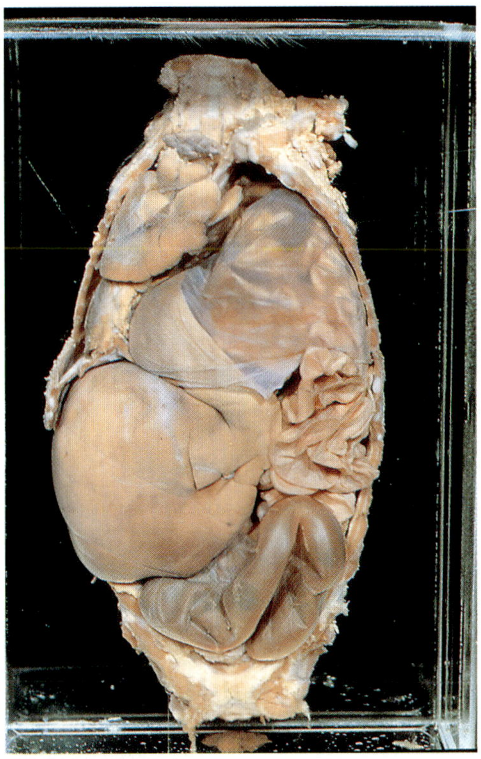

5.67 Fetus: Congenital Rubella Syndrome

This infant was delivered at term by a 26-year-old woman who had unknowingly suffered a rubella infection in the 10th week of pregnancy. The child weighed 6lb and showed no external abnormality but died after only 15 minutes.

The trunk of this infant has been dissected to show a large left-sided diaphragmatic hernia, containing the left lobe of the liver, the stomach and some of the small bowel. The heart is displaced to the right. Other findings at autopsy included a persistent ductus arteriosus and an atrial septal defect.

The fetus is at risk of developing congenital malformations if the mother suffers rubella infection at any time from conception to about 16 weeks gestation. In particular, if infection occurs prior to 8 weeks then there is up to a 60 per cent likelihood of fetal abnormalities. The classical major defects include cataracts, congenital heart disease and deafness. Other possible findings include microcephaly and hepatosplenomegaly. The value of inoculating pre-pubescent schoolgirls against rubella is therefore self-evident.

BREAST

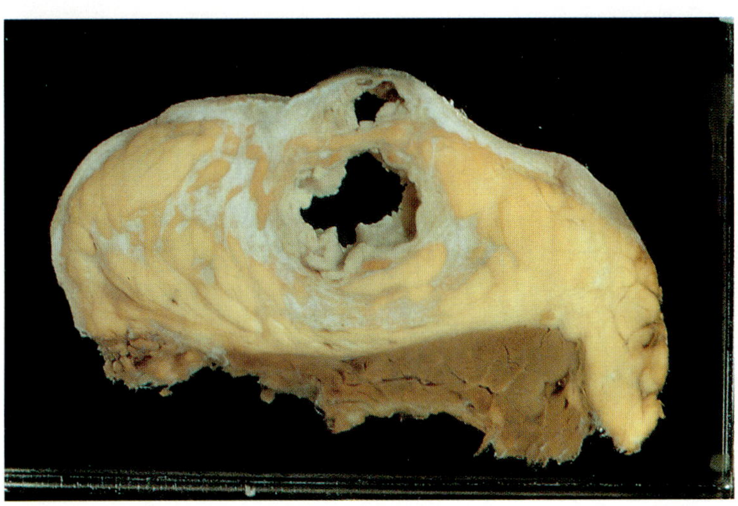

5.68 Chronic Abscess

This specimen was excised from a 42-year-old woman who had noticed a lump in the left breast for 18 months. On examination there was a hard, fixed mass above the nipple and a number of axillary lymph nodes were palpable.

A section through the breast shows a large abscess cavity containing inspissated pus which has extended almost as far as the skin surface.

Breast abscesses most commonly occur as a result of bacterial infection, particularly due to *Staphylococcus aureus*, during lactation. It may also complicate a mammary fistula. Tuberculous or fungal infections of the breast may result in a similar appearance but are extremely rare in the British Isles.

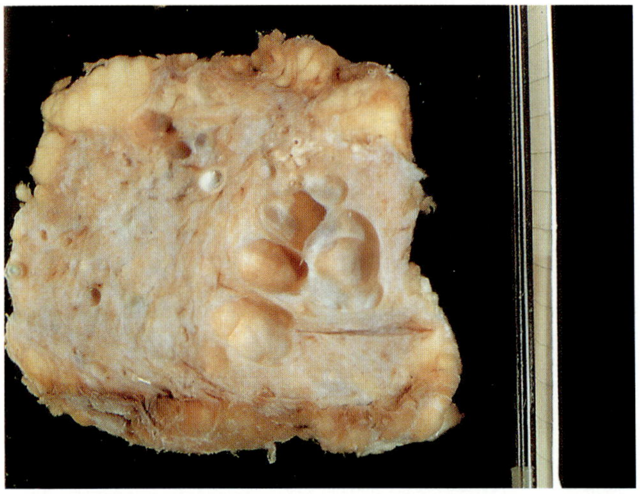

5.69 Fibrocystic Disease

This specimen was excised from a 41-year-old woman who had noticed lumpiness and pain in both breasts for several years, which was aggravated during menstruation. She had previously had a benign lump removed from the left breast, since when numerous cyst aspirations had also been performed.

The breast tissue shows numerous irregular cysts, some of which contain creamy-white material, admixed with excessive connective tissue.

Fibrocystic disease, also known as fibroadenosis, cystic mastopathy, cystic hyperplasia and cystic mastitis, may affect up to 5 per cent of females and usually presents in the 3th or 4th decades, almost always before the menopause. It is more common in nulliparous women or in patients with menstrual irregularity and is thought to result either from hormonal imbalance during the childbearing years or from altered sensitivity of the breast tissue to the normal hormonal cycle. The typical histological changes of fibrosis, adenosis, cyst formation, apocrine metaplasia and epitheliosis may each be present to a varying degree. Of these, epitheliosis (epithelial hyperplasia) is the only feature which may occasionally be associated with the development of carcinoma.

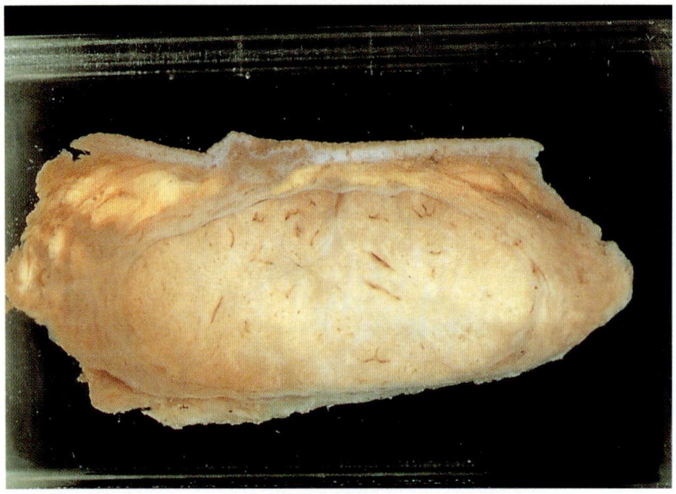

5.70 Fibroadenoma

No clinical details are available.

A section through the breast tissue shows an ovoid, well-circumscribed tumour, measuring 5 x 3cm, which is lobulated and contains irregular cleft-like spaces.

Fibroadenomas occur most often in young women in the 2nd and 3rd decades and are the most common benign breast tumours. They may be multiple and are soft, rubbery and mobile – occasionally being referred to as 'breast mice'. Despite their apparent neoplastic nature, these tumours are responsive to the hormonal cycle and, since histologically identical foci may be found in fibrocystic disease, the pathogenesis of fibroadenomas is thought also to be related to an altered hormonal response. Histologically they may be divided into pericanalicular and intracanalicular subtypes, the latter being supposedly more common in older women, but most often these tumours are mixed and therefore subclassification is of doubtful value. They have no known potential to undergo malignant change.

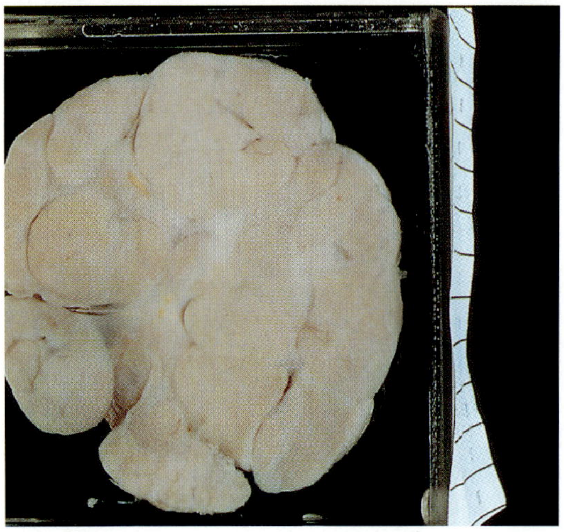

5.71 Fibroadenoma

This specimen was excised from a 28-year-old woman who had noticed a slowly growing lump in the right breast for 3 years. The mass was tender during menstruation. Examination revealed a smooth, discrete mass which, at operation, was easily separated from the adjacent compressed breast tissue.

A rounded, coarsely lobulated tumour, measuring 8cm in diameter, is surrounded by a smooth fibrous capsule.

These are the classical macroscopical appearances of a fibroadenoma.

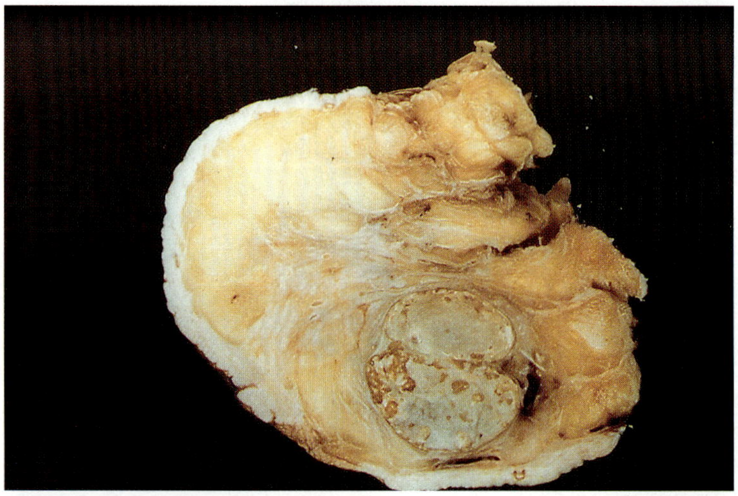

5.72 Calcified Fibroadenoma and Carcinoma

This specimen was excised from a 70-year-old woman with a hard rounded mass in the breast. She developed metastatic disease and died 16 months later.

A section through the breast shows a rounded, encapsulated and partly calcified tumour, 3cm in diameter in the upper half of the picture. Beneath this is a quite separate neoplasm which has spread diffusely through the breast tissue and filled the main ducts beneath the nipple.

In older post-menopausal women, a fibroadenoma may commonly undergo regressive changes which include hyalinisation and calcification. The finding of an invasive adenocarcinoma in the same breast is purely coincidental and serves to reiterate the ubiquity of both benign and malignant breast tumours.

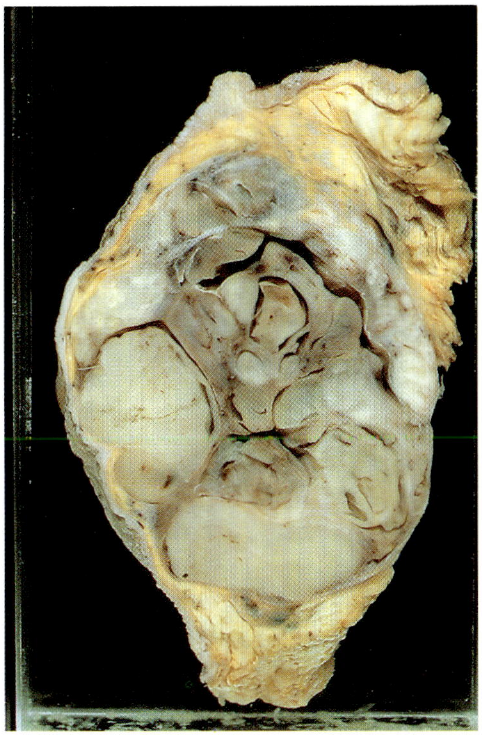

5.73 Phyllodes Tumour

No clinical details are available.

This enlarged breast has been sectioned to show an encapsulated tumour, 10cm in diameter, which is composed of irregular masses of almost translucent fibrous tissue projecting into ill-defined cystic spaces.

The phyllodes tumour, also known as a giant fibroadenoma, cystosarcoma phyllodes and Brodie's tumour, is an uncommon variant of a fibroadenoma which most often affects elderly women and typically grows rapidly to a large size. It may induce discoloration of the skin and eventually fungate. It is distinguished from conventional fibroadenomas by the extensive myxoid change and fibrous stromal proliferation which is usually seen, such that it may mimic a sarcoma. However, a large proportion of these tumours are benign and only about 5 per cent undergo true sarcomatous change giving rise to metastases and resulting in death. Histological distinction between benign and malignant variants of phyllodes tumours can be extremely difficult.

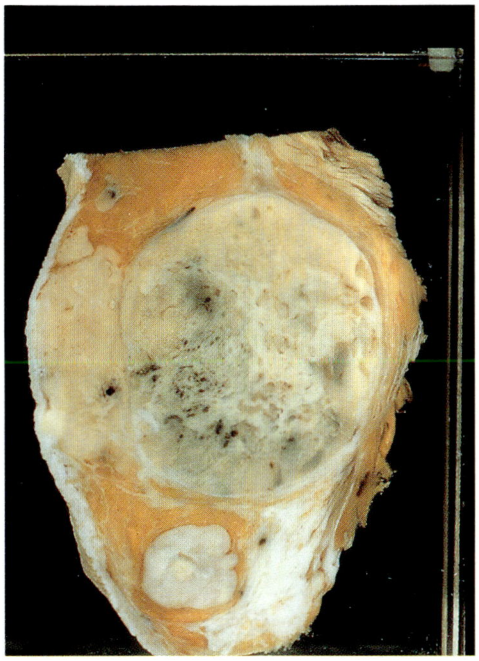

5.74 Malignant Phyllodes Tumour

This specimen was excised from a 55-year-old woman who had noticed a lump in the left breast for 18 months which had rapidly enlarged and was associated with redness of the overlying skin. Within a year of mastectomy she developed pulmonary and skeletal metastases and died.

A section through the breast shows a well-circumscribed tumour, measuring 5cm in diameter, which is focally necrotic and haemorrhagic. Superficially the tumour has extended through the capsule and has infiltrated the skin. A separate, smaller tumour nodule is seen in the lower part of the specimen.

Histologically, foci of this tumour were so undifferentiated and pleomorphic that the diagnosis of malignancy presented no difficulty.

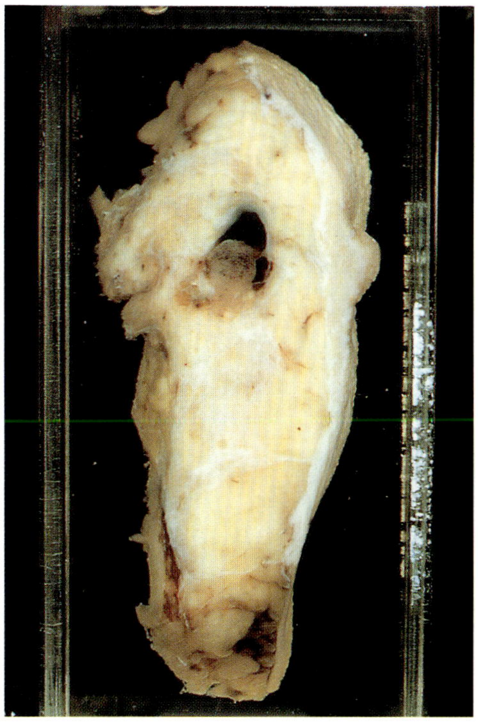

5.75 Duct Papilloma

This specimen was excised from a 49-year-old woman who complained of a blood-stained discharge from the nipple for two weeks. Examination revealed a cystic swelling deep to the nipple, from which blood-stained fluid could be expressed.

A section through the breast shows, beneath the nipple, a cyst into which projects a polypoid tumour measuring 1cm in diameter. The adjacent breast tissue shows evidence of fibrocystic disease.

Duct papillomata arise most often in middle-aged women and are the commonest cause of a discharge from the nipple. Identification of the discharging duct may be the most reliable way of detecting a small impalpable papilloma. These lesions usually originate in a major duct close to the nipple and tend to be solitary. If the duct becomes obstructed then cystic dilatation may occur. It is considered most unlikely that duct papillomata may progress to the development of papillary carcinoma.

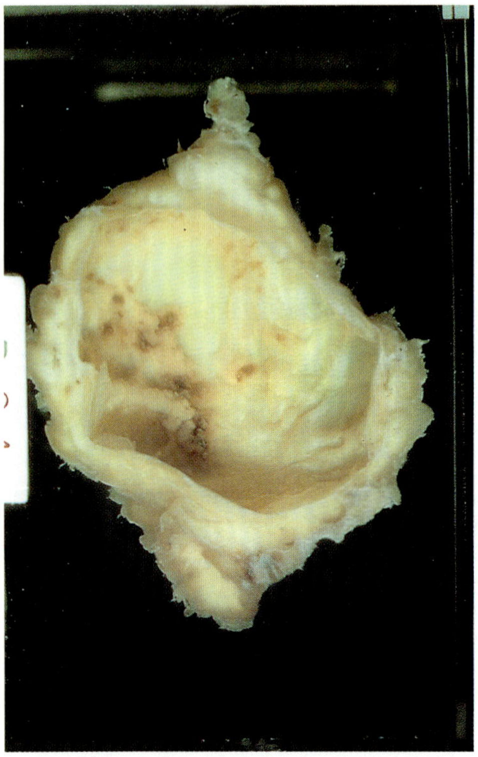

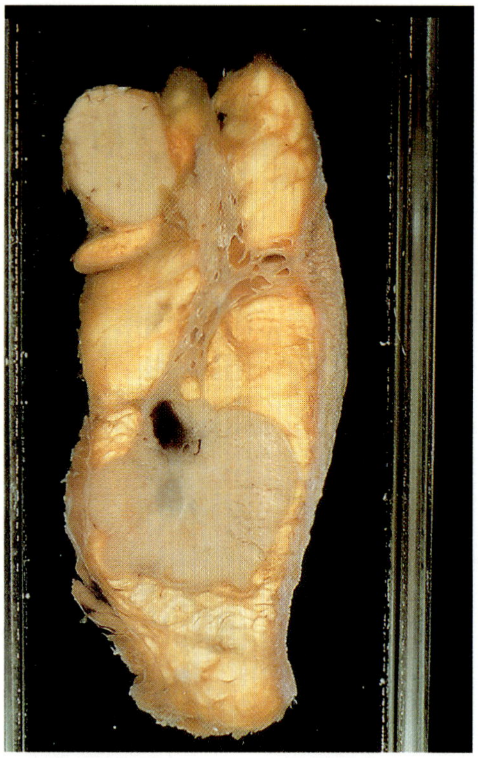

5.76 Intracystic Papillomatosis

This specimen was excised from a 57-year-old man who complained of a painless swelling in the left breast which had been present for 7 months.

Beneath the nipple (left), a thin-walled cyst measuring 3cm in diameter, can be seen. The lining shows several papillary excrescences.

This lesion represents multiple, small duct papillomata which, in obstructing the lactiferous duct, have resulted in cystic dilatation as a secondary phenomenon. Duct papillomata are extremely rare in men.

5.77 Adenocarcinoma

This specimen was excised from a 55-year-old woman with a 3 month history of a firm painless enlarging lump in the right breast. At presentation, firm axillary lymph nodes were palpable.

A section through the breast shows an irregular, rounded tumour, measuring 4cm in diameter. The tumour is adherent to both the skin and pectoral fascia. At the top left of the picture an enlarged lymph node replaced by metastatic tumour is seen.

Carcinoma of the breast is the commonest cause of death from malignant disease in women in the British Isles. The incidence has been increasing steadily throughout this century and up to 6 per cent of the female population may be affected at one time, of whom at least one third will die of the disease. Women of any age may develop breast carcinoma but it is increasingly common from about the age of 30. The aetiology remains uncertain but the following factors have been noted:
1) there is a clear inherited tendency;
2) breast carcinoma is more common in nulliparous women, late age at first parturition and women who have not breast fed;
3) bilateral oöphorectomy may be protective;
4) pre-existing epitheliosis in fibrocystic disease may occasionally predispose to carcinoma, and
5) the Bittner agent (RNA mammary tumour virus) has been identified as a cause of carcinoma in mice.

Adenocarcinoma of the breast may be of lobular or ductal origin, the latter group constituting at least 90 per cent. Lobular carcinoma has a particular tendency both to multicentricity in one breast and to bilaterality. Up to 50 per cent of carcinomas develop in the upper, outer quadrant of the breast, which therefore spread to axillary lymph nodes, and approximately 50 per cent of all cases show metastatic involvement of lymph nodes at presentation. It is the fact that dissemination of these tumours appears to occur so early in the course of the disease that explains why, despite all the recent advances in treatment, the prognosis of breast cancer has not changed over the last 30 years. Early detection of breast cancer, perhaps by self-examination, remains the principal hope for improving prognosis. Blood-borne spread usually involves primarily the lungs, liver, bone and adrenals.

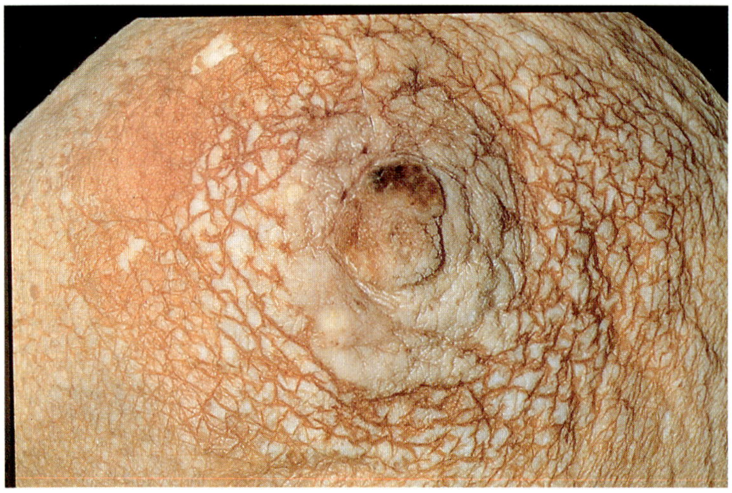

5.78 Peau D'Orange

No clinical details are available.

This mastectomy specimen shows thickening and pitting of the skin, so that it resembles the rind of an orange. The nipple is enlarged and ulcerated and the areola shows irregular nodularity.

In the substance of the breast there was an invasive adenocarcinoma, showing extensive infiltration of dermal lymphatics. This appearance is a result of widespread lymphatic obstruction such that cutaneous oedema occurs.

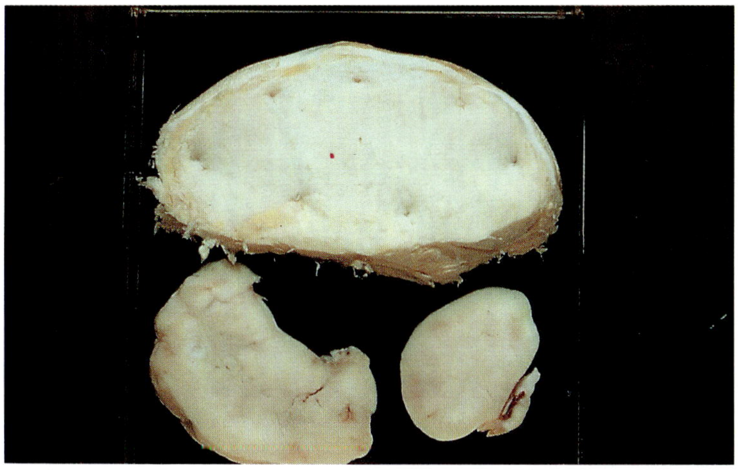

5.79 Paget's Disease of the Nipple

This specimen was excised from a 59-year-old woman who complained of a discharging, encrusted nipple for 3 months with associated pain in the breast. Examination revealed a palpable mass in the upper inner quadrant of the breast.

The breast has been sectioned to show that the nipple is flattened and surrounded by a nodular, encrusted area, 3cm in diameter. A small tumour mass can be seen occupying the central part of the nipple and underlying breast tissue. Deeper in the breast, smaller ducts are obstructed and distended by inspissated, purulent material.

Paget's disease represents carcinomatous infiltration of the skin and constitutes a very small proportion of all breast cancers. Irrespective of the duration of the nipple lesion, *in every case an underlying intraduct or invasive adenocarcinoma of a major duct is present*, whether or not it is clinically detectable. Skin biopsy of any such suspicious lesion is mandatory since mistaken treatment for dermatitis can only have a deleterious effect on prognosis.

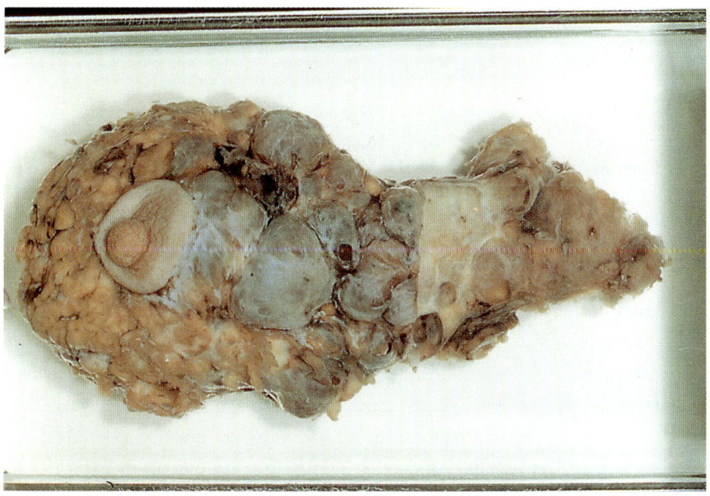

5.80 Mucoid ('Colloid') Carcinoma

This specimen was excised from a 42-year-old woman who had noticed an enlarging area of lumpiness in the breast for one year. On examination there appeared to be generalised cystic change involving most of the breast.

The breast and axillary tail, from which most of the skin has been removed, shows virtual replacement by a mass of soft, rounded nodules, measuring up to 3cm in diameter. Several of these nodules in the axillary tail have been sectioned to show their mucoid cystic nature.

This variant of breast carcinoma, in which there is massive mucus secretion, is comparatively uncommon and tends to affect more elderly women. Clinically it may easily be confused with a benign cystic lesion. It is believed by some to carry a better prognosis than the more usual variants of breast cancer.

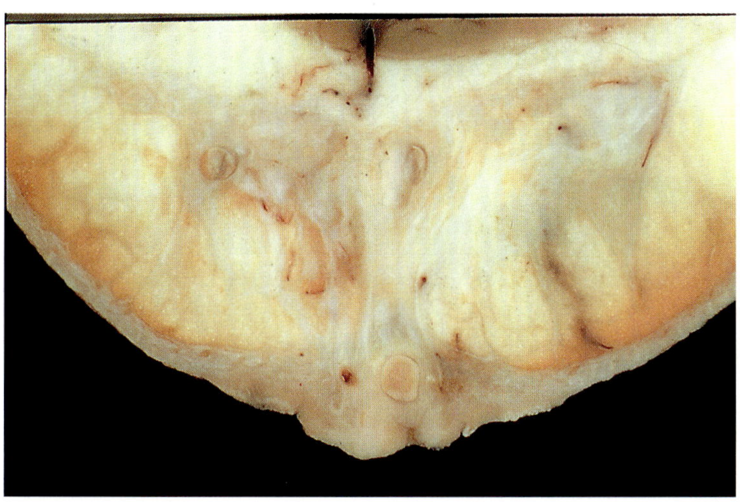

5.81 Carcinoma in Pregnancy

These specimens were excised from a 23-year-old woman who had given birth one month previously. Post-partum both breasts were engorged but, in the absence of lactation, continued to enlarge rapidly. It became evident that the condition was due to bilateral carcinoma and within 3 weeks there were obvious pulmonary metastases and a mass was present in the lower abdomen. Bilateral oöphorectomy and adrenalectomy were performed at which operation metastases were found in intra-abdominal lymph nodes, both kidneys and both ovaries. The patient soon died.

Sections through the right breast (above) and both ovaries (below) show almost complete replacement by pale tumour.

Carcinomas of the breast that present during pregnancy or lactation commonly enlarge and spread rapidly, carrying a very grave prognosis. This appalling clinical course is attributed to the high levels of circulating oestrogens.

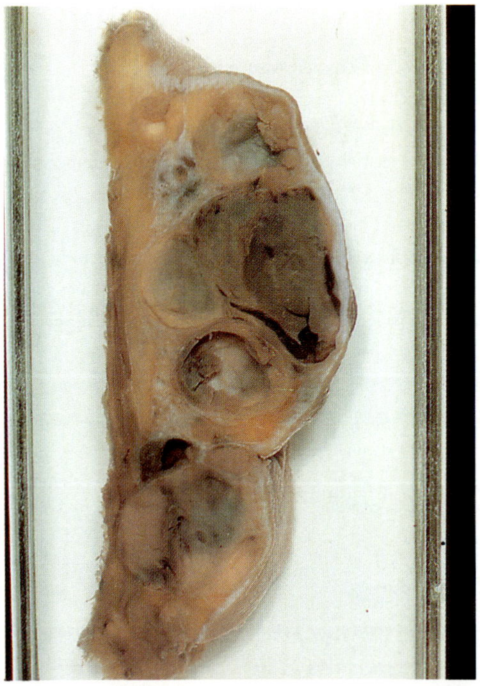

5.82 Intracystic Papillary Carcinoma

This specimen was excised from a 45-year-old woman who had noticed a slow growing lump in the breast for 5 years which had recently ulcerated through the skin. On examination the mass was adherent to the skin and pectoral muscles and had a fluctuant consistency.

A section through the breast shows virtual replacement by a collection of cysts, measuring up to 3cm in diameter. Numerous papillary nodules of tumour project into the cyst cavities.

Papillary carcinoma of the breast is very uncommon and most often arises in the major ducts beneath the nipple, as a result of which it may give rise to a blood-stained discharge. Cyst formation is again a secondary phenomenon as a consequence of duct obstruction (see Legend 5.75). The usual superficial origin of these tumours predisposes them to early ulceration.

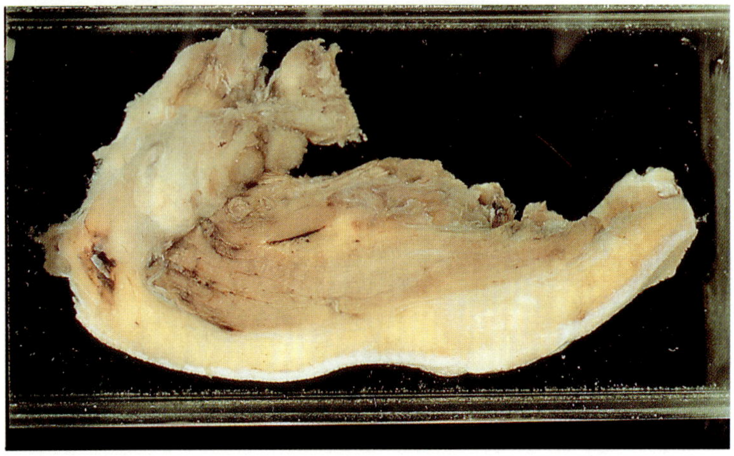

5.83 Carcinoma of Male Breast

This specimen was excised from a 48-year-old man with a one year history of a painful lump in the left breast.

The breast and axillary tail have been sectioned to show retraction of the nipple, beneath which there is a firm, white tumour measuring 2cm in diameter. Several axillary lymph nodes containing pale metastatic tumour can also be seen.

Approximately 1 per cent of breast cancers arise in men, most often in the elderly, and pre-existent gynaecomastia is not uncommon. The histological variants are the same as in the female breast. Involvement of overlying skin, underlying pectoral structures and axillary lymph nodes occurs even earlier than in women and is responsible for the tumour's worse prognosis in men.

MALE GENITAL SYSTEM

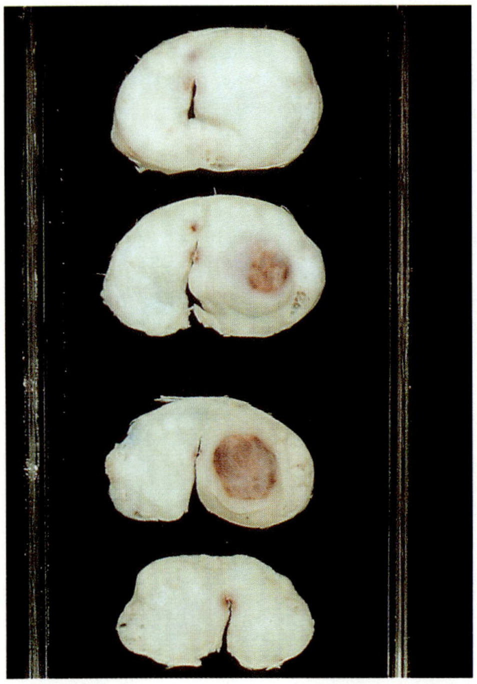

5.84 Prostate: Infarct

No clinical details are available.

This enlarged prostate has been serially sectioned to show a rounded, haemorrhagic infarct, measuring 2cm in diameter, in the centre of the lateral lobe.

Prostatic infarction is not uncommon and usually occurs in glands showing benign nodular hyperplasia, particularly if very large. The precise cause is unknown.

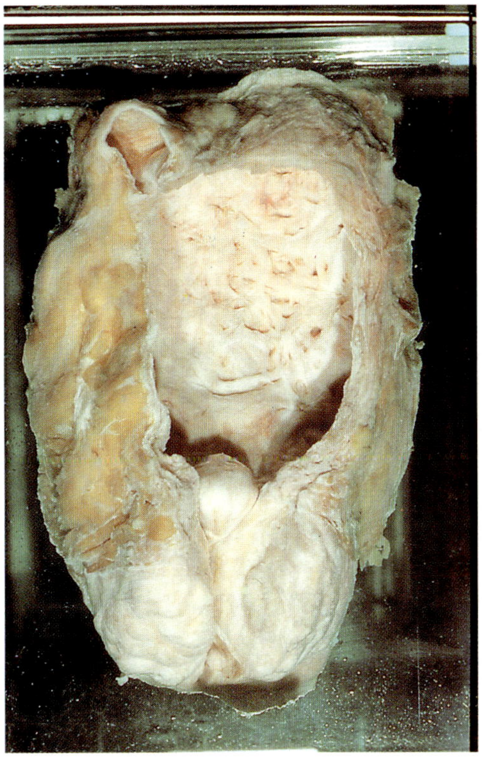

5.85 Prostate: Benign Hypertrophy

This was an incidental finding at post-mortem in a 76-year-old man who died of a cerebral infarct.

The bladder has been opened to show a symmetrically enlarged prostate gland at its base, with a prominent 'middle lobe' which projects into the trigone and obstructs the bladder neck. The prostate shows marked nodularity and the bladder is trabeculated. In addition, a small diverticulum is apparent in the fundus.

This is the typical appearance of benign, prostatic, nodular hyperplasia which is increasingly common with age and is almost universal in men in the 8th and 9th decades. It results from proliferation of both the connective tissue and glandular components, usually of the inner group of glands in the middle and lateral lobes. It only occurs in the presence of normal testes and is thought to be due to an imbalance in the androgen/oestrogen ratio. The principal complications are those of urinary obstruction. This condition does not predispose to carcinoma of the prostate, but in view of the frequency of both lesions, they may occur in the same patient.

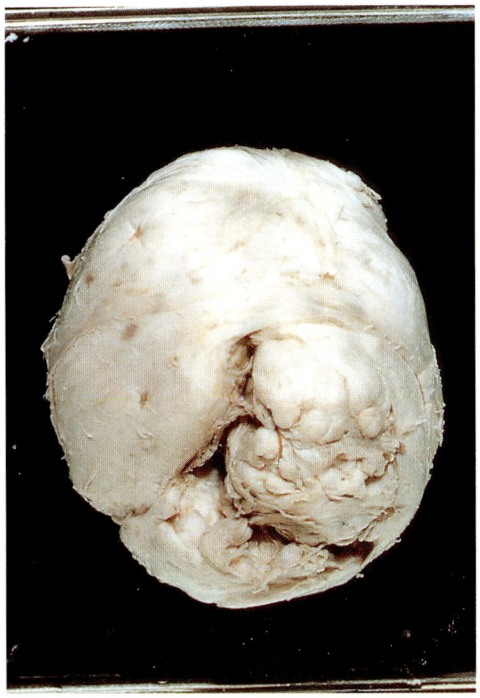

5.86 Prostate: Benign Hypertrophy

This is a retropubic prostatectomy specimen from a 77-year-old man who complained of dysuria and frequency. On examination the bladder was distended in keeping with chronic urinary retention.

This enlarged prostate weighed 305g and measured 9 x 7 x 5cm. The lateral lobes are principally enlarged. Note the consequent slit-like narrowing of the urethra.

This is a typical surgical specimen of benign nodular hyperplasia of the prostate.

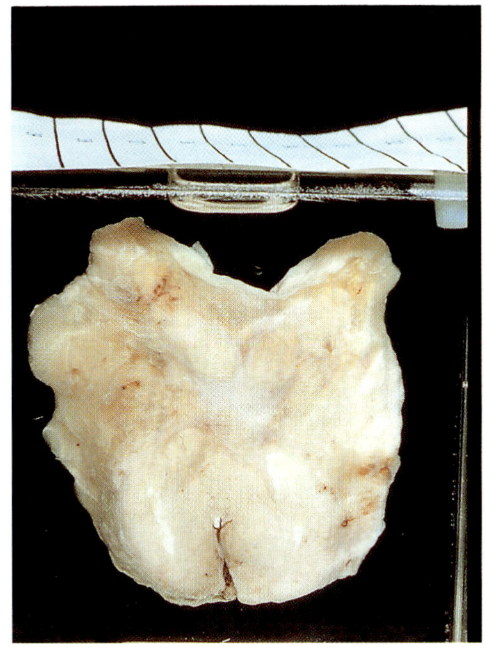

5.87 Prostate: Adenocarcinoma

This is a post-mortem specimen from a 60-year-old man who had been treated with stilboestrol for carcinoma of the prostate 6 years previously. He was lost to follow-up but represented with extensive skeletal and pulmonary metastases, and died shortly afterwards.

The enlarged prostate has been sectioned transversely to show diffuse, irregular infiltration by pale, scirrhous tumour, which is extending into the adjacent soft tissues. Note that the appearance is quite different from that of benign nodular hyperplasia.

Adenocarcinoma is much the commonest epithelial malignancy of the prostate, although transitional cell carcinoma and squamous cell carcinoma also occur, arising from major prostatic ducts. Adenocarcinoma, like benign hyperplasia, is increasingly common with age and it is said that microscopic foci are virtually always present in the prostate of patients over the age of 80. It principally affects the outer group of glands, particularly the posterior lobe (cf. benign hyperplasia) and is often multifocal. It has a particular tendency to metastasise to bone, giving rise to osteosclerotic secondaries. Survival is dependent upon staging and histological grading of the tumour, ranging from 90 per cent at 5 years for small, well-differentiated tumours to only 15 per cent for extensive, poorly differentiated cases. The aetiology is unknown but hormonal factors are thought to be important and, interestingly, prostatic adenocarcinoma is especially common in the Western world.

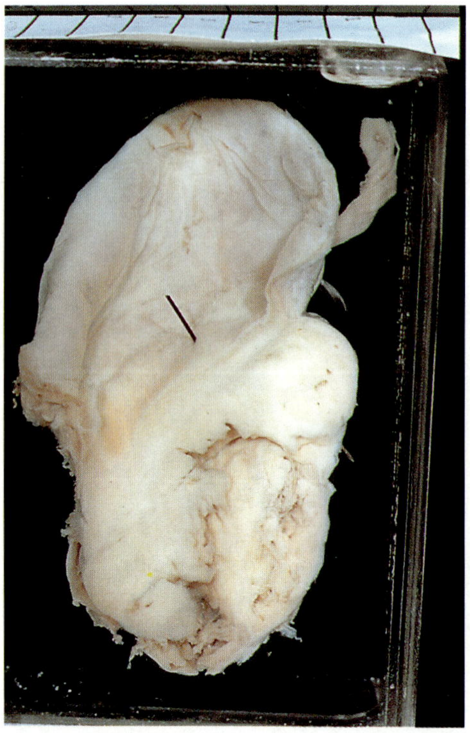

5.88 Prostate: Embryonal Rhabdomyosarcoma

This is a post-mortem specimen from an 11-month-old boy.

A vertical section through the prostate and base of the bladder shows a lobulated neoplasm, measuring 4cm in diameter, arising in the prostate. The tumour shows extensive necrosis and is infiltrating the bladder neck causing urinary retention and dilatation of the bladder. Note that the base of the bladder has been pushed up by the tumour. The thin black probe is located in one of the ureteric orifices.

Embryonal rhabdomyosarcoma, although the commonest genito-urinary tumour in childhood, is rare and is virtually confined to young children. It may often have a botryoid appearance, giving rise to grape-like masses due to subepithelial proliferation of tumour. Prostatic tumours commonly present with urinary obstruction by which time there is frequently lymphatic or vascular invasion. While the prognosis remains very poor, improved survival is being obtained with modern multimodal therapy.

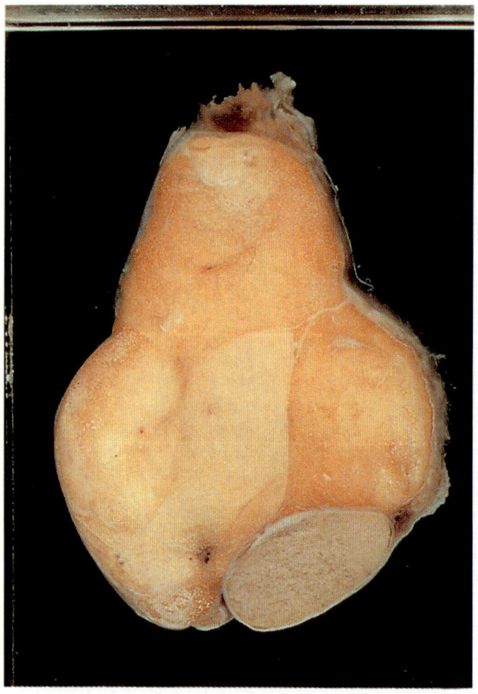

5.89 Spermatic Cord: Lipoma

This specimen was excised from a 62-year-old man who had noticed a soft, slowly-enlarging swelling in the scrotum for some time.

The testis and cord have been sectioned to show a well-circumscribed, lobulated tumour, composed of adipose tissue, situated in the lower cord and displacing the testis and epididymis downwards.

Lipomas of the spermatic cord are the most common paratesticular soft tissue tumour.

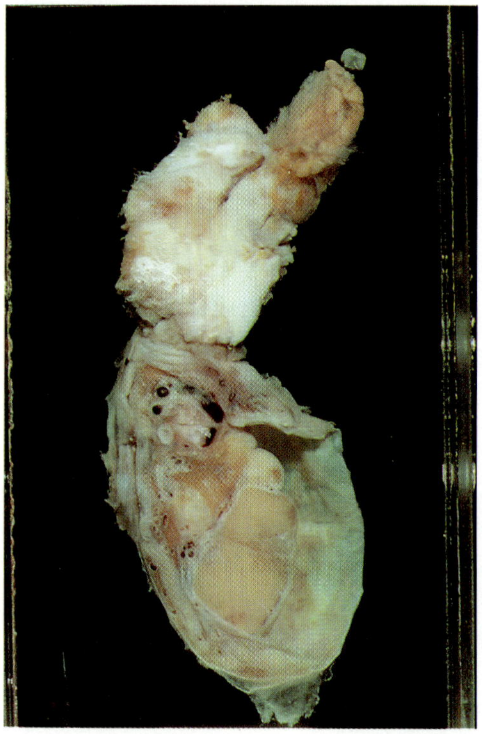

5.90 Spermatic Cord: Sclerosing Liposarcoma

This specimen was excised from a 70-year-old man who presented with an irreducible left inguinal hernia. On examination, there was a firm, partly mobile mass in the left spermatic cord.

The testis with part of the cord is shown. There is a hydrocele and the testis is somewhat atrophic. In addition, the lower part of the cord is replaced and surrounded by a dense mass of pale neoplastic tissue, measuring 3cm in diameter.

Liposarcoma of the spermatic cord is very rare but, like liposarcomas elsewhere, usually occurs in the elderly. Sclerosing liposarcoma is a variant of the well-differentiated group and, as such, is prone to local recurrence but very seldom metastasises.

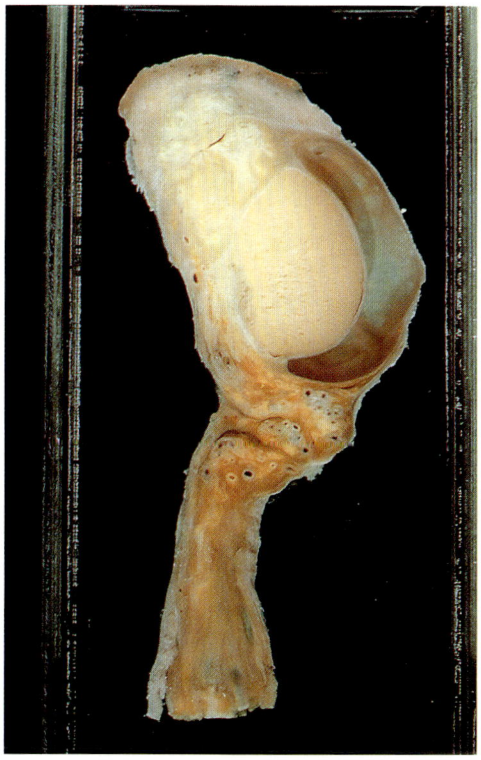

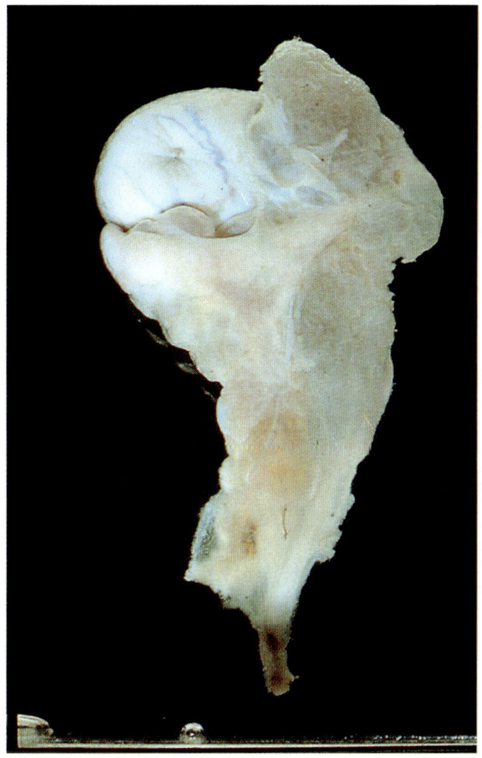

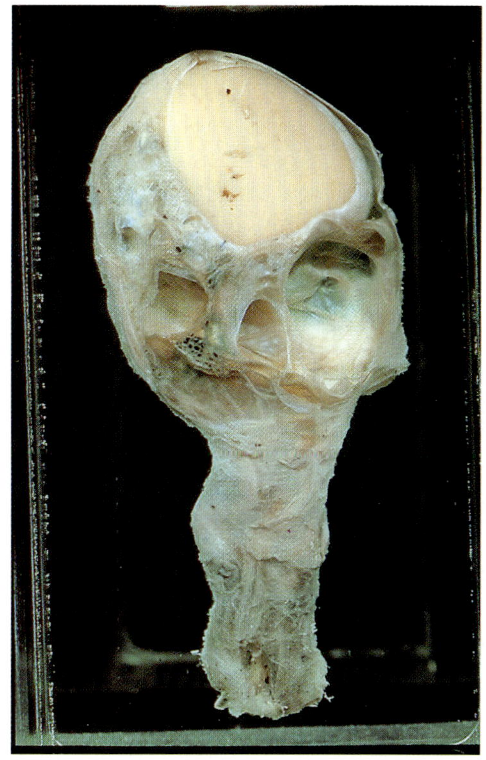

5.91 Epididymis: Tuberculous Epididymitis

This specimen was excised from a 28-year-old man who had noticed swelling of the testis for 12 months. He finally presented when the lesion burst, leaving a discharging scrotal sinus.

The testis has been sectioned to show a tuberculous cold abscess in the epididymis with adherence of the overlying tunica and scrotal skin (bottom right). The testis itself appears unaffected.

The majority of patients presenting with genital tuberculosis have primary tuberculous infection elsewhere, especially in the lungs. In males, infection of the prostate or seminal vesicles occurs due to haematogenous or urinary spread, from which retrograde spread to the epididymis may then follow. It is commonest in early adulthood and may sometimes be bilateral. Nowadays, with the incidence of tuberculosis declining in Caucasians, the painless irregular swelling may be mistaken for a testicular tumour.

5.92 Epididymis: Spermatocele

This was an incidental post-mortem finding in a 72-year-old man who died of a myocardial infarct.

The epididymis shows almost complete replacement by numerous thin-walled cysts, which contain pale, slightly turbid fluid. The testis appears small but is otherwise normal.

Spermatoceles are cysts containing spermatozoa which result either from distal obstruction or from aberrant blind-ending tubules. They are commonest in middle age and are never seen before puberty.

5.93 Epididymis: Inflamed Spermatocele

This specimen was excised from an 83-year-old man who had recently undergone prostatectomy for benign enlargement. He developed a painful swollen testis, which initially was thought to be due to acute orchitis.

The testis has been sectioned to show a multiloculated cyst in the epididymis, measuring 2cm in diameter. The cyst lining is focally congested. The compressed testis appears normal but is adherent to the lower margin of the cyst.

Haemorrhage or infection in any type of epididymal cyst is not uncommon; only if prolonged or particularly severe is testicular exploration warranted.

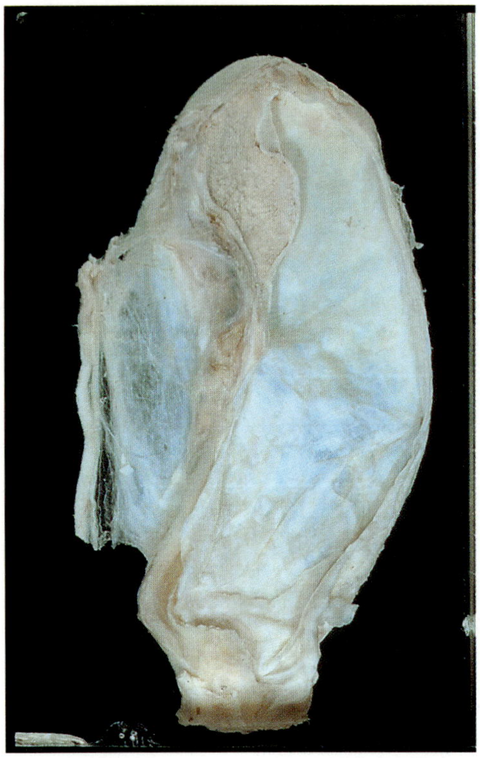

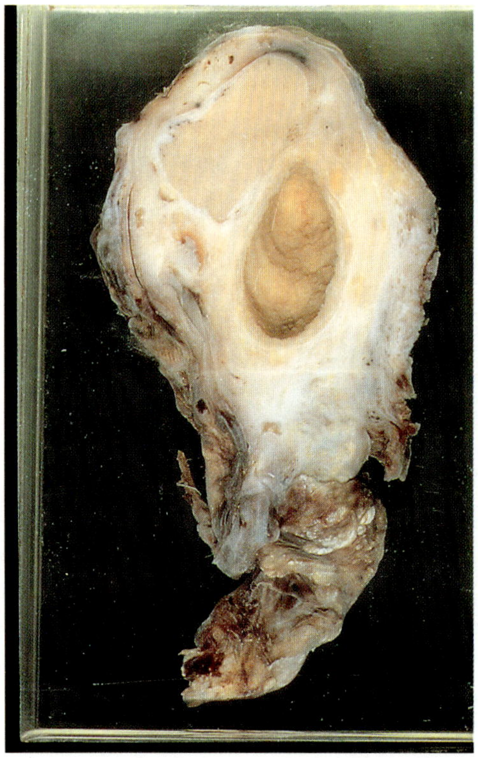

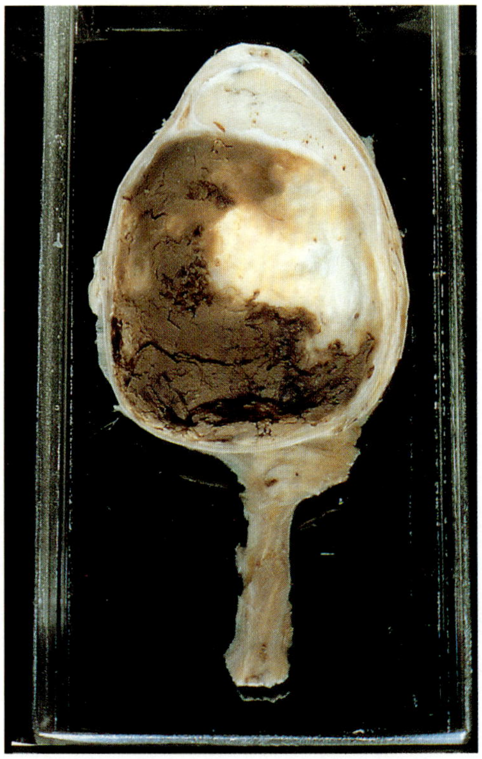

5.94 Tunica Vaginalis: Hydrocele

This was an incidental post-mortem finding in a 78-year-old man who died of bronchopneumonia.

The testis with its coverings has been sectioned to show marked distension of the tunica vaginalis to form a thin-walled sac, measuring 10cm in maximum diameter. The sac has a smooth lining and the testis (bottom centre) is atrophic.

A hydrocele represents a collection of fluid between the layers of the tunica vaginalis or within the processus vaginalis. Most are idiopathic in origin but some are thought to develop as a consequence of the peritoneal end of the processus failing to close. Hydroceles are common, usually occur in adulthood and may be bilateral. Inflammation or infection occasionally occurs and a degree of associated testicular atrophy is to be expected.

5.95 Tunica Vaginalis: Chronically Inflamed Hydrocele

This specimen was excised from a 58-year-old man who had a long-standing hydrocele which had been repeatedly tapped but had recently become swollen and tender.

The testis and epididymis have been sectioned to show a thick-walled abscess cavity in the position of the tunica vaginalis, measuring 3cm in diameter. The testis is compressed and rather atrophic.

Chronic hydroceles are particularly prone to infection if tapped. They may also be the presenting feature of underlying tuberculous or filarial epididymo-orchitis.

5.96 Tunica Vaginalis: Haematocele

No clinical details are available.

The testis has been bisected to show gross distension of the tunica vaginalis, which has a thickened fibrous wall and contains recent blood clot. The compressed testis is visible at the lower end of the sac.

A haematocele represents haemorrhage either into a previously normal tunica or into a hydrocele. It most often results from local trauma, but some cases appear to arise spontaneously and others may be the presenting feature of an underlying tumour.

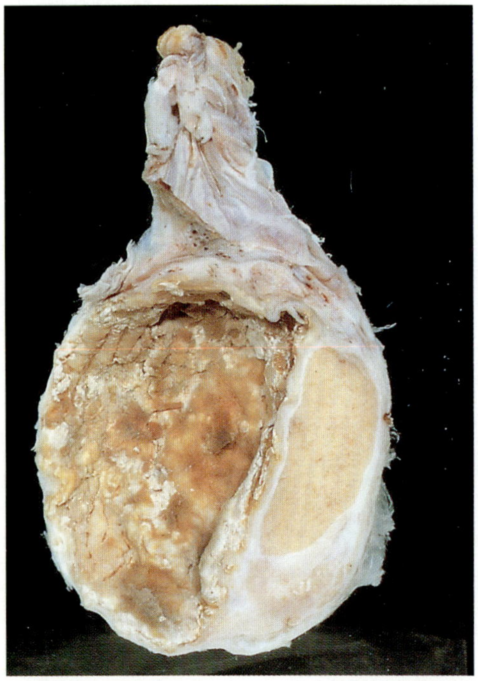

5.97 Tunica Vaginalis: Chronic Haematocele

This specimen was excised from a 44-year-old man who had noticed testicular swelling for the past 30 years, following a blow from a football. On examination, the testis was palpable at the back of a hard, opaque, non-fluctuant mass.

The testis has been sectioned to show marked thickening and dilatation of the tunica vaginalis. The walls of the sac are extensively calcified and there is adherent blood clot. The body of the testis and the fibrotic epididymis are compressed.

This is the typical appearance of a long-standing haematocele in which the blood clot has organised and the wall has undergone fibrosis and dystrophic calcification. Clinically the firmness and irregularity of such a lesion may easily be confused with a neoplasm.

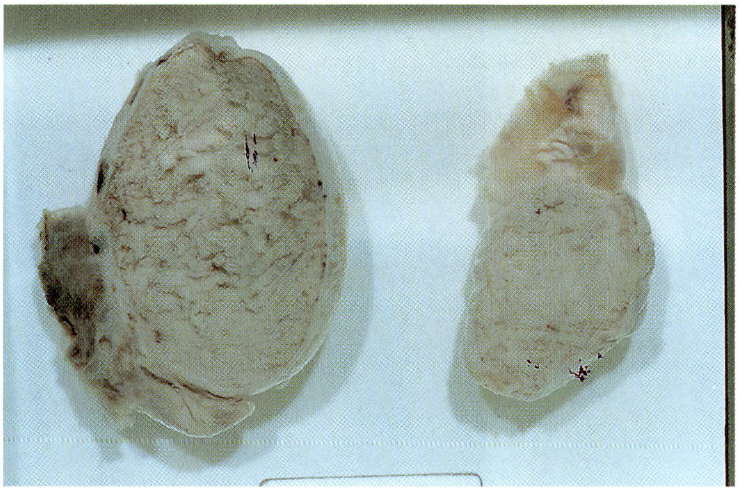

5.98 Testis: Maldescent

This was an incidental finding at post-mortem in a 69-year-old man who died of a cerebral haemorrhage. At autopsy the left side of the scrotum was noted to be empty and the corresponding testis was found in the left inguinal canal, at the head of a hernial sac.

Both testes have been sectioned to contrast the normal right testis with the imperfectly descended left one, which is markedly atrophic and appears rather fibrotic.

Testicular maldescent may be divided into either the more common arrest in the normal path or true ectopia. The incidence is about 4 per cent in male neonates and about 1 per cent in all males over the age of 1. The commonest sites of arrest in the normal path are high in the scrotum, the superficial inguinal pouch, the inguinal canal or within the abdomen. Ectopic sites include above the pubis, the femoral canal and above the inguinal ligament. If brought down into the scrotum by the age of 4-6 years, such testes can retain normal function. If left, the affected testis will fail to show spermatogenesis and there is an increased risk of developing a testicular neoplasm, most commonly a seminoma.

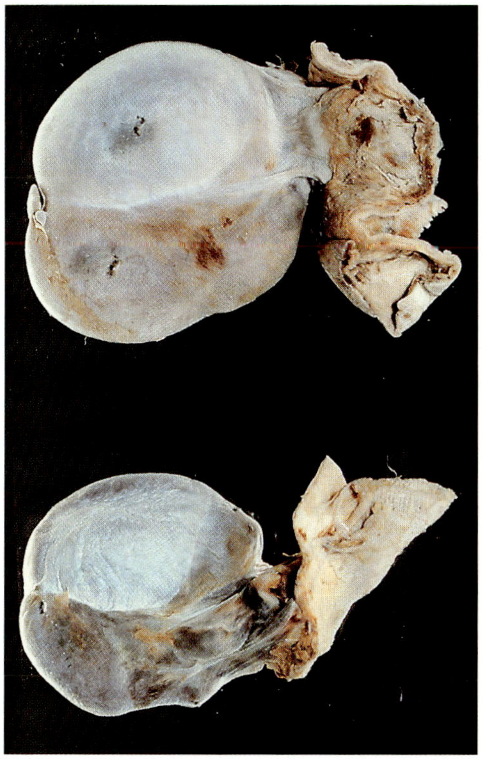

5.99 Testis: Torsion

No clinical details are available in either of these cases.

Complete torsion of the spermatic cord has resulted in intense haemorrhagic swelling of both these testes, both of which are infarcted.

Torsion of the spermatic cord most often occurs in adolescence and may sometimes be associated with local trauma. It is more common in testes having an elongated mesorchium or an abnormally inserted tunica vaginalis. If torsion is complete and remains untreated for 6 hours or more then infarction of the testis is likely to occur. Lesser degrees or shorter duration of torsion may give rise to ischaemic fibrosis or atrophy. The causative abnormality may sometimes be bilateral and there is, therefore, an increased risk of torsion on the unaffected side, leading some surgeons to perform bilateral orchidopexy at the outset.

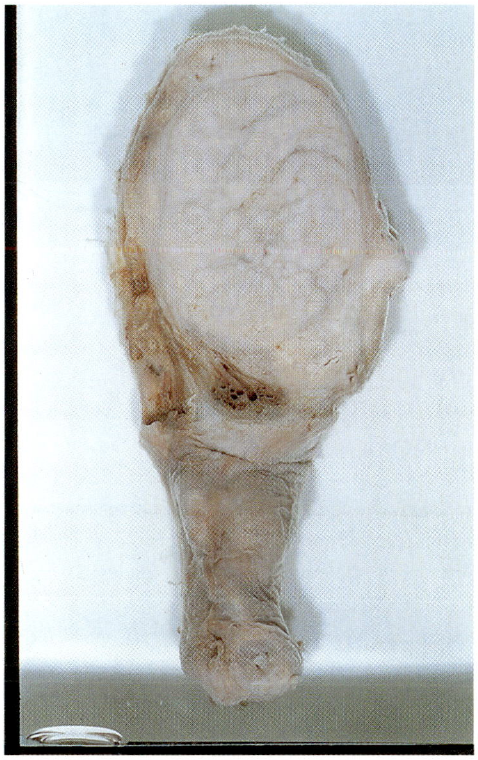

5.100 Testis: Tuberculous Epididymo-orchitis

This specimen was excised from a 59-year-old man who had long-standing pulmonary tuberculosis. He presented with a tense hydrocele and a discharging scrotal sinus.

The testis and cord have been sectioned to show total replacement of the body of the testis by caseous material. The adjacent epididymis is similarly involved and the skin sinus is apparent on the left.

This degree of testicular involvement is very unusual and is probably related to the long duration of infection in this case.

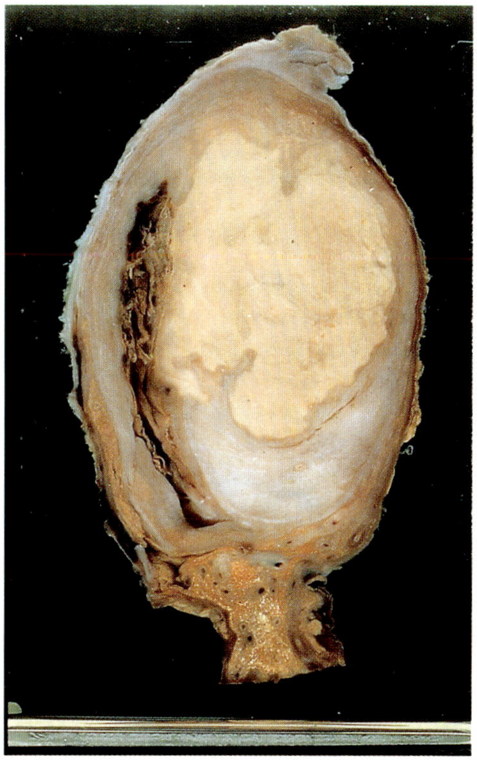

5.101 Testis: Syphilitic Gumma

No clinical details are available.

The testis has been sectioned to show diffuse fibrosis and enlargement, associated with an irregular, yellowish gummatous area involving the greater part of the organ. The tunica is thickened and fibrotic and on the right there is a haematocele containing recent blood clot.

Syphilitic infection of the testis may be congenital or acquired. Gummatous involvement represents the tertiary stage of infection and may rarely be complicated by scrotal involvement and sinus formation. It should be noted that, occasionally, tertiary infection is manifest only by diffuse fibrosis with no testicular enlargement.

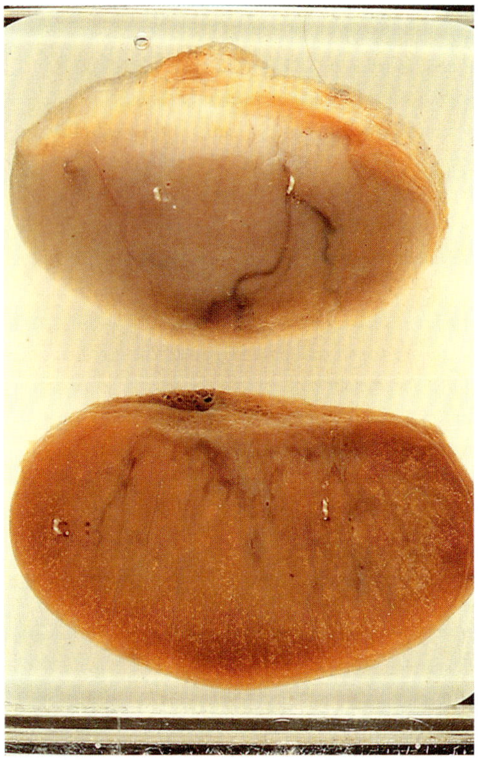

5.102 Testis: Mumps Orchitis

This specimen was excised from a 32-year-old man who had suffered a severe attack of mumps, complicated by orchitis, 4 months previously. Testicular enlargement persisted and excision was performed to exclude malignant disease.

The enlarged testis has been bisected and the cut surface shows loss of the normal structural pattern associated with numerous very small, pale areas of necrosis.

Orchitis may occur in up to 20 per cent of adult cases of mumps and the epididymis may also be involved. The condition is important since the necrosis and scarring may lead to infertility in many cases. The use of pre-operative modern serological techniques, not available in the case here, facilitates the avoidance of unnecessary orchidectomy.

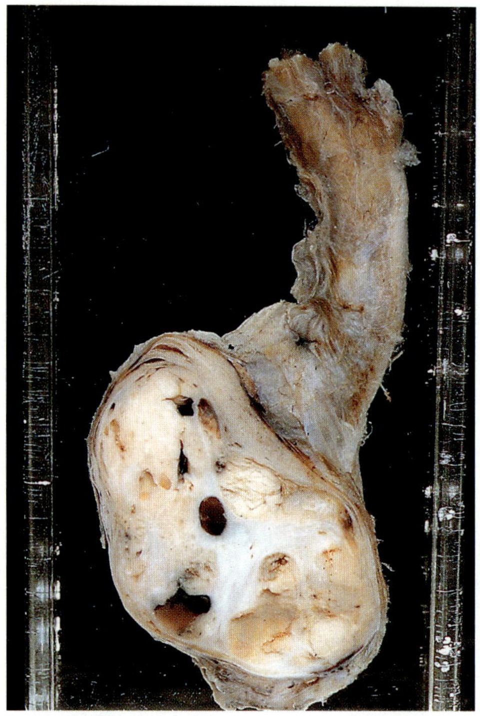

5.103 Testis: Seminoma

This specimen was excised from a 31-year-old man who had noticed gradual enlargement of the testicle for 6 months.

The testicle has been sectioned to show a pale solid ovoid tumour, measuring 4cm in diameter, which has replaced the entire body of the testis. The tumour shows rather more nodularity than is usual. The tunica vaginalis is closely adherent over most of the testis, the remaining space containing some recent blood clot. Note that the tumour has invaded the epididymis, a particular feature in seminomas.

Seminoma is the most common primary malignant tumour of the testis and arises most often in patients 30-40 years of age. It is classically a well-circumscribed tumour of uniform greyish-pink colour, which occasionally shows foci of necrosis but is only extremely rarely haemorrhagic. It spreads largely by lymphatics. These tumours are very radiosensitive such that 5-year-survival is now at least 95 per cent. Tumour staging and serum estimations of tumour markers, both pre- and post-operatively, are essential in the assessment of prognosis.

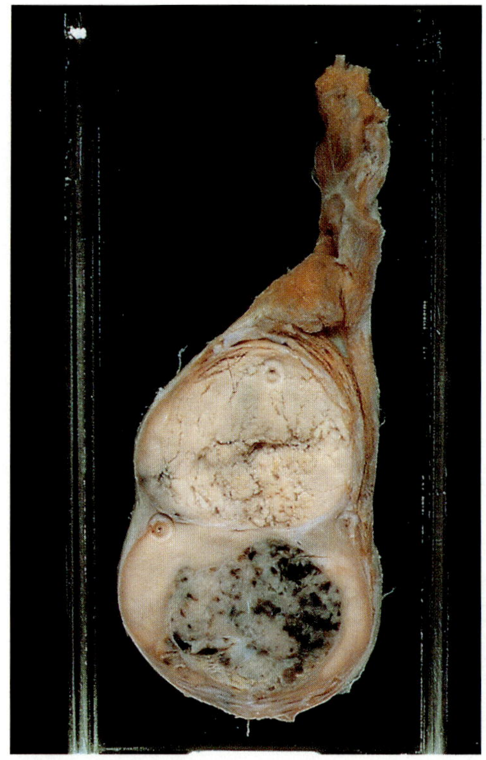

5.104 Testis: Teratoma with Seminoma

This specimen was excised from a 43-year-old man who presented with a 9 month history of painless enlargement of the testis.

The enlarged testis, measuring 9cm from upper to lower pole, has been sectioned to show a bilobed appearance, the upper part consisting of a pale, encapsulated mass while the lower part is largely replaced by haemorrhagic tumour.

The upper tumour shows the typical features of a seminoma, while the lower one is a teratoma showing both differentiated and malignant components. While seminomatous areas may be found in all teratomas other than the differentiated ones, they are usually very small and in this case it would appear, therefore, that these are two genuinely separate neoplasms. Such an occurrence is extremely rare and the prognosis would be that of the teratoma.

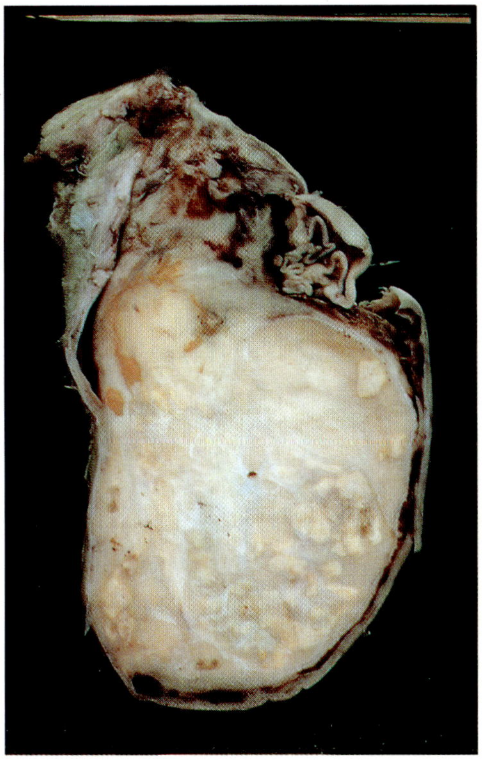

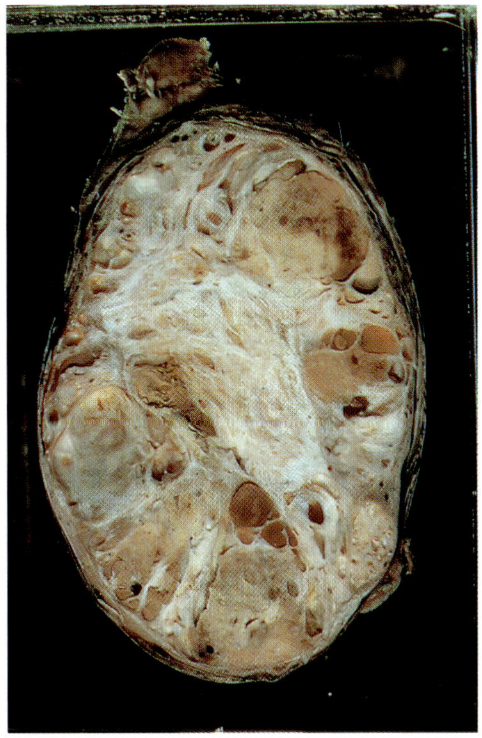

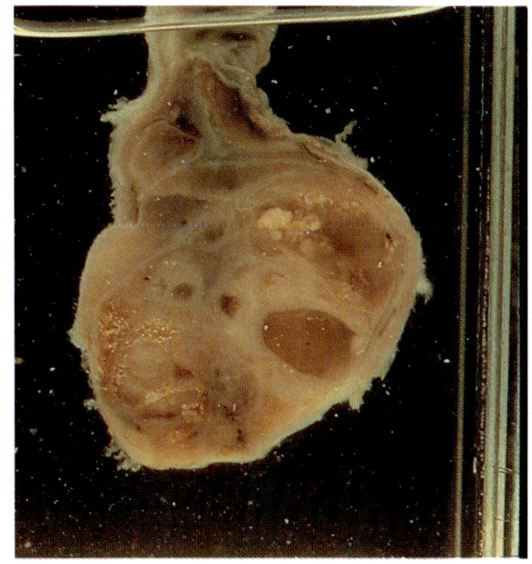

5.105 Testis: Malignant Teratoma Intermediate

This specimen was excised from a 27-year-old man who presented with a one month history of a painless swollen testis.

The testis is enlarged and contains a well-defined tumour, composed largely of solid pale tissue with cystic foci. There is a rim of residual normal testis at the upper pole and the cord shows no evidence of invasion.

In Britain, teratomas are divided into teratoma differentiated (TD), malignant teratoma intermediate (MTI), malignant teratoma undifferentiated (MTU), malignant teratoma trophoblastic (MTT). Teratomas account for about 30 per cent of primary testicular tumours and are most common in the 3rd decade. A small proportion arise in undescended testes. Spread is both lymphatic and haematogenous and the prognosis is related to the histological subtype, TD having the best prognosis and MTT the worst. At least 15 per cent of patients present with metastases, these usually being the more malignant tumours. Five-year-survival has improved dramatically in recent years with the addition of sophisticated chemotherapy to radiotherapy, and the figure quoted nowadays for MTI is about 55 per cent. Tumour markers may be of value in follow-up.

5.106 Testis: Malignant Teratoma Undifferentiated

No clinical details are available.

This grossly enlarged testis has been sectioned to show almost total replacement of the body by an ovoid tumour, measuring 10cm in maximum dimension. The tumour is partly cystic and partly solid and has invaded the spermatic cord.

MTU shows no differentiated or organoid areas but rather is composed of carcinomatous or sarcomatous tissue. MTU tends to present at a more advanced stage than MTI and 5-year-survival is of the order of 35 per cent.

5.107 Testis: Teratoma Differentiated

This specimen was excised from a 3-year-old boy who had been noticed to have an enlarged testis for 3 months.

The testis has been sectioned to show a well-circumscribed tumour, measuring 2cm in diameter, which has solid and cystic areas. There is no evidence of necrosis or haemorrhage. A rim of normal testicular tissue is apparent over the upper pole of the tumour.

Teratoma differentiated is typified by ectodermal, endodermal and mesodermal elements of many types, showing completely normal differentiation. It is most common in young children and carries much the best prognosis of all testicular teratomas, 5-year-survival being of the order of 95 per cent.

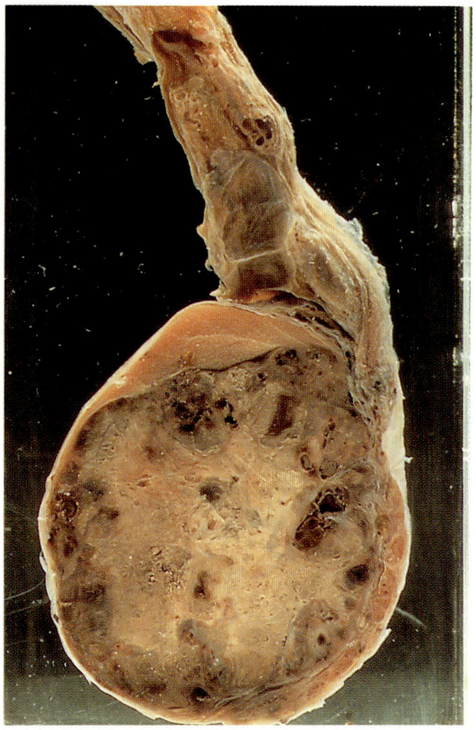

5.108 Testis: Malignant Teratoma Trophoblastic

This specimen was excised from a 28-year-old man who presented with haemoptysis and was found to have multiple pulmonary metastases. The enlarged testis was excised in the hope of retarding the course of the disease but he died 2 months later.

The testis has been sectioned to show a rounded, haemorrhagic and focally necrotic tumour, measuring 5cm in diameter.

This is the typical appearance of an MTT, also known as choriocarcinoma, which contains foci of syncytio- and cyto-trophoblast located within any of the histological subtypes of teratoma already mentioned. It constitutes the smallest subset of testicular teratomas but carries the worst prognosis, although with modern multimodal therapy the survival rate is constantly improving.

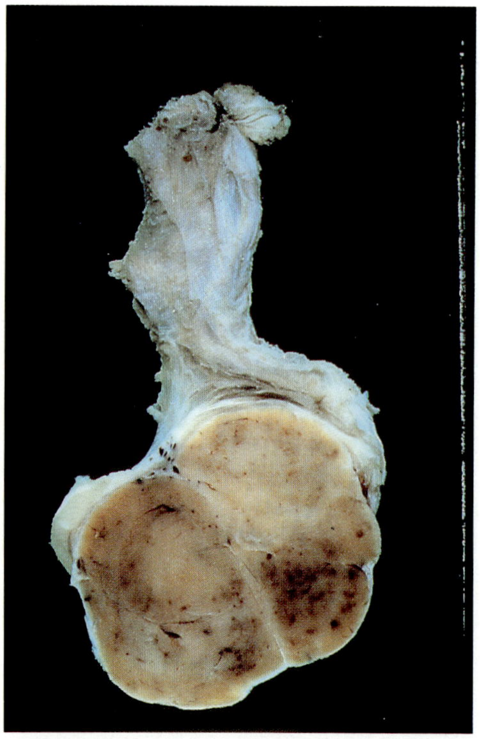

5.109 Testis: Leydig Cell Tumour

This specimen was excised from a 12-year-old boy. At the age of 6 he had required psychiatric treatment for aggressive behaviour. At the age of 8 he showed signs of precocious puberty. Eventually enlargement of the right testis became manifest and the urinary oxosteroid concentration was grossly elevated.

The testis has been sectioned to show virtual replacement by a classically well-circumscribed, solid yellow-brown tumour measuring 3cm in diameter.

Leydig (interstitial) cell tumours account for about 2 per cent of testicular neoplasms and are most common in adulthood. Younger patients, as in this case, almost invariably have endocrine abnormalities, in particular precocious puberty. In adults, symptoms of feminisation, especially gynaecomastia, are more common. The majority of these tumours run a benign course, but up to 10 per cent metastasise. Criteria for recognising the malignant subgroup are, unfortunately, imprecise.

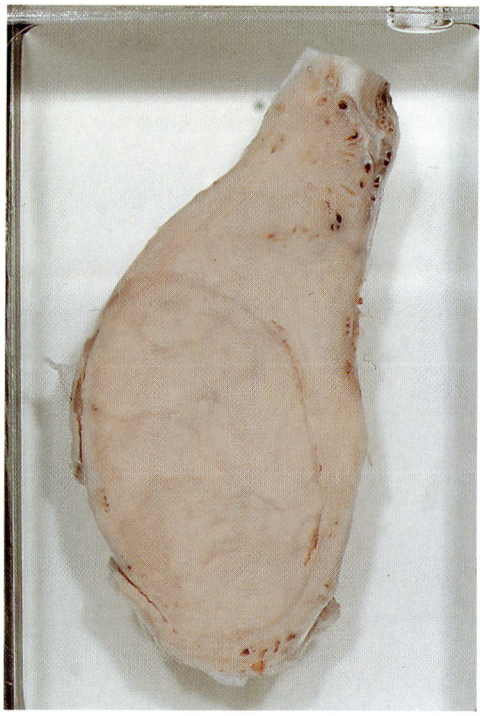

5.110 Testis: Non-Hodgkin's Lymphoma

This specimen was excised from a 69-year-old man who presented with a 6 month history of painless testicular enlargement. On examination the testis was smoothly enlarged with a coincident hydrocele, and the epididymis and distal spermatic cord were hard and enlarged.

The enlarged testis, epididymis and lower end of the spermatic cord have been sectioned to show total replacement by a pale diffuse neoplasm.

Primary malignant lymphoma of the testis is not uncommon but metastatic involvement by a disseminated lymphoreticular neoplasm is more frequent. Primary tumours arise most often in elderly males and there may be bilateral involvement. The most common histological type is poorly-differentiated non-Hodgkin's lymphoma: Hodgkin's disease of the testis is extremely rare. The prognosis in general is very poor. It should be noted here that leukaemic patients, particularly children, very often show testicular infiltration.

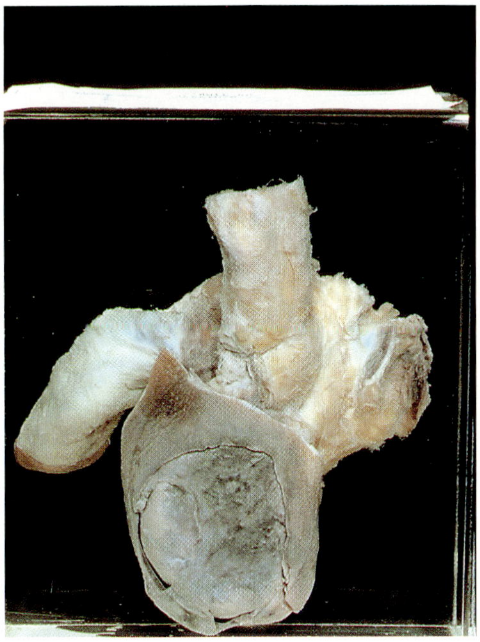

5.111 Scrotum: Fournier's Gangrene

This is a post-mortem specimen from a 67-year-old man who had an inoperable carcinoma of the sigmoid colon invading the pelvic wall and bladder. Shortly after an exploratory laparotomy the scrotum became swollen, painful and ulcerated: the condition spread rapidly but the patient died suddenly of a pulmonary embolism.

The penis and scrotum have been partially dissected to show a swollen haemorrhagic testis lying within the necrotic oedematous scrotum.

Fournier's gangrene is extremely rare and usually occurs in adults. Gangrenous necrosis spreads rapidly from the scrotum through adjacent peritesticular and perineal soft tissues, sometimes affecting the penis. It is thought to arise as a consequence of vascular thrombosis followed by invasion of the overlying tissues by anaerobic organisms, particularly *Bacteroides fragilis*. Even with modern antibiotics, some cases are fatal due to endotoxaemia.

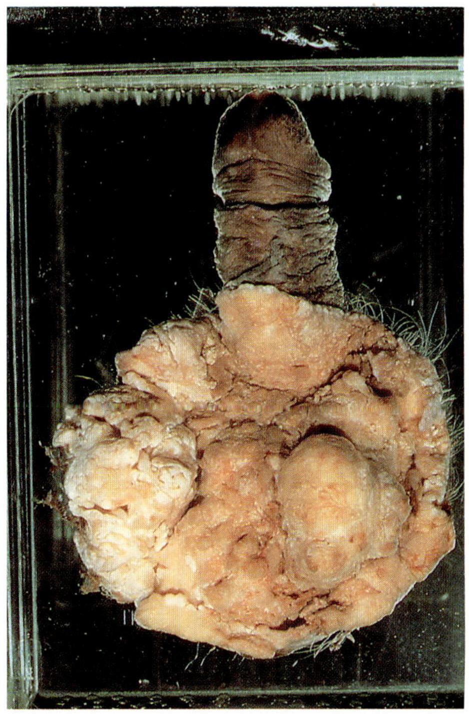

5.112 Scrotum: Squamous Carcinoma

This specimen was excised from a 63-year-old man who had noticed scrotal ulceration for 18 months before consulting a doctor. He had worked with pitch for 24 years.

The scrotum is destroyed by a large ulcerated neoplasm which has extended to involve the base of the penis. On the right, a testis and epididymis are visible but are encased in tumour.

Carcinoma of the scrotum is very uncommon but has become famous since Percival Pott recognised its frequency in chimney sweeps in 1775, the first example of occupational cancer. It occurs in elderly males and currently those at risk due to their occupation include workers with mineral oil, tar or pitch. It is thought that rugosity of the scrotal skin, by making adequate cleaning difficult, allows prolonged contact with any carcinogen. These tumours frequently ulcerate and it may be difficult to distinguish between reactive and metastatic inguinal lymphadenopathy. Spread is virtually confined to lymphatics and in general the prognosis is quite good.

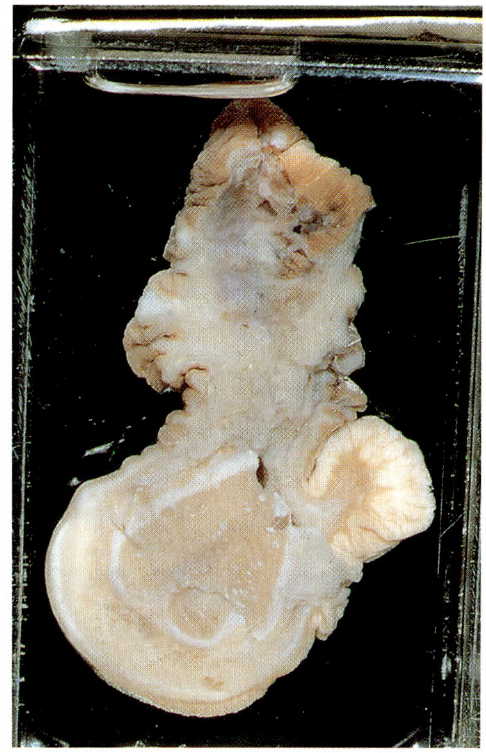

5.113 Penis: Condyloma Acuminatum

This specimen was excised from a 50-year-old man who had noticed a warty nodule on the glans penis, which had been present for 1 month and had rapidly increased in size. A mistaken diagnosis of carcinoma was made and a partial penile amputation performed.

The amputation specimen has been bisected parasagittally to show a warty, papilliferous lesion, measuring 2.5 × 2 × 1cm, projecting from the surface of the glans. The lesion is well demarcated and shows no evidence of infiltration.

Condylomata acuminata (viral warts) of the penis are common and are due to infection with human papillomavirus. They are more common in young adults and are probably sexually acquired. They are usually quite small and typically develop over a short period of time. Extremely rarely, progression to squamous carcinoma may occur.

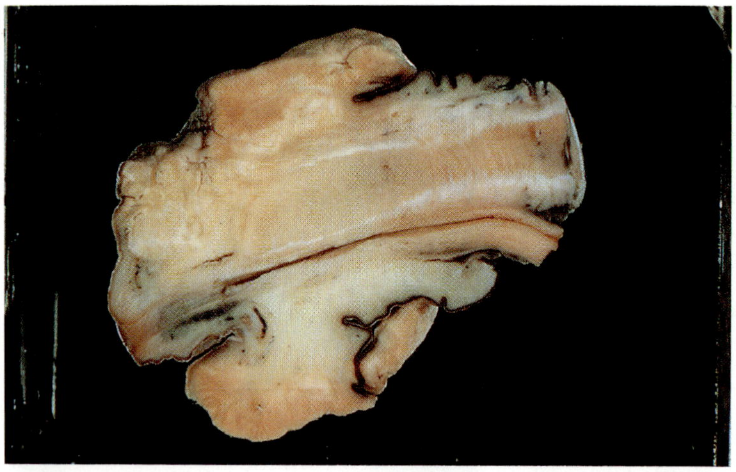

5.114 Penis: Squamous Carcinoma

This specimen was excised from a 32-year-old African, who had a past history of gonorrhoea and syphilis, and presented with an 8 month history of a penile growth. Partial penile amputation and radiotherapy were carried out and the patient was clinically free of tumour 2½ years later.

The amputation specimen has been bisected to show a large fungating mass involving the glans and prepuce.

In the Western world, carcinoma of the penis is uncommon but in parts of the Far East and Africa it is one of the commonest malignancies in males. It is virtually confined to uncircumcised men and known predisposing conditions include Bowen's disease, erythroplasia of Queyrat and balanitis xerotica obliterans. Typically the lesions are fungating and may become infected but spread tends to be delayed by the penile fascia.

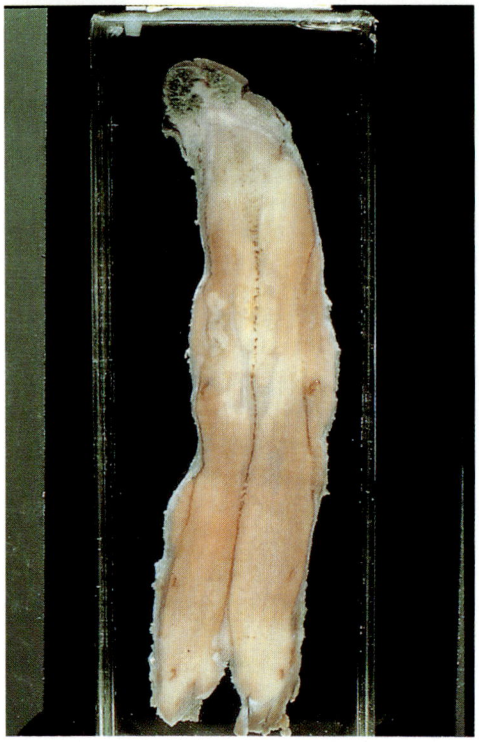

5.115 Penis: Leiomyosarcoma

This specimen was excised from a 32-year-old West Indian who had noticed a gradual thickening at the base of the penis. Urethroscopy revealed an annular growth half way along the cavernous urethra and penile amputation was performed.

The penis has been bisected in the coronal plane to show diffuse infiltration of the corpora cavernosa by a pale, yellowish neoplasm. The urethra has been opened to demonstrate an area of stricture formation.

While malignant soft tissue tumours of the penis are very rare, leiomyosarcoma is one of the commonest. It most often arises in the penile shaft and is usually of comparatively low grade, tending principally to local recurrence only.

6. ENDOCRINE SYSTEM

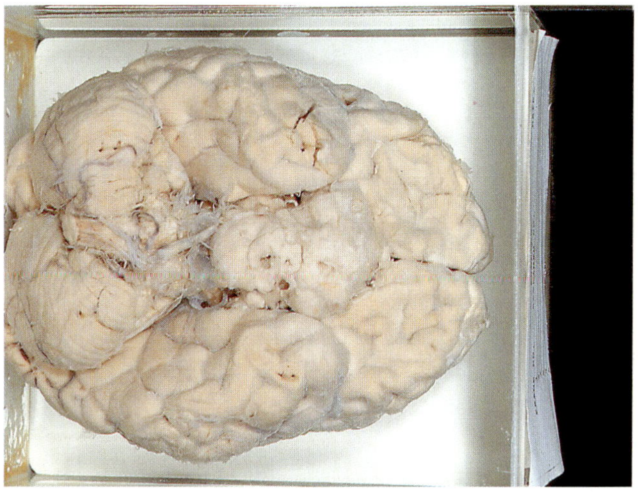

6.1 Base of Brain: Craniopharyngioma

This is a post-mortem specimen from a 72-year-old blind, diabetic female who died suddenly at home.

The base of the brain is shown and, arising adjacent to the pituitary gland, there is a large, pale multinodular tumour extending over the inferior surface of both frontal lobes. The optic tracts and pituitary gland are compressed above the tumour and are therefore not visible.

Craniopharyngiomas are most often suprasellar and are said to arise from Rathke's pouch, a derivative of the stomatodaeum, from which the anterior pituitary develops. They may be found at all ages but are commonest in childhood. They are slow growing and may present due to pressure either on the optic tracts or pituitary. Histologically they are very similar to oral ameloblastomas and calcification of these tumours is common.

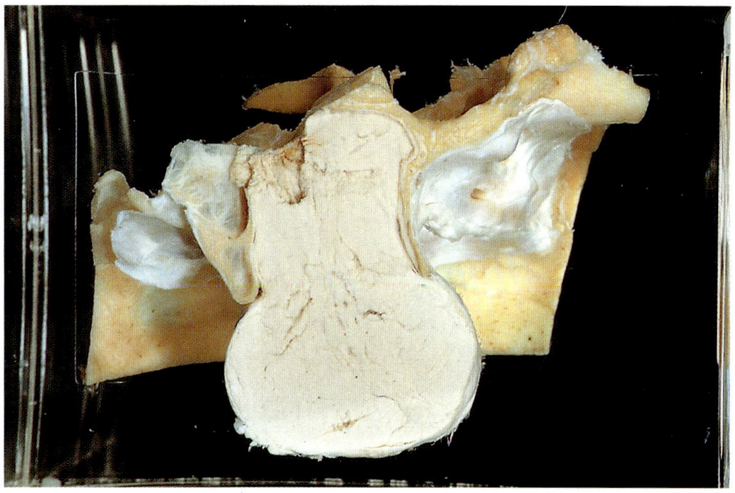

6.2 Pituitary: Acidophil Adenoma

This is a post-mortem specimen from a 41-year-old woman with long-standing acromegaly and amenorrhoea, who latterly became blind and developed diabetes insipidus. Finally she died of pneumonia.

This a sagittal section through the base of the skull and pituitary gland. The pituitary is markedly enlarged measuring 5 × 4 × 4cm, and forms a rounded projection into the cranial cavity. The tumour is enclosed in a fibrous capsule and the pituitary fossa is expanded.

About one-third of pituitary adenomas are composed of acidophils, the cells which normally secrete growth hormone and prolactin. They may arise at any age and are usually small, the case here being unusually large. As a result of their increased hormone production these tumours may present with gigantism, acromegaly, amenorrhoea or galactorrhoea. In the case described here, blindness and diabetes insipidus most probably resulted from the pressure effects on the optic chiasma and posterior pituitary, respectively.

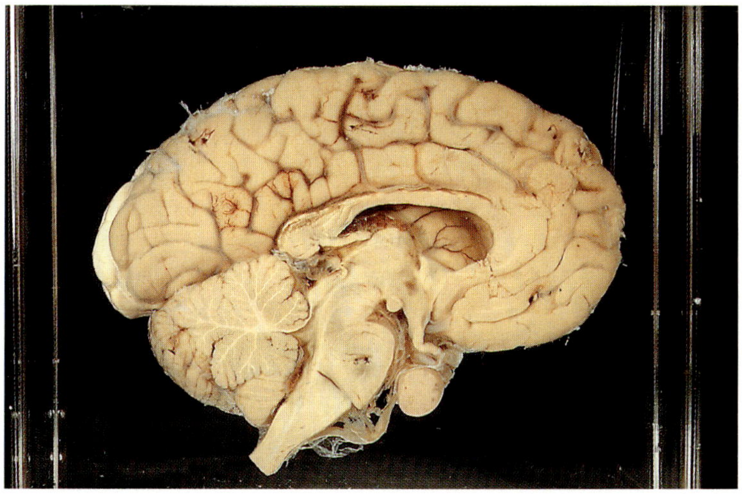

6.3 Pituitary: Acidophil Adenoma

This is a post-mortem specimen from a 64-year-old woman who presented with a 2 year history of visual disturbance and occipital headaches. She was found to be grossly acromegalic and to have a fasting blood glucose of 15mmol/l with a severely abnormal glucose tolerance curve. Over the succeeding 2 years she developed severe congestive cardiac failure and persistent hyperglycaemia, unresponsive to insulin. She became comatose and died.

A sagittal section through the brain shows a well-demarcated, rounded, pituitary tumour, anterior to the mid-brain, which measures 1.5cm in diameter.

Since growth hormone antagonises the actions of insulin by inhibiting glucose uptake and stimulating lipolysis, patients with acromegaly commonly have impaired glucose tolerance and up to 50 per cent of such cases may develop frank diabetes mellitus. Congestive cardiac failure associated with cardiomegaly is also a frequent feature of acromegaly.

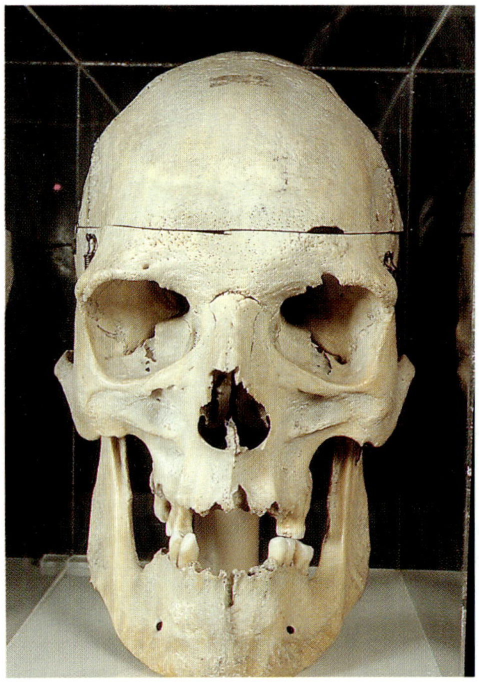

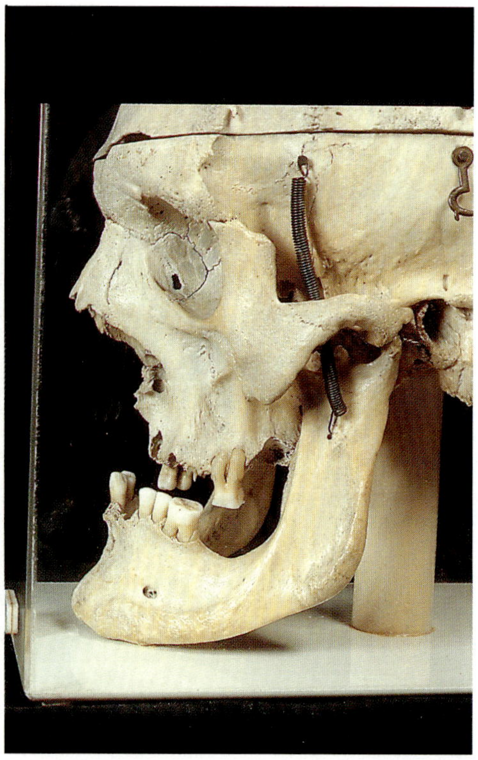

6.4 Skull: Acromegaly

This specimen was obtained from a man with proven long-standing acromegaly.

The vertical measurement of the face is markedly increased (6.4a) with lengthening of the superior maxillae and rami of the lower jaw. There is bony thickening of the upper orbital margins, lateral angular processes and zygomatic arches. In the lateral view (6.4b), note the marked prognathism which results in dental malocclusion.

The facial changes in acromegaly result from enlargement of soft tissues and cartilaginous structures, associated with irregular osteoblastic activity which leads to bony thickening. Note that there is only an increase in the patient's height if there is excessive growth hormone secretion prior to epiphyseal fusion (gigantism).

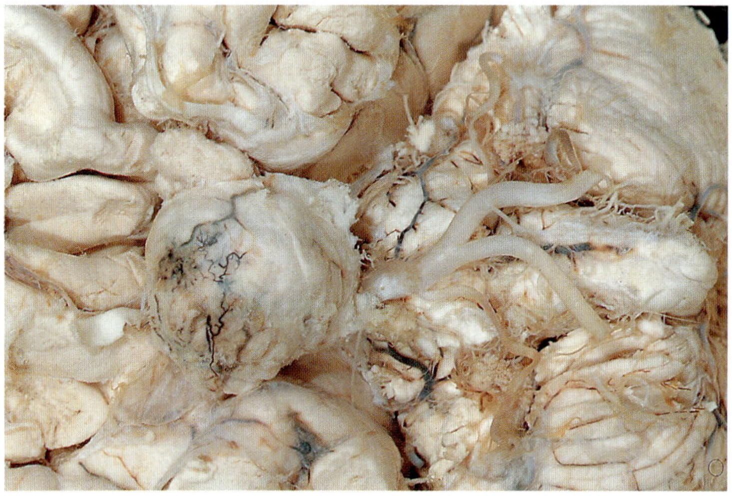

6.5 Pituitary: Chromophobe Adenoma

This was an incidental finding at post-mortem in a 53-year-old woman who committed suicide. She also was found to have multiple intracranial meningiomas.

Attached to the base of the brain is a large smooth tumour, measuring 2.5cm in diameter, which is impinging on the optic chiasma.

About 60 per cent of pituitary adenomas are derived from chromophobe cells and, as such, these form the commonest group of pituitary tumours. Chromophobe cells are thought to represent actively secreting, and therefore degranulated, cells. These tumours commonly attain a large size giving rise to pressure effects; the hormone that they most often produce is prolactin leading to sterility in either sex, and amenorrhoea with or without galactorrhoea in females. Occasionally these neoplasms undergo cystic change or calcification. It should be noted here that basophil adenomas, which may give rise to Cushing's disease, are rare and are usually so small as to be undetectable macroscopically.

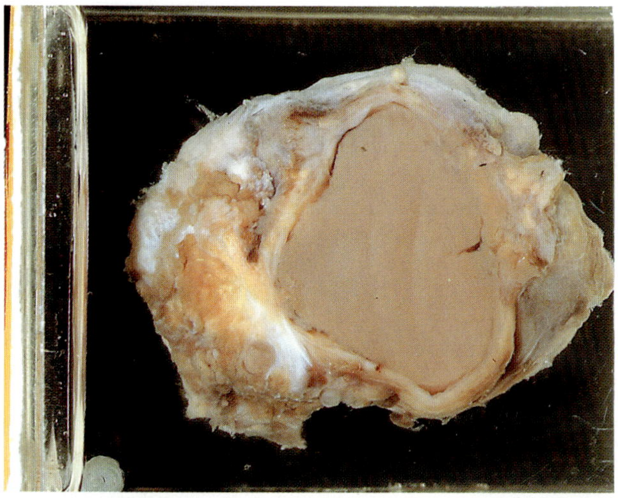

6.6 Hyoid Bone: Thyroglossal Cyst

This specimen was excised from a 58-year-old man who had noted a slowly enlarging swelling in the mid-line beneath his chin for 13 years. At operation the lesion was found to extend both posterior to the thyroid cartilage and upwards into the hyoid bone.

A portion of the hyoid bone (top) is shown to which is attached a unilocular, thick-walled cyst measuring 4cm in diameter. The cavity of the cyst contains blood clot.

A thyroglossal cyst represents a remnant of the thyroglossal duct along which the thyroid migrates embryologically from the base of the tongue. Such cysts are most often found close to the hyoid bone in the mid-line of the neck and they may occasionally contain vestigial thyroid follicles.

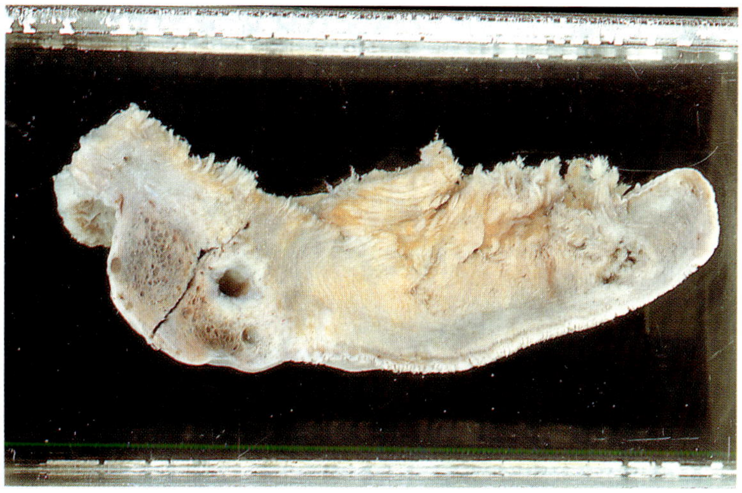

6.7 Tongue: Aberrant Thyroid Tissue

This was an incidental finding at post-mortem in a 69-year-old man who died of a cerebral haemorrhage.

This is a sagittal section through the tongue which shows a smooth, ovoid swelling, measuring 2cm in diameter, projecting from the posterior third. Within the mass numerous small and large cysts with surrounding reddish-brown thyroid tissue are apparent.

This is an example of the so-called lingual thyroid and represents ectopic thyroid tissue remaining at the foramen caecum from whence the thyroid gland is derived. Ectopic thyroid tissue may be found at any site along the course of the thyroglossal duct and occasionally this represents the sole source of thyroid hormone in the absence of a normally located gland.

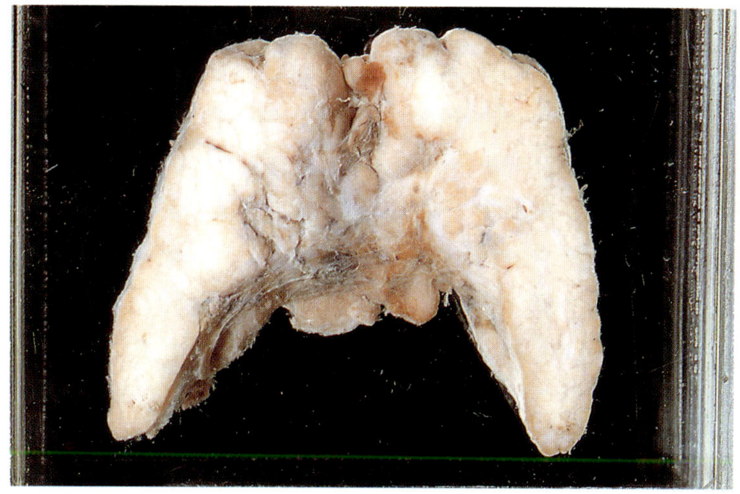

6.8 Thyroid: Hashimoto's Disease

This specimen was excised from a 69-year-old woman who had noticed a gradually enlarging mass in the neck for 9 years. The mass was firm, simulating a carcinoma, and there were no symptoms of altered thyroid function.

The thyroid is grossly enlarged, weighing nearly 3 times the normal size (normal 15-30g). It has a pale, irregularly nodular appearance and macroscopically appears to contain little colloid.

Hashimoto's disease represents a chronic autoimmune thyroiditis and most often presents in the 4th and 5th decades, predominantly in females. This condition is closely related to Graves' disease and antibodies to thyroglobulin and a microsomal antigen are commonly found. There may be other coexistent autoimmune conditions, for example, pernicious anaemia or Addison's disease. Up to 50 per cent of cases may develop myxoedema as a consequence of extensive fibrosis.

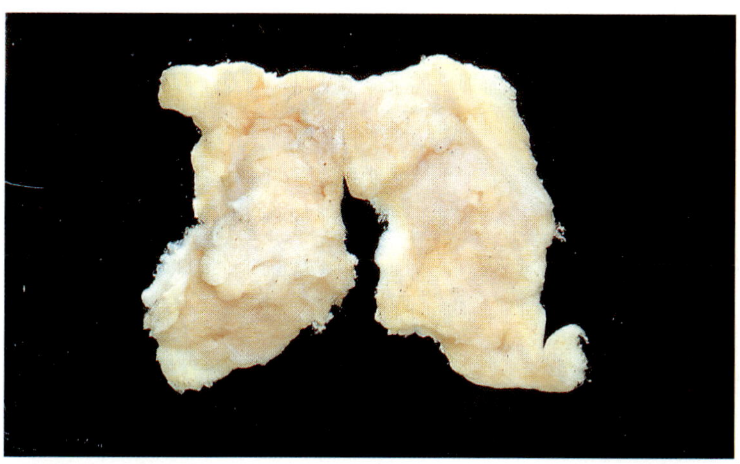

6.9 Thyroid: Myxoedema

This was an incidental post-mortem finding in a 66-year-old woman who died of carcinomatosis of the breast. There was no evidence of pituitary metastasis at autopsy.

The thyroid has retained its normal shape but is atrophic and virtually replaced by fibrous tissue. No colloid is apparent.

Myxoedema in adults is most often due to chronic autoimmune thyroiditis and probably represents an exaggerated form of Hashimoto's disease. Women are predominantly affected and there may be associated congestive cardiac failure, extensive atheroma and other autoimmune diseases. Other causes of myxoedema include an end-stage toxic goitre, iodine deficiency, ablation by surgery or radiotherapy and genetic dyshormonogenesis.

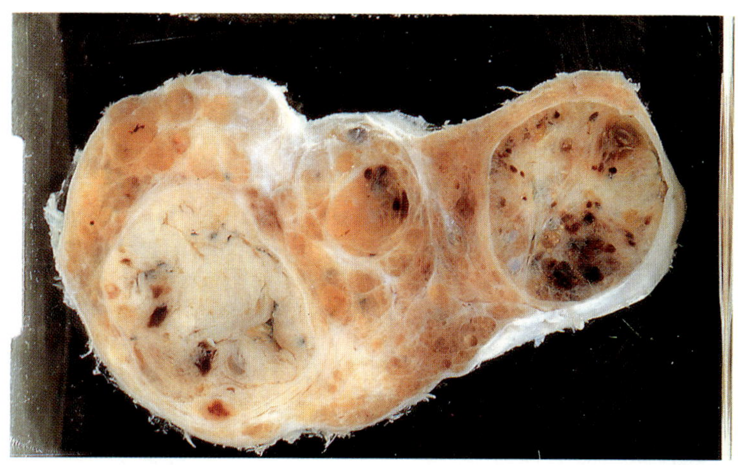

6.10 Thyroid: Multinodular Goitre

No clinical details are available.

This is one of the lateral lobes of a thyroid gland which has been sectioned to show multiple, well-circumscribed nodules of varying size and appearance, measuring up to 3cm in diameter. Note the irregular bands of fibrosis and foci of cystic change.

A multinodular goitre represents the commonest form of thyroid disease and is simply the end-stage of a diffuse non-toxic goitre. Non-toxic goitres may be endemic, usually due to iodine deficiency, or sporadic, due to a combination of environmental (e.g. excessive ingestion of Brassicas or neck irradiation in childhood) and genetic factors (e.g. dyshormonogenesis or abnormalities of thyroxine-binding globulin) with or without iodine deficiency. TSH stimulation leads to diffuse parenchymal hyperplasia but with time, colloid nodules representing foci of involution appear thus giving rise to the mixed pattern seen here. Such patients are usually euthyroid but occasionally nodules may autonomously secrete excessive thyroid hormone, leading to Plummer's syndrome (see Legend 6.15). A very small proportion of cases may develop carcinoma in a multinodular goitre, particularly in endemic areas.

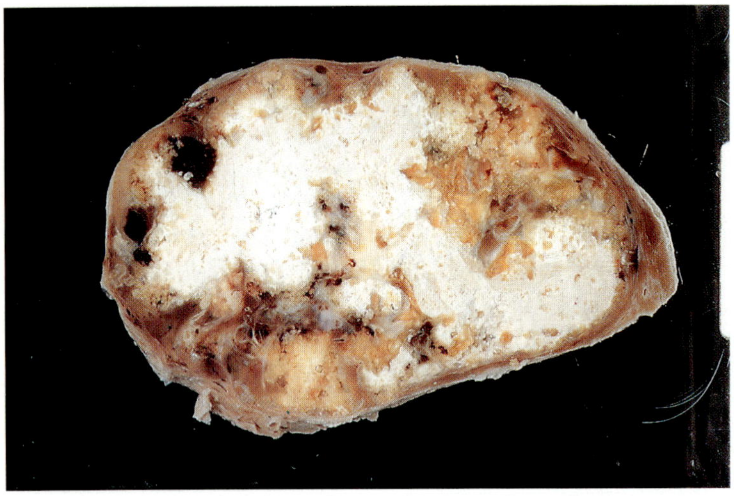

6.11 Thyroid: Calcified Goitre

This was an incidental finding at post-mortem in a 75-year-old man who died of a myocardial infarct.

The thyroid, which was irregularly enlarged, has been sectioned to show extensive replacement of the parenchyma by dense calcified tissue. There are also foci of haemorrhage and a thin rim of normal thyroid tissue remains (bottom).

Dystrophic calcification is a common feature in multinodular goitres and usually occurs at the site of either extensive scarring or haemorrhage. However, calcification occurring to this degree is extremely rare.

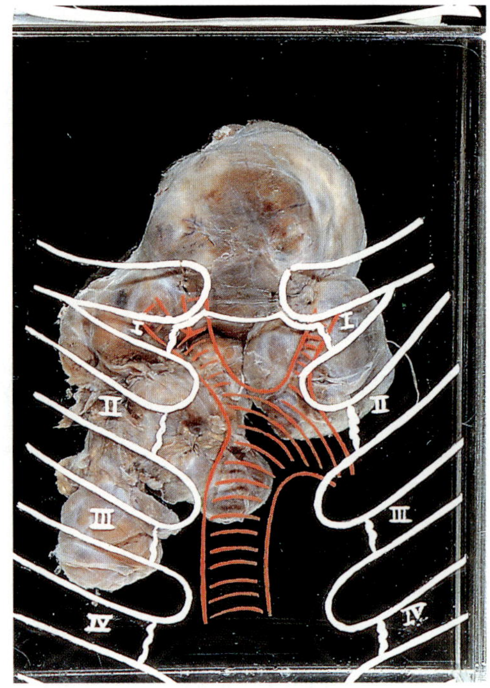

6.12 Thyroid: Retrosternal Multinodular Goitre

No clinical details are available.

This thyroid gland is grossly and asymmetrically enlarged with a coarsely multinodular appearance. At operation this goitre was largely retrosternal and an outline of the sternum, ribs and arch of the aorta have been superimposed to demonstrate its anatomical relations.

This case serves to demonstrate the very large size that multinodular goitres may attain, particularly in endemic areas. Retrosternal extension, or particularly large goitres in the neck, may lead to distortion of the trachea with resultant dyspnoea or even stridor.

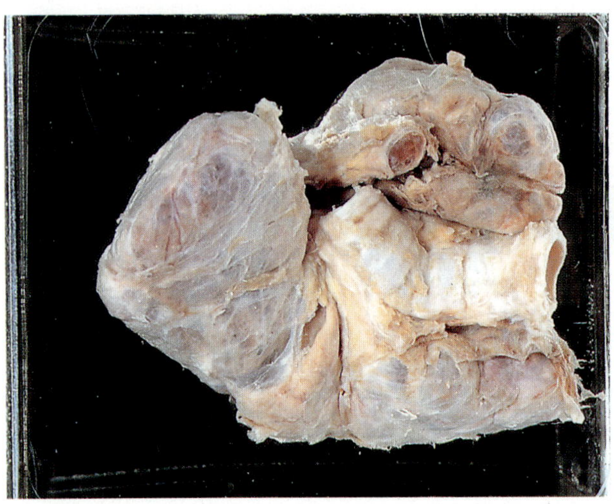

6.13 Thyroid: Multinodular Goitre causing Tracheal Compression

This was an incidental finding at post-mortem in an 83-year-old woman. Much of the goitre was intrathoracic.

The thyroid shows gross multinodular enlargement, most particularly of the left lobe. The trachea has been irregularly compressed on both sides but, surprisingly, has remained patent.

It is not hard to appreciate that a goitre such as this could lead to marked respiratory difficulty.

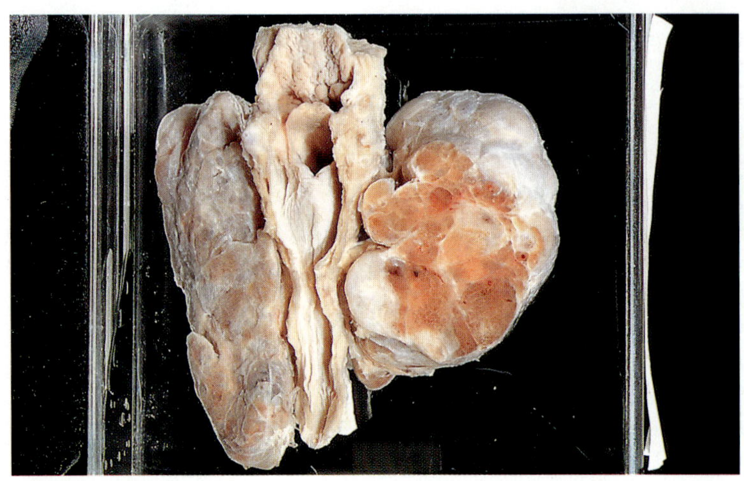

6.14 Thyroid: Multinodular Goitre causing Oesophageal Compression

This was an incidental finding at post-mortem in an 81-year-old woman who died following a fractured neck of femur.

This large multinodular goitre has encircled the trachea and is compressing the oesophagus posteriorly.

Dysphagia resulting from a large goitre, while less common than a degree of respiratory obstruction, is well recognised.

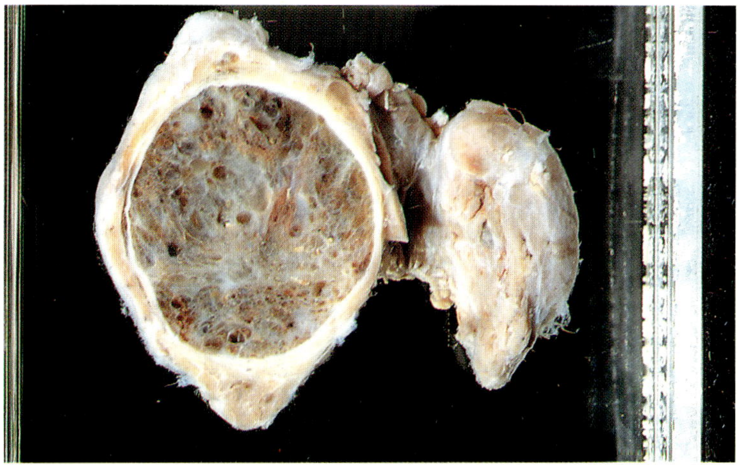

6.15 Thyroid: Plummer's Disease

This specimen was excised from a 56-year-old woman who had a non-toxic goitre for 14 years. In the last 2 years she developed florid thyrotoxicosis and the right lobe of the thyroid increased in size.

Within this normal-sized, rather nodular thyroid gland is a large solitary, well-circumscribed lesion, measuring 5cm in diameter.

Plummer's disease may represent either the development of an autonomous toxic nodule in a multinodular goitre or simply a toxic adenoma in the absence of any other thyroid disease. Differentiation between the two is sometimes only possible by histological examination of thyroid tissue away from the toxic nodule.

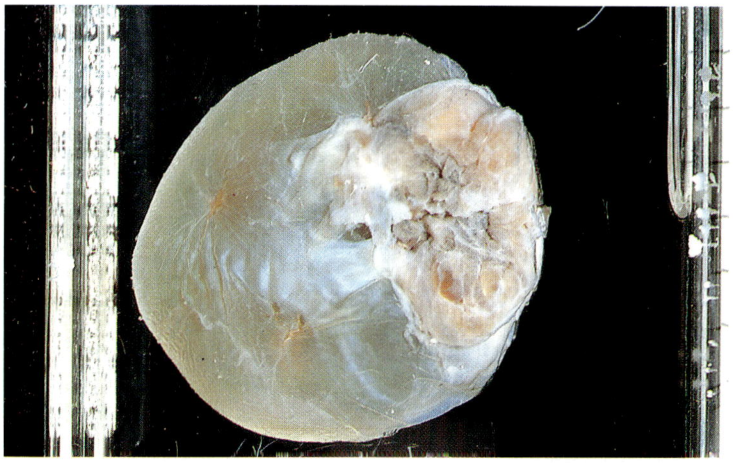

6.16 Thyroid: Simple Cyst

This specimen was excised from a 46-year-old woman who had noticed a swelling in the neck for 3 years which was not responsive to Lugol's iodine. The remainder of the thyroid gland appeared normal at operation.

The cyst is translucent and thin-walled, measuring 5cm in diameter. On the right there is a fragment of normal thyroid tissue excised with the cyst.

Cysts in the thyroid gland are common and most often represent a part of a multinodular goitre. Solitary cysts, within an apparently normal gland, may represent degeneration of a follicular adenoma (see Legend 6.21). Clinically they may cause confusion when presenting as a solitary cold nodule in the thyroid.

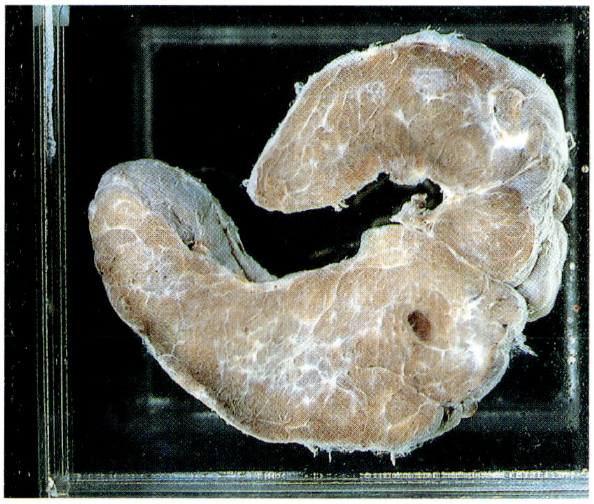

6.17 Thyroid: Graves' Disease

This specimen was excised from a 22-year-old man who presented with weight loss, tremor, excessive sweating and exophthalmos. He had noticed these symptoms for one year, during the course of which his neck had gradually become swollen.

The thyroid is greatly enlarged, most particularly on the left, and weighed 378g in the fresh state. The cut surface is uniform, with no nodularity, and has a rather 'beefy' appearance. This degree of enlargement is unusual in Graves' disease.

Graves' disease, or diffuse toxic goitre, affects mainly young adults, particularly females. The condition is autoimmune in origin, the most important autoantibodies being those which mimic the action of TSH (previously known as long-acting thyroid stimulator, LATS). Antibodies to thyroglobulin and a microsomal antigen may also be found, as in Hashimoto's disease. In true Graves' disease, ophthalmopathy is very commonly present and there may be associated thymic and lymph node enlargement, pretibial myxoedema and neutropenia. The action of LATS leads to unopposed thyroid hormone production and thus thyrotoxicosis. Histologically, the presence of foci more typical of Hashimoto's disease should raise the possibility of post-operative hypothyroidism in cases treated by subtotal thyroidectomy.

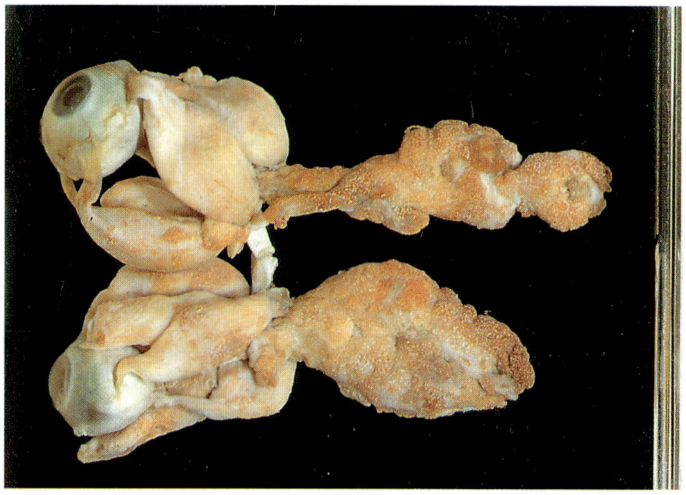

6.18 Eyes: 'Malignant' Exophthalmos

This is a post-mortem specimen from a 74-year-old man who developed rapidly progressive exophthalmos and died of an intercurrent infection.

The orbital contents show tense swelling with a marked increase in volume of the soft tissues and extra-ocular muscles. The resulting forward displacement of the globes has led to inflammation of the sclerae.

Exophthalmos in Graves' disease is thought to be due to a separate but specific autoantibody which binds to extraocular soft tissues and leads to the local production of excessive mucopolysaccharides with an associated inflammatory response. Alternatively, some believe it is a consequence of the deposition of immune complexes (antithyroglobulin bound to thyroglobulin). Most often it takes only a mild form of slow onset but severe cases, such as the one here, are well recognised.

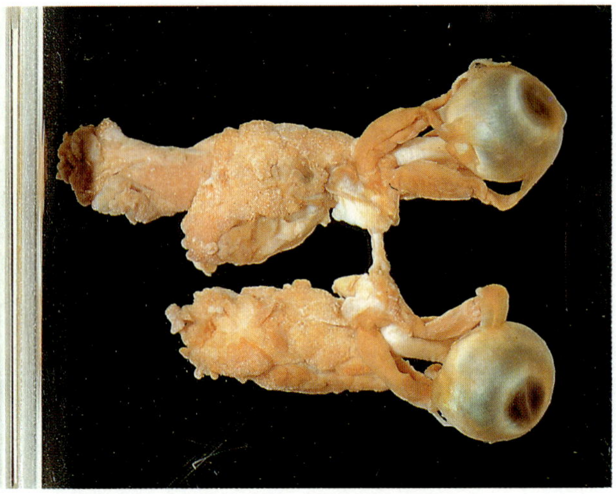

6.19 Eyes: Apparent 'False' Exophthalmos

This is a post-mortem specimen from a 54-year-old woman who died of congestive cardiac failure while awaiting thyroidectomy. She had suffered from long-standing thyrotoxicosis with marked lid retraction.

The orbital contents show a relatively normal appearance and are mounted for comparison with Legend 6.18.

Lid retraction or lid lag, commonly seen in thyrotoxicosis, may be easily mistaken for true exophthalmos.

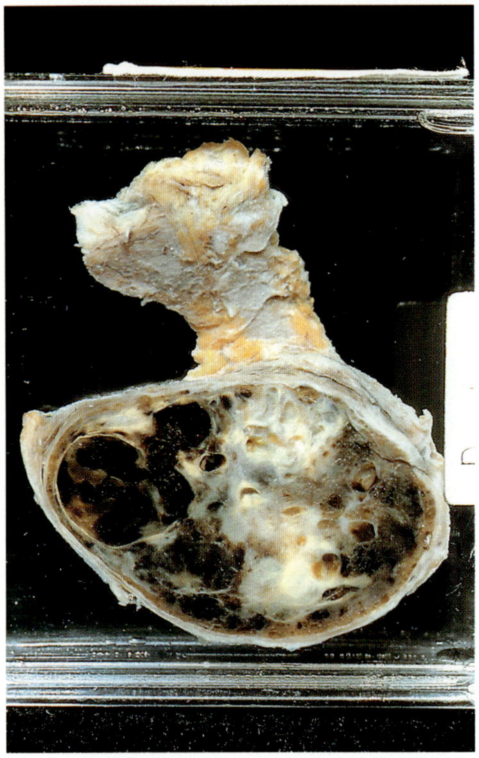

6.20 Thyroid: Solitary Adenoma

This was an incidental finding at post-mortem in an elderly woman who died of cor pulmonale.

The majority of the thyroid gland appears normal but, in the left lobe, there is a large, well-circumscribed mass, measuring 6cm in maximum diameter, into which there has been extensive haemorrhage.

Adenomas of the thyroid gland may arise asymptomatically at any age in up to 15 per cent of the normal population and can only be reliably recognised either in the absence of a multinodular goitre or by showing a distinctive histological pattern. Their complications are similar to those of a colloid nodule within a multinodular goitre, including hyperfunction, degenerative changes and the occasional development of carcinoma.

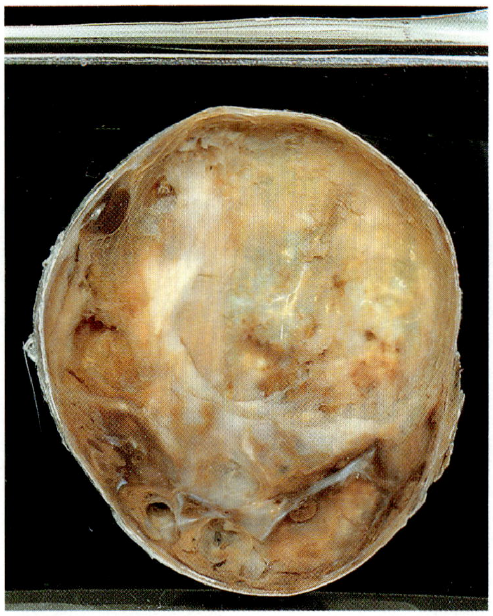

6.21 Thyroid: Adenoma with Cystic Degeneration

This specimen was excised from a 62-year-old woman who had non-toxic enlargement of the thyroid for 40 years. The thyroid had increased in size in recent years and, at operation, this lesion in the right lobe was found to be displacing the larynx laterally.

The tumour is rounded and encapsulated, measuring 9cm in maximum diameter. At the lower pole, traces of the original adenoma are apparent but the remainder has undergone extensive cystic degeneration. Note also foci of previous haemorrhage.

Adenomas of the thyroid are particularly prone to degenerative changes, including haemorrhage, cyst formation and dystrophic calcification. As such, taken in isolation, they may be difficult to differentiate from a nodule within a goitre.

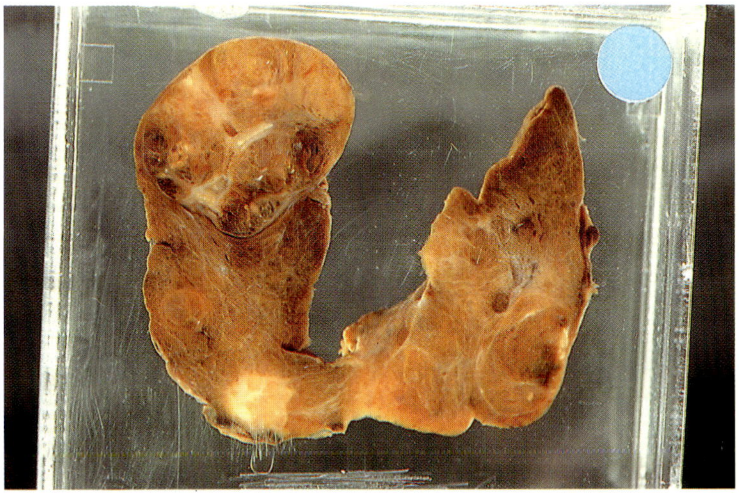

6.22 Thyroid: Papillary Carcinoma

This specimen was excised from a 54-year-old woman who presented with a 6 month history of a mass just above the manubrium sterni. Examination revealed right-sided cervical lymphadenopathy and a biopsy specimen was diagnosed as papillary carcinoma. A thyroidectomy was performed.

A section through the thyroid gland reveals a small, whitish tumour, with irregular margins, situated in the lower pole of the left lobe. In addition, the cut surface of the thyroid has a multinodular appearance and there are foci of cystic change.

Papillary carcinoma is by far the commonest malignant tumour of the thyroid, accounting for about 65 per cent of such neoplasms. It is commonest in the 3rd and 4th decades and shows a marked predilection for females. Some cases are aetiologically related to previous irradiation of the head and neck region in childhood. It is not uncommon for cervical lymph node metastases to become apparent before the primary tumour, as in this case, and because of the usually well-differentiated histological appearances, such deposits were often erroneously labelled 'lateral aberrant thyroid' in the past. From the microscopical point of view it should, however, be noted that *any* thyroid neoplasm showing a papillary pattern (even if only focally) should be regarded as malignant. Papillary carcinoma tends to rather indolent lymphatic spread and 5-year-survival is at least 90 per cent: younger age at presentation confers a prognostic advantage. (Courtesy of St. Bartholomew's Hospital Medical School Museum)

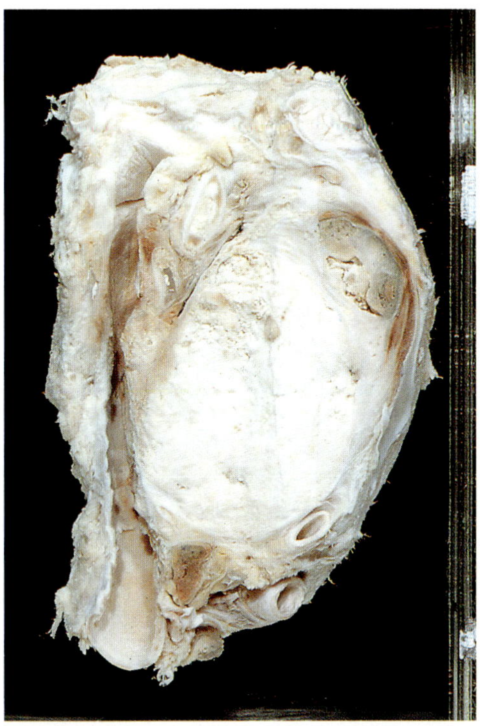

6.23 Thyroid: Follicular Carcinoma

This is a post-mortem specimen from a 67-year-old woman who had a known goitre for about 30 years. Latterly, it had increased markedly in size and at operation the tumour was found to be inoperable. She died post-operatively.

A sagittal section through the larynx, trachea and thyroid shows that the bulk of the thyroid gland is replaced by a rounded, pale neoplasm, measuring 7.5cm in diameter. There is extensive infiltration of adjacent soft tissues and the anterior tracheal wall, resulting in considerable tracheal stenosis.

Follicular carcinoma accounts for about 25 per cent of primary malignant tumours of the thyroid. Middle-aged adults, predominantly females, are most often affected. These tumours may be divided into an encapsulated micro-invasive group and a macroscopically obviously invasive group, the latter carrying a worse prognosis. In general, follicular carcinomas tend to haematogenous spread and the overall 5-year-survival is of the order of 60 per cent.

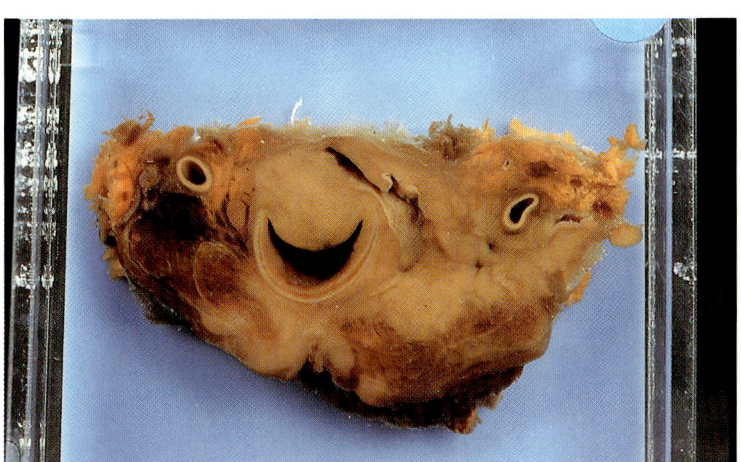

6.24 Thyroid: Anaplastic Carcinoma

This is a post-mortem specimen from a 76-year-old man who had noticed a lump in the neck only 10 weeks previously. Thereafter he developed rapidly progressive hoarseness, dyspnoea and dysphagia and he died. At autopsy the tumour extended from the right clavicle to the hyoid bone and there were metastases in cervical lymph nodes, the mediastinum, both lungs, the liver, heart and adrenals.

A horizontal section through the thyroid, trachea and both carotid arteries shows massive, irregular replacement of the thyroid gland by a pale, ill-defined, infiltrative neoplasm. The trachea is invaded posteriorly and the right carotid artery is grossly distorted.

Approximately 10 per cent of thyroid carcinomas are anaplastic in nature; these tumours arise almost exclusively in the elderly and extensive local invasion, as in this case, is characteristic. The prognosis is generally appalling, the average survival being about 6 months. (Courtesy of St. Bartholomew's Hospital Medical School Museum)

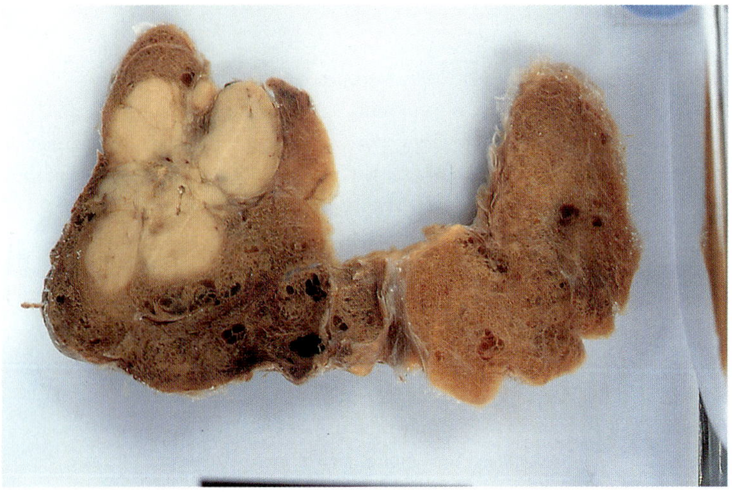

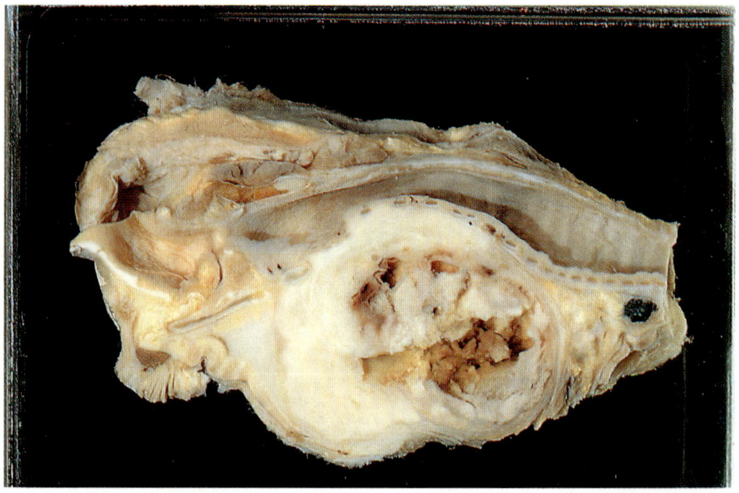

6.25 Thyroid: Medullary Carcinoma

This specimen was excised from a 61-year-old man who had noticed a swelling in the neck for the previous 10 months. A thyroidectomy was performed.

Within the right lobe of the thyroid there is a fairly well-circumscribed, pale, oval tumour which is partly encapsulated.

Medullary carcinoma of the thyroid is derived from parafollicular 'C' (calcitonin-secreting) cells and constitutes rather less than 10 per cent of primary thyroid malignancies. It is therefore a neuro-endocrine tumour of the APUD system and up to 15 per cent of cases are familial. These latter have an autosomal dominant inheritance and may form part of the Type II Multiple Endocrine Neoplasia (Sipple) syndrome. The 5-year-survival is about 50 per cent. (Courtesy of St. Bartholomew's Hospital Medical School Museum)

6.26 Thyroid: Squamous Carcinoma

No clinical details are available.

A sagittal section through the larynx, trachea and thyroid gland shows an irregular, pale tumour, measuring 5cm in diameter, arising in the thyroid and displacing the trachea posteriorly. The tumour, which shows central necrosis, is infiltrating adjacent soft tissues and the anterior wall of the trachea.

Squamous carcinoma of the thyroid is very rare and may represent either malignant change in a vestigial remnant of the ultimobranchial body or extensive metaplasia in a poorly-differentiated follicular or papillary carcinoma.

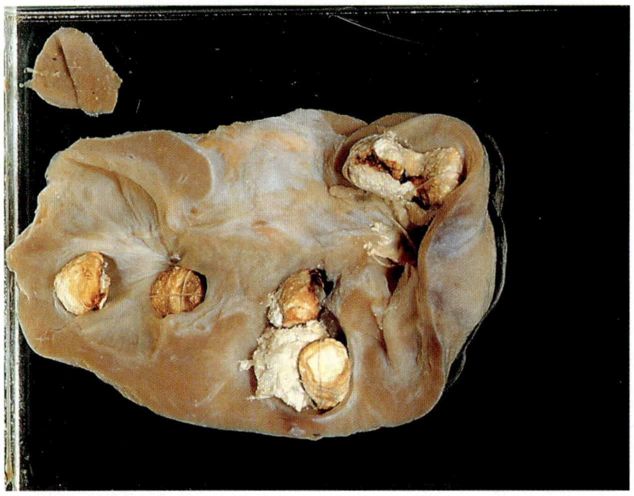

6.27 Parathyroid: Adenoma with Renal Calculi

These are post-mortem specimens from a 50-year-old woman who died in chronic renal failure. Three years previously she had a calculus removed from the left kidney. At autopsy, in addition to the parathyroid tumour, there was bilateral pyonephrosis with staghorn calculi.

On the left is an enlarged parathyroid gland, measuring 3 × 2 × 2cm and weighing 10g. On the right, one of the kidneys is mounted and shows intrarenal hydronephrosis, fragments of a staghorn calculus and extensive parenchymal scarring.

A parathyroid adenoma is much the commonest cause of hyperparathyroidism, accounting for at least 80 per cent of cases. Other causes include primary parathyroid hyperplasia, tertiary hyperparathyroidism, parathyroid carcinoma and ectopic production of parathyroid hormone by other tumours, particularly renal adenocarcinoma and bronchial carcinoma.

Parathyroid adenomas present most commonly in middle age and are more frequent in females than males. They are most often found in the lower parathyroid glands and show great variation in size, the average weight being between 2-10g (normal adult parathyroid 30mg). In general, larger tumours give rise to more severe hyperparathyroidism with consequently more marked bone involvement and hypercalcaemia. Elevated parathyroid hormone levels, by increasing osteoclastic activity in bone and tubular reabsorption of calcium in the kidney, may give rise to nephrocalcinosis or nephrolithiasis, the latter being seen here. Excessive bone resorption gives rise to changes known as osteitis fibrosa cystica or von Recklinghausen's disease of bone. This is typified by rarefaction of bone, destruction with cyst formation and cortical erosions (particularly in the phalanges).

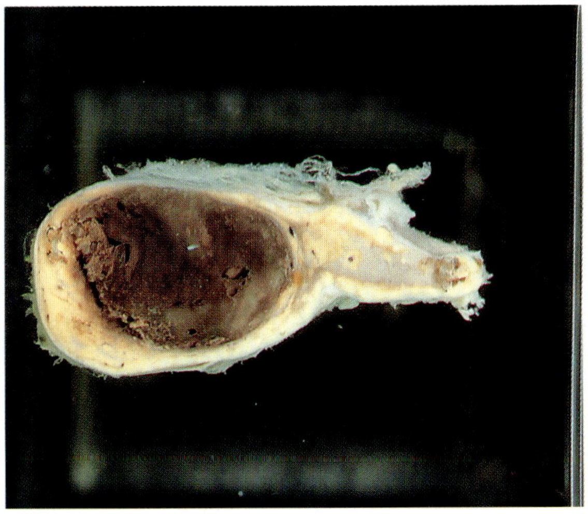

6.28 Adrenal: Medullary 'Haemorrhage'

No clinical details are available.

A section through this adrenal gland shows extensive haemorrhage into the medulla with complete sparing of the cortex.

Pure medullary haemorrhage with cortical sparing is exceptionally rare since even medullary vein thrombosis will lead to some cortical involvement. It seems far more likely that this specimen represents the effects of haemorrhage into a medullary tumour, most likely a phaeochromocytoma.

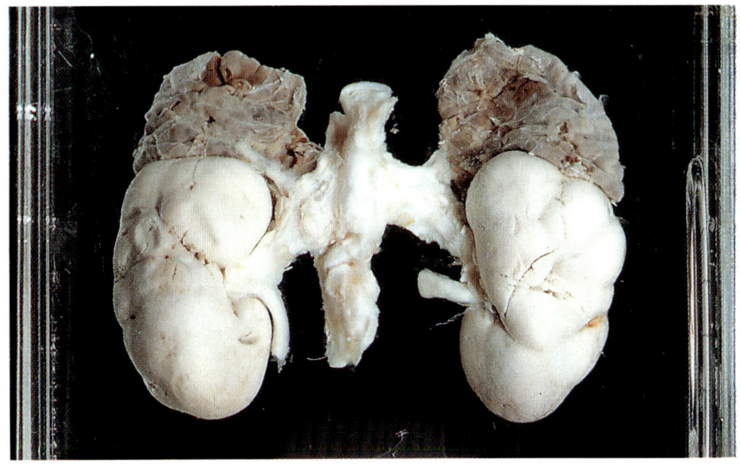

6.29 Adrenal: Waterhouse-Friderichsen Syndrome

This is a post-mortem specimen from an 8-week-old boy who developed a fulminating pyrexial illness associated with extensive purpura. He was found to have meningococcal meningitis and died rapidly.

Both kidneys and adrenals are mounted with the aorta and their vessels. The adrenal glands are swollen and uniformly haemorrhagic although their normal shape has been retained. Note the persistent fetal lobulation of the kidneys.

Waterhouse-Friderichsen syndrome refers specifically to the occurrence of adrenal haemorrhage associated with a fulminant septicaemic illness. The commonest culpable organism is *Neisseria meningitidis* but other organisms, including *Haemophilus influenzae* and the pneumococcus, may occasionally be implicated. It is thought that the adrenal haemorrhage, which principally affects the cortex, results from a combination of 'stress', the action of endotoxins and a variable degree of disseminated intravascular coagulation. A similar appearance, not included in the clinical syndrome of Waterhouse-Friderichsen, may be seen in various complications of pregnancy (e.g. retroplacental haemorrhage and eclampsia) and also in neonates suffering perinatal trauma or asphyxia.

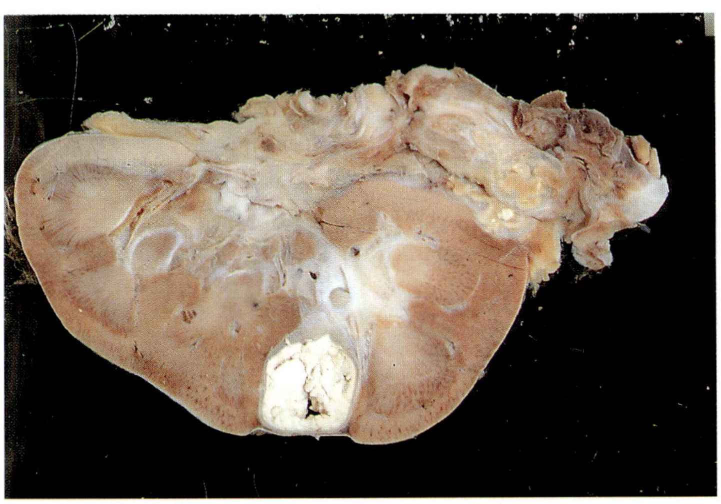

6.30 Adrenal: Addison's Disease due to Tuberculosis

This is a post-mortem specimen from a 36-year-old woman who had suffered from long-standing spinal tuberculosis (Pott's disease). More recently she had become weak, nauseated and had developed bronze pigmentation over her entire skin surface, particularly the face and breasts and in the buccal mucosa. She rapidly deteriorated and died.

At the upper pole of this kidney the adrenal gland shows dense fibrosis with irregular foci of caseation. No identifiable normal adrenal tissue remains. The kidney has been bisected to show a well-circumscribed, caseous focus, measuring 2cm in diameter involving one renal pyramid.

Addison's disease, which refers to primary chronic adrenocortical insufficiency, may arise at any age in either sex and was first described in 1855. For many years, the commonest cause was tuberculous destruction of the adrenal gland. However, with the marked decrease in incidence of tuberculosis in Caucasians, the commonest cause in the Western world is now primary autoimmune adrenalitis leading to adrenal atrophy. This condition is comparable in nature to primary myxoedema. Other causes include replacement of the adrenal by metastatic tumour, amyloidosis and fungal infection, particularly histoplasmosis. Tuberculous adrenalitis is most often found in association with infection elsewhere in the body and classically results in diffuse involvement of the entire adrenal gland. Whatever the cause, it is generally accepted that there has to be destruction of at least 90 per cent of the cortical tissue before clinical insufficiency develops.

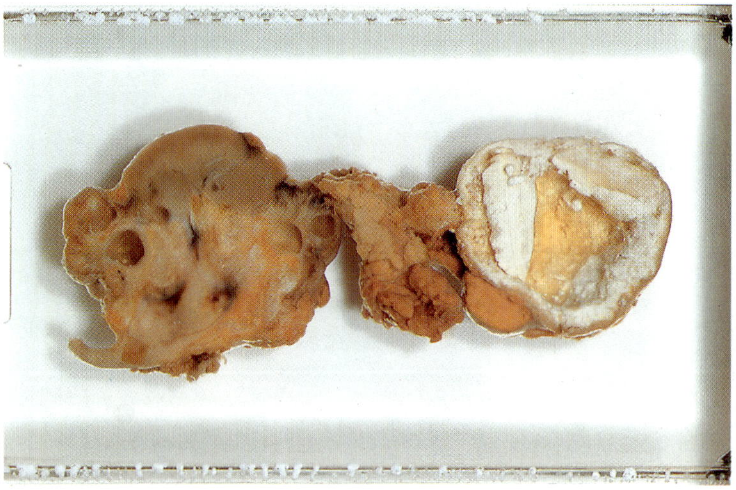

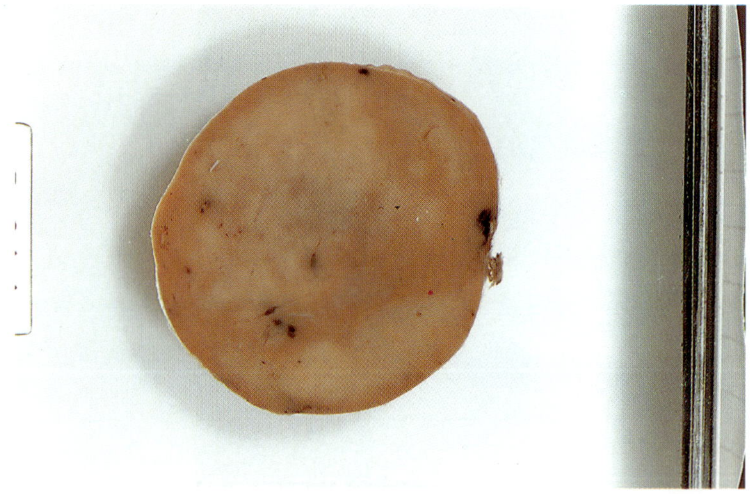

6.31 Adrenal: Calcified Cyst and Adenoma

This specimen was excised from a 52-year-old woman who presented with a 2 month history of loin pain. Radiological examination revealed a calcified lesion in the adrenal and a small kidney with an apparently abnormal calyceal system. There was no evidence whatever of tuberculous infection and a unilateral nephrectomy and adrenalectomy were performed.

The adrenal and kidney, with intervening adipose tissue, have been coronally sectioned. The adrenal gland is distorted by a fibrous-walled cyst showing irregular calcification. Adjacent to its infero-medial aspect is a small, ovoid yellowish nodule, measuring 1cm in diameter. The kidney is dysplastic (see Chapter 4) with a fairly normal middle segment but aberrant development of the upper and lower poles. The pelvis is rather dilated and congested.

Adrenal cysts are comparatively uncommon and usually represent either undetected parasitic infection (e.g. hydatid disease) or degeneration in a previous haematoma or tumour. The presence of a cortical adenoma may be coincidental or may suggest that the cystic degeneration has occurred in an adjacent area of nodular hyperplasia. The association with the dysplastic kidney must be regarded as a chance observation of no significance.

6.32 Adrenal: Cortical Adenoma with Virilism

This specimen was excised from a 19-year-old woman who presented with a one year history of lassitude, decreased libido, amenorrhoea and excessive growth of body hair. Urinary 17-oxosteroid levels were markedly elevated and an adrenalectomy was performed.

This adrenal tumour is spherical and encapsulated, measuring 4cm in diameter. The cut surface shows a uniform yellowish-brown appearance with a few small, haemorrhagic foci but no evidence of necrosis.

True adrenal adenomas, as opposed to hyperplastic nodules, are classically solitary and the adjacent cortical tissue is either normal or may be atrophic as a consequence of pituitary suppression. Functioning adenomas may be of variable size and most often give rise to Cushing's syndrome. Rarely, as in the case here, they may elaborate excessive androgens, in particular dehydroepiandrosterone and androstenedione. Virilism, as a consequence of adrenal disease, is more often seen in young children with a deficiency of either 21- or 11-hydroxylase (congenital adrenal hyperplasia).

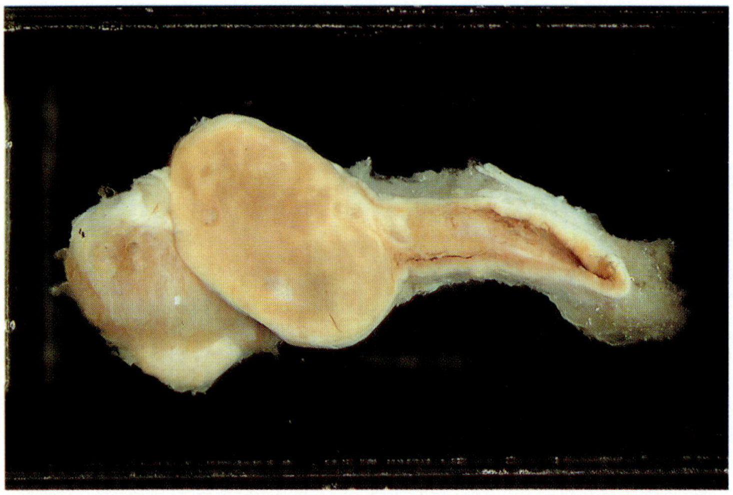

6.33 Adrenal: Non-Functioning Cortical Adenoma

This was an incidental finding at post-mortem in a 62-year-old woman who died of carcinoma of the stomach.

The adrenal gland has been sectioned to show a well-circumscribed, ovoid tumour, measuring 1.5cm in maximum diameter. Note that the cut surface has the typical yellow colour with smaller brownish areas.

This lesion can be classified as a true adenoma since the remainder of the adrenal is normal with no evidence of nodular hyperplasia. Non-functioning adrenocortical adenomas are not uncommon incidental findings at post-mortem and they may show extreme variation in size. They are thought to arise from small foci of cortical hyperplasia, in the absence of any endocrinological disturbance, and their incidence increases with age.

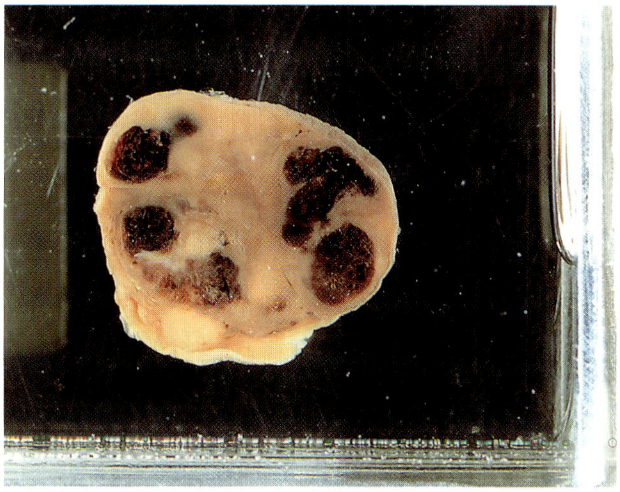

6.34 Adrenal: Cortical Adenoma and Metastatic Carcinoma of the Bronchus

This specimen was found at post-mortem in an 80-year-old man who died of carcinomatosis of bronchial origin.

The adrenal gland is virtually replaced by a rounded, haemorrhagic lesion measuring 3.5cm in maximum diameter. On the right a small fragment of normal adrenal gland remains, within which is a small, pale nodule, measuring 0.5cm in diameter.

Surprisingly, the larger lesion is the non-functioning adenoma, showing degenerative change. The tiny nodule on the right is a deposit of anaplastic carcinoma similar to the primary tumour in the patient's lung. The adenoma was, therefore, a chance finding and the metastasis confirms the propensity of bronchial carcinoma to spread to the adrenal.

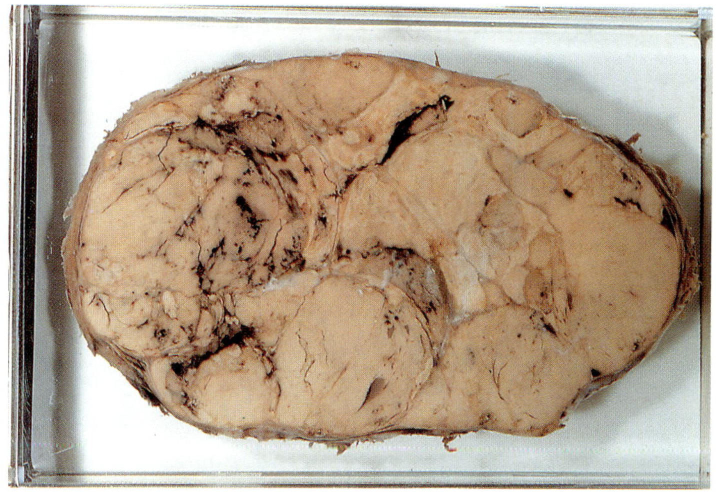

6.35 Adrenal: Cortical Carcinoma

This specimen was excised from a 27-year-old man who had first noticed an abdominal swelling 2 months previously. At laparotomy, small deposits of metastatic tumour were noted in the liver. The patient died of bronchopneumonia shortly after the operation.

This adrenal gland is completely replaced by a very large tumour, which measures 20 × 12 × 12cm and weighed 2120g in the fresh state. The cut surface shows a coarsely lobulated structure with numerous foci of haemorrhage and necrosis.

Adrenocortical carcinoma is comparatively uncommon and shows no predilection for age or sex. These tumours commonly attain a very great size, the case here being quite average. This is probably because their steroid production, if any, is usually inefficient such that the carcinoma may remain asymptomatic for some considerable time. Histologically, it is almost impossible to distinguish reliably between benign and malignant adrenocortical lesions and metastasis is the only incontrovertible reliable indicator. These carcinomas do show a particular tendency to invade the adrenal or renal veins, giving rise to early haematogenous dissemination and the prognosis, in general, is very poor.

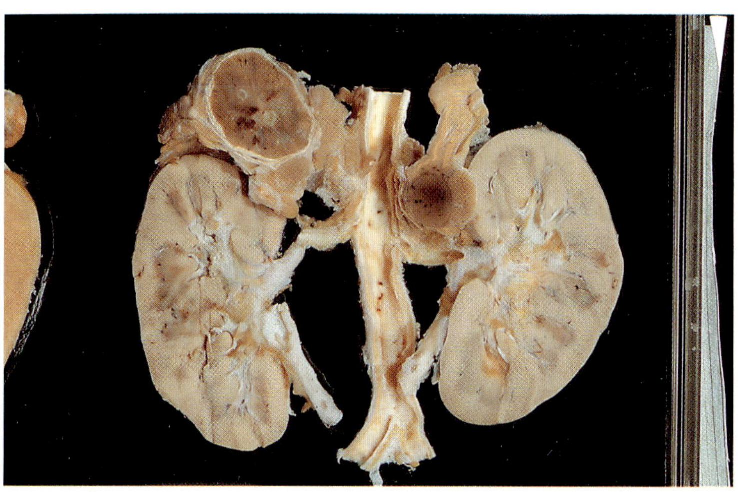

6.36 Adrenal: Bilateral Phaeochromocytoma

This is a post-mortem specimen from an 11-year-old boy who presented with a 5 year history of intermittent attacks of acute abdominal pain associated with sweating and tachycardia. He also complained of failing vision and was found to have florid hypertensive retinopathy. Further examination revealed marked, but variable, hypertension and left ventricular hypertrophy. Laparotomy revealed bilateral adrenal tumours but the patient died intra-operatively before anything could be done.

Both adrenals, with the kidneys, their vessels and the aorta, are shown. In the medulla of each adrenal there is a typical rounded, dark brown tumour over which is stretched a rim of normal, yellow cortical tissue. Note also the atheromatous plaques in the aorta and at the origins of the renal arteries.

Phaeochromocytomas arise from the chromaffin cells either in the adrenal medulla or in the sympathetic chain, the former being more usual. These tumours are comparatively uncommon but most often arise in young adults of either sex. There may be a familial tendency and some cases occur either in the Multiple Endocrine Neoplasia Syndrome Type II (Sipple) or in association with von Recklinghausen's neurofibromatosis. While the vast majority are benign, their principal importance lies in their ability to give rise to paroxysmal hypertension due to excessive secretion of catecholamines. This secretion, however, facilitates their diagnosis since the urinary metabolite of adrenaline and noradrenaline, vanillylmandelic acid, is usually elevated. Bilaterality in phaeochromocytoma is not infrequent but is most often seen in familial cases. As with adrenocortical tumours, there are no reliable histological criteria for differentiating between benign and malignant cases.

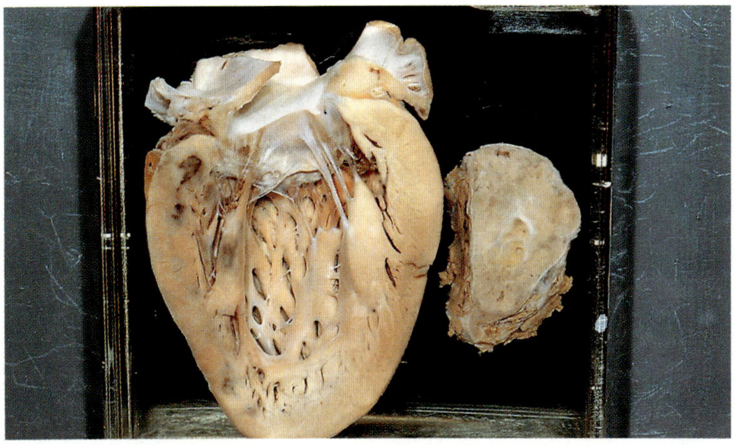

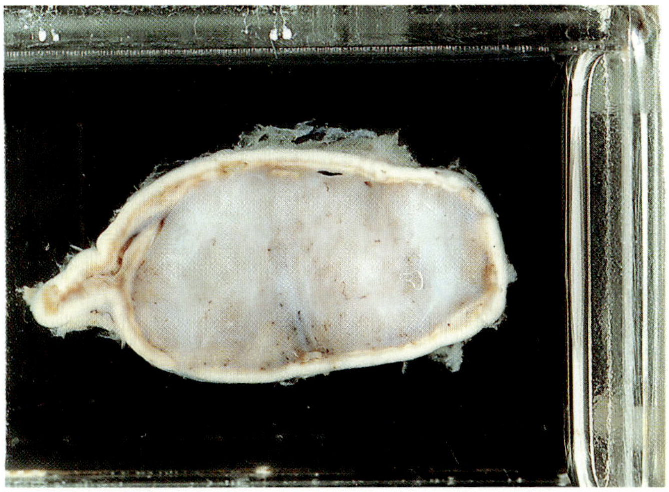

6.37 Adrenal: Phaeochromocytoma with Myocardial Infarction

These are post-mortem specimens from a 22-year-old man who presented with intermittent severe headaches which were found to be associated with paroxysmal hypertension. He began to have attacks of profuse sweating and suddenly collapsed. A diagnosis of myocardial infarction with left ventricular failure was made and he died soon after.

On the right, an adrenal gland containing an ovoid, brownish tumour measuring 4 × 2.5 × 2cm is shown. Around the tumour is a thin rim of apparently normal adrenocortical tissue. On the left a sagittal section through the young man's left ventricle, adjacent to the interventricular septum, is shown. There is extensive recent infarction in the posterior wall and note also the marked left ventricular hypertrophy and dilatation.

The consequences of severe hypertension are precisely the same, whatever the aetiology. As a result, phaeochromocytoma is a well-recognised cause of accelerated atheroma, left ventricular hypertrophy and myocardial infarction in comparatively young people.

6.38 Adrenal: Ganglioneuroma

This was an incidental finding at post-mortem in a 55-year-old man who died of bronchopneumonia.

The adrenal gland has been sectioned to show a well-circumscribed, greyish tumour measuring 3 × 15 × 1.5cm, expanding and replacing the medulla. A thin layer of normal cortical tissue is easily visible around the neoplasm.

A ganglioneuroma is a benign adrenal medullary tumour derived from the non-chromaffin neural element. It arises more commonly elsewhere in the sympathetic chain but, at either site, most often occurs in the 3rd and 4th decades. In principle it represents the fully differentiated end of the spearum from neuroblastoma (an embryonal tumour) with the rare, intermediately differentiated ganglioneuroblastoma lying between the two extremes. Occasionally, ganglioneuromas may synthesise catecholamines but usually they are asymptomatic.

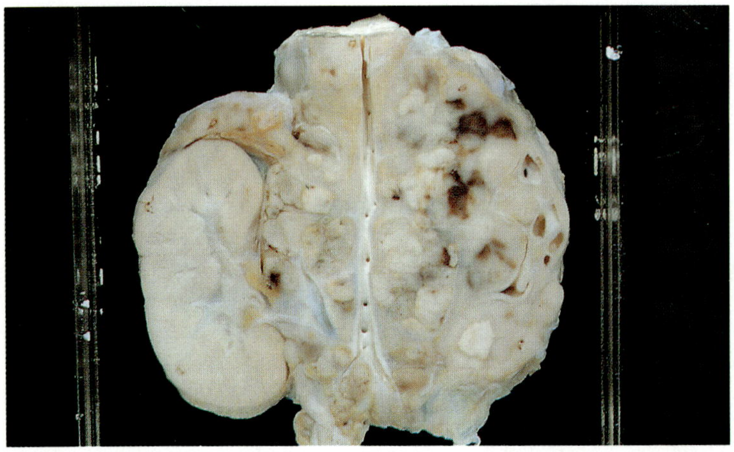

6.39 Adrenal: Neuroblastoma

This is a post-mortem specimen from a 2½-year-old boy who presented with non-specific symptoms and was found to have a large tumour adjacent to the left kidney and widely disseminated metastases. He died rapidly.

This is a block of tissue from the retroperitoneum, which has been sectioned to show both kidneys, both adrenals, the aorta and numerous para-aortic lymph nodes. Arising in the adrenal gland on the right is a large, pale, nodular mass showing focal haemorrhage which has replaced the entire adrenal and has compressed the ipsilateral kidney leaving only a small hydronephrotic remnant (far right). The kidney and adrenal gland on the left appear normal. Numerous para-aortic nodes bilaterally are completely replaced by similar tumour.

Neuroblastomas are derived from non-chromaffin cells in the neural crest. They arise most often in the adrenal medulla but may also be found anywhere along the sympathetic chain. These tumours occur almost universally in small infants and children, occasionally being congenital. They are highly malignant, tending to early metastasis, but modern multimodal therapy has led to a greatly improved survival, and even cure, rate. It should be noted that these tumours may occasionally secrete catecholamines.

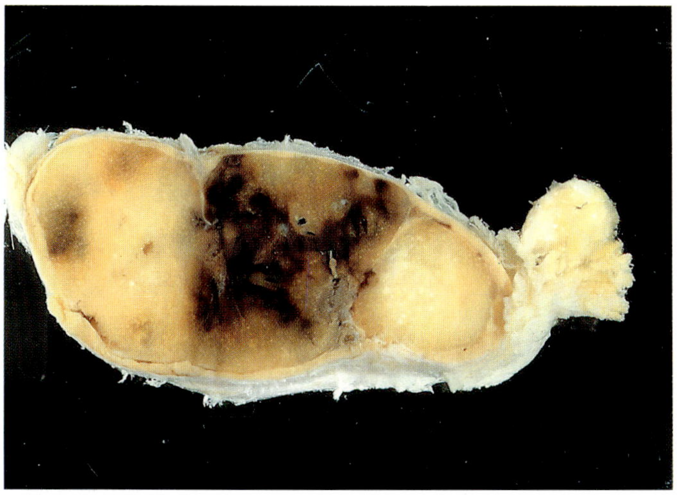

6.40 Adrenal: Myelolipoma

This was an incidental finding at post-mortem in a 46-year-old woman who committed suicide.

This enlarged adrenal gland, which measures 4 × 2 × 2cm, has been sectioned to show an attenuated rim of adrenal tissue around a well-circumscribed mass of fatty tissue in which there are dark red haemorrhagic areas. The latter correspond histologically to myeloid nodules.

Adrenal myelolipomas are rare, usually asymptomatic, lesions. The case here shows the typical macroscopic features. They do not represent true neoplasms but, rather, are thought to be hamartomatous malformations composed of adipose and haemopoietic tissue. There may be a familial tendency.

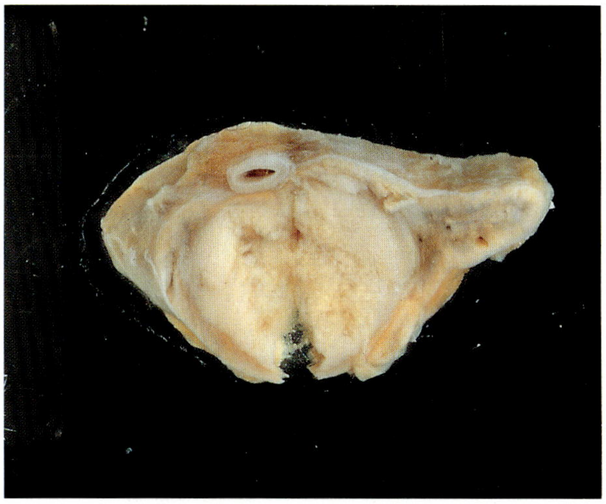

6.41 Adrenal: Metastatic Bronchial Carcinoma

This was a post-mortem finding in a 75-year-old man who died of carcinomatosis due to oat cell carcinoma of the bronchus.

The adrenal has been sectioned to show replacement of the medulla by a focally necrotic, pale nodule of metastatic tumour, over which the cortex is stretched.

Carcinoma of the bronchus is by far the commonest source of adrenal metastases. While any primary tumour may occasionally be responsible, other common sources include carcinoma of the breast and malignant melanoma. In general, adrenal metastases are bilateral and most often appear first in the medulla. However, cortical involvement is very common and, rarely, such metastatic spread may give rise to Addison's disease (see Figure and Legend 6.30).

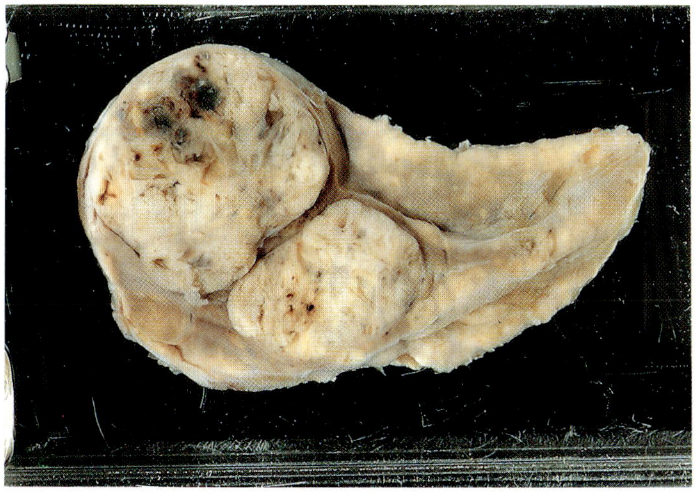

6.42 Adrenal: Metastatic Renal Adenocarcinoma

This is a post-mortem specimen from a 68 year-old man who died of carcinomatosis from a renal adenocarcinoma.

The adrenal gland is greatly enlarged and contains two large nodules, measuring up to 2cm in diameter, of metastatic carcinoma which have the typical variegated appearance of renal adenocarcinoma. The adrenal cortex is preserved but attenuated over these deposits.

As already stated, any malignant tumour may occasionally metastasise to the adrenal gland. Adrenal metastases, in the case here, were bilateral thus ruling out the possibility of local spread from the kidney.

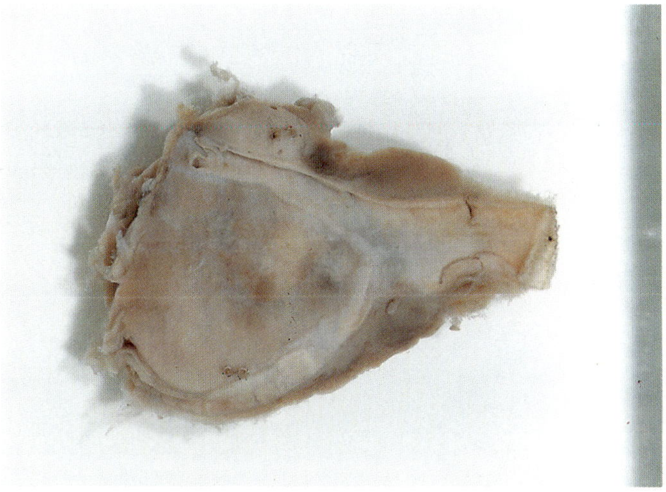

6.43 Carotid Body: Chemodectoma

This specimen was excised from a 47-year-old woman who had noticed a slow-growing tumour in the right side of the neck for 3 years.

An encapsulated, brownish tumour, measuring 3cm in maximum diameter, is seen firmly adherent to a portion of the carotid artery.

Chemodectomas (synonym: carotid body tumours) are the commonest tumour of the extra-adrenal paraganglionic system and as such are derived from the neural crest. They may occur at any age but are significantly more common in populations living at high altitudes; this is thought to be due to hyperplasia of the carotid body as a consequence of prolonged hypoxia. They are very vascular lesions and usually arise, and are adherent to, the bifurcation of the common carotid artery. Whereas, in the past, surgical intervention was thought rather hazardous with the risk of cerebral ischaemia, the operative risk with modern techniques is very low. As with phaeochromocytoma, there are no reliable histological criteria for determining malignancy but up to 10 per cent of cases may behave in a malignant fashion.

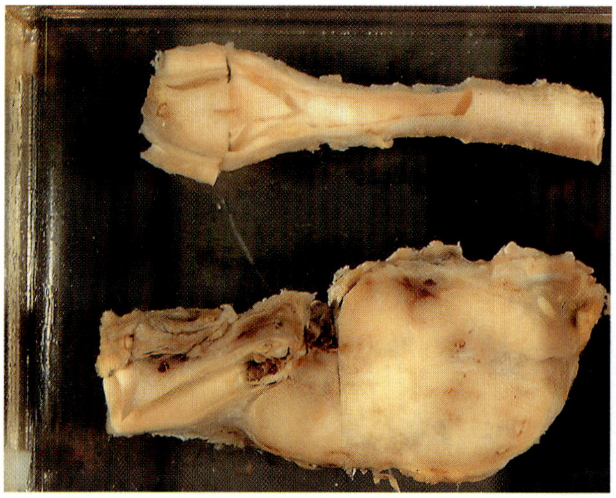

6.44 Carotid Body: Bilateral Chemodectoma

These are post-mortem specimens from a 34-year-old man who was admitted to hospital with numerous enlarged cervical lymph nodes. Biopsy revealed metastatic tumour. He died shortly afterwards.

The bifurcations of both carotid arteries are mounted. On the left, there is an infiltrative tumour, measuring 3cm in diameter, which has completely enveloped much of the common carotid artery. On the right, lying in the angle of the bifurcation, is a small well-circumscribed tumour measuring 0.7cm in diameter.

Bilaterality is well-recognised in chemodectomas. Similarly these tumours may be associated with paragangliomas at other sites and they may also represent part of a multiple endocrine neoplasia syndrome. In the case here, at least one of these tumours (probably that on the left) had behaved in a malignant fashion. Death was due to virtual occlusion of the common carotid artery.

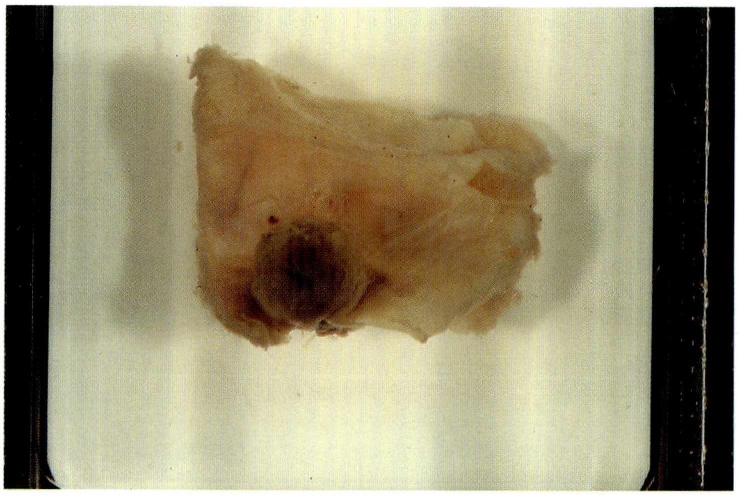

6.45 Temporal Bone: Glomus Jugulare Tumour

This is a post-mortem specimen from a 76-year-old woman who died of bronchopneumonia. She had been known to have a middle ear neoplasm, probably a glomus jugulare tumour, for 18 years, but this had been treated with radiotherapy alone.

A portion of the right petrous temporal bone is shown from which protrudes a small, rounded, pinkish tumour measuring 1cm in diameter.

Glomus jugulare tumours are the second commonest extra-adrenal paraganglioma and occur most often in adults. There is a marked female preponderance. Commonly, they arise laterally in the temporal bone and erode into the middle ear but, occasionally, they may be found adjacent to the jugular bulb and present as a mass at the base of the skull. Up to 40 per cent of cases show extension into the cranial cavity. While the vast majority are benign, their vascularity and inaccessibility often make surgical excision difficult. Since residual tumour may give rise to a local recurrence, post-operative radiotherapy is often indicated.

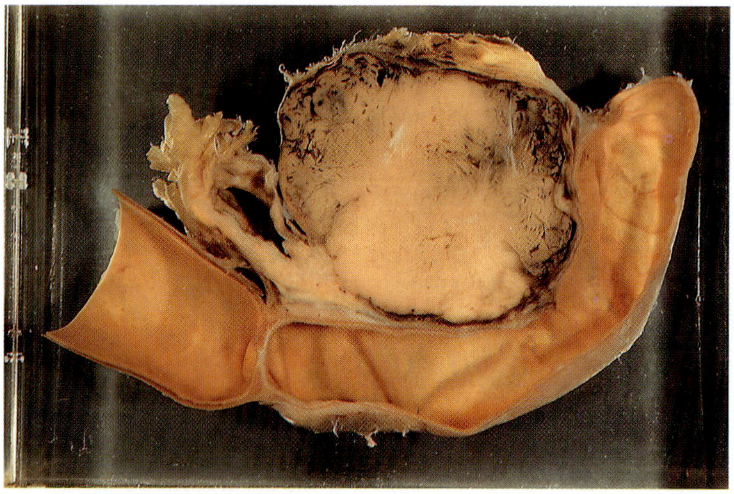

6.46 Pancreas: Islet Cell Tumour

This specimen was excised from a 35-year-old woman who presented with an 8 month history of backache and intermittent abdominal pain. Post-operatively she developed hepatorenal failure and died.

The pyloric canal, proximal duodenum and head of the pancreas are shown. The head of the pancreas is completely replaced by a circumscribed tumour, measuring 7cm in diameter, which is focally necrotic and haemorrhagic. There is no infiltration of the duodenal wall. Note the cystic dilatation of the pancreatic duct in the body of the pancreas (right) due to obstruction by the tumour.

Small islet cell tumours are common incidental findings at post-mortem and are often asymptomatic. However, they may present with excessive hormone production or pressure effects as a result of increasing size. Of the functioning lesions, up to 70 per cent are ß-cell tumours which secrete insulin. A further 15 per cent are of α-cell origin (glucagon) and δ-cell tumours account for up to 10 per cent (gastrin and somatostatin). A much smaller group may secrete pancreatic polypeptide or vaso-active intestinal peptide, the latter giving rise to the Verner-Morrison syndrome. Pancreatic islet cell tumours may be multiple or may form part of the Multiple Endocrine Neoplasia Syndrome Type I (Wermer). These neoplasms are only rarely malignant, although histological criteria are imprecise; the commonest malignant islet cell lesions are of probable δ-cell origin, up to 60 per cent of gastrinomas are malignant. The tumour here is unusually large and appears to have been non-functioning.

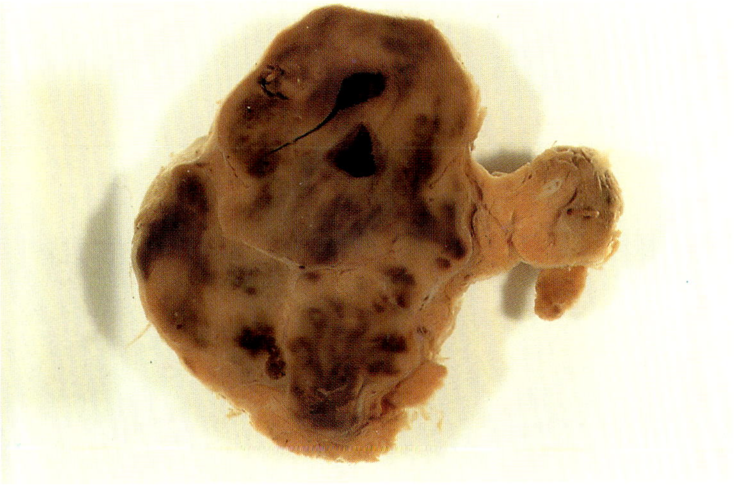

6.47 Pancreas: Insulinoma

This specimen was excised from a 70-year-old man who presented as an emergency in a semiconscious state. He was found to be hypoglycaemic and, when more rational again, was able to give a 3 year history of hypoglycaemic attacks associated with fits, particularly after exercise. He suffered 2 subsequent attacks both of which were rapidly relieved by the administration of glucose. At laparotomy, a small tumour was found in the tail of the pancreas.

In the tail of the pancreas is a well-circumscribed, highly vascular tumour, measuring 3cm in diameter. It has a distinctly lobulated appearance.

This patient presented with the classical Whipple's triad of hyperinsulinism: hypoglycaemia, neurological symptoms associated with exercise or fasting, and prompt relief of symptoms by glucose. About 70 per cent of such cases are due to a solitary ß-cell adenoma but other causes include multiple adenomata, ß-cell carcinoma, diffuse ß-cell hyperplasia or ectopic hormone production.

7. HAEMOPOIETIC AND LYMPHORETICULAR SYSTEMS

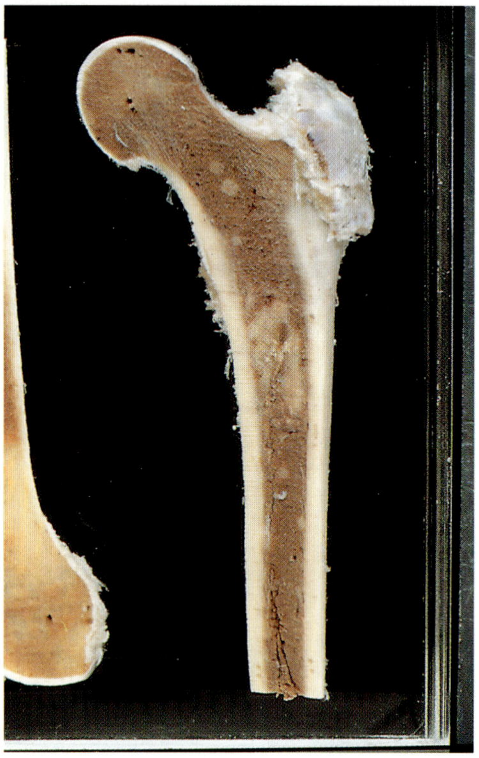

7.1 Bone Marrow: Erythroblastic Hyperplasia

No clinical details are available.

This femur, sectioned in the coronal plane, shows extensive replacement of the normally fatty marrow by red haemopoietic tissue.

In a normal adult femur there should only be macroscopical evidence of haemopoiesis in the head and neck. The appearance seen here may be the result of a primary disorder, such as polycythaemia rubra vera, or it may be compensatory, as in secondary polycythaemia, severe haemolytic anaemia or pernicious anaemia.

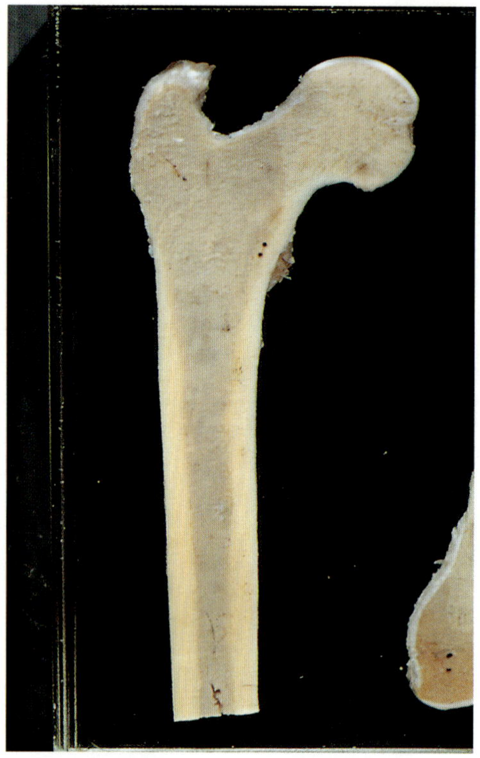

7.2 Bone Marrow: Myeloid Hyperplasia

No clinical details are available.

This femur, sectioned in the coronal plane, shows extensive replacement of the normal marrow cavity by pinkish-grey leucoblastic tissue.

This appearance is most often seen in either an acute leukaemia or chronic myeloid leukaemia. However, it may rarely be associated with a leukaemoid reaction, as is occasionally found with fulminant bacterial pneumonia and meningitis, widespread sepsis, tuberculosis, or certain malignant neoplasms, in particular of the kidney and bronchus.

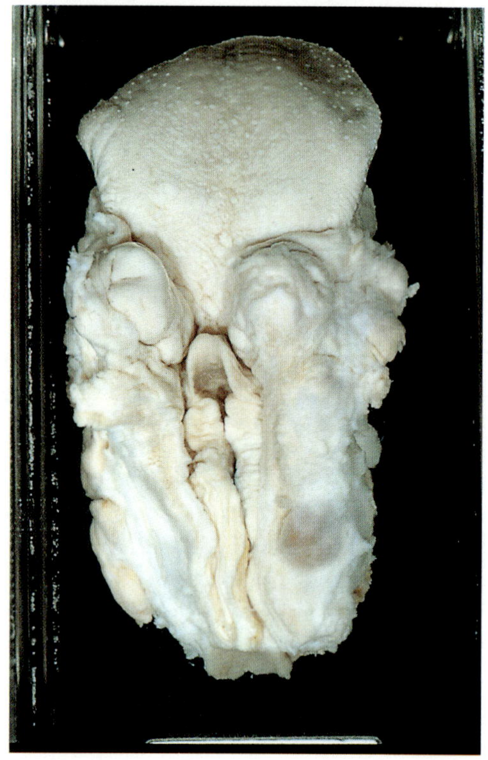

7.3 Tonsils: Hyperplasia

This specimen was taken from a 3-year-old boy who died as a result of a road traffic accident.

The tongue, with pharynx and larynx opened from behind, shows a pair of considerably enlarged, hyperplastic faucial tonsils.

Faucial lymphoid tissue, which forms part of Waldeyer's ring, may enlarge either acutely, due to bacterial tonsillitis, or chronically as a result of colonisation by upper respiratory tract viruses which induce reactive hyperplasia of the lymphoid follicles.

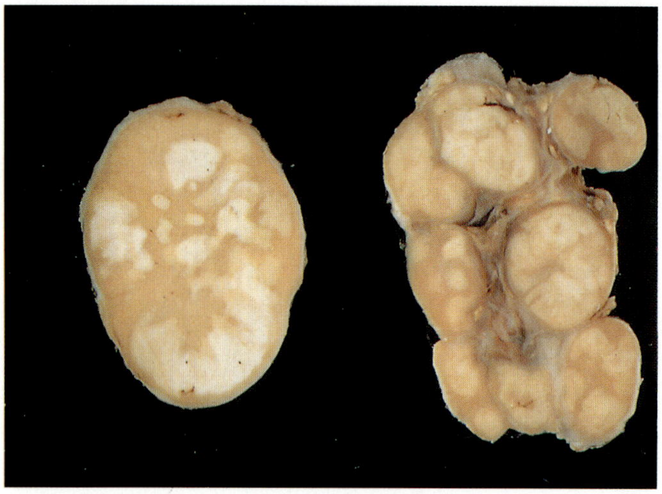

7.4 Lymph Nodes: Tuberculosis

No clinical details are available.

The specimen consists of a group of enlarged lymph nodes, measuring 4cm in diameter, removed from the patient's neck. The tissue has been sectioned (top) to show opaque, white caseous foci, in different stages of coalescence, within the darker granulomatous areas. The nodes are adherent to each other ('matted') owing to fibrosis of the adjacent soft tissues.

Tuberculous infection of cervical nodes most often occurs in association with primary tonsillar infection and, not uncommonly, may lead to formation of a sinus tract with the skin surface.

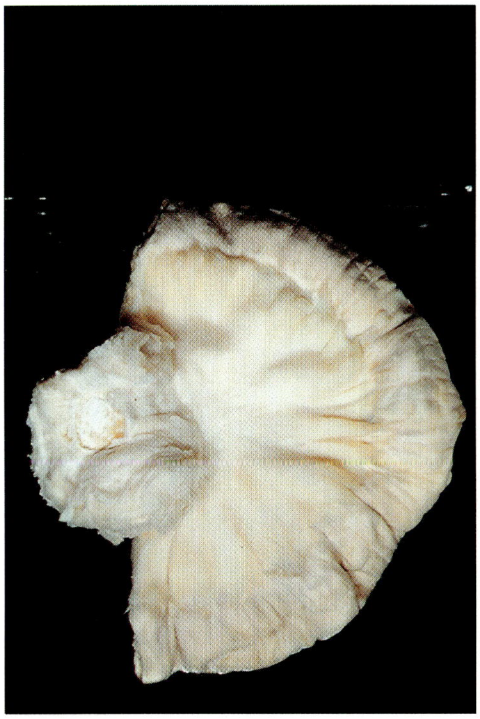

7.5 Lymph Node: Dystrophic Post-Tuberculous Calcification

This was an incidental post-mortem finding in a 75-year-old woman who died of myocardial infarction.

A loop of small bowel with attached mesentery, is seen. At the root of the mesentery there is a hard, calcified lymph node measuring 1.5cm in diameter.

Dystrophic calcification often occurs in tuberculous nodes forming part of the primary complex but this does not always imply resolution of the infection. Calcified nodes may also occur in association with fungal infection. When found in the mesentery, such nodes usually signify previous intestinal tuberculosis resulting from the ingestion of unpasteurised milk. Radiologically they may cause confusion with stones in the gall bladder or urinary tract.

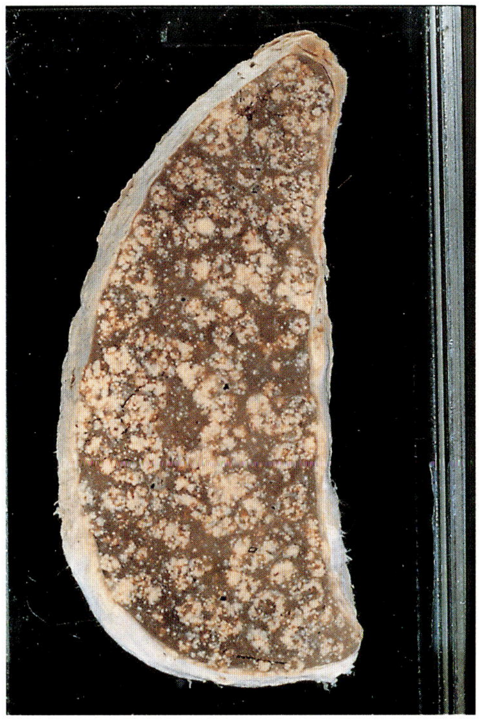

7.6 Spleen: Miliary Tuberculosis

This specimen was removed at post-mortem from a 30-year-old African from Zimbabwe who died with acute miliary tuberculosis.

The spleen shows numerous discrete caseous nodules distributed throughout the deeply congested pulp. In some areas the lesions have coalesced to form nodules up to 0.5cm in diameter.

Splenic involvement is almost invariable in miliary tuberculosis, which usually occurs due to haematogenous spread of the primary infection. Acute miliary tuberculosis remains a common cause of death in underdeveloped countries, but in the British Isles is rarely seen and is more often associated with advanced cases of post-primary infection (see Chapter 2).

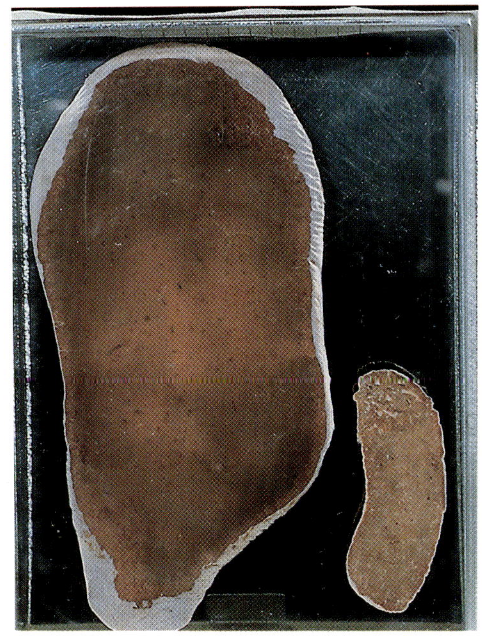

7.7 Spleen: Malaria

These specimens were both collected at post-mortem from Africans living in Zimbabwe.

Both spleens show thickened capsules. The spleen on the left is enlarged, measuring 16 × 8cm, and is from a 30-year-old man. The spleen on the right is shrunken, measuring 6 × 3cm, and is from a 60-year-old man. Both are greyish in colour due to the extensive deposition of malarial pigment.

Chronic malaria commonly results in massive splenomegaly due to proliferation of macrophages, responsible for the removal of parasitised erythrocytes, and to an increase in fibrous tissue. Splenic atrophy is unusual in malaria and, in this case, is more likely to have been a result of co-existent sickle cell trait.

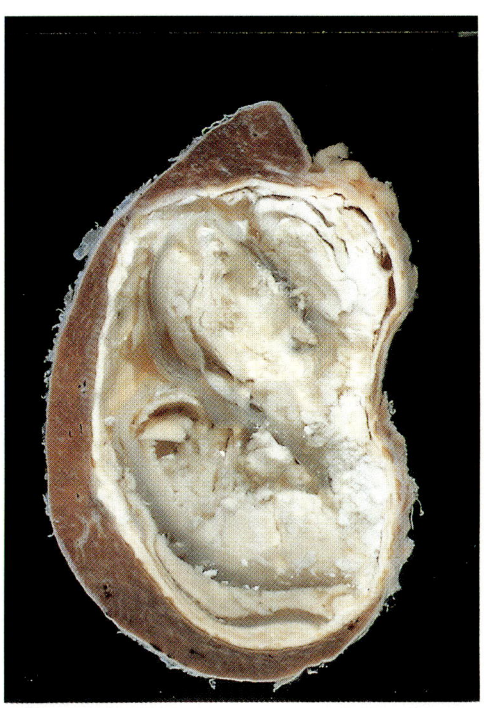

7.8 Spleen: Hydatid Cyst

This specimen was excised from a 54-year-old woman, who had a hydatid cyst of the liver marsupialised at the age of 12. More recently she had suffered attacks of abdominal pain and plain X-rays revealed a partially calcified cyst of the spleen. At operation the spleen was adherent to the diaphragm and kidney.

A section through the spleen shows an ovoid cyst, 8cm in diameter. The fibrous cyst wall is focally calcified and the cavity contains necrotic material in which the folded remnants of a laminated membrane can be seen.

Hydatid disease is due to infestation by the tapeworm, *Echinococcus granulosus*, and is most often seen in sheep-farming communities. The cysts are typically multilocular, containing numerous daughter cysts within which the brood capsules are formed. The cyst shown here appears, to a large extent, to be 'burnt out', there being little evidence of activity. The diagnosis may be made by demonstration of cutaneous hypersensitivity to hydatid antigen, the Casoni test.

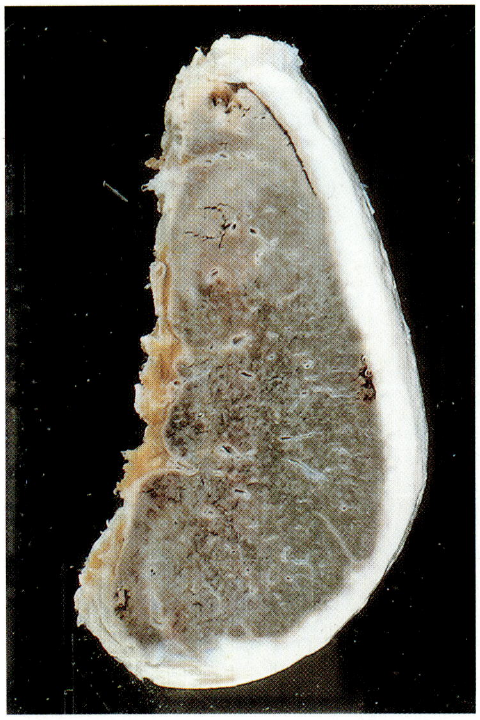

7.9 Spleen: Perisplenitis

This specimen was removed at post-mortem from an 89-year-old woman who died of basal pneumonia. Apart from the spleen, the peritoneal surfaces were normal.

A section through this normal size spleen shows gross thickening of the capsule over the convex surface, due to the deposition of fibrous tissue.

Perisplenitis results in the pale external appearance, known as 'sugar-icing' spleen. It is a common incidental finding at post-mortem and may involve a variable area of the splenic capsule. While this appearance may be found in people who have died from almost any disease, it is particularly common in association with either chronic splenomegaly or underlying infarction.

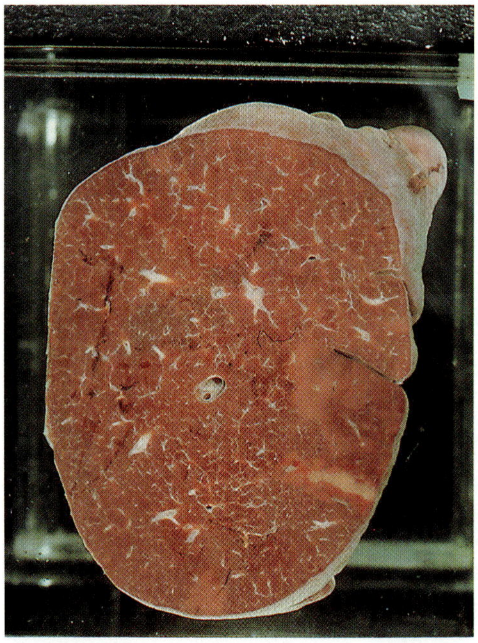

7.10 Spleen: Chronic Venous Congestion

This was an incidental finding at post-mortem in a 55-year-old man with a long history of ischaemic heart disease who developed congestive cardiac failure. Death was due to myocardial infarction and at autopsy all the principal organs were engorged.

This section of spleen shows the mild enlargement and deep red colour typical of chronic venous congestion. The organ is firm and its fibrous framework stands out against the engorged red pulp. On the right hand side there is a narrow strip of pale infarction.

This appearance is due solely to passive venous engorgement consequent upon impaired myocardial function. There is usually much greater enlargement of the spleen when the congestion is secondary to portal hypertension.

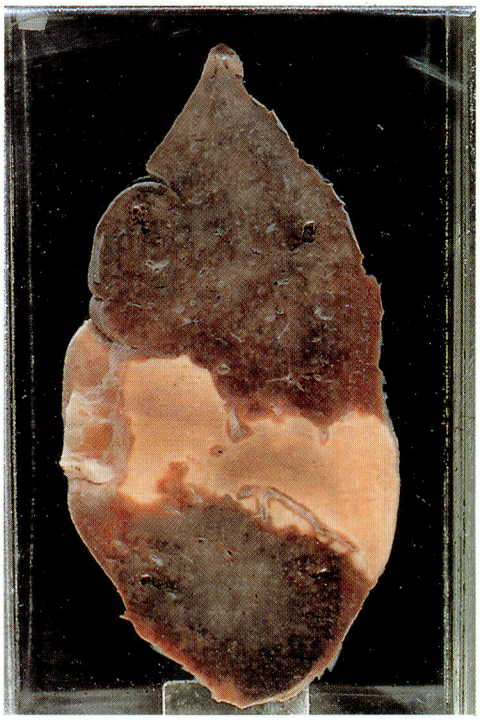

7.11 Spleen: Infarct

This was an incidental finding at post-mortem in a 72-year-old woman who died of carcinoma of the rectum with extensive hepatic metastases.

A section through the spleen shows a recent yellowish, well-defined infarct traversing the middle of the organ.

Splenic infarction most commonly results from embolism complicating such conditions as mural thrombus in the heart or infective endocarditis. It may also occur in almost any form of splenomegaly, especially if massive, due to thrombosis or ischaemia. In this case it is most probable that encroachment of hepatic tumour deposits on the origin of the splenic artery led to a diminution of the splenic blood supply.

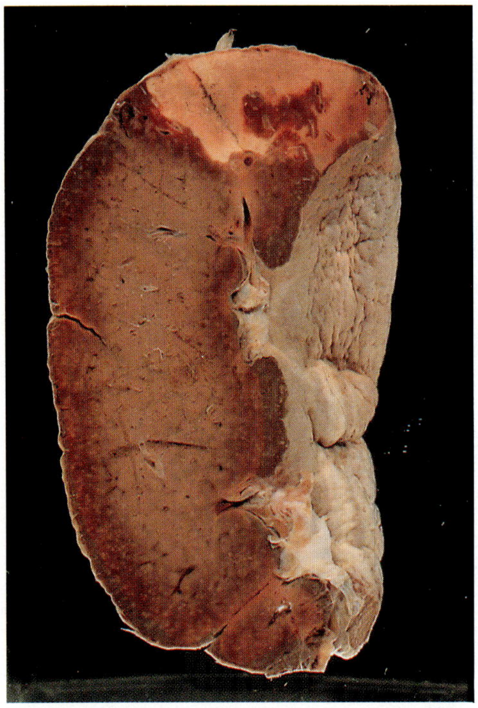

7.12 Spleen: Infarct

This spleen was removed at post-mortem from a 54-year-old woman who died of myocardial infarction. She had a long history of progressive ischaemic heart disease and autopsy revealed an old left ventricular infarct with overlying mural thrombosis.

A section through the spleen shows a wedge-shaped infarct at the upper pole. It is pale pink in colour, suggesting a fairly recent origin, and over the surface the capsule is thickened.

The wedge shape of the infarct is more typical than that in Figure 7.11 and results from occlusion of an end-artery.

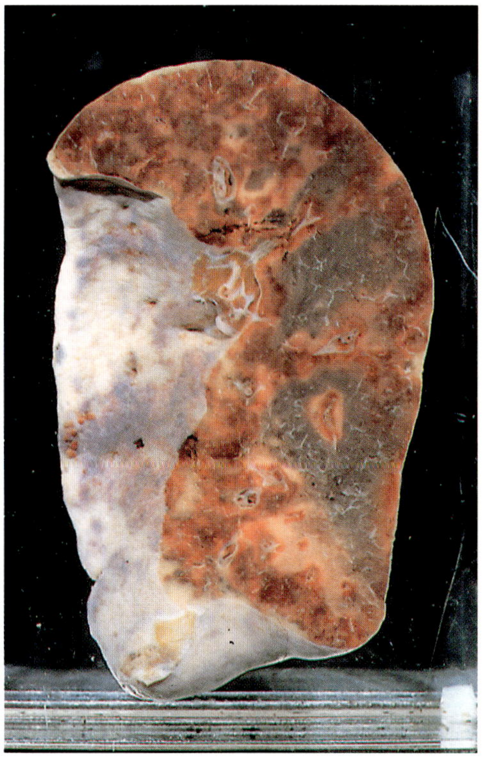

7.13 Spleen: Haemorrhagic Infarction

This specimen was removed from a 69-year-old man who developed disseminated intravascular coagulation after retroperitoneal leakage of bladder irrigation fluid. He died with bronchopneumonia and acute renal tubular necrosis.

The spleen has been sectioned to show that both the outer and cut surfaces have a red and pale yellow mottled appearance, which is due to zones of diffuse haemorrhage interspersed with well-defined areas of pale infarction. The splenic vein at the hilum is thrombosed.

In this case the rapid consumption of coagulation factors was probably initiated by entry of irrigation fluid into the bloodstream. More common causes of disseminated intravascular coagulation include peri-partum haemorrhage, Gram-negative septicaemia and incompatible blood transfusions.

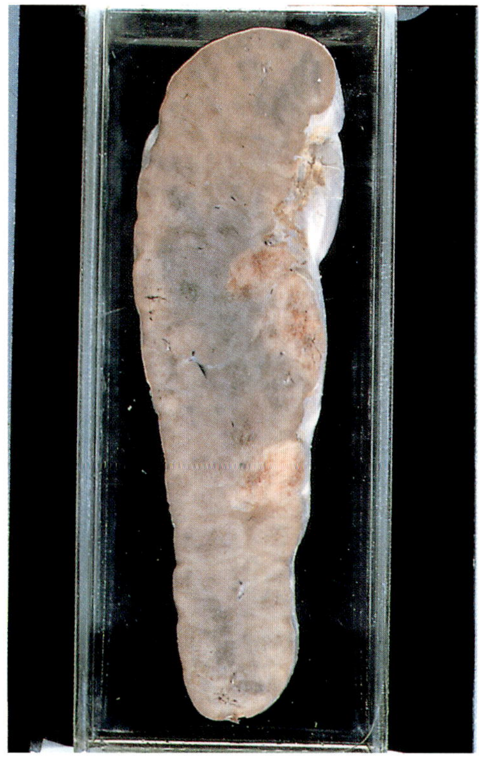

7.14 Spleen: Sarcoidosis

This specimen was excised from a 35-year-old woman who had noticed an enlarging mass in the left side of the abdomen for 18 months. The peripheral blood count and bone marrow were normal. It was 18 months after splenectomy before she developed signs of pulmonary disease, associated with lymphadenopathy and conjunctivitis.

A section through this moderately enlarged spleen, measuring 24 × 6.5 × 4cm, shows almost complete replacement of the pulp by coarse pale nodules.

Splenomegaly is usually only found in advanced sarcoidosis, an idiopathic generalised disease of the lymphoreticular system which results in chronic granulomatous inflammation. Common presenting features are respiratory symptoms, lymphadenopathy, skin involvement or eye involvement. Investigations frequently reveal bilateral hilar lymph node enlargement and occasionally osteolytic bone lesions. The disease probably represents an unusual host reaction to a foreign antigen or antigens, the nature of which are unknown. Steroids may accelerate the natural tendency to healing.

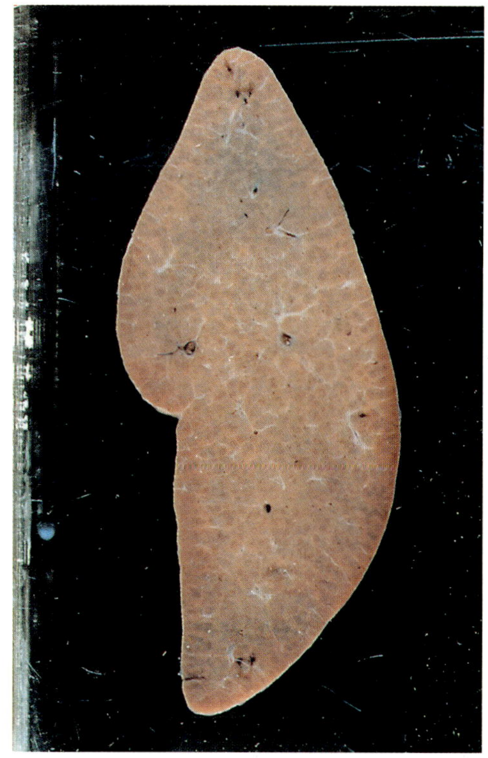

7.15 Spleen: Amyloidosis

No clinical details are available.

A section through the spleen shows numerous, rounded, waxy nodules scattered throughout the splenic pulp.

This appearance is known as 'sago spleen'. Involvement of the spleen is more common in secondary amyloidosis than in primary and is usually more extensive. Amyloid is a fibrillary protein, arranged in ß-pleated sheets, which is derived from immunoglobulin light chains in primary, or myeloma-associated, disease and from a naturally occurring serum amyloid A protein in secondary disease. Common causes of secondary amyloidosis include tuberculosis, bronchiectasis, rheumatoid arthritis and almost any chronic inflammatory disease.

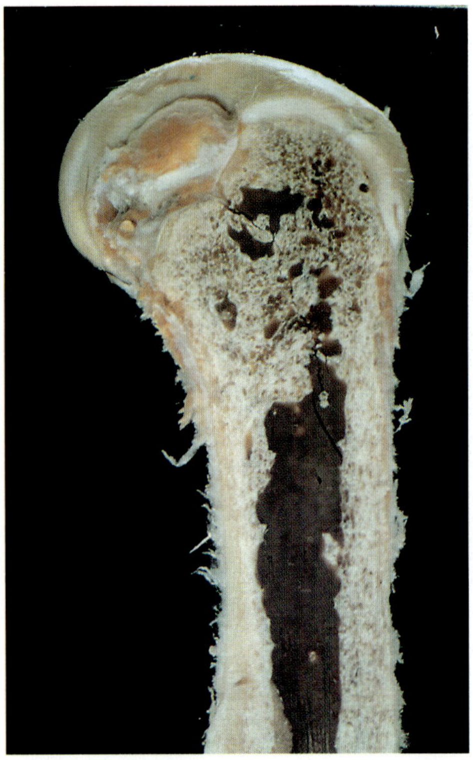

7.16 Bone Marrow: Myelosclerosis

This specimen was taken from a 67-year-old man who had a 10 year history of purpura, haemoptysis, bone pain and weight loss. Investigation revealed increased density and coarse trabeculation of bone throughout the skeleton, moderate anaemia, thrombocythaemia and a neutrophil leukocytosis. In addition, there was cryoglobulinaemia and the neutrophil alkaline phosphatase was elevated. He became progressively anaemic and leucopenic and finally died in congestive cardiac failure with a chest infection. At autopsy there was extreme skeletal sclerosis and moderate splenomegaly (624g).

This coronal section of the upper end of the femur shows extensive obliteration of the medullary cavity by dense bony trabeculae, the remaining spaces are filled with red haemopoietic marrow.

This is an example of a myeloproliferative disorder and is a variant of myelofibrosis, in which the marrow is more commonly replaced by fibrous tissue. It is a chronic disorder of insidious onset and is most often seen in the elderly. Extramedullary haemopoiesis, which forms part of the disease process and is not compensatory, is often found in the spleen (see Figure and Legend 7.18) and liver. Death usually results from the complications of impaired haemopoiesis, in particular infections or haemorrhage. The cryoglobulinaemia in this case appears to be coincidental and is more usually found in association with multiple myeloma or Waldenstrom's macroglobulinaemia. Splenomegaly is usually more marked than in this case.

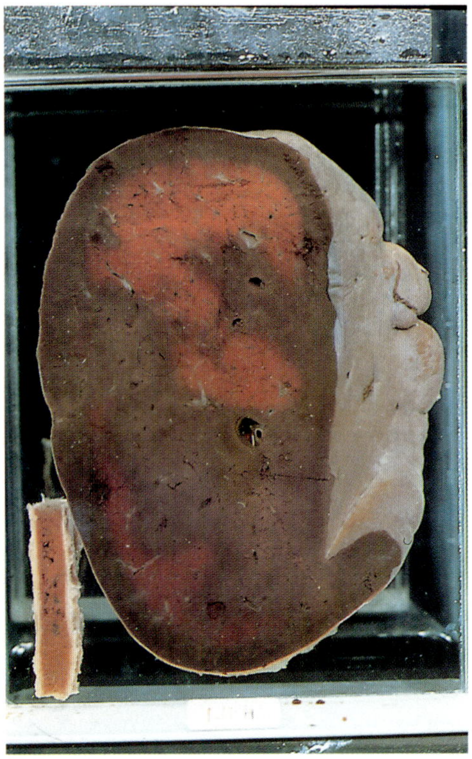

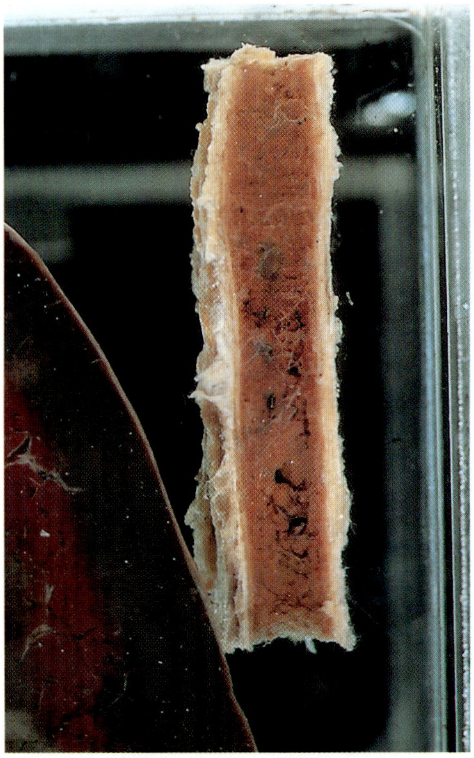

7.17 Spleen and Bone Marrow: Polycythaemia Rubra Vera

These specimens were taken from a 70-year-old man with a 15 year history of polycythaemia rubra vera, who died suddenly of a myocardial infarction.

The spleen is markedly enlarged (7.17a) and deeply congested. The sternal bone marrow, seen in close up (7.17b), is expanded in width and is largely replaced by red haemopoietic tissue.

Polycythaemia rubra vera, another of the myeloproliferative disorders, usually occurs in the elderly. It results in a marked predisposition to vascular thrombosis. An accompanying leucocytosis or thrombocythaemia is common, and occasionally it may be complicated by the development of myelofibrosis (Legend 7.18).

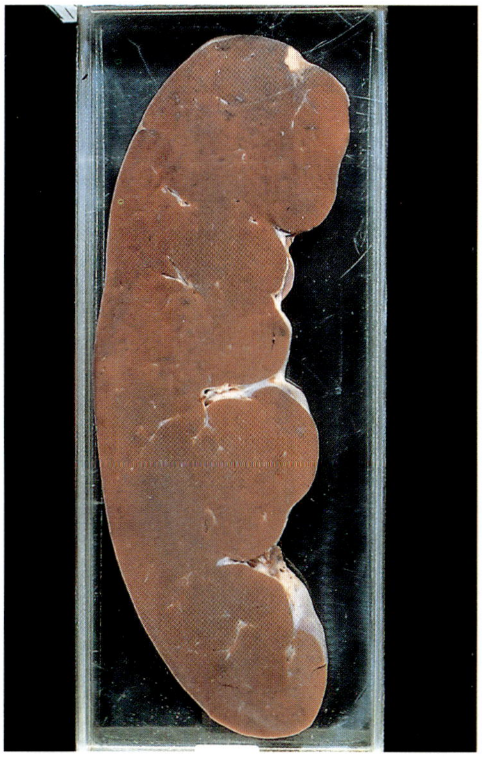

7.18 Spleen: Myeloproliferative Disorder

This specimen was excised from a 53-year-old man who presented initially with polycythaemia rubra vera 30 years previously. He had been treated with radioactive phosphorous and radiotherapy but latterly he developed myelofibrosis with splenomegaly. He also suffered frequent attacks of gout.

A section through this massively enlarged spleen, weighing 5270g, shows it to have a brownish-red, beefy appearance. There is an old healed infarct at the upper pole.

Either polycythaemia rubra vera or essential thrombocythaemia may progress to myelofibrosis and because the 3 conditions are closely interrelated they are all labelled as myeloproliferative disorders. The great proliferation of blood cell precursors and the subsequent destruction of the increased circulating cells may lead to frequent attacks of gout following the breakdown of nucleic acids to uric acid. Any of the myeloproliferative disorders may be complicated by acute myeloblastic leukaemia. In this case the early age of presentation and prolonged survival are unusual.

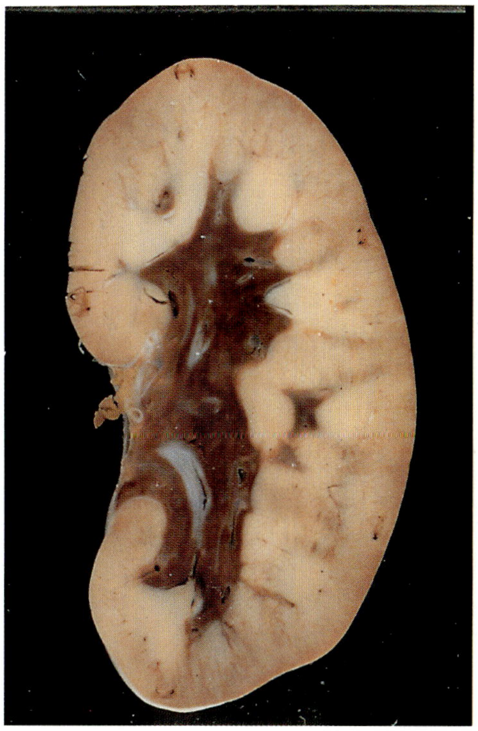

7.19 Kidney: Haemorrhage associated with Aplastic Anaemia

This specimen was taken from a 3-year-old boy who died after a 6 month history of progressive pancytopenia. At autopsy there was marked hypoplasia of the bone marrow and widespread visceral purpura were present.

The kidney shows extensive haemorrhage into the peripelvic connective tissue. The adjacent medulla and cortex are pale and anaemic by contrast.

Aplastic anaemia may either be idiopathic in origin or may result from exposure to drugs, such as chloramphenicol or cytotoxics, or to ionising radiation. The course of this condition is dependent upon the severity of the aplasia. However only about 50 per cent of patients will survive more than one year. Death often results from either overwhelming infection or internal haemorrhage.

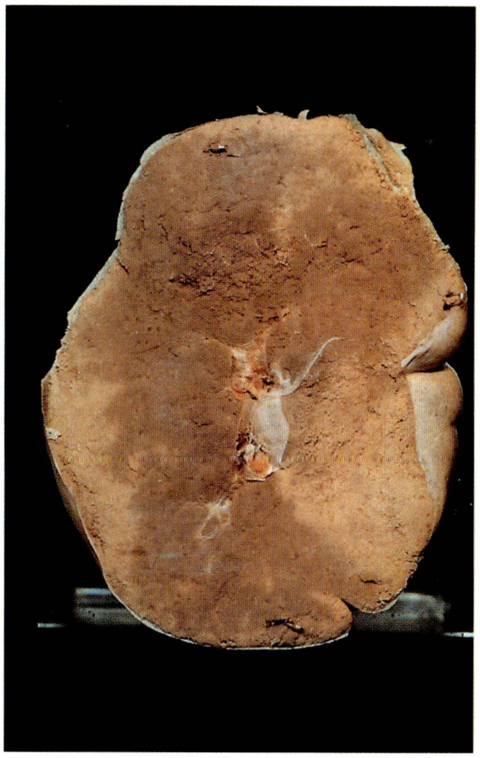

7.20 Spleen: Acute Lymphoblastic Leukaemia

This specimen was taken from a 49-year-old woman who complained of headache and malaise for a fortnight and then deteriorated rapidly. A blood count revealed acute leukaemia. She died shortly after admission to hospital. At autopsy there was a mass of enlarged mediastinal lymph nodes and splenomegaly.

The spleen is only moderately enlarged (cf. Figure 7.23) and its cut surface has a uniform grey-brown appearance. There is loss of the normal splenic architecture.

Acute lymphoblastic leukaemia is most common in children and may conceivably have a viral aetiology. Lymph node involvement is much more common than in acute myeloblastic leukaemia. There may be an associated anaemia or thrombocytopenia. Common complications include raised intracranial pressure due to involvement of the central nervous system, a bleeding tendency, and infection.

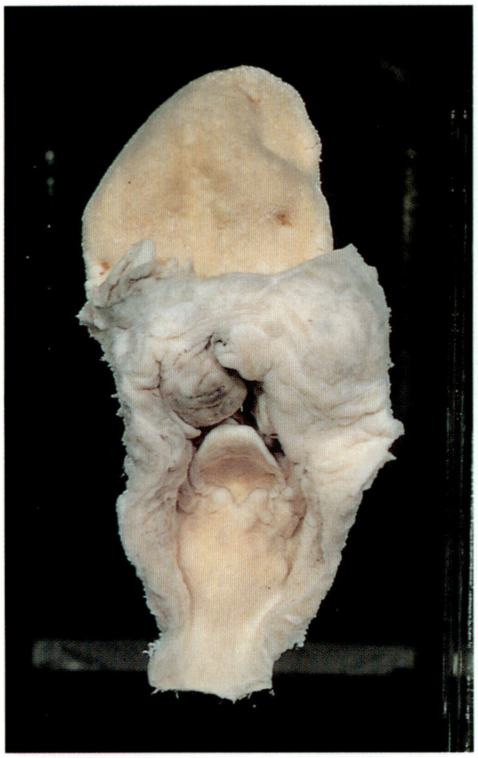

7.21 Pharynx: Acute Leukaemia

No clinical details are available.

The tongue with the larynx and pharynx are dissected to show massive enlargement of the tonsils and pharyngeal lymphoid tissue with almost complete obstruction of the lumen. There is extensive necrosis and sloughing.

Infiltration of the tonsils and mucous membranes may occur in any of the acute leukaemias.

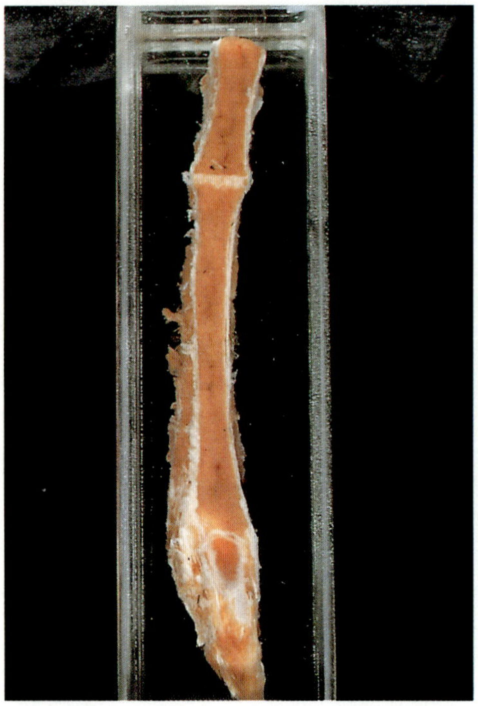

7.22 Bone Marrow: Chronic Myeloid Leukaemia

This specimen was taken from a 67-year-old woman who died suddenly. She had a history of recurrent chest infections and a recent episode of herpes zoster infection. At autopsy the spleen was enlarged, weighing 1200g, and there was bronchopneumonia.

This sagittal section of the sternum shows virtual replacement of the normal marrow by soft, pale pinkish tissue.

Chronic myeloid leukaemia most often affects middle-aged or elderly people and is invariably fatal, commonly terminating in metamorphosis to acute myeloblastic leukaemia. In the majority of cases a specific chromosomal abnormality, known as the Philadelphia chromosome, is found which results from a translocation between chromosomes 22 and 9. Chronic myeloid leukaemia is one of the more common causes of massive splenomegaly (greater than 1kg).

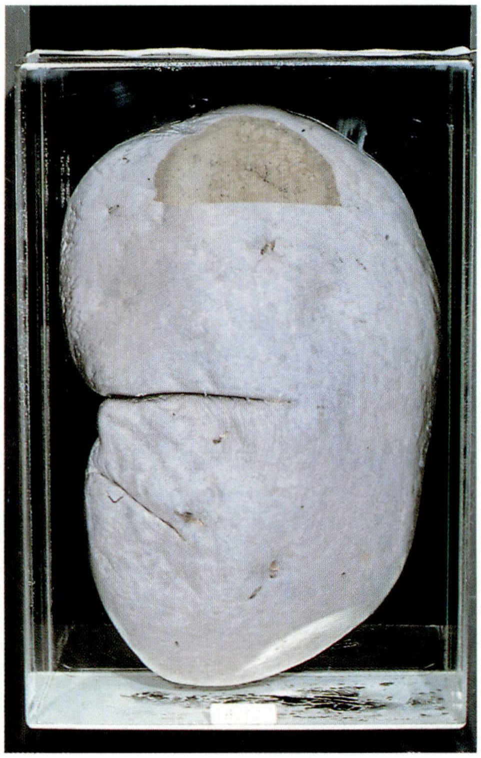

7.23 Spleen: Chronic Myeloid Leukaemia

This specimen was taken from a 75-year-old man who had been treated for chronic myeloid leukaemia for 7 years. He died with bronchopneumonia.

The spleen is massively enlarged, weighing 2890g. A portion of the anterior surface has been removed to show the uniform pinkish-grey appearance of the cut surface.

Chronic myeloid leukaemia is one of the more common causes of massive splenomegaly, which may lead to secondary thrombocytopenia.

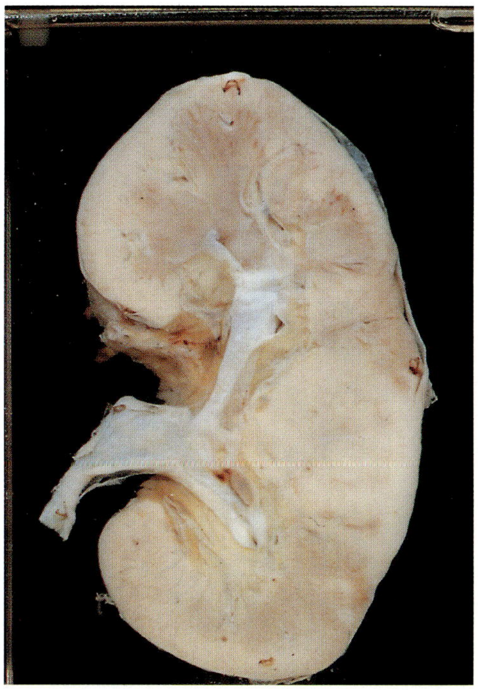

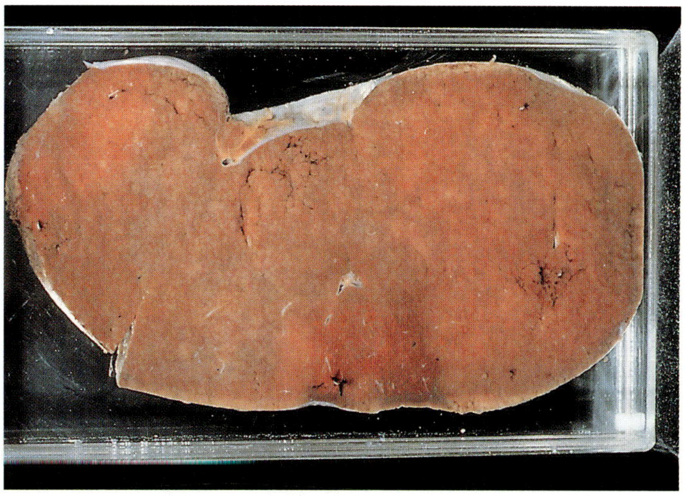

7.25 Spleen: Chronic Lymphatic Leukaemia

This was an incidental finding at post-mortem in a 64-year-old man who died of myocardial infarction.

The specimen consists of a massively enlarged spleen, weighing 2460g, which has been sectioned to show numerous enlarged, lymphoid follicles presenting as small irregular white nodules against a red background of splenic pulp. An intensely congested, wedge-shaped area of incipient infarction is apparent beneath the capsule in the mid-portion of the specimen.

Chronic lymphatic leukaemia occurs predominantly in males and most often presents in old age. Clinically there is usually a generalised lymphadenopathy associated with a very high circulating lymphocyte count. The degree of splenomegaly in this case is unusual, most cases showing only moderate enlargement (less than 1000g). Involvement of the skin is not uncommon. The condition is often complicated by hypogammaglobulinaemia and recurrent infections. The clinical outcome is very variable but, in older patients, life expectancy may not be affected.

7.24 Kidney: Chronic Myeloid Leukaemia

This specimen was removed from a 79-year-old woman who presented with abdominal pain and anorexia. There was hepatosplenomegaly; a blood film revealed occasional myeloid cells. A sternal marrow aspirate showed chronic myeloid leukaemia. Despite treatment, she developed bronchopneumonia and congestive cardiac failure and died. At post-mortem there was generalised enlargement of lymph nodes and leukaemic deposits in the liver and kidneys.

This section through the kidney is abnormally pale and shows ill-defined areas of leukaemic infiltration, where the normal renal architecture is destroyed. There is a small submucosal haemorrhage in the pelvis.

The blood film and post-mortem findings suggest that, terminally, acute blast transformation occurred.

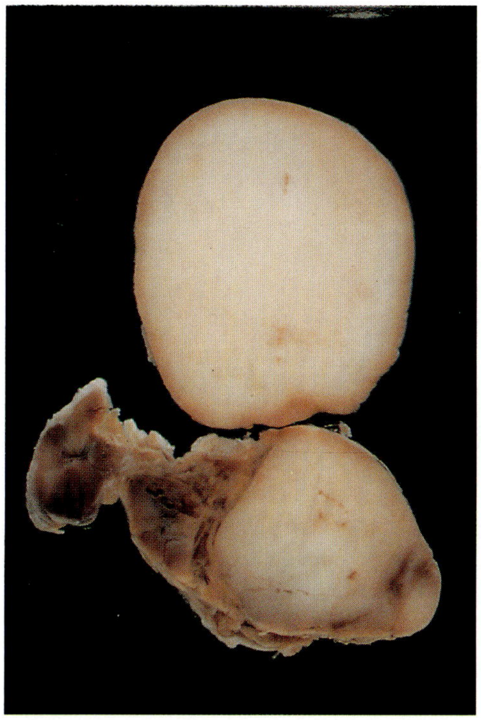

7.26 Lymph Nodes: Hodgkin's Disease

This specimen was excised from a 40-year-old man who complained of a swelling in the left side of the neck which had been present for 9 months. There had been no pain, cough, or increase in size of the mass. Post-operatively, he was treated with radiotherapy and made a good recovery.

A group of 4 lymph nodes is shown, two of which are grossly enlarged and replaced by pale, uniform tumour. The nodes are discrete and there is no evidence of inflammatory adhesions (cf. tuberculosis).

Hodgkin's disease is a lymphoma of uncertain histogenesis but which has the Reed-Sternberg cell as its diagnostic *sine qua non*. It affects males more often than females and has a bimodal age distribution with peaks in the 2nd-3rd and 6th-7th decades. The Rye classification, which is universally applied, divides Hodgkin's lymphoma into 4 histological types, which have a progressively worse prognosis: lymphocyte-predominant, nodular sclerosing, mixed cellularity, and lymphocyte-depleted. The Ann Arbor system of staging also correlates well with prognosis. Epidemiological studies have suggested that this disease may possibly have an infective aetiology.

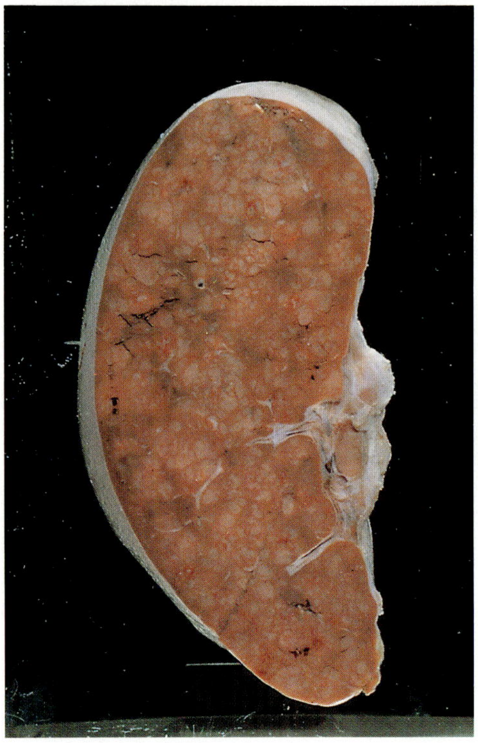

7.27 Spleen: Hodgkin's Disease

This specimen was removed from a 48-year-old man who had presented with large masses of lymph nodes in the neck, groins and axillae one year previously. Mixed cellularity Hodgkin's disease was diagnosed but, despite treatment, he became cachectic and died.

This section through the enlarged spleen shows numerous pale, semi-translucent nodules scattered throughout the pulp. These nodules have resulted in the so called 'German sausage' or 'hardbake' (almond toffee) appearance. In addition, a group of enlarged, firm, white nodes is present in the hilum.

Splenic involvement in generalised Hodgkin's disease is common and may be detected at staging laparotomy. Primary extranodal Hodgkin's disease arising in the spleen is, however, extremely rare.

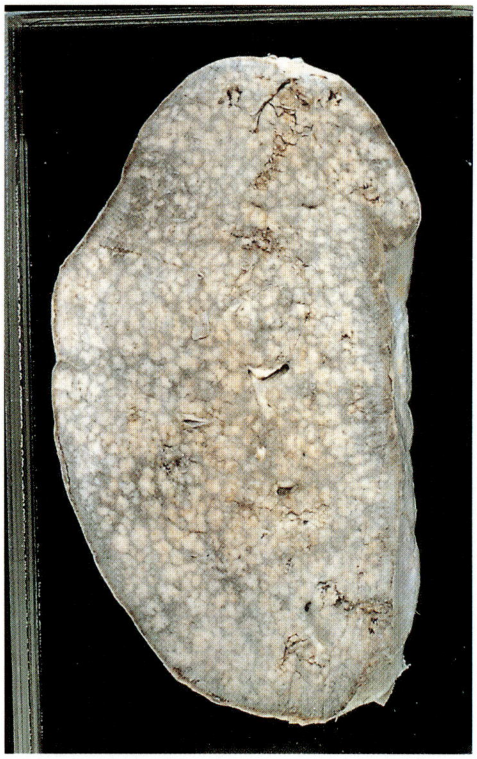

7.28 Spleen: Non-Hodgkin's Lymphoma

This specimen was removed from a 78-year-old woman who died 3 months after having a hip fracture pinned. She was not known to have lymphoma prior to death. At autopsy, degenerating cutaneous lesions were found and the entire abdominal cavity was covered with tumour deposits. Numerous lymph nodes, the spleen and the liver were also infiltrated.

A section through this enlarged spleen shows numerous white tumour deposits, up to 0.5cm in diameter, uniformly scattered throughout the pulp.

Non-Hodgkin's lymphoma is more common than Hodgkin's disease and occurs predominantly in the 6th decade onwards. Known predisposing factors include autoimmune disease and iatrogenic immunosuppression. The classification of non-Hodgkin's lymphoma, based on histological grounds, is a source of confusion to all but experts in the field. The best known classifications are those of Rappaport, Kiel, and Lukes and Collins, to which reference should be made. Dependent upon the extent of the disease, non-Hodgkin's lymphoma may involve any organ in the body and may result in both decreased resistance to infection and disturbances of the blood picture. This particular case was classified as well-differentiated, lymphocytic lymphoma (Rappaport).

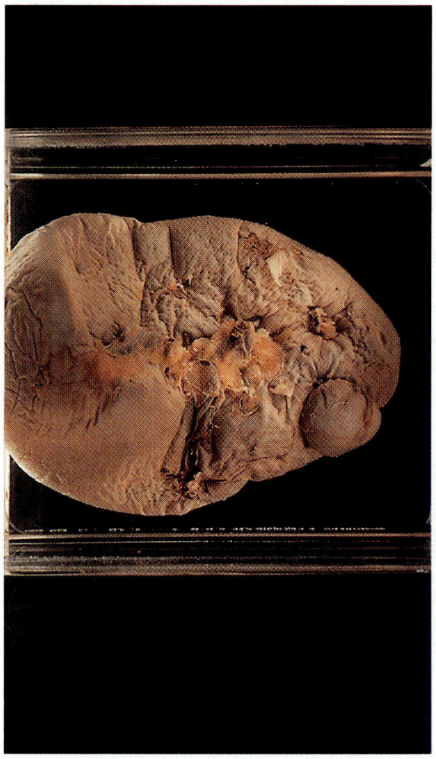

7.29 Spleen: Attached Splenunculus

This was an incidental finding at post-mortem in a middle-aged man who died of myocardial infarction.

There is an ovoid nodule of accessory splenic tissue, measuring 2.5 × 1.5cm, attached to the anterior border of the visceral surface of the spleen.

Splenunculi, also known as accessory spleens or spleniculi, are common congenital anomalies found in up to 10 per cent of the population. They are most often found either at the hilum of the spleen or in the tail of the pancreas and very rarely exceed 1.5cm in diameter. Their only clinical significance lies in the fact that, if not identified at the time of therapeutic splenectomy, they may grow to replace the original spleen and therefore recapitulate the problem for which it was removed.

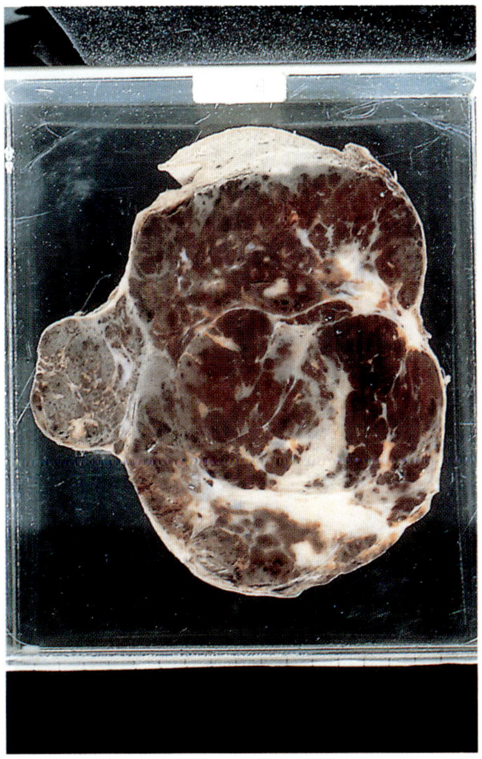

7.30 Spleen: Hamartoma

This specimen was removed from a 54-year-old woman with a short history of upper abdominal pain and a sensation of swelling. She had also noticed a tendency to bruise easily. Examination revealed an enlarged spleen and numerous cutaneous petechiae and bruises. There was also severe thrombocytopenia. She underwent splenectomy, after which she remained well and the platelet count returned to normal.

A grossly enlarged spleen, weighing 1430g, is seen consisting almost entirely of a solid, dark, tumour-like mass with irregular projections, within which are irregular bands of pale fibrous tissue. A portion of attenuated normal splenic tissue is seen at the bottom of the specimen and is well demarcated from the haemorrhagic tumour tissue.

Splenic hamartomas are uncommon and very rarely attain this size. They are clinically benign but may result in hypersplenism.

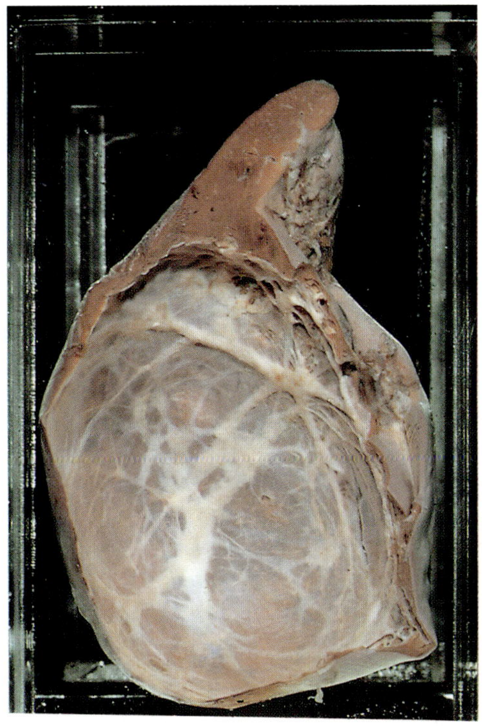

7.31 Spleen: Cystic Lymphangioma

This specimen was excised from a 22-year-old woman who had a 2 year history of fullness in the left side of the abdomen, more recently associated with pain.

The spleen is grossly enlarged, being almost entirely replaced by an ovoid cystic mass, 13 × 11cm in diameter. The cyst is smooth-walled and numerous pale, fibrous strands can be seen traversing it.

Lymphangiomas of the spleen are hamartomatous malformations and are exceedingly rare.

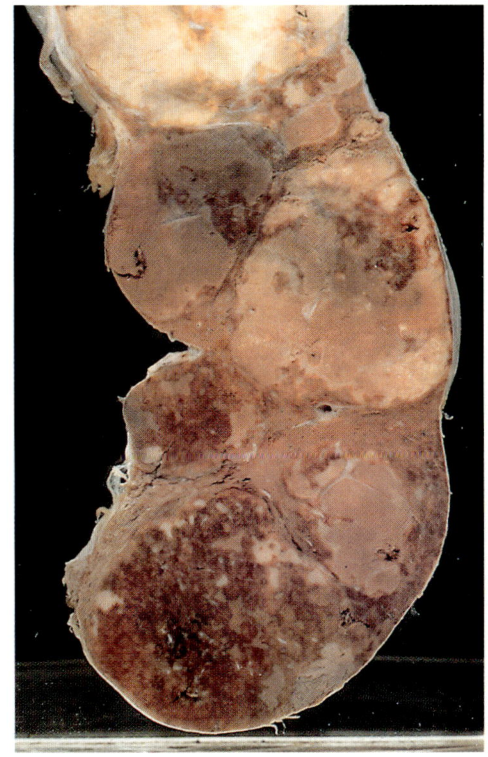

7.32 Spleen: Haemangiosarcoma

No clinical details are available.

A section through this enlarged spleen, measuring 19 × 6.5 × 5.5cm, shows nodules surrounded by surviving normal splenic pulp. The nodules are largely necrotic, but the large deposit in the lower pole is better preserved, and shows the contrast between the bright red neoplastic tissue and the brownish colour of the adjacent splenic pulp.

The spleen is not an uncommon site for this rare visceral tumour and there may be an associated haemolytic anaemia. The prognosis is invariably very poor.

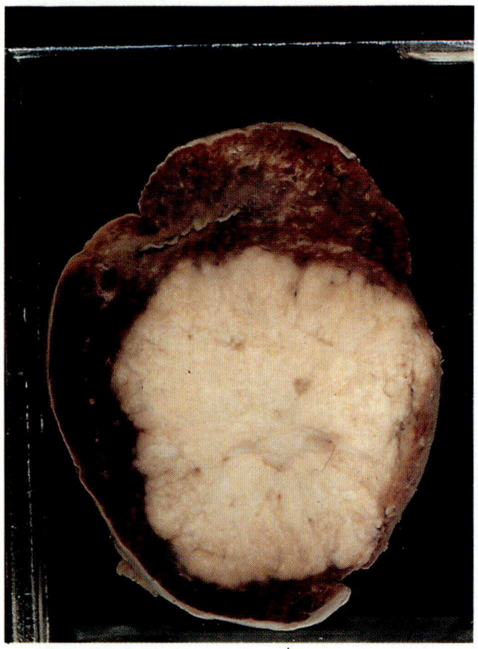

7.33 Spleen: Metastatic Carcinoma

This specimen was removed at post-mortem from an 82-year-old man who died from adenocarcinoma of the rectum.

This spleen, of normal size, has been sectioned to show replacement of much of its substance by a large deposit of pale tumour, 5cm in diameter.

Secondary deposits of tumour in the spleen are uncommon, although not rare. It remains unknown whether the immunological role of the spleen may be in part responsible for this relative sparing.

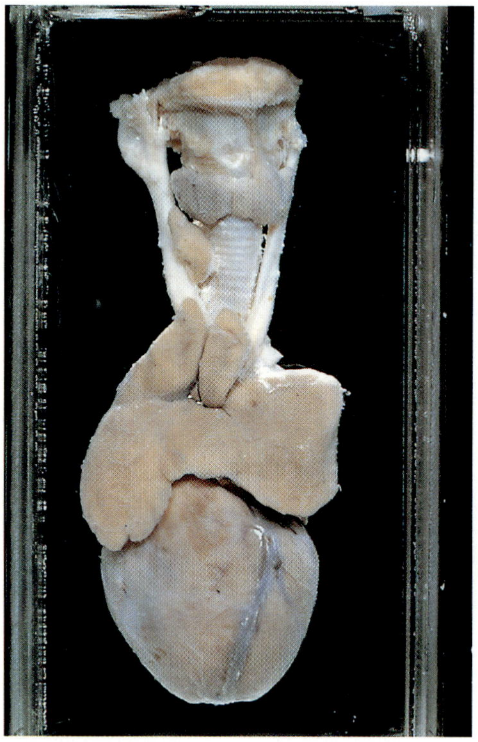

7.34 Thymus: Accessory Gland

No clinical details are available regarding this child.

The neck and part of the thorax, including the heart, have been dissected to show a normally located thymus gland, above the heart, measuring 12 × 7 × 4cm. In addition, adjacent to the infero-lateral border of the right lobe of the thyroid, a nodule of ectopic cervical thymic tissue is visible, measuring 2 × 2 × 1cm.

Such ectopic thymic tissue is not uncommon and results from partial failure of the downward migration, *in utero*, of thymic tissue derived from the 3rd and 4th branchial pouches. It has no clinical significance and, post-pubertally, it would involute with the normally sited thymus. On rare occasions, thymic tumours may develop in such accessory tissue.

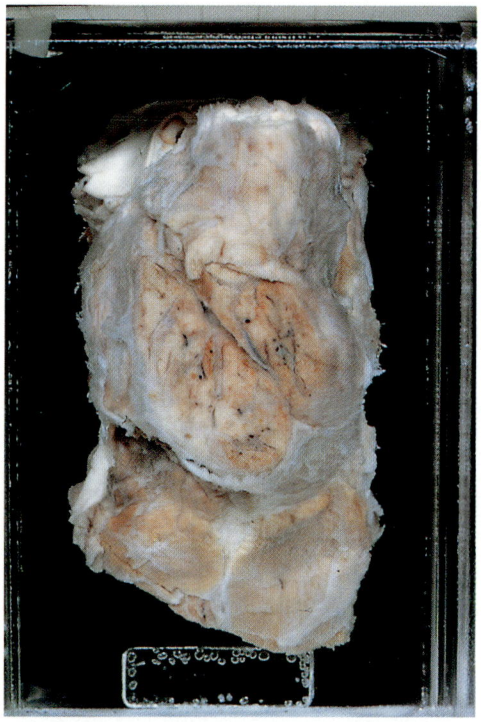

7.35 Thymus: Hyperplasia

This was an incidental finding at post-mortem in a 14-year-old boy who died after being involved in a road traffic accident. At autopsy, the thyroid gland was found to be enlarged.

The thymus is symmetrically enlarged and of uniform consistency and appearance. It weighed approximately 100g in the fresh state, which is about twice the normal weight for an individual of this age.

Thymic hyperplasia is extremely uncommon and is most often associated with endocrine diseases, the best recognised of which is thyrotoxicosis. Increased circulating levels of thyroxine are known to result in lymphoid hyperplasia throughout the body. Other known associations include acromegaly and Addison's disease. The so-called thymic hyperplasia sometimes seen in myasthenia gravis refers, in fact, to increased numbers of active lymphoid follicles and not to a true increase in the size or weight of the thymus.

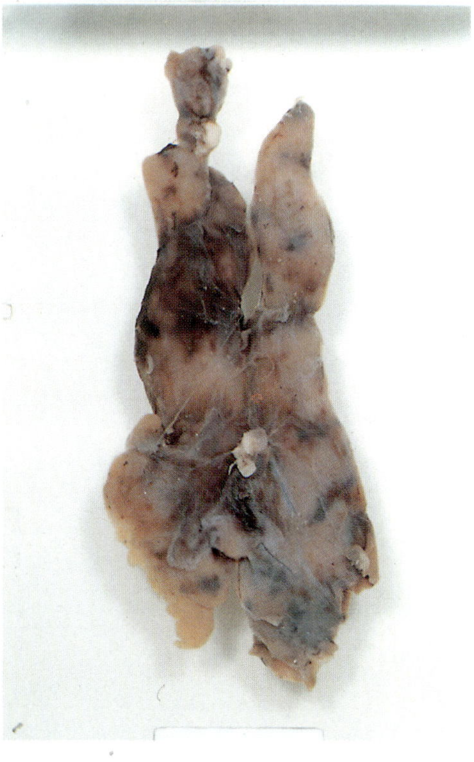

7.36 Thymus: Thymoma with Myasthenia Gravis

This specimen was excised from a 34-year-old man who presented 2 months previously with myasthenia gravis. Despite thymectomy his condition deteriorated and he died 3 months later. At autopsy, there was no evidence of residual tumour.

The thymus gland, weighing 66g, contains a firm, pale multinodular tumour which is more apparent on the left. The tumour is encapsulated and contains several minute cysts.

Thymomas are not uncommon and most often present in middle age. The majority are composed of a mixture of lymphoid and epithelial components. They are usually slow-growing and may be locally invasive; however, metastasis is extremely rare. In general these lesions are radiosensitive and the prognosis is good. Their most interesting feature is that about 30 per cent of cases are associated with other systemic illnesses; the commonest of these is myasthenia gravis but others include systemic lupus erythematosus, red cell aplasia, hypogammaglobulinaemia and Cushing's syndrome. It is thought that the thymomas may give rise to an altered cell-mediated autoimmune response in myasthenia, but the exact nature of this relationship remains uncertain. Up to 15 per cent of patients with myasthenia gravis are found to have a thymoma. Thymectomy often leads to a substantial improvement in their condition and, not infrequently, a complete cure. It should be noted, however, that elderly patients often derive less benefit from thymectomy.

8. SKIN

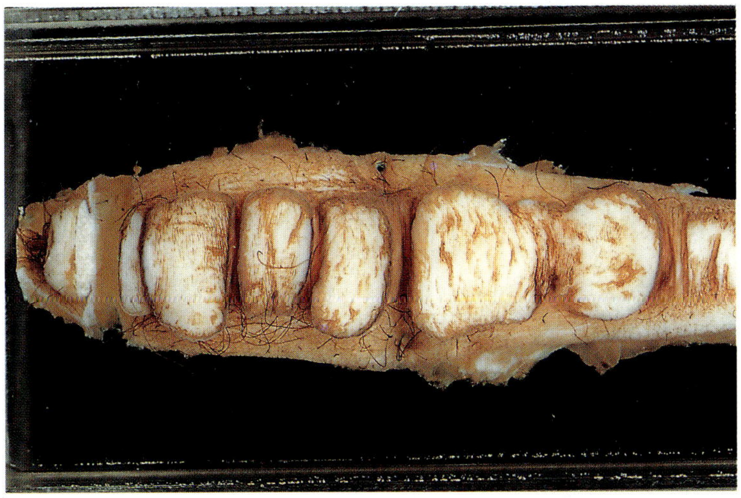

8.1 Keloid

This specimen was excised from a woman, aged 40, who had had an abdominal operation some years previously.

It consists of a strip of skin taken from the site of the healed surgical incision. The scar is deeply pigmented and is partly covered with a series of firm, pale rounded nodules measuring up to 1cm in diameter.

Keloids represent excessive collagen production at the site of tissue trauma. They are particularly common in the Negroid population but are occasionally found in Caucasians. Keloids may sometimes be itchy or painful and typically extend beyond the margins of the original site of damage. While they are cosmetically disfiguring, they should be regarded as reactive, rather than neoplastic, lesions. Local recurrence after excision (which is common), reflects the individual patient's tendency to form keloidal scars.

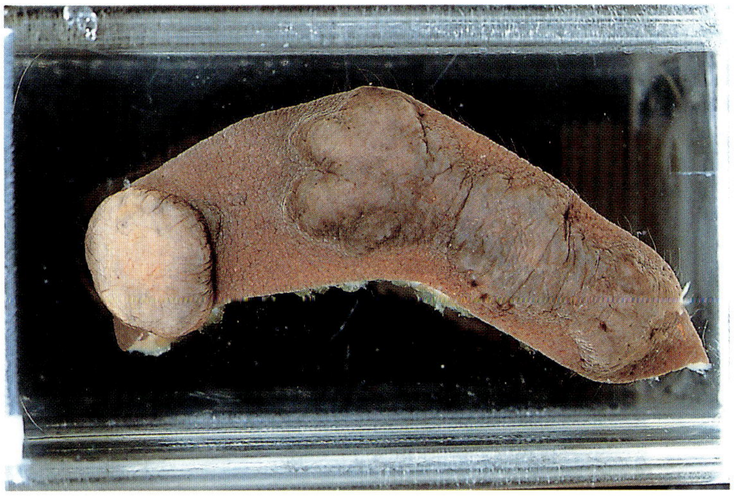

8.2 Keloid at Vaccination Site

This specimen was excised from the left shoulder of a 16-year-old Jamaican girl who had been vaccinated against smallpox at this site.

An ellipse of skin is shown bearing two separate areas of exuberant keloid formation, one rounded and the other irregularly linear.

In general, keloid scars are most often seen in the head and neck region or on the trunk.

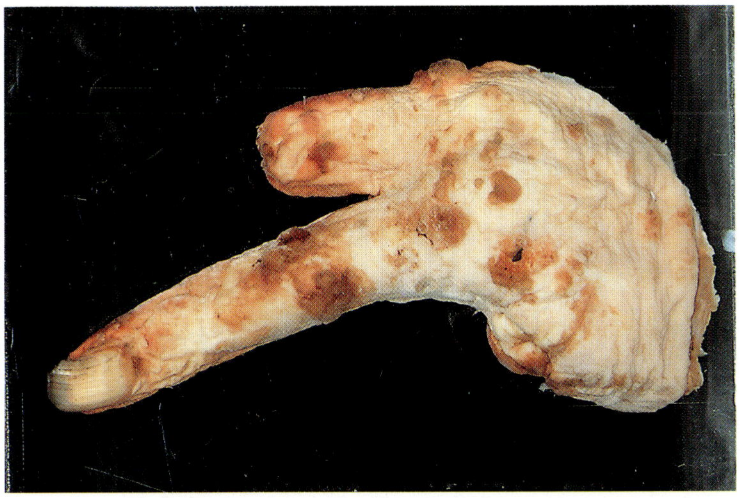

8.3 Radiodermatitis

No clinical details are available.

The skin of the hand is scarred, puckered and studded with warty excrescences.

Radiodermatitis most often complicates repeated therapeutic doses of radiotherapy. The clinical manifestations are essentially an exaggeration of the ageing process. The epidermis is typically atrophic and radiation keratoses (as seen in this case), basal cell and squamous cell carcinomata are not uncommon complications.

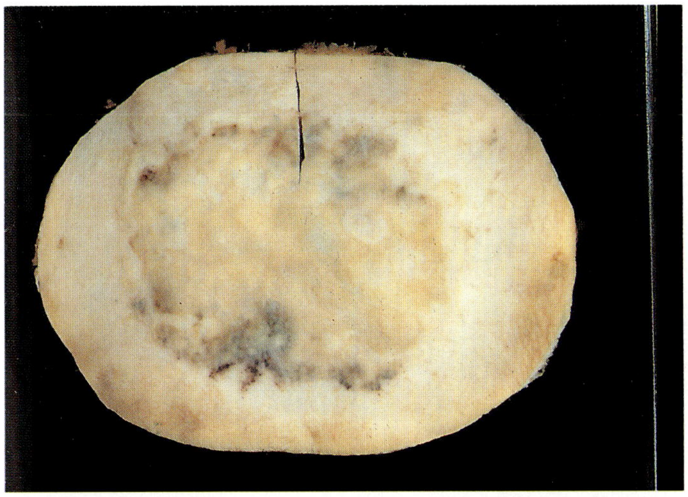

8.4 Radiation Ulcer

This specimen was excised from a 67-year-old woman who had undergone long-term radiotherapy for arthritis of the knees. After 5 years of weekly treatment she developed a large ulcer on the medial aspect of the thigh which was excised and grafted.

The specimen consists of a piece of skin with an oval area of necrosis measuring 8 × 6cm. The margin of the ulcer is heaped up and the surrounding rim shows telangiectasia.

Ulceration is an occasional complication of radiodermatitis, resulting from a combination of cutaneous atrophy and ischaemia, due to damage to the underlying dermal blood vessels.

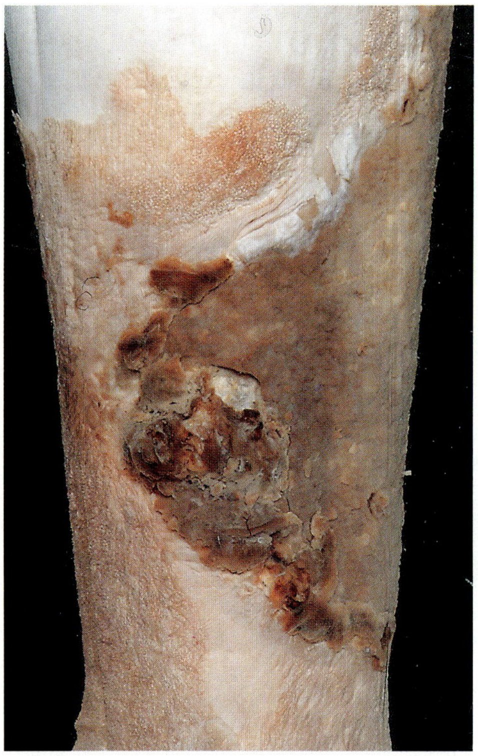

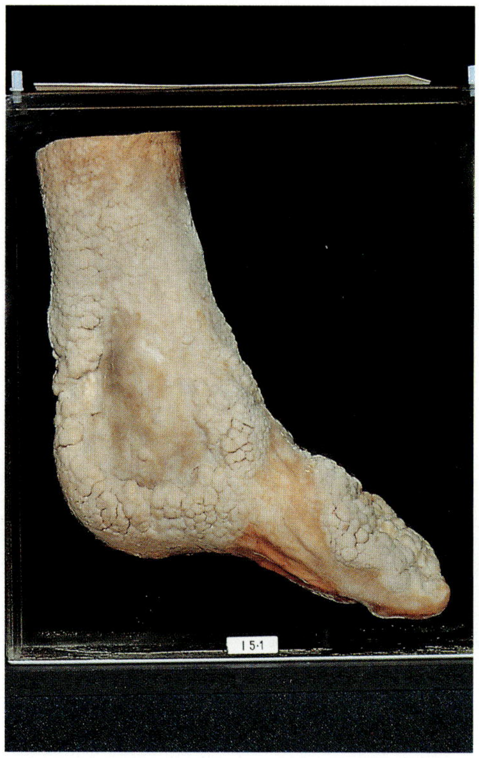

8.6 Leg: Lymphoedema

This is a below-knee amputation specimen from a 58-year-old woman who had suffered recurrent swelling and ulceration of the lower leg for 20 years. Examination revealed massive oedema, numerous papillomatous warts which discharged foul pus and an indurated chronic ulcer over the medial malleolus. There was no evidence of lymphadenopathy or varicose veins.

The skin and subcutaneous tissues of the leg (8.6a) are thickened and oedematous, and are covered with flat warty papillomata. There is an indurated ulcer over the medial malleolus (8.6b), around which the papillomata appear more exuberant.

Lymphoedema most often occurs as a secondary phenomenon due to lymphatic spread of malignant tumours, surgical removal of draining lymph nodes, filariasis or as a result of inflammatory fibrosis. More rarely it may be idiopathic, occurring either from birth (Milroy's disease) or in adolescents and young adults (lymphoedema praecox). Irrespective of the aetiology, chronic lymphoedema results in subcutaneous fibrosis and oedematous thickening of the skin. It may be complicated by lymphangitis, cellulitis, ulceration and, rarely, the development of lymphangiosarcoma (see Chapter 9).

8.5 Varicose Ulceration

This is a below-knee amputation specimen from a patient with long-standing varicose veins.

The skin of the lower leg shows extensive and severe ulceration with adjacent scarring.

The process of varicose ulceration is thought to be due to tissue hypoxia induced by fibrin deposition around venules and veins, which occurs because chronic venous stasis results in abnormally increased vascular endothelial permeability.

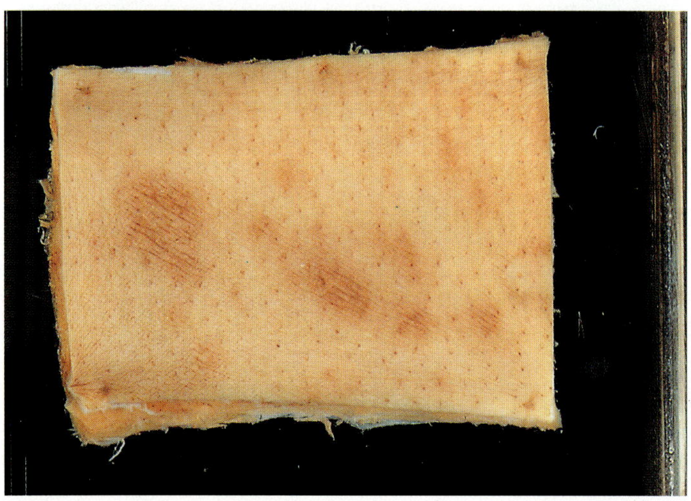

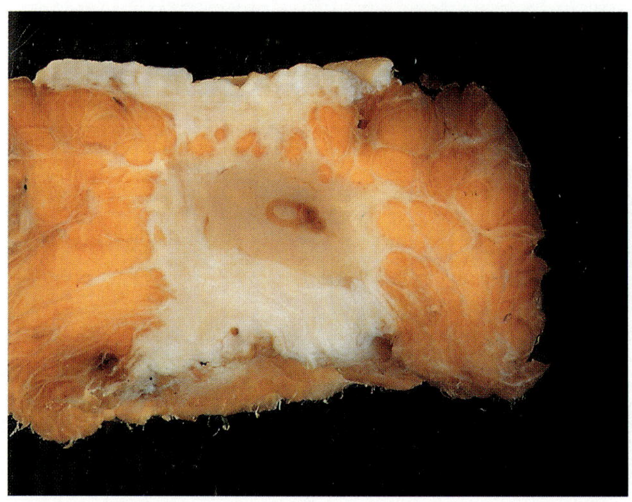

8.7 Arsenical Pigmentation

This is a post-mortem specimen taken from a man who developed a skin eruption which was treated with arsenic. When the eruption did not improve, the dose was increased and he finally died from arsenical poisoning.

This piece of skin shows ill-defined patches of brown pigmentation.

Arsenical pigmentation often has a raindrop configuration with the heaviest staining at the peripheries of the drops. Arsenic therapy may also be complicated by the development of keratoses (particularly on the soles and palms) which may progress to squamous carcinomata. It is also associated with the development of multiple basal cell carcinomata at other sites.

8.8 Stitch Abscess

This specimen was excised from a 59-year-old woman who developed a painful abscess at the site of previous cholecystectomy.

A sagittal section through the skin and subcutaneous tissue from the abdominal wall at the site of the surgical incision shows strands of fibrous tissue extending down from the operation scar into the underlying fatty tissue. Within the scar there is an indurated area containing an irregular cavity lined by granulation tissue in which a knotted ligature is embedded.

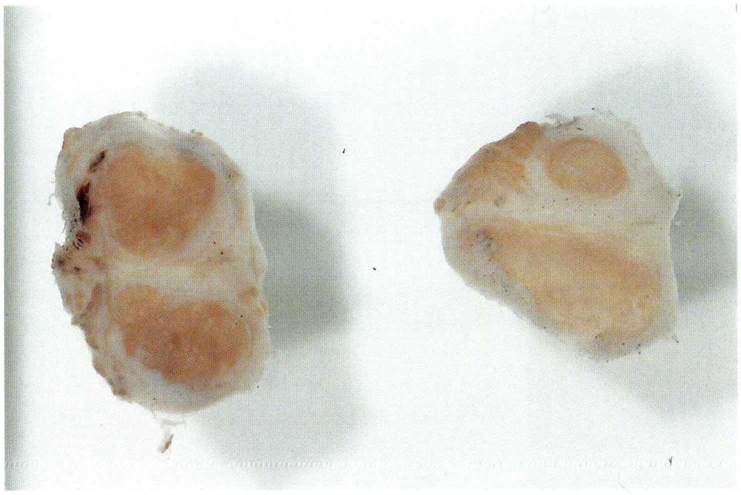

8.9 Subcutaneous Onchocercal Nodule

This specimen was excised from the subcutaneous tissue over the iliac crest of a young Nigerian adult.

A section through the excised subcutaneous nodule reveals a capsule of dense fibrous tissue surrounding an orange-coloured mass in which the sinuous tracks of the adult worms may be seen.

Onchocerciasis is due to infestation by the roundworm, *Onchocerca volvulus*, which is transmitted by the buffalo gnat, *Simulium damnosum*. Lesions develop at the site of the insect bite. The condition is endemic in tropical Africa and Central America. Cutaneous and subcutaneous involvement is characteristic and is due to the presence of adult worms in the upper dermis. Microfilaria often spread to the eye and this frequently results in blindness.

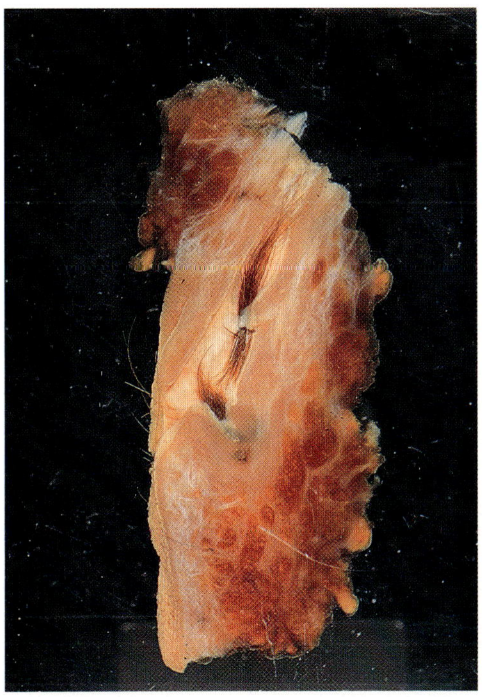

8.10 Perineum: Pilonidal Sinus

This specimen was taken from a 30-year-old man who complained of a recurrent discharging sinus over the mid-line of the sacrum, approximately 2cm above the anus.

A section through the skin shows a smooth-walled sinus containing a number of hairs.

While this is the commonest site for the development of pilonidal sinuses, they may also occur in the axillae and interdigital spaces. They are caused by the impaction of shed hairs in the orifice of sebaceous or sweat glands: young adults, particularly males, are most often affected.

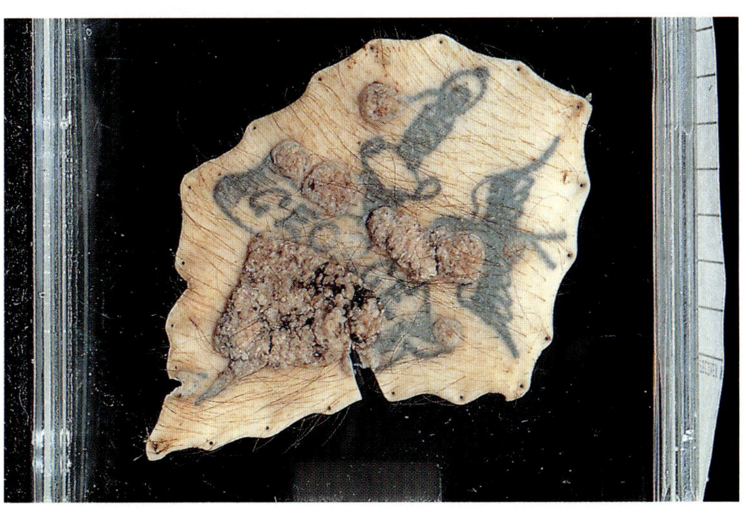

8.11 Papilloma arising in a Tattoo

No clinical details are available.

A piece of skin is shown bearing a tattoo. Much of the design is obscured by numerous warty excrescences (of probable viral aetiology).

Tattoos may also be complicated by pyogenic infections, syphilis and hepatitis B due to the use of contaminated needles. Warts such as these are due to infection with human papillomavirus.

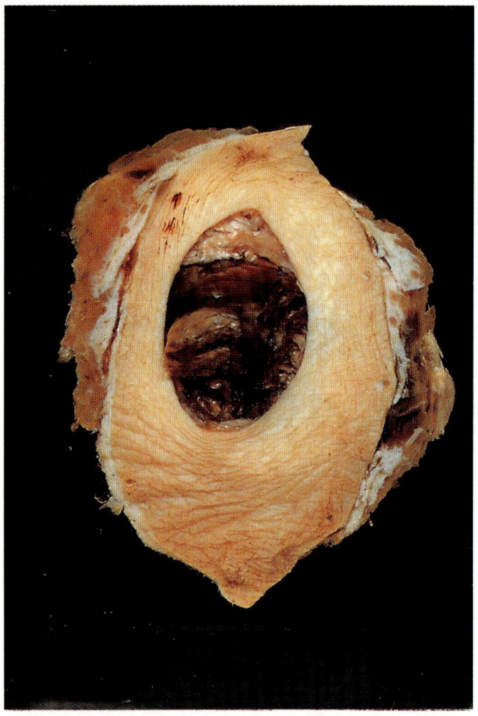

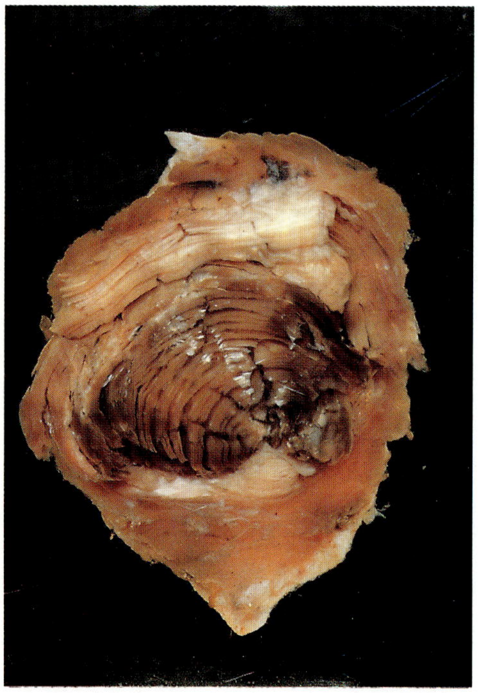

8.12 Keratin Horn

This specimen was excised from a 67-year-old woman who had noticed a discharging swelling over the left iliac crest for 35 years.

It consists of an oval piece of skin with a round opening, 2cm in diameter, through which protrude a number of irregular, brown horny processes (8.12a). The back of the specimen shows a fibrous-walled, epidermoid cyst packed with concentric layers of keratin (8.12b).

Keratin horns represent exuberant hyperkeratosis, typically overlying a solar keratosis or seborrhoeic wart. They may also be associated with viral warts, Bowen's disease or squamous carcinoma.

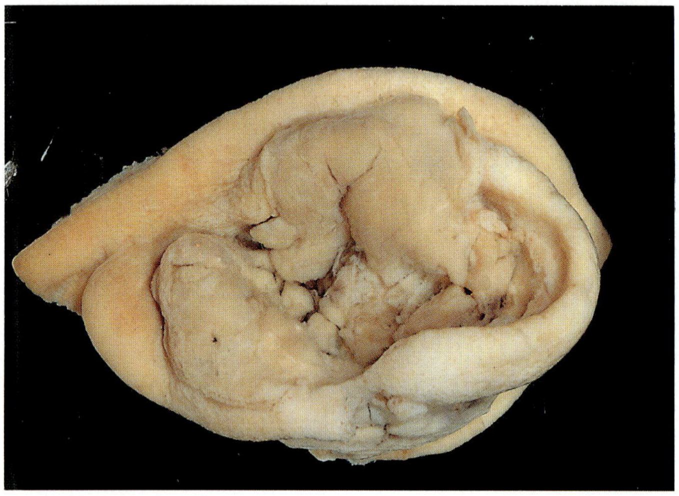

8.13 Squamous Cell Carcinoma

No clinical details are available.

The left external ear shows an extensively ulcerated carcinoma involving the greater part of the inner surface. The tumour has perforated the organ and has formed an ulcerated swelling posteriorly.

Squamous cell carcinoma is the second most common malignant skin tumour in the British Isles (basal cell carcinoma being the commonest). Nowadays it most often arises on sun-damaged skin and precursor lesions include solar keratosis and Bowen's disease. A small percentage of cases are still due to ingested arsenicals. It may also arise at the site of varicose eczema, a chronic sinus (e.g. osteomyelitis), burns, irradiation or occupational exposure to polyhydrocarbons (e.g. tar). In addition it may complicate various congenital conditions such as xeroderma pigmentosum, albinism and poikiloderma congenitale, and may very rarely occur in lupus vulgaris, cutaneous syphilis and leprosy. The clinical course is very variable but, in contrast to basal cell carcinoma, there is a definite risk of metastasis.

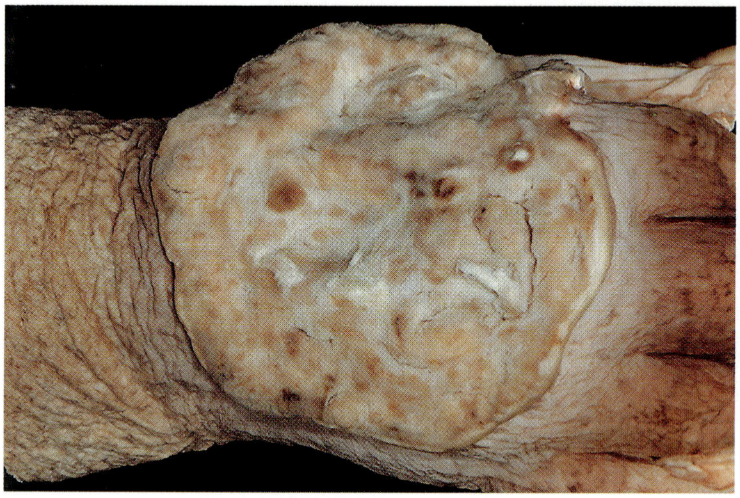

8.14 Hand: Squamous Cell Carcinoma

This specimen was excised from a confused 79-year-old lady who had persistently refused treatment for an ulcer on her right hand which had been present for 5 years. When she was eventually seen at a hospital the tumour was no longer amenable to conservative treatment and an amputation was performed.

The dorsal aspect of the right hand is almost completely replaced by a large, ulcerated squamous carcinoma. The edges of the ulcer are raised and everted; the surface is infected and the purulent and sloughing areas are clearly visible.

This case demonstrates that cutaneous squamous cell carcinoma may be slow growing and show extensive local invasion without always metastasising.

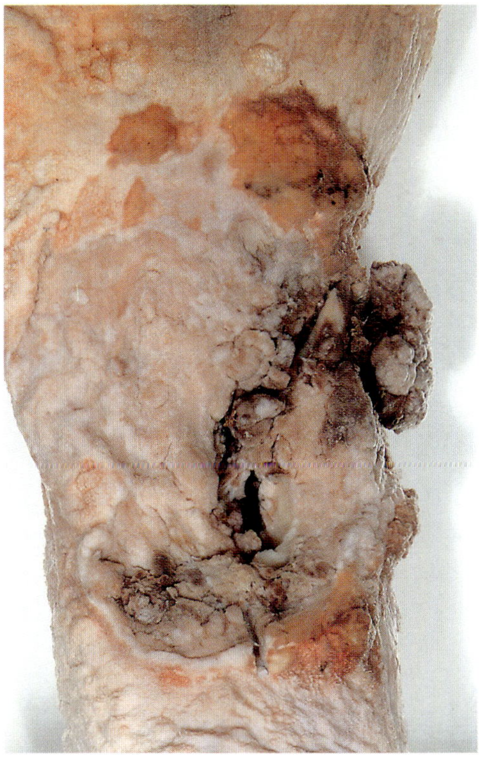

8.15 Squamous Cell Carcinoma arising in a Chronic Venous Ulcer

This specimen was taken from an 80-year-old woman who had suffered from varicose ulceration over the medial aspect of the right shin for approximately 50 years. She was admitted to hospital with a pathological fracture due to bone destruction by a tumour which had arisen in the ulcer.

A close-up view of the below-knee amputation specimen shows a fungating, ulcerated squamous cell carcinoma over the medial malleolus and the anterior surface of the lower leg.

A small proportion of squamous carcinomata are well known to develop at the site of long-standing cutaneous ulceration, the latter usually being varicose or tropical in origin. Such an occurrence is known as Marjolin's ulcer. Basal cell carcinomata may also, although more rarely, be seen.

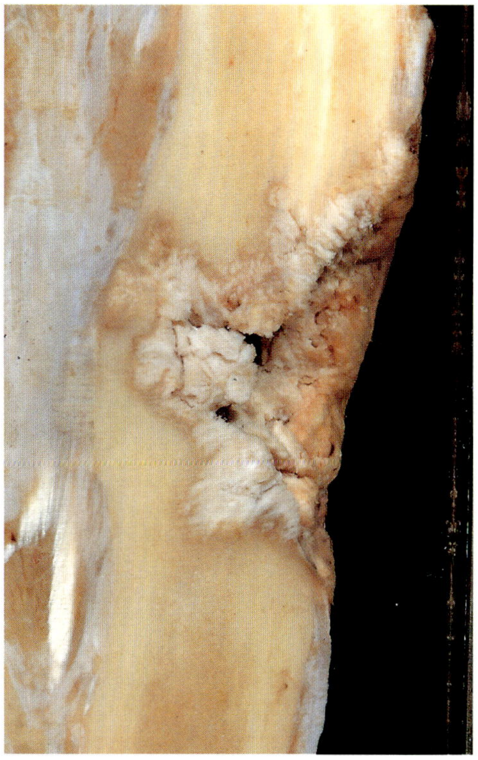

8.16 Squamous Cell Carcinoma arising in a Chronic Osteomyelitis Sinus

This specimen was excised from a man with a 5 year history of osteomyelitis with bone abscess and sinus formation, which developed at the site of a compound fracture of the tibia and fibula. Amputation was performed after biopsy of the ulcer revealed malignant change.

A sagittal section through a portion of the leg below the knee shows a deeply ulcerated area surrounded by pale tumour which has penetrated the shaft of the tibia.

Chronic osteomyelitic sinuses are also a well recognised site at which squamous carcinoma may arise.

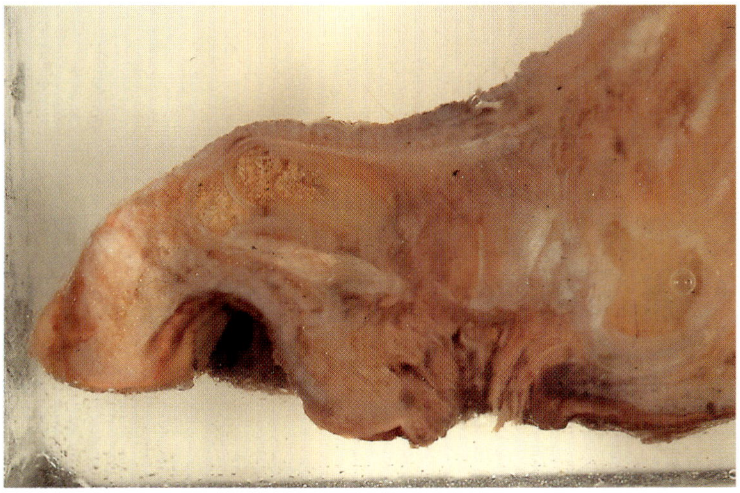

8.17 Sole of Foot: Carcinoma Cuniculatum

This specimen was excised from a 50-year-old man who had noticed a wart on the sole of his right foot for 25 years. Both he and a chiropodist had trimmed it repeatedly. On examination there was a very large warty lesion, situated below the metatarsal arch, with a surrounding hyperkeratotic collar. Despite frequent curettage, the lesion recurred on numerous occasions over the ensuing 2 years. Complete excision was performed but pain and incomplete healing of the wound led to the decision to perform a Syme's amputation.

A sagittal section through the foot (8.17a) shows an ulcer of the skin in the region of the metatarsal arch; seen in close up (8.17b) it has a ragged base and everted edges. It penetrates into the fascial and tendinous tissues to a depth of 1cm.

This tumour is a rare variant of squamous cell carcinoma, coming into the category of verrucous carcinoma. This is a slow-growing, fungating tumour that may penetrate deeply into the tissues but metastasises only very late, if at all. Such tumours are often not recognised histologically as malignant since they are characteristically very well-differentiated. Verrucous carcinoma occurs on the oral mucosa as oral florid papillomatosis, on the external genitalia and perianal skin as a giant condyloma acuminatum, and on the sole of the foot as epithelioma cuniculatum. The tumours at the latter site are frequently associated with pre-existing viral warts, which may be of aetiological importance.

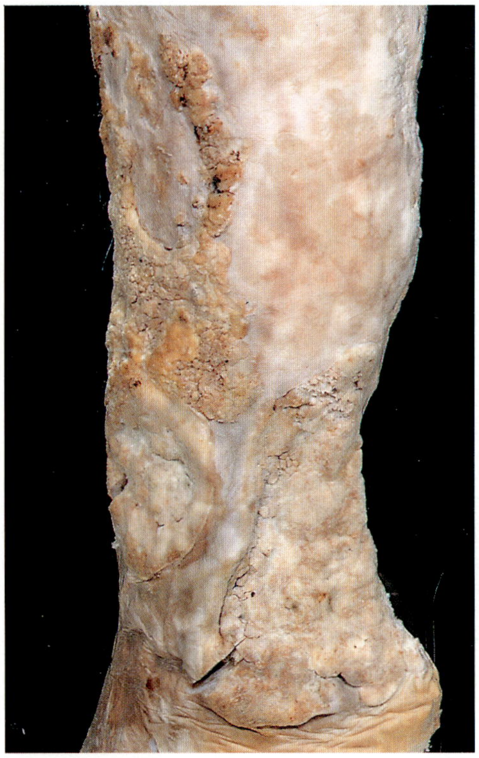

8.18 Squamous Cell Carcinoma complicating Dermolytic Epidermolysis Bullosa

This specimen was taken from a 38-year-old woman with a long history of a bullous skin eruption diagnosed as dermolytic (dystrophic) epidermolysis bullosa. This variant of epidermolysis bullosa has an autosomal recessive inheritance. The patient developed large areas of ulceration on the left lower leg which clinically were considered to be malignant and therefore an above-knee amputation was performed.

The lower part of the leg shows multiple, variably sized ulcers with heaped-up irregular edges. Histologically these proved to be squamous cell carcinomata. Much of the residual skin is discoloured and scabbed while other areas are pale and atrophic.

Epidermolysis bullosa is a rare inherited condition characterised by the development of cutaneous blisters at the site of trauma. There are several clinically distinct subtypes, of which the dermolytic (dystrophic) variant is known to predispose to squamous cell carcinoma.

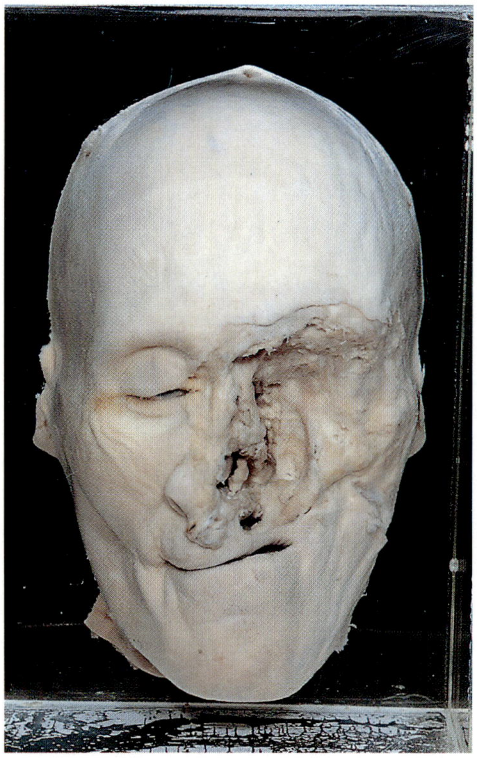

8.19 Basal Cell Carcinoma

This is the head of an elderly man who had attended hospital repeatedly for a progressive rodent ulcer on the left side of his face.

The eye, the orbit and the nasal fossa have been completely destroyed; the lower part of the right nasal fossa is exposed and there is a perforation in the anterior portion of the right side of the palate.

Basal cell carcinoma is the commonest primary malignant neoplasm of the skin and typically affects middle-aged or elderly adults. The majority arise in the head and neck region and known aetiological factors include solar or irradiation damage, industrial exposure to polyhydrocarbons and the ingestion of arsenicals. Occasional cases have a genetic basis. These tumours tend to relentless local invasion if untreated (as in this case) but metastatic spread is exceedingly uncommon.

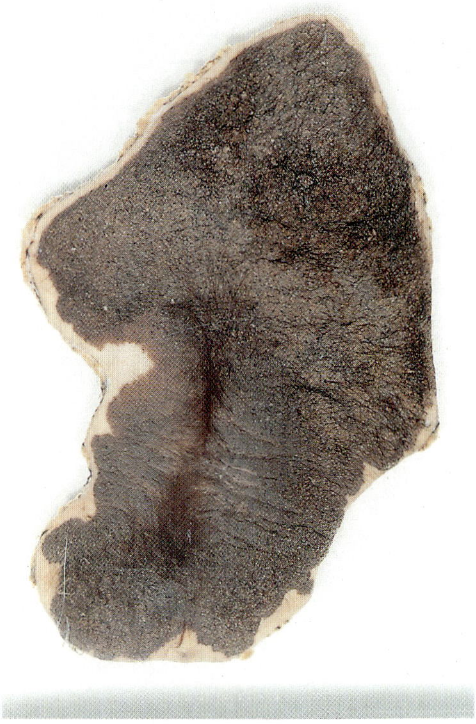

8.20 Skin of Chest: Congenital Giant Pigmented (Bathing Trunk) Naevus

This lesion was excised from a 28-year-old man who presented with a pigmented lesion on the left side of the chest which had been noticed since birth. There had been no increase in size but it was prone to superficial ulceration after minor injury. The area was excised down to deep fascia and grafted.

The specimen consists of skin and subcutaneous tissue from the chest, the former being deeply pigmented and covered with small warty nodules.

Congenital giant pigmented naevi are benign melanocytic lesions which are by definition present from birth. While the skin around the limb girdles is most often affected, the site and size of these tumours is very variable. These naevi may be complicated by the development of malignant melanoma in between 5 and 10 per cent of cases.

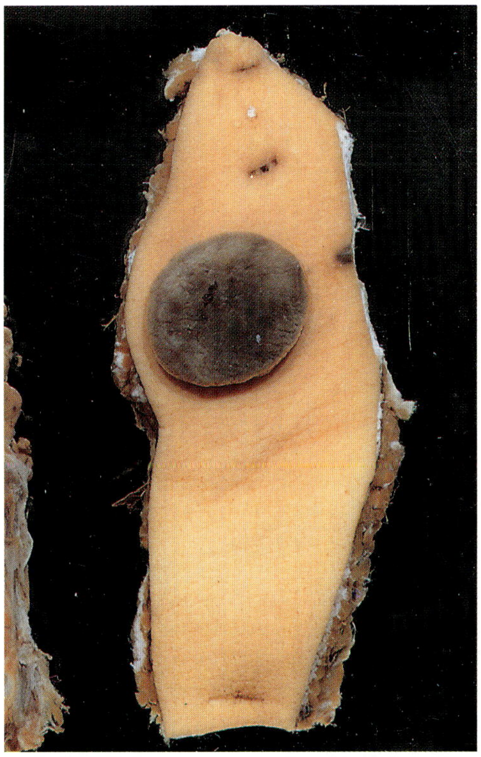

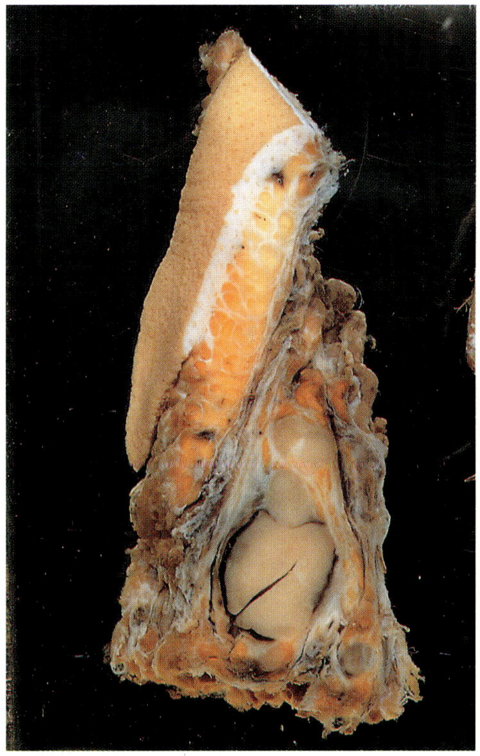

8.21 Skin of Back: Malignant Melanoma with Axillary Lymph Node Metastases

These specimens were excised from a 25-year-old woman who had first noticed a pigmented skin lump below the right shoulder blade 2 months previously. One week before presentation, a painful swelling developed in the right axilla. The tumour with the axillary nodes and the intervening skin was excised in one piece down to deep fascia and the area was grafted.

An oval piece of skin shows a rounded pigmented tumour 2cm in diameter, which projects from the skin surface (8.21a). Close by there is a similar tumour, 0.25cm in diameter, which represents a satellite nodule. A section through the axillary tissue shows enlargement and infiltration of the lymph nodes by metastatic tumour (8.21b).

Malignant melanoma is an increasingly common cutaneous neoplasm, which in most instances, is directly related to excessive exposure to solar irradiation. Only a very small proportion arise in a pre-existing benign lesion. The most indolent form, Hutchinson's freckle (lentigo maligna), is a slow-growing pigmented macule which arises most often on the face or dorsum of the hand and carries a relatively good prognosis. Superficial spreading melanoma, the commonest form, presents typically on the trunk or limbs and has a poorer prognosis, similar to that of the third type, acral lentiginous melanoma, which arises most frequently on the hands, feet or mucous membranes. Finally, nodular malignant melanoma, which appears to arise without a preceding horizontal growth phase, presents at almost any cutaneous site and is associated with the worst prognosis. The commonest symptoms are increasing size of a pigmented lesion, change in colour, itching or bleeding. The most significant prognostic factor in malignant melanoma is tumour thickness, those greater than 0.76mm having an appreciably worse prognosis.

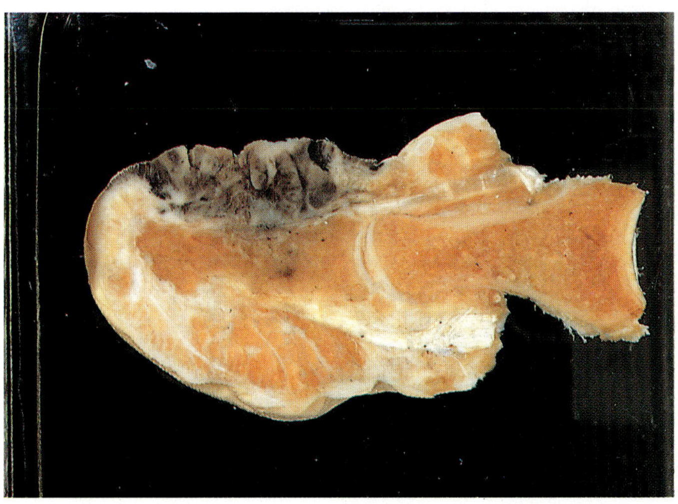

8.22 Subungual Malignant Melanoma of the Great Toe

This toe was amputated from a 55-year-old woman who had noticed blackening of the nail for 2 years. This was followed by loss of the nail which exposed a pigmented tumour.

The outer half of the right great toe shows a melanotic tumour, 1cm in diameter, arising from the nail-bed and invading the underlying bone. The surface of the tumour is extensively ulcerated.

Malignant melanoma arising in a nail bed (acral lentiginous melanoma) is an uncommon but well-recognised phenomenon, which may be confused clinically with a haematoma.

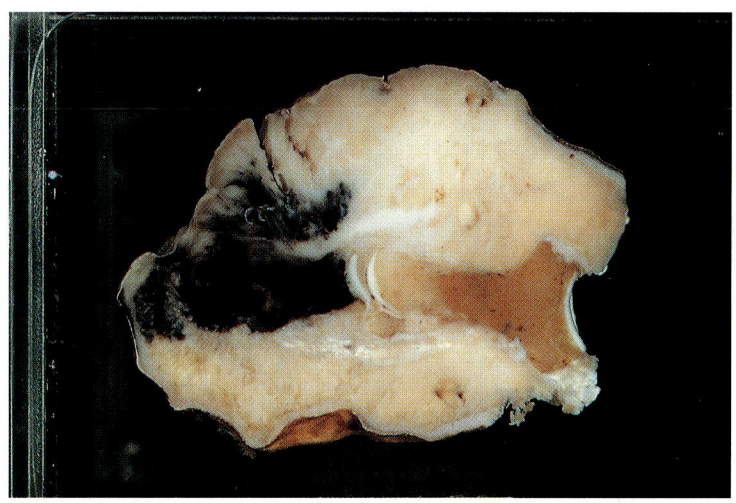

8.23 Great Toe: Malignant Melanoma

This specimen was excised from a 45-year-old African male, living in Malawi, who presented with a mass occupying most of the left great toe.

The enlarged and distorted great toe has been sectioned to show an extensive mass of tumour infiltrating the skin, soft tissue and phalanges. Note that the tumour replacing the distal phalanx shows heavy melanotic pigmentation, while much of the adjacent tumour is amelanotic.

While malignant melanoma is uncommon in the negroid population, the most frequent sites of origin are the sole of the foot and the nail folds.

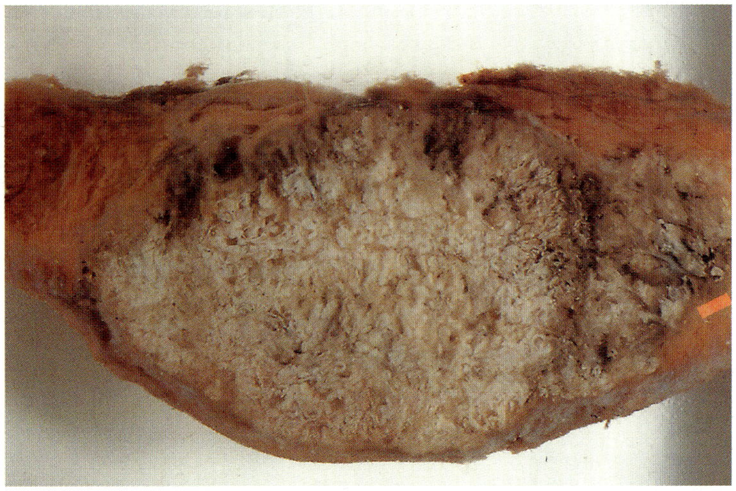

8.24 Calcifying Epithelioma of Malherbe

This specimen was excised from the right shoulder of a 63-year-old woman who had noticed a slowly growing lump for 4 years.

A section through skin and subcutaneous tissue shows a circumscribed, ovoid mass, measuring 4 × 2cm, which is covered by attenuated epidermis. The cut surface of the tumour has an opaque, white granular appearance due to irregular dystrophic calcification.

The calcifying epithelioma (synonym: pilomatrixoma) is a benign tumour of follicular origin. It usually arises in children and young adults, affects females more than males, and most often presents as a dome-shaped nodule on the face or neck.

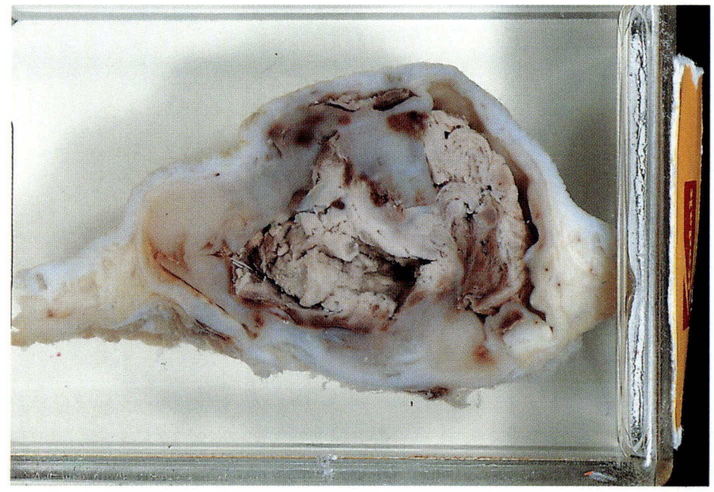

8.25 Chondroid Syringoma (Mixed Tumour of Skin)

No clinical details are available.

The specimen consists of a fairly well-circumscribed, subcutaneous tumour, measuring 5cm in diameter and covered by a thin layer of normal skin. The tumour has undergone extensive cystic change and there is a prominent myxoid component.

Chondroid syringomas are benign tumours of probable eccrine sweat gland origin. They are usually small and arise most often on the head and neck.

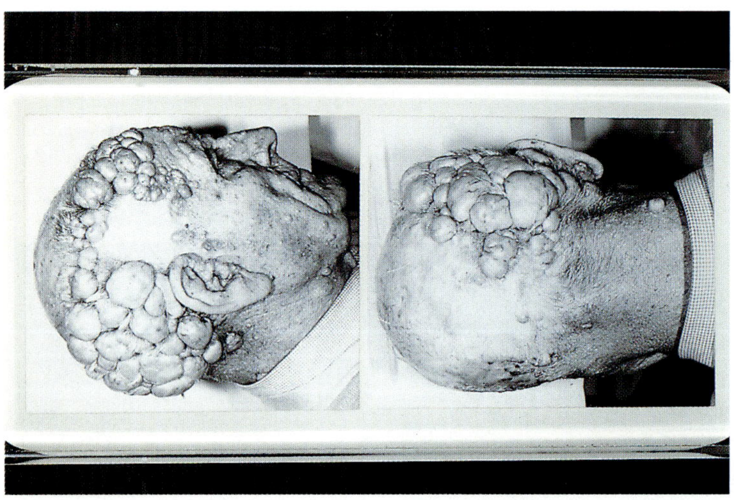

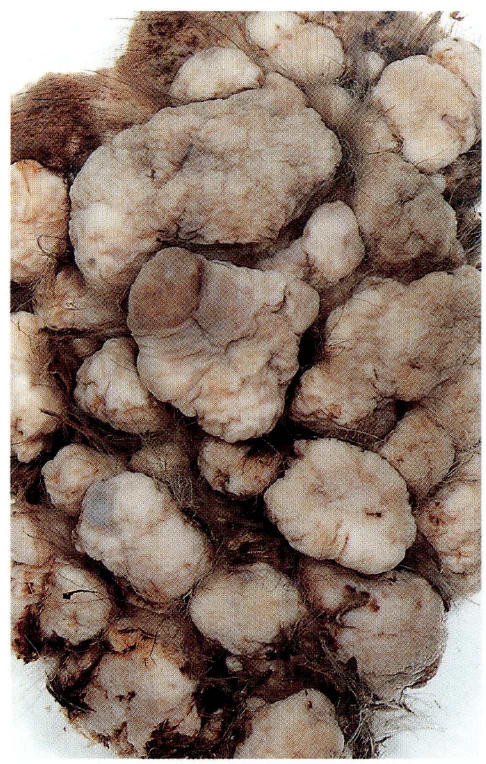

8.26 Multiple Cylindromata of the Scalp ('Turban' Tumours)

The clinical photograph (8.26a) shows a 76-year-old man who first developed a tumour of the scalp at the age of 19. Over the succeeding 40 years he developed multiple tumours on the scalp and trunk which were intermittently excised. At the age of 60 a crop of small tumours around the left ear were irradiated but radionecrosis occurred and the ear was amputated.

Further excision was required for radionecrosis of the mastoid and zygomatic areas. The appearance of yet more tumours precipitated excision of a large area of the scalp, seen on the right (8.26b).

The syndrome of multiple cylindromata has an autosomal dominant inheritance and, in this case, there was a strong family history, the patient's grandmother, mother and three out of five siblings being affected. Cylindromata are benign tumours of probable eccrine sweat gland origin, which almost exclusively arise in the scalp and typically are first noticed in childhood.

9. SOFT TISSUES

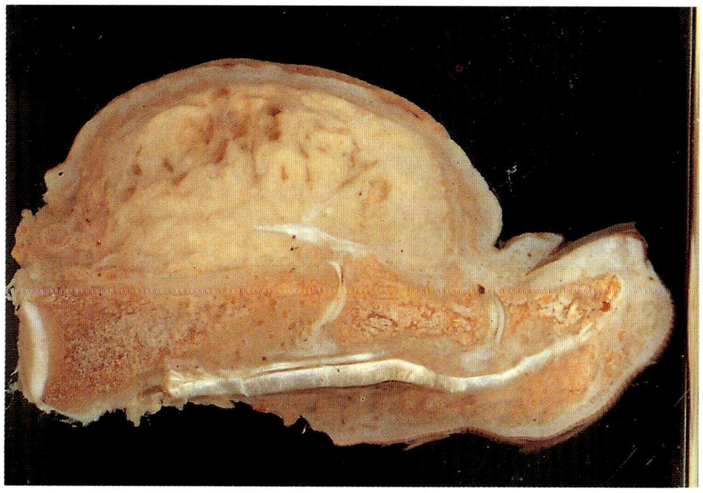

9.1 Toe: Gouty Tophus

This toe was amputated from a 52-year-old man who had suffered from gout for 8 years. There had been progressive swelling of the toe for 9 months but X-rays revealed no damage to the underlying bone.

A longitudinal section through the toe shows an ovoid mass, measuring 3cm in length, beneath the skin of the dorsal surface. The mass is fibrous in appearance but contains yellowish areas and small cystic spaces.

Gout is a clinical disorder which results from alterations in purine metabolism causing hyperuricaemia. It is sometimes a primary condition, which is commonest in older individuals, may have a familial tendency, and may be precipitated by a high alcohol intake. These individuals commonly show either an idiopathic increase in purine synthesis or a decrease in urate excretion. Secondary cases are principally due to increased nucleic acid turnover; e.g. in malignant tumours (multiple myeloma is the classic example), cytotoxic treatment or psoriasis, or to decreased urate excretion, e.g. in glomerular disease or acidosis. Attacks of gout lead to urate deposition in joints and juxta-articular tissues, and the gouty tophus is composed of a nidus of urate crystals surrounded by scar tissue showing a foreign body reaction.

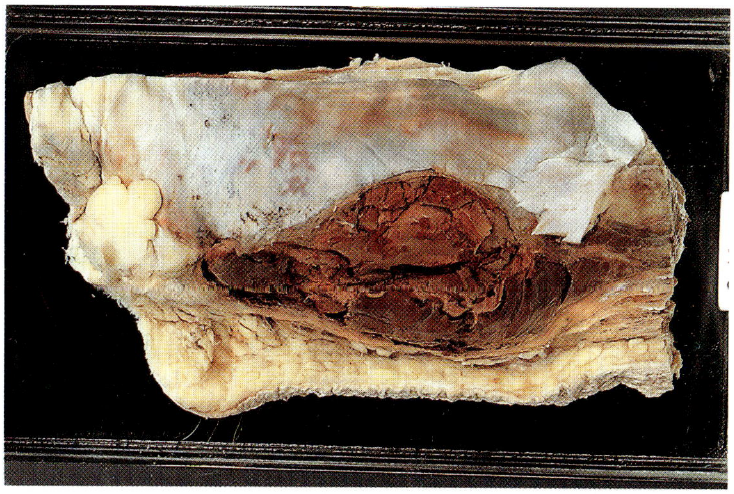

9.2 Abdomen: Ruptured Rectus Muscle

This was an incidental finding at post-mortem in an elderly man who died with cor pulmonale due to chronic obstructive airways disease.

A section through the anterior abdominal wall shows a large haematoma enclosed within the ruptured belly of the rectus abdominis muscle.

Rupture of a rectus muscle with consequent development of a rectus sheath haematoma usually occurs after prolonged or excessive straining and, in this case, was probably due to severe coughing.

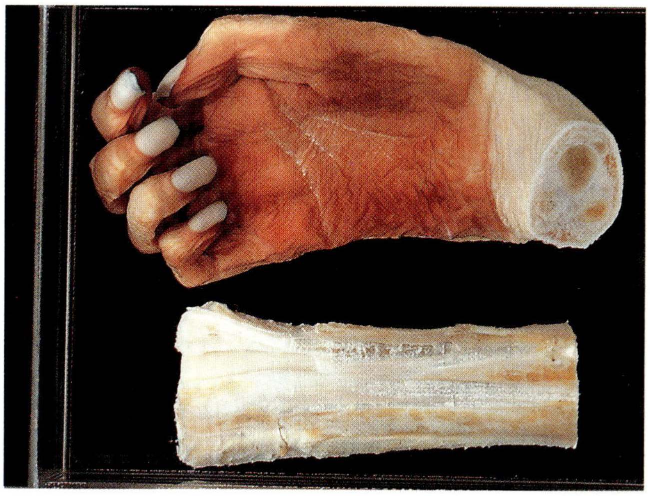

9.3 Forearm: Volkmann's Ischaemic Contracture

This is an amputation specimen from a 26-year-old man who had fractured his right wrist 3 years previously. This was reduced and fixed in plaster but painful swelling developed followed by prolonged sepsis of the forearm. Over a period of months an ischaemic contracture developed and, despite intensive physiotherapy, the lower arm became quite useless.

The right hand shows marked muscle wasting with flexion of the wrist, fingers and thumb. A longitudinal section through the soft tissues of the forearm shows complete fibrous replacement of the muscles.

Volkmann's ischaemic contracture most often results from the application of excessively tight plaster or bandaging. It is argued whether venous or arterial obstruction is the principal culprit but, whichever the case, infarction of muscle occurs followed by necrosis and replacement of muscle bundles by fibrous scar tissue.

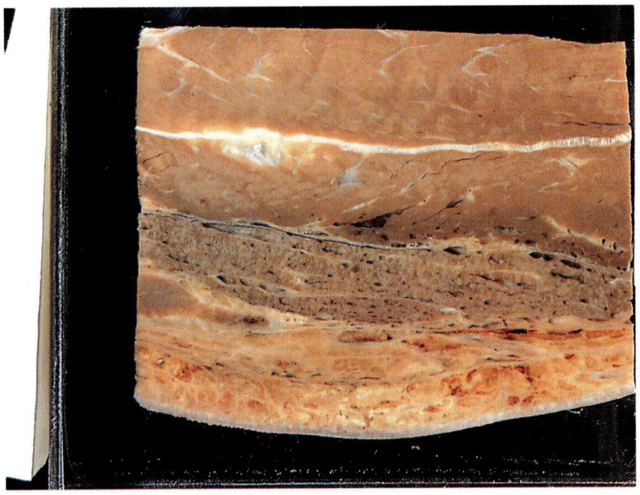

9.4 Muscle: Gas Gangrene

This is a post-mortem specimen from a soldier who was shot in the thigh during the First World War. On admission to hospital in Rouen, the wound was foul-smelling and there was interstitial oedema and gas formation extending up to the abdominal wall. He died a few hours later.

The soft tissues of the thigh have been sectioned to show greyish discolouration of the muscle, and the presence of numerous bubbles of gas.

Gas gangrene is most commonly due to infection by the anaerobe *Clostridium welchii* which grows rapidly in damaged muscle and produces a variety of lethal toxins which spread through adjacent viable tissue, destroying it and thereby providing ideal conditions for further bacterial multiplication. The infection usually results from contamination of a wound, either traumatic or surgical, with soil, other dirt or skin from areas commonly colonised by intestinal bacteria. Ischaemic tissue, of whatever origin, provides the necessary low oxygen tension required for multiplication of clostridial organisms.

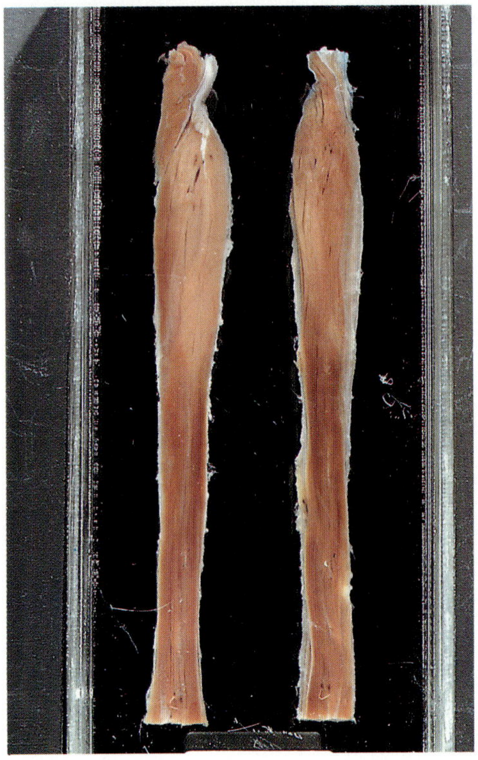

9.5 Rectus Muscle: Zenker's Hyaline Degeneration

This is a post-mortem specimen from a 34-year-old soldier who developed a pyrexial illness while in Cairo. Over a period of 6 weeks he deteriorated with a swinging fever, delirium, diarrhoea and splenomegaly. Blood cultures were positive for *Salmonella typhi* and he died rapidly.

Two vertical sections have been taken through the rectus abdominis muscle to show a pale, swollen area near the uppermost end.

Zenker's hyaline degeneration occurs in several septicaemic illnesses but most especially in typhoid fever. There is necrosis of muscle with adjacent regeneration. This condition is thought not to be due to direct bacterial invasion but rather to the effects of endotoxaemia.

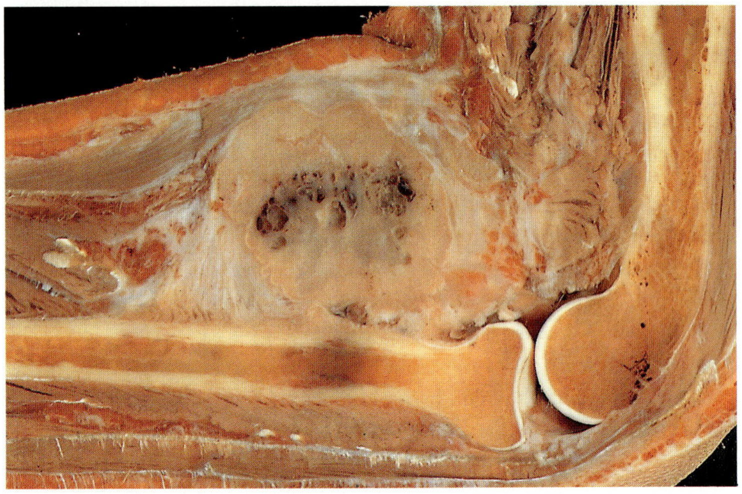

9.6 Forearm: Myositis Ossificans

This specimen was excised from a 47-year-old woman who had noticed a painful swelling of the proximal forearm for several weeks. The lesion was explored and a biopsy taken from the mass was reported as sarcoma. The arm was then amputated above the elbow.

The elbow and forearm have been sectioned to show fibrosis of the muscles around a circumscribed bony mass, measuring 3cm in diameter. The adjacent radius shows subperiosteal thickening and a small medullary haemorrhage.

Myositis ossificans may either be idiopathic or occasionally traumatic in origin. It is a benign reactive condition consisting of peripheral ossification around a florid spindle cell proliferation and is usually associated with a chronic inflammatory reaction. The condition may occur in almost any skeletal muscle and it is not uncommon for both surgeon and pathologist to make a mistaken diagnosis of malignancy.

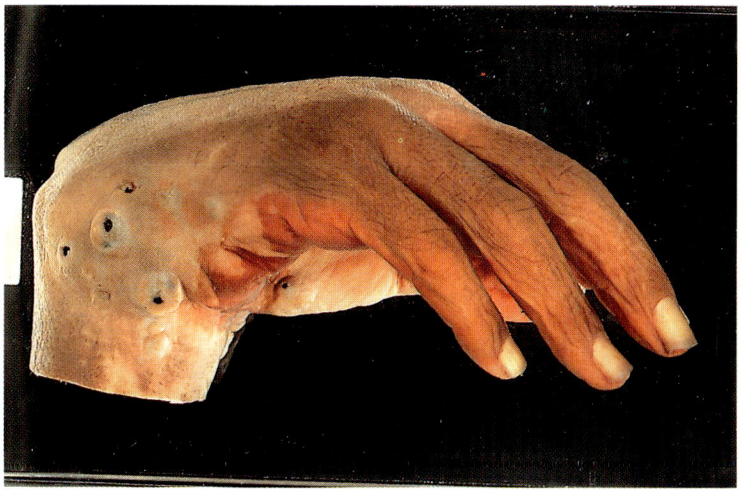

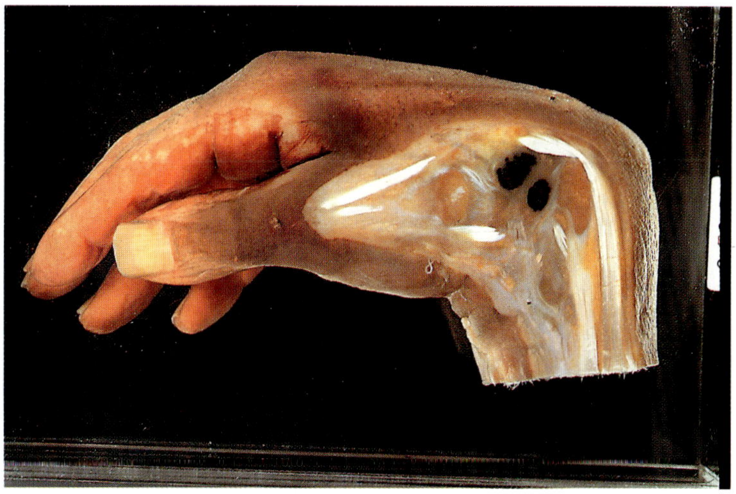

9.7 Hand: Mycetoma

This is an amputation specimen from a 47-year-old Sudanese man who had complained of swelling of the right hand, with multiple sinuses which discharged pus containing black granules, for 17 years.

The contracted and deformed hand (9.7a) shows multiple sinuses, in some of which black granular masses are visible. A section through the radial aspect (9.7b) shows widespread involvement of the deeper tissues.

Mycetoma, also known as maduromycosis, is almost exclusively a tropical disease which most often affects the extremities. The combination of chronic suppuration, pigmented granules, sinus formation and extensive scarring are typical of this condition. It may result from infection by either fungi or actinomycetes. This particular case was due to the fungus *Madurella sp.*

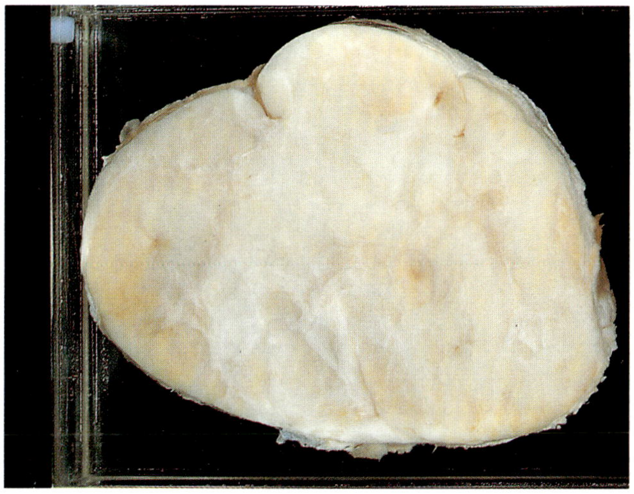

9.8 Subcutaneous Tissue: Lipoma

This was an incidental finding in the neck of an 86-year-old man who died from ischaemic heart disease.

The specimen consists of a soft lobulated tumour, measuring 8 × 5 × 5cm, with a well-defined capsule. The cut surface has the typical pale yellow colour of mature adipose tissue.

Benign lipomas are ubiquitous and affect females more than males. They are slow-growing lesions, which are sometimes multiple, and have no tendency to undergo malignant change.

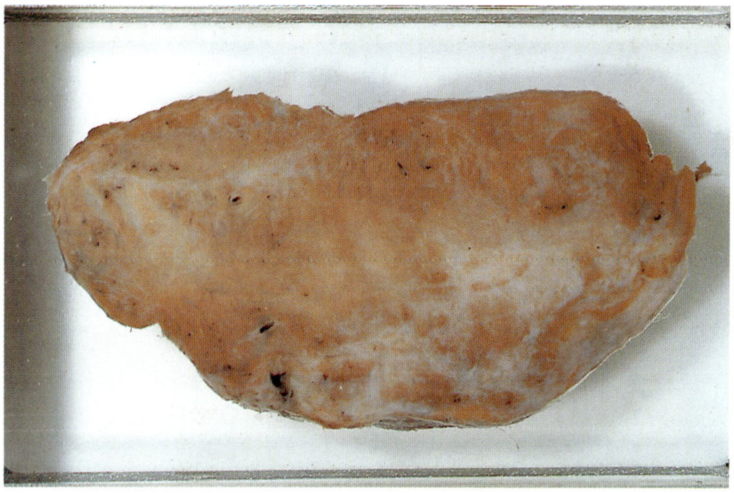

9.9 Subcutaneous Tissue: Hibernoma

This slowly enlarging, firm tumour was excised from the thigh of a 61-year-old woman. It had been present for 40 years. At operation it was found to be only loosely attached to the underlying muscle and adjacent neurovascular bundles.

A section of this solid tumour shows it to be well circumscribed. It has a variegated appearance, the bulk having a brownish colour (typical of hibernoma) interspersed by yellowish areas and strands of pale fibrous tissue.

Hibernomas are exceedingly rare tumours which are thought to arise from vestigial foci of brown fat. They are found most often around the neck and shoulders. They are sometimes very vascular and pre-operative angiography may lead to a mistaken diagnosis of malignancy.

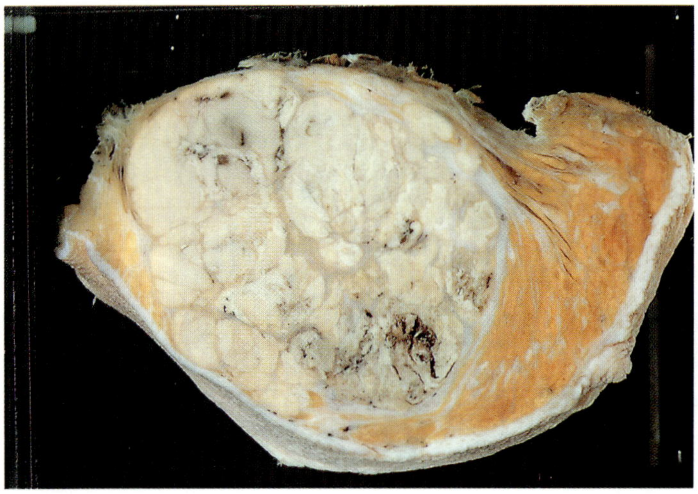

9.10 Breast: Pleomorphic Liposarcoma

This specimen was excised from a 54-year-old woman who complained of very rapid, painless enlargement of the right breast over the preceding 5 months. Local excision was performed but 6 weeks later she developed abdominal metastases and 14 months after operation she died with disseminated tumour.

The breast has been sectioned through the nipple to show a circumscribed, solid tumour measuring 8cm in diameter. The tumour is composed of lobules of yellowish tissue interspersed by bands of fibrous tissue, and shows patchy haemorrhage and necrosis. Note also the small nodules on the deep aspect of the tumour.

Liposarcoma most often presents in the 6th and 7th decades and affects males more than females. The commonest sites of origin are the thigh and retroperitoneum but the breast is by no means an unusual location. Typically these tumours are large and surprisingly, tend to be well circumscribed. However, adjacent separate nodules, as seen in this case, are common and wide excision is most important. Histologically, pleomorphic liposarcoma constitutes about 10 per cent of all liposarcomas and carries the gravest prognosis, largely due to its propensity to metastasise.

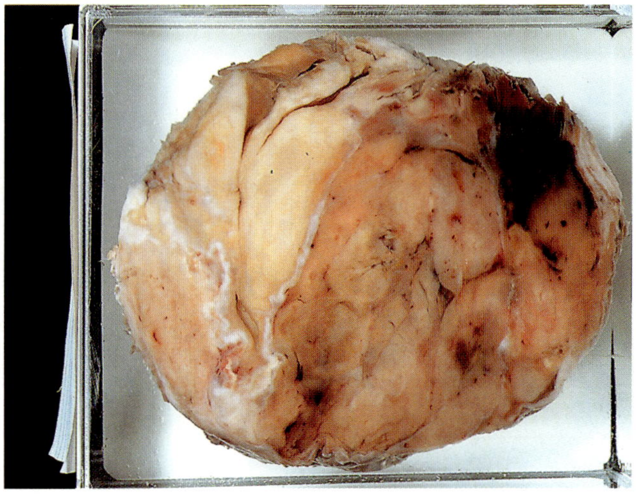

9.11 Subcutaneous Tissue: Myxoid Liposarcoma

This tumour, which was excised from the thigh of a 68-year-old woman, had been present for 6 years. Shortly before presentation, the tumour had rapidly increased in size and ulcerated. At operation it was found to be infiltrating muscle.

A section through the tumour shows a homogeneous pinkish mucoid mass which is locally infiltrative.

Myxoid liposarcoma is the commonest histological variant. All liposarcomas have a tendency to recur and up to 50 per cent may metastasise and result in death.

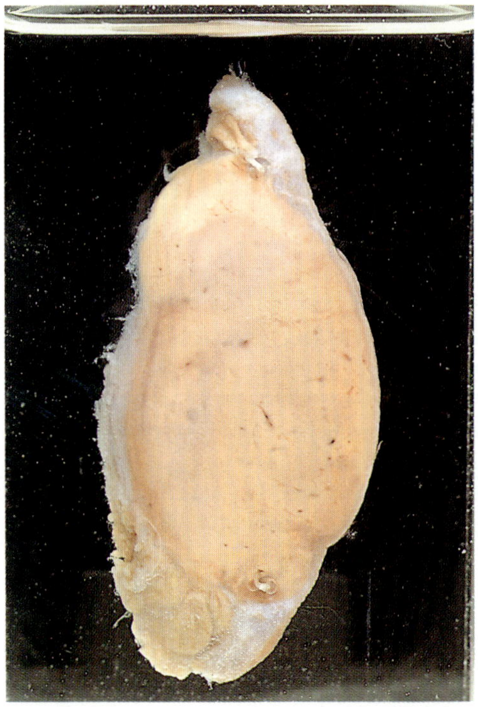

9.12 Skin: Fibrous Histiocytoma

This specimen was taken from a 54-year-old woman who had noticed a small swelling on the right flank. Clinically this was thought to be a sebaceous cyst.

An ellipse of skin overlies an oval, circumscribed tumour which occupies the dermis and superficial subcutaneous fat, and forms a nodule on the skin surface.

Fibrous histiocytoma (synonyms: dermatofibroma, sclerosing haemangioma) is a common benign cutaneous tumour which most often presents on the lower limb. Middle-aged adults, particularly females, are typically affected. Occasionally the tumour contains abundant haemosiderin pigment which may lead to clinical diagnostic confusion with malignant melanoma.

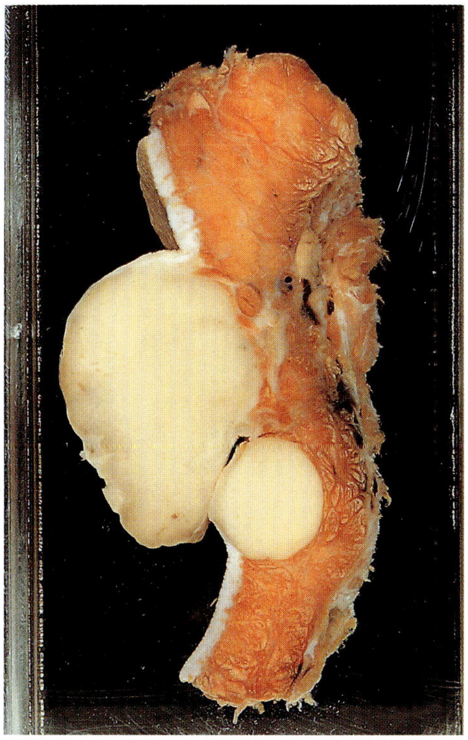

9.13 Skin: Dermatofibrosarcoma Protuberans

This specimen, which was excised from the chest wall of a 38-year-old woman, had been present for some time. It had recently increased in size and had shown a tendency to bleed. During 5 years of follow-up there had been no evidence of a recurrence.

The specimen shows a multinodular tumour arising in the dermis, extending deeply into subcutaneous fat. The skin is superficially ulcerated. Note that this tumour gives the misleading impression of being well circumscribed.

Dermatofibrosarcoma protuberans, formerly known as low-grade fibrosarcoma of skin, most commonly arises on the trunk or lower limbs of young adults. Typically it is slow growing, multinodular and induces a reddish-blue discoloration of the overlying skin. While up to one-third of these tumours may recur locally, metastasis is extremely rare and there is therefore no indication for radical treatment.

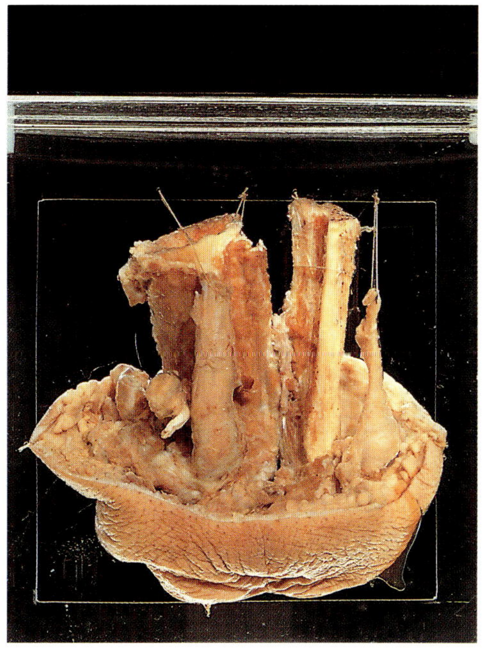

9.14 Amputation Stump: Traumatic Neuroma

No clinical details are available.

This below-knee amputation stump has been dissected to show several large neuromata, attached to both the tibia and skin.

Traumatic neuromata are regenerative nodules arising at the site of an injured or transected nerve. They may become painful when traumatised as a consequence of either their superficial site, their adherence to other mobile structures, or an ill-fitting prosthesis.

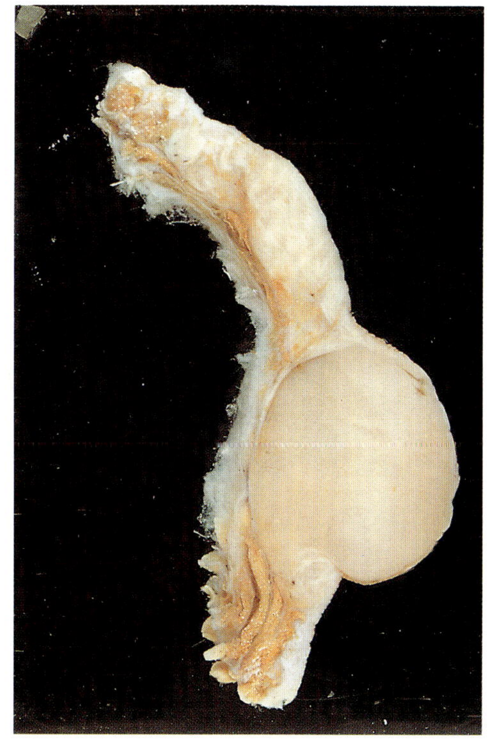

9.15 Subcutaneous Tissue: Neurofibroma

This specimen was excised from the thigh of a 51-year-old man who had first noticed the tumour 12 years previously.

A section through the skin and subcutaneous tissue shows a rounded tumour, measuring 3cm in diameter.

Neurofibromas are benign tumours of nerve sheath origin. They most often arise in the head and neck or extremities and principally affect adults. Solitary neurofibromas are quite common but the tumours may also be multiple, as seen in von Recklinghausen's neurofibromatosis.

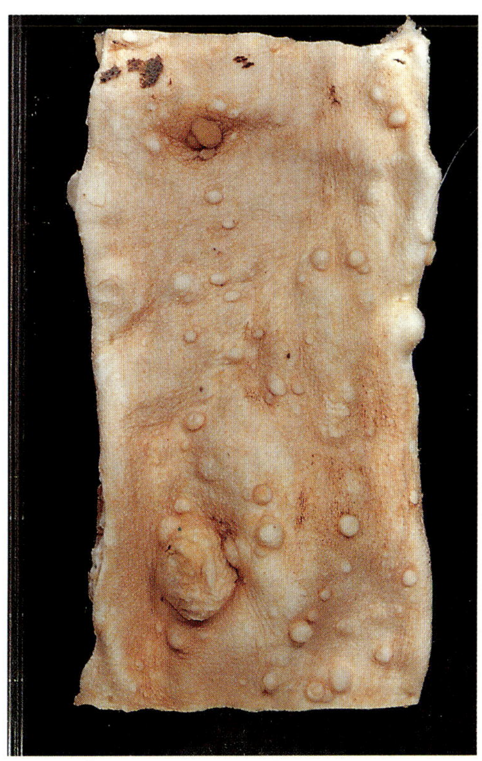

3.16 Skin: Multiple Neurofibromata

This is a post-mortem specimen from a 53-year-old man, with known von Recklinghausen's disease, who died of bronchopneumonia.

A portion of skin from the anterior chest wall shows multiple, discrete, rounded tumours projecting upwards from the dermis.

This appearance is diagnostic of von Recklinghausen's neurofibromatosis.

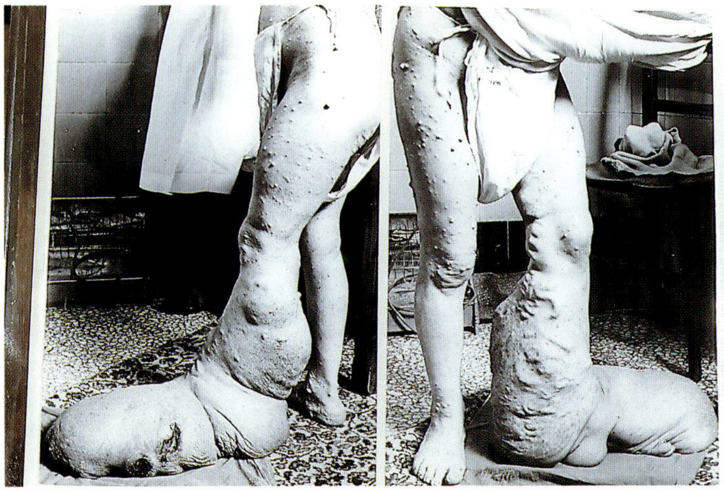

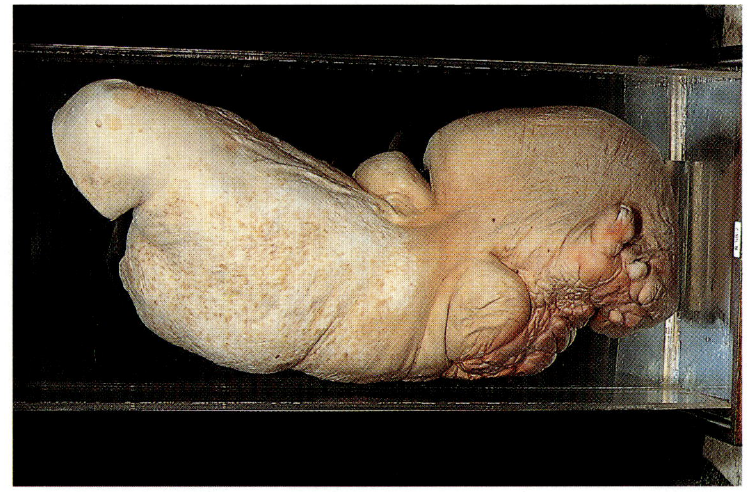

9.17 Leg: Diffuse ('Elephantiasiform') Neurofibroma

This is an amputation specimen from a 57-year-old woman with von Recklinghausen's neurofibromatosis, who had developed progressive swelling and deformity of the lower left leg (9.17a). Despite this she had managed to work in domestic service until ulceration of the left foot became intractable.

The lower part of the left leg (9.17b), amputated below the knee, is grossly swollen and expanded by diffuse (focally nodular) neurofibromatous tissue. Note also the café-au-lait macules. The lateral border of the foot (bottom left) is ulcerated.

Diffuse neurofibromata may arise in isolation but at least 10 per cent present in patients with von Recklinghausen's disease; these lesions are typically found about the head, neck or trunk of young adults. Von Recklinghausen's disease is an autosomal dominantly inherited condition, characterised by multiple neurofibromata and cutaneous café-au-lait macules. There may be associated hamartomas of the iris, tumours of the central nervous system, phaeochromocytoma and a constellation of other lesions. There is a significantly increased incidence of malignant nerve sheath tumours.

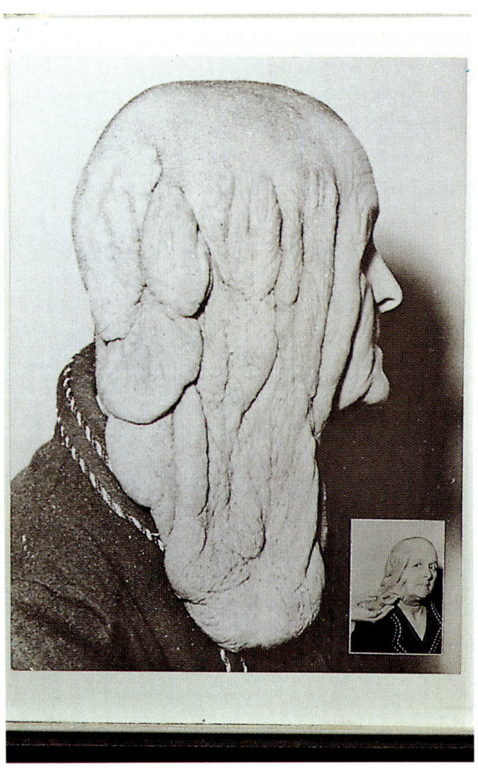

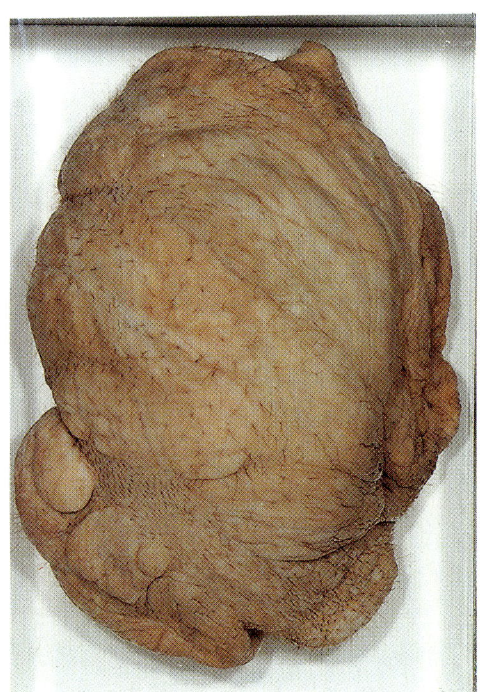

9.18 Scalp: Plexiform Neurofibroma

This specimen was excised from a 48-year-old woman who had had a tumour of the scalp since childhood. The lesion had progressively enlarged becoming pendulous (9.18a) and a source of embarrassment. She also had numerous cutaneous neurofibromata (of nodular appearance) over the rest of her body.

The excised specimen (9.18b) appears as an irregular, pendulous and focally nodular piece of skin. The dermis and subcutaneous tissue (not visible in this view) are diffusely infiltrated by neurofibromatous tissue.

Plexiform neurofibromata, which are almost invariably a feature of von Recklinghausen's disease, tend to arise in the limbs or head and neck region and are characterised by large, redundant folds of skin.

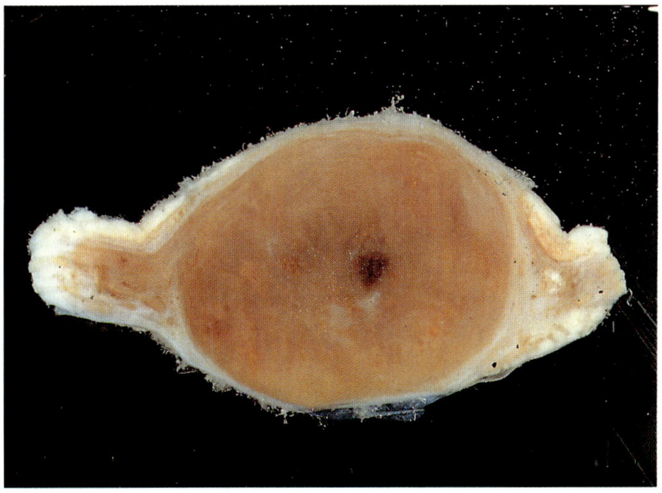

9.19 Subcutaneous Tissue: Neurilemmoma (Schwannoma)

This specimen was excised from a 64-year-old man, who had noticed a lump on the left elbow for many years. Recently he had developed pain and paraesthesia in the forearm and hand. At operation the tumour was found to arise from the ulnar nerve.

This is a segment of the ulnar nerve which is expanded by an ovoid, encapsulated tumour, measuring 4 × 2.5 × 2cm. The cut surface is tan-coloured and shows foci of haemorrhage and translucent myxoid degeneration.

Neurilemmomata (Schwannomata) are common benign tumours of nerve sheath origin which typically present in the limbs or head and neck region of middle-aged adults. They are usually solitary and are only occasionally associated with von Recklinghausen's disease. Benign neurilemmomata are only rarely associated with neurological symptoms: in contrast to neurofibromata, malignant change is exceedingly rare.

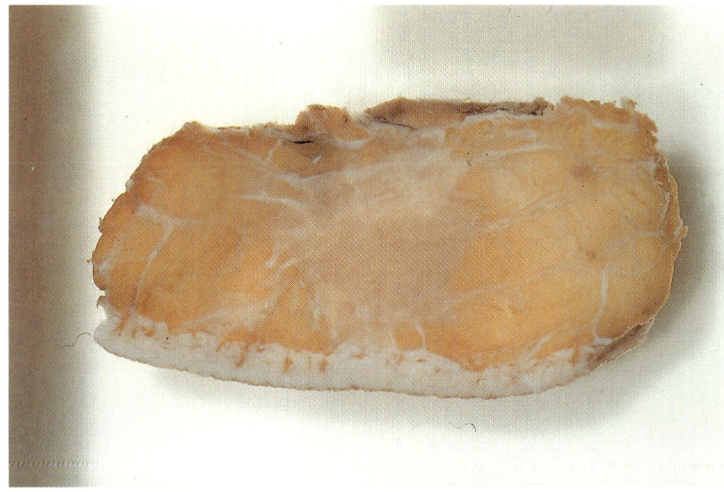

9.20 Skin of Hip: Granular Cell Tumour

This specimen was excised from a 57-year-old woman who for 2 years had noticed a slowly growing lump over the left hip.

A cross-section shows a reasonably circumscribed, but unencapsulated, cream-coloured neoplasm.

Granular cell tumours, previously known as granular cell myoblastomas, are benign lesions of Schwann cell origin. They may arise at any site, but are particularly common in the tongue and breast; young or middle-aged adults are most often affected.

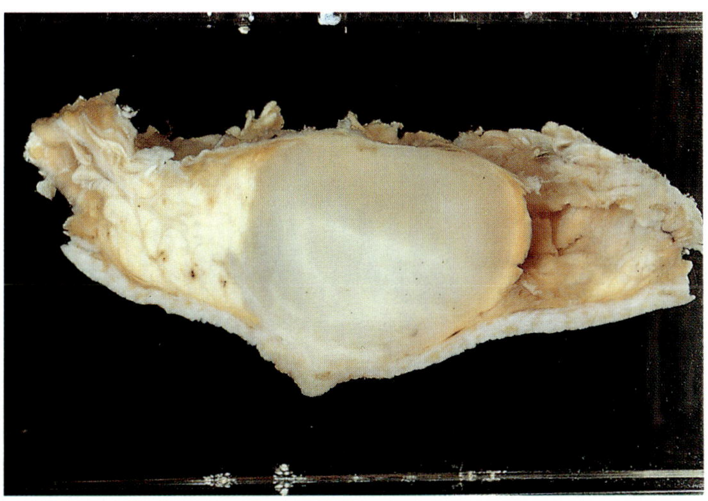

9.21 Male Breast: Ganglioneuroma

This specimen was excised from a 65-year-old man who had noticed a small, firm nodule medial to the left nipple for 4 years. More recently the whole breast had increased in size. Examination revealed a mass in the breast which was fixed to the skin but not to the pectoral fascia.

The left breast has been bisected to show a well-circumscribed, pale tumour, measuring 5cm in diameter, and situated deep to the nipple.

Ganglioneuromata are uncommon benign tumours of the sympathetic nervous system and most often arise from major autonomic nerve trunks. The commonest sites are the mediastinum and retroperitoneum where these tumours often attain a large size; young adults are typically affected. Very rarely these tumours may occur at sites quite separate from the major sympathetic trunks and it is assumed, as in this case, that such neoplasms have originated in small autonomic nerves. The degree of circumscription seen here is characteristic.

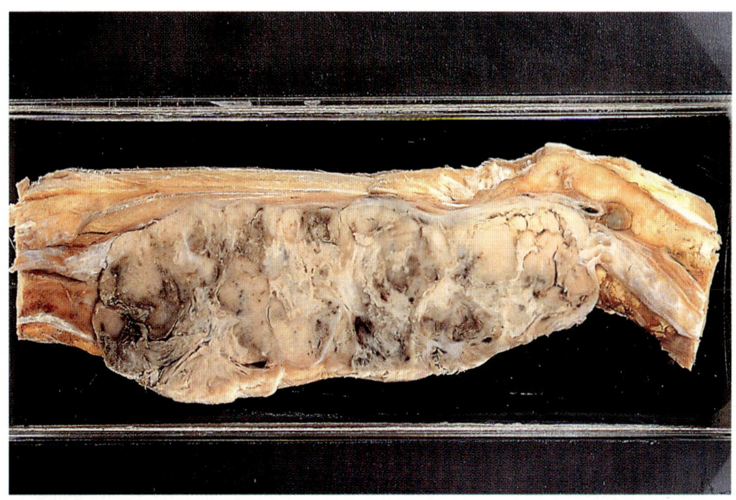

9.22 Leg: Malignant Nerve Sheath Tumour

This is an amputation specimen from a 22-year-old man, who presented with a 2 month history of pain and swelling in the right calf. Examination revealed, in addition to a mass, numerous café-au-lait macules which had been present since birth.

Arising from the tibial nerve, which is markedly thickened (top centre), is a large fusiform mass, measuring 22 × 8 × 8cm. The cut surface is lobulated and haemorrhagic but the tumour appears relatively well circumscribed.

Malignant nerve sheath tumours (synonyms: neurofibrosarcoma, malignant Schwannoma) comprise about 5 per cent of soft tissue sarcomas. Adults in the 5th and 6th decades are more often affected; however, up to 50 per cent of cases are associated with pre-existent neurofibromatosis (as in this case) in which circumstance patients tend to present in the 3rd and 4th decades and show a male predominance. This tumour most commonly arises in the limbs, sometimes within a pre-existent neurofibroma, and may give rise to neurological symptoms if a major nerve is involved. The 5-year-survival is about 50 per cent, but this figure is halved in patients with neurofibromatosis.

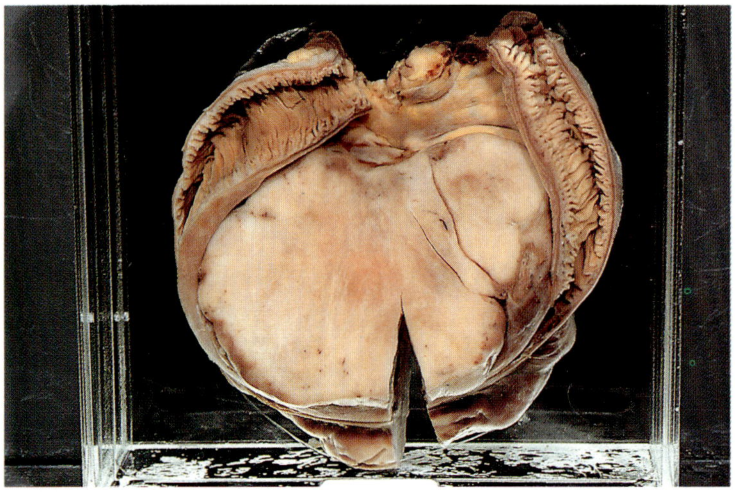

9.23 Small Bowel Mesentery: Malignant Fibrous Histiocytoma

This specimen was excised from a 35-year-old woman, who presented with a vague history of malaise, anorexia and weight loss. Laparotomy revealed a large tumour in the mesentery of a loop of ileum.

Situated in the mesentery is a large, pale, multinodular tumour, which measures 12cm in maximum diameter. The cut surface is fleshy and shows focal areas of necrosis.

Malignant fibrous histiocytoma is the commonest sarcoma of adulthood and presents most often in the 6th and 7th decades, affecting males more than females. It arises most frequently in the deep soft tissues of the limbs or retroperitoneum, but has been reported at almost any site. There are 5 well-defined, but not mutually exclusive, histological subtypes: pleomorphic, myxoid, giant cell, inflammatory, and angiomatoid. Of these, the latter is distinguished by its almost invariable occurrence in childhood. Overall, the pleomorphic variant is by far the most common, accounting for about 70 per cent of cases. In general, malignant fibrous histiocytomas are very prone to local recurrence and up to 60 per cent metastasise with fatal consequences, usually within 5 years.

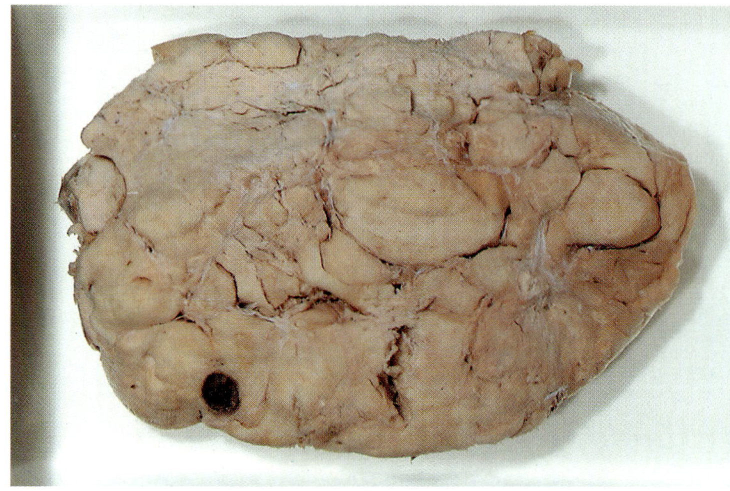

9.24 Retroperitoneum: Leiomyosarcoma

This specimen was excised from a 44-year-old woman who had suffered left-sided abdominal pain for 3 months. At operation a very large retroperitoneal tumour was found filling the left side of the abdomen from the pelvic brim to the left kidney. The mass was densely adherent to the lower pole of the kidney such that partial nephrectomy was also required.

A large mass is seen which consists of retroperitoneal fat intersected by coarse trabeculae of pinkish-grey tissue. Small foci of fat necrosis can be seen in the lower part of the tumour.

The retroperitoneum is by far the commonest site for soft tissue leiomyosarcoma, which arises most often in females in the 6th and 7th decades. Frequently these tumours attain a very great size such that complete resection is impossible. The prognosis is very poor both due to metastatic spread and the lethal effects of extensive local invasion.

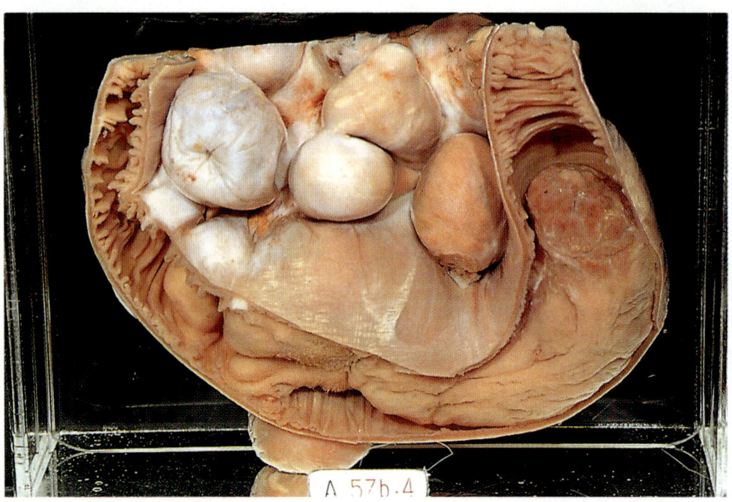

9.25 Small Bowel Mesentery: Leiomyosarcoma

This specimen was excised from a 42-year-old woman, who presented with a 2 week history of colicky abdominal pain and was found to have a mass in the right iliac fossa. Laparotomy revealed a large mesenteric mass which projected into the lumen of the ileum.

The resected loop of ileum and mesentery shows a multinodular pale mass, arising in the mesentery, which has protruded into the bowel lumen (top right) and has extended as a banana-shaped mass along the ileum. The tumour has retained a mucosal covering.

The peritoneal cavity, including the mesentery, is a common site for leiomyosarcomas. It should by noted that distinction between benign and malignant smooth muscle tumours on histological grounds, is notoriously difficult on occasions, but the most useful guide is the degree of mitotic activity.

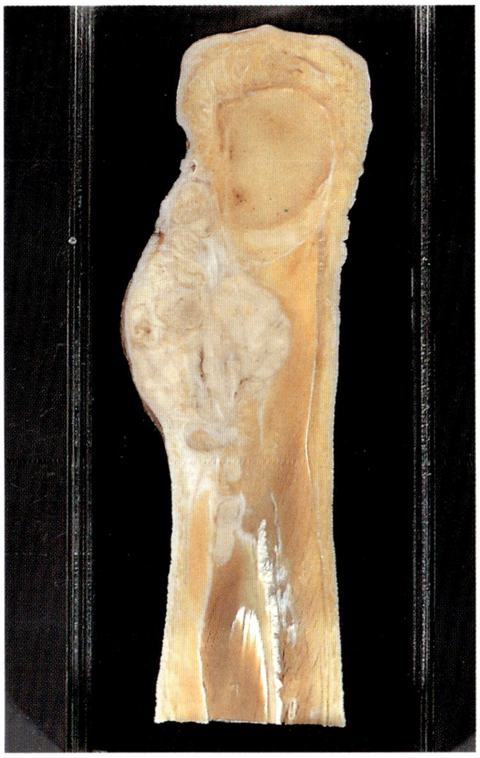

9.26 Subcutaneous Tissue: Leiomyosarcoma

This is an amputation specimen from a 72-year-old man, who presented with an 8 month history of a swelling in the region of the left ankle which had recently shown a rapid increase in size. Biopsy revealed a sarcoma and below-knee amputation was performed.

The lower part of the leg and ankle have been bisected coronally and are viewed from the anterior surface. Arising supero-laterally to the ankle joint is a pale, multinodular neoplasm which shows extensive necrosis. The tumour has infiltrated both beneath the overlying skin and into the adjacent muscle.

Leiomyosarcoma arising in the limbs may be cutaneous (originating from arrector pili muscle) or subcutaneous (originating from the vascular smooth muscle). Adults in the 5th-7th decades are typically affected. The overall mortality is about 25 per cent and is largely attributable to the subcutaneous lesions.

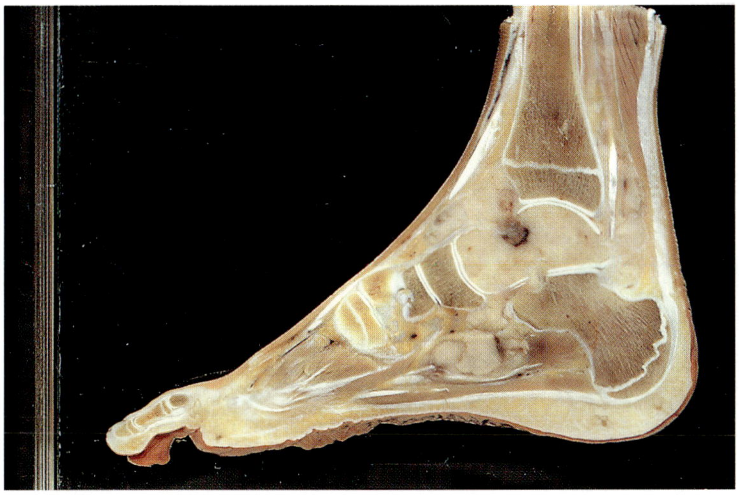

9.27 Foot: Synovial Sarcoma

This is an amputation specimen from a 13-year-old boy who complained of a painful right ankle for 2½ years. The discomfort had become progressively worse and, during the last 6 months, rapid swelling developed.

The right foot has been sectioned to show ill-defined, pale tumour masses, which were in continuity *in vivo*, but are now apparent in the sole of the foot beneath the tendo calcaneus and on the upper surface of the talus. The tumour has invaded bone and soft tissues widely.

Synovial sarcoma (synonym: malignant synovioma) is predominantly a tumour of adolescents and young adults and is substantially more common in males than females. It most often arises in the extremities, particularly around the knee. The prognosis is proportional to the size of the primary tumour; lethal metastases may supervene in up to 70 per cent of cases.

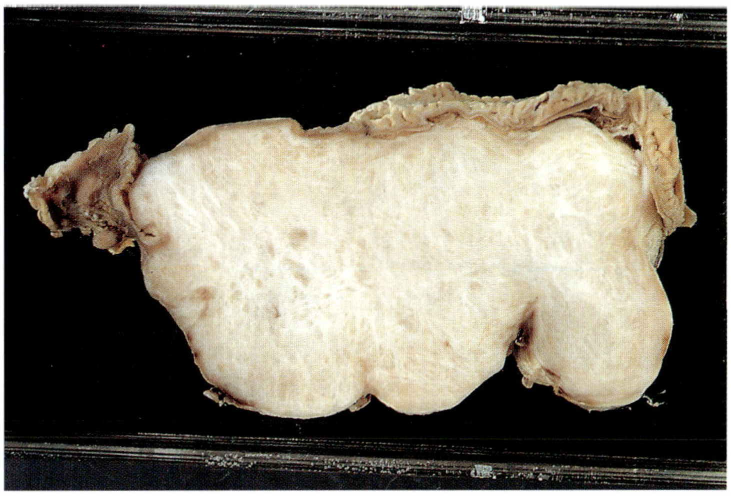

9.28 Retroperitoneum: Desmoid-Type Fibromatosis

This specimen was excised from an 11-year-old girl, who presented with lassitude and was found to have a large mass in the right side of the abdomen. At laparotomy there was a large retroperitoneal tumour, over which the terminal ileum, ascending colon and hepatic flexure were adherent.

Beneath the adherent loop of bowel is a pale, lobulated tumour, which measures 24 × 9 × 6cm. The cut surface of the lesions reveals a whorled, fibrous appearance, not dissimilar to a uterine fibroid.

The desmoid-type fibromatoses may arise either in the anterior abdominal wall musculature (the most common site), skeletal muscle elsewhere (particularly the limb girdles), or within the peritoneal cavity. Retroperitoneal origin is well recognised. The disease is commonest in young adults, particularly females, and may be associated with Gardner's syndrome. Metastasis *does not* occur, therefore the old designation of low-grade fibrosarcoma is inappropriate.

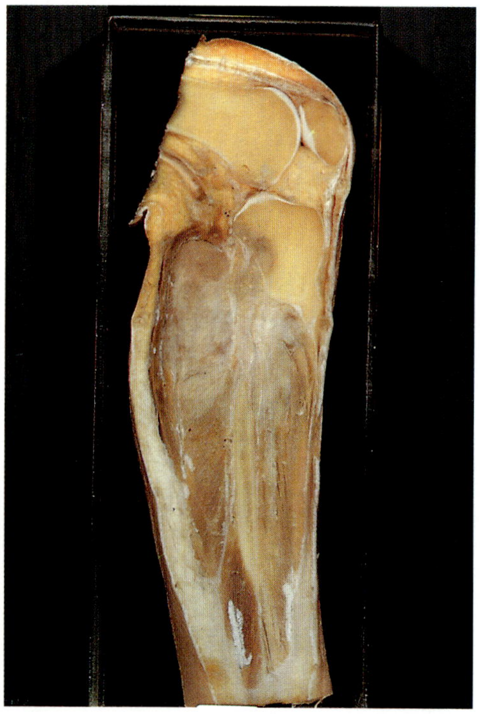

9.29 Lower Leg: Fibrosarcoma

This is an amputation specimen from a 37-year-old woman who had a slowly growing tumour adjacent to, and invading, the upper end of the right fibula. One year after local excision and curettage, there was extensive local recurrence and X-rays revealed pulmonary metastases. The limb was amputated as a palliative measure.

A section through the knee and lower leg shows a firm, pale mass surrounding and eroding the head of the fibula. The tumour has invaded the tibia and there is diffuse infiltration of the adjacent soft tissues.

While many malignant soft tissue neoplasms were designated as fibrosarcoma in the past, modern techniques of determining histogenesis have allowed more accurate diagnosis and reclassification of the majority of such tumours. Fibrosarcoma affects males more than females and usually presents in the 5th or 6th decades. It most commonly arises in the extremities, particularly the leg, and recurs locally in up to 50 per cent of cases. Bloodborne metastases, particularly to the lung, are common and result in a 5-year survival of about 40 per cent.

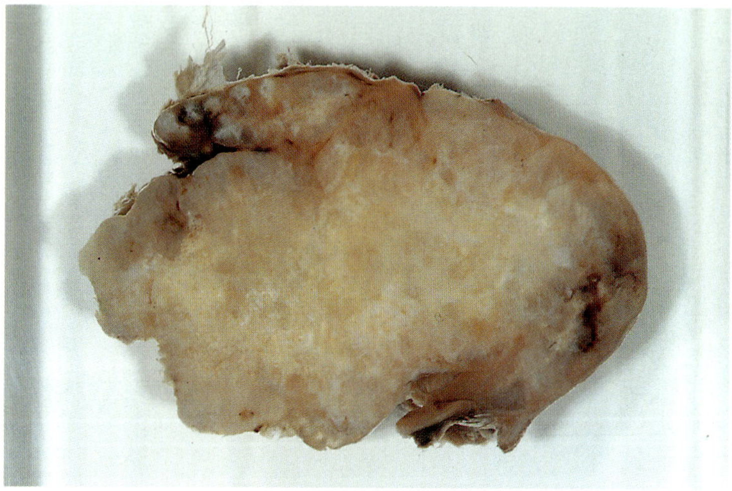

9.30 Nasal Septum: Chondrosarcoma

This specimen was excised from a 66-year-old woman who had noticed progressive swelling of the nose for 4 years, which had resulted in lateral displacement of her eyes and gradual loss of vision. A radical excision was carried out and she made an uneventful recovery with rapid return of her eyesight.

A sagittal section through the tumour shows a nodular cartilaginous mass with focal calcification and ossification. The attenuated skin of the nose is tightly stretched over the anterior surface of the tumour.

Chondrosarcoma occurs most often in the 4th or 5th decades and affects males more than females. It most often arises in the axial skeleton or proximal portion of long bones; while the nasal septum is a well-recognised primary site, such tumours are very rare. Chondrosarcoma carries a better prognosis than most primary skeletal malignancies since metastasis usually occurs late in the clinical course. Most complications usually arise from extensive local invasion or recurrence.

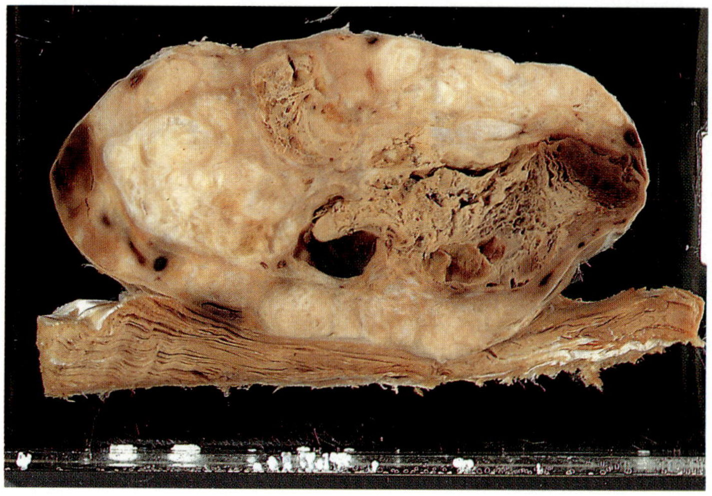

9.31 Thigh Pleomorphic Rhabdomyosarcoma

This is part of an amputation specimen from a 76-year-old woman who complained of swelling and pain in the right thigh for 9 months. A biopsy was reported as sarcoma and, therefore, amputation through the hip joint was performed.

A portion of the biceps femoris has been sectioned to show a reasonably well-defined, ovoid tumour, measuring 11 × 6cm, which is firmly attached to the muscle. The cut surface of the tumour has a variegated appearance being focally fibrous, necrotic and cystic.

Rhabdomyosarcoma is currently thought to affect children in the vast majority of cases, and is usually embryonal in type; most of the cases diagnosed in adults in the past are thought more likely to have been examples of pleomorphic malignant fibrous histiocytoma (see Legend 9.23). However, there remain a few cases of true pleomorphic rhabdomyosarcoma which most often arise in the limbs of older adults. While 5-year-survival has improved dramatically in recent years with the benefit of multimodal therapy, these tumours still carry a grave prognosis, particularly in adults.

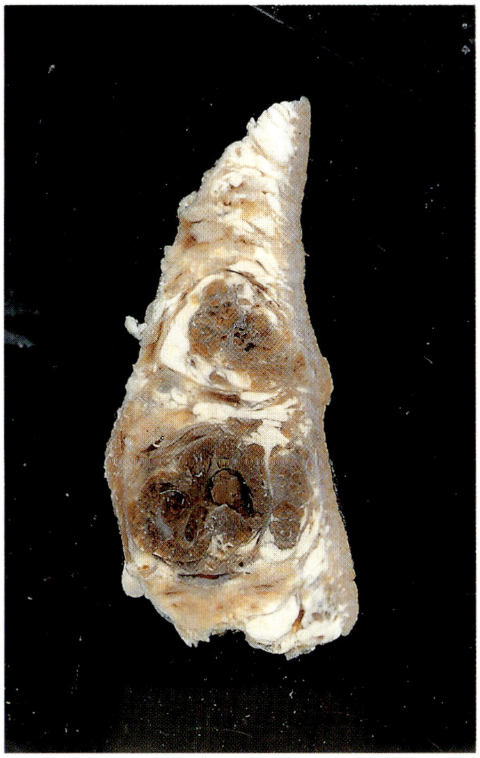

9.32 Subcutaneous Tissue: Cavernous Haemangioma

This specimen was excised from the left flank of a small child. No further clinical details are available.

A section through the skin and subcutaneous tissue shows a bilobular mass composed of numerous vascular spaces of varying size. Many of these spaces are filled with thrombus. Note that, owing to the age of the specimen, the subcutaneous fat has adopted a white, chalky appearance.

Cavernous haemangiomas are common benign lesions, which are most often seen in neonates and young children. They may arise at any site but are most common about the head and neck and tend to show a slight predilection for females. They tend to be larger than capillary haemangiomas, often exceeding 5cm in diameter and are frequently diffuse. They show little, if any, tendency to spontaneous involution. Clinically, cavernous haemangiomas may be associated with multiple enchondromas (Maffucci's syndrome), haemangiomas in the alimentary tract (blue rubber-bleb naevus syndrome), or within a consumption coagulopathy due to platelet deposition with the lesion (Kasabach-Merritt syndrome).

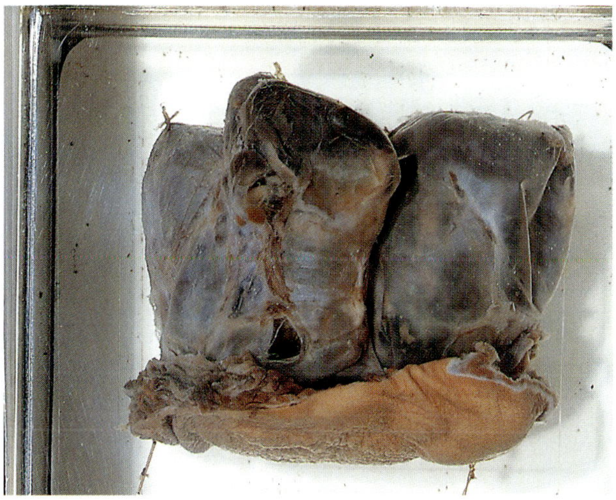

9.33 Subcutaneous Tissue: Cystic Hygroma

This specimen was excised from the back of the neck of a young infant; it had been present from birth.

Beneath attenuated skin, there is a thin-walled, multilocular cystic tumour, which measures 8cm in maximum diameter. In the fresh state it contained clear fluid.

Cystic hygromas are benign lesions of infancy, which may be hamartomatous in nature and are thought to represent ectatic variants of a cavernous lymphangioma. They present typically as a large, cystic mass in the neck, axillae or groin. Local recurrence is not infrequent unless wide excision is performed.

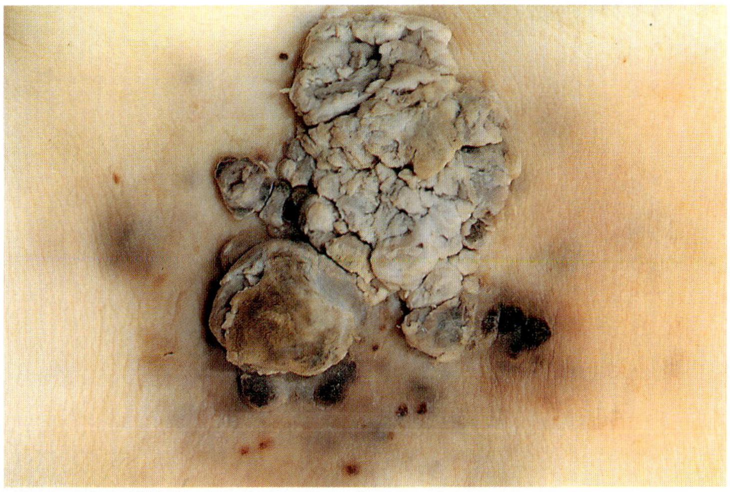

9.34 Skin of Arm: Post-Mastectomy Angiosarcoma

This specimen was excised from a 52-year-old woman who had undergone left radical mastectomy 9 years previously. Massive lymphoedema of the left arm had been present since the operation and in recent months she had noticed purplish, ulcerated nodules appearing in the skin of the upper arm.

The skin shows a cluster of lesions, measuring up to 2cm in diameter, projecting from an irregular area of dusky discoloration.

Post-mastectomy angiosarcoma (Stewart-Treves-syndrome) is a malignant tumour of vascular epithelium. While there is no conclusive proof, it is assumed to arise from lymphatics in the arm following axillary lymph node clearance. This complication of radical mastectomy is comparatively rare and usually arises more than 10 years after the development of lymphoedema. The prognosis is generally poor with repeated local recurrence and eventual dissemination being the rule.

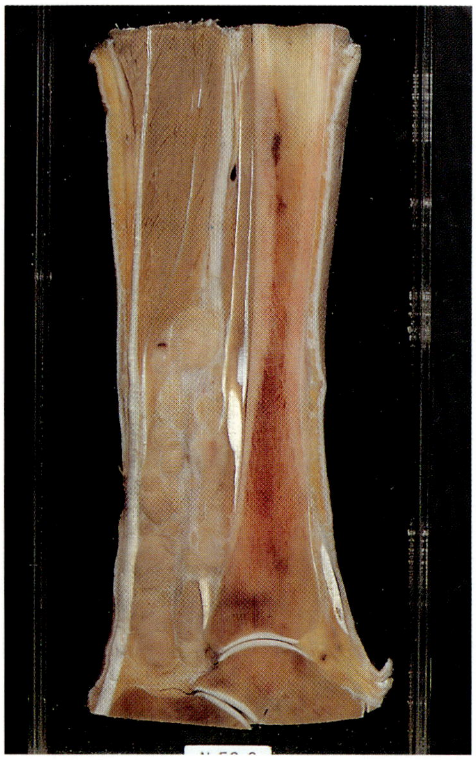

9.35 Subcutaneous Tissue: Malignant Haemangiopericytoma

This is an amputation specimen from a 38-year-old man, who had presented 6 months earlier with a swelling in the calf. Initially a tenosynovitis was suspected but the lump continued to enlarge so local excision was performed. Two months post-operatively the mass recurred so the leg was amputated.

A vertical section through the lower part of the leg shows a reasonably circumscribed, lobulated mass deep to the Achilles tendon. The tumour, which is tan-coloured, is invading muscle superiorly and the ankle joint inferiorly.

Haemangiopericytomas are fairly uncommon soft tissue tumours which most often present in the lower limb or retroperitoneum of middle-aged adults. Histological distinction between benign and malignant examples is often very difficult. While benign lesions are most common, malignant haemangiopericytomas pursue a fatal course in at least 70 per cent of cases.

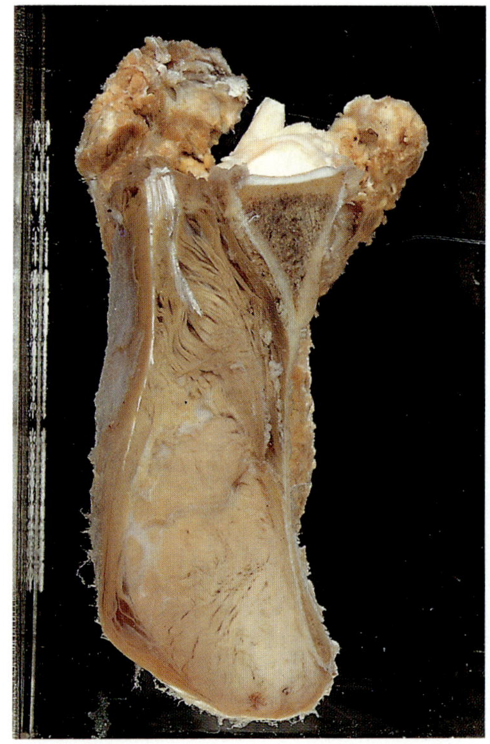

9.36 Infraspinatus Muscle: Extraskeletal Ewing's Sarcoma

No clinical details are available.

The right scapula with attached musculature has been sectioned to show a pale ovoid mass, measuring 5cm in diameter situated within the belly of infraspinatus. The tumour is ill-defined and infiltrates the muscle but there is no invasion of the underlying bone.

Extraskeletal Ewing's sarcoma is an extremely rare tumour of unknown histogenesis. It most often presents in young adults and commonly arises in the lower limb or paravertebral region. Its clinical course is characterised by rapid dissemination and death in most cases.

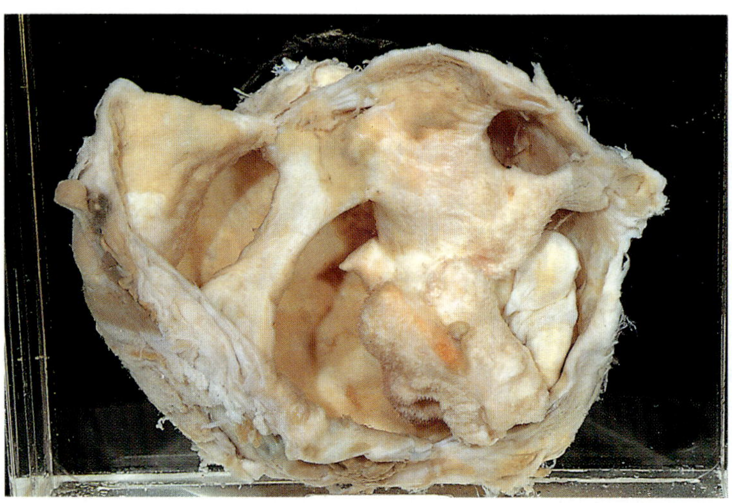

9.37 Retroperitoneum: Benign Cystic Teratoma

This specimen was excised from a 9-year-old boy whose mother had noticed a lump in his abdomen one week previously. Investigation suggested a partly cystic, partly calcified soft tissue mass adjacent to the right kidney and behind the ascending colon. At operation the tumour was densely adherent to adjacent viscera.

A section of part of the tumour, which in its entirety measured 14cm in maximum diameter, shows irregular cystic spaces bridged by solid tissue. Other parts of the tumour (not shown) contained copious hair and sebaceous material.

Benign teratomata are well recognised in the retroperitoneum and commonly arise in the sacrococcygeal and perirenal areas. These tumours are principally found in young children and may attain a large size, very often being cystic. They are identical in nature to those cystic teratomata found in the ovary, mediastinum and thymus. Their frequent firm adherence to other structures is often suggestive of malignancy to the surgeon, but this is entirely due to a fibrous reaction to extravasated cyst contents.

10. OSTEOARTICULAR SYSTEM

BONES

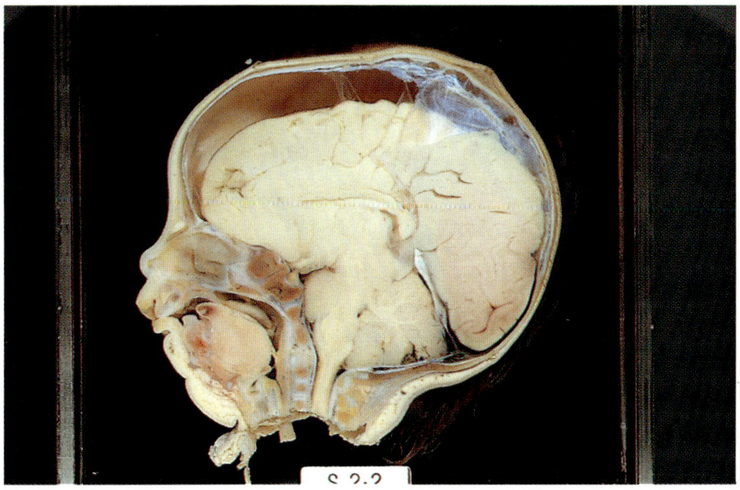

10.1 Lower Jaw: Bilateral Hypoplasia

No clinical details are available.

A sagittal section through this infant's head shows symmetrically retarded growth of the mandibles. The symphysis is displaced posteriorly and, consequently, the tongue has been forced backwards to completely obstruct the upper laryngeal orifice.

Mandibular hypoplasia (synonym: micrognathia) is sometimes seen to a minor degree as a familial phenomenon. When severe and associated with glossal recession, as here, it is known as the Pierre-Robin syndrome; malformations of the ears typically coexist. Micrognathia may also be seen in association with other congenital anomalies, for example Potter's syndrome.

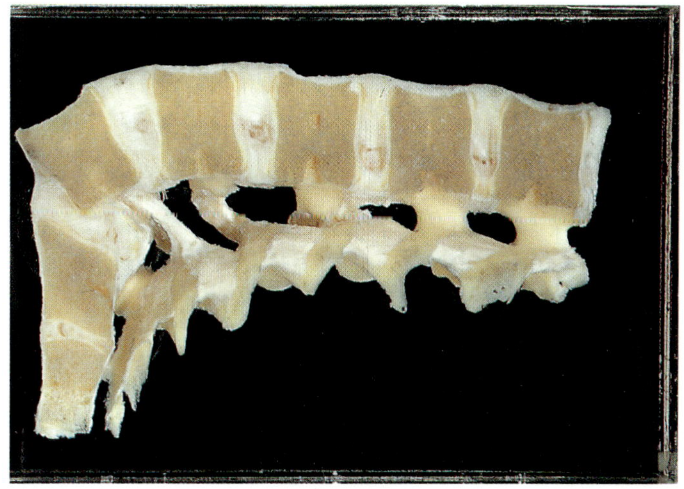

10.2 Vertebral Column: Spondylolisthesis

This was an incidental finding at post-mortem in a 16-year-old girl who died of tetanus infection following a puncture wound of the foot.

A sagittal section through the lumbosacral region of the spine shows that the body of the sacrum is displaced posteriorly, such that the 5th lumbar vertebra projects 2cm anteriorly. The neural arches of the distal 3 lumbar vertebrae show abnormal pedicles with fibrous replacement at L4 and L5.

Spondylolisthesis is most often due to a congenital defect in the pars interarticularis at L5/S1 and may also be a result of trauma, associated with degenerative disc disease at L3/L4. Typically patients present with non-specific low backache and lordosis, sometimes associated with entrapment of spinal nerve roots. The spinal canal and cord are unaffected because the laminae remain normally situated.

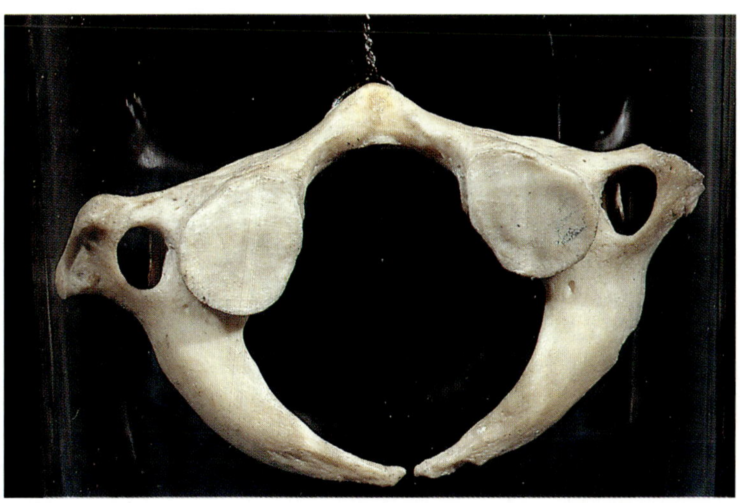

10.3 Spine: Incomplete Fusion of Laminae (Spina Bifida Occulta)

No clinical details are available.

This atlas vertebra shows incomplete posterior fusion of the laminae, which are slender and tapering.

Minor anomalies of the vertebral column are not uncommon and result mainly from failed or abnormal fusion of the two posterior spinal ossification centres that develop behind the notochord *in utero*. Wide separation of the posterior rami, which is commonest in the lumbosacral region, is a feature of spina bifida with its associated neurological complications (see Chapter 11).

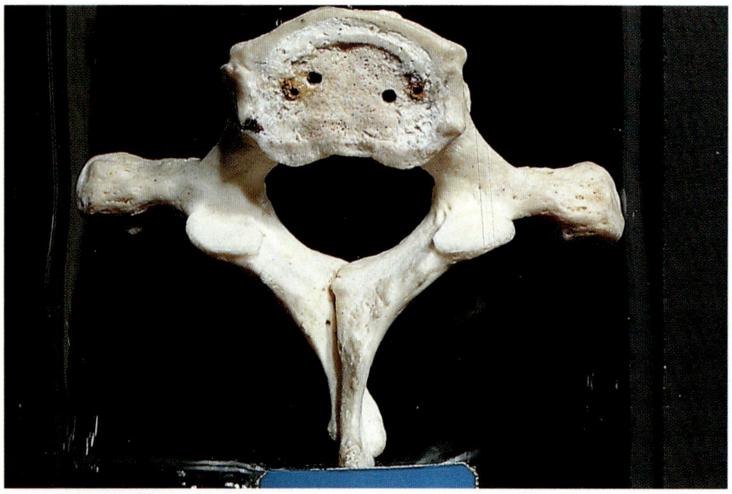

10.4 Spine: Incomplete Fusion of the Posterior Arch

No clinical details are available.

The dorsal laminae of this thoracic vertebra have failed to unite but their spinous processes overlap, thus closing the neural canal. Note also the irregular contour of the vertebral body, suggesting a coexistent degenerative process.

Significant spinal defects, associated with a meningocele or meningomyelocele, are very uncommon in the cervicothoracic portion except in cases of anencephaly in which craniorrhachischisis often occurs.

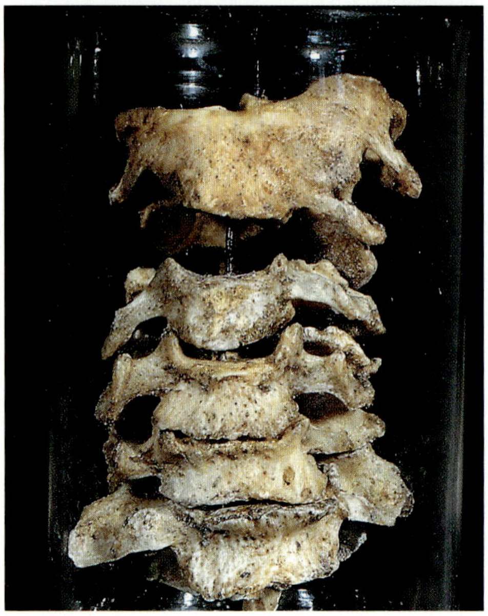

10.5 Spine: Vertebral Fusion

No clinical details are available.

These are the cervical vertebrae of an adult, the first two of which are fused into a single bone (so-called 'block vertebra'). There are two transverse processes and intervertebral foraminae on the patient's left side but only one on the right. Note that the remainder of the cervical spine shows degenerative arthritis.

Partial or complete fusion of adjacent vertebrae due to incomplete segmental separation *in utero* is another well-recognised anomaly, which may also be associated with other spinal abnormalities, including vertebral hypoplasia and neural arch defects.

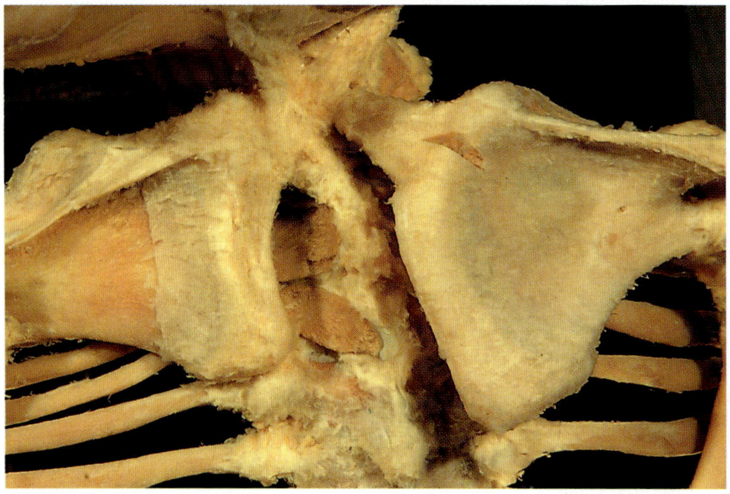

10.6 Shoulder: Congenitally Elevated Scapulae (Sprengel's Deformity)

This was an incidental finding at post-mortem in a female child who died of malnutrition.

The thoracic skeleton (viewed posteriorly) shows both scapulae to be located higher than is usual. That on the left (patient's right) is bound to the vertebral column by cartilage, while that on the right is attached by a fibrous band.

Sprengel's deformity represents a failure of descent of the scapulae from the neck *in utero.* It may be associated with marked shortening of the neck due to severe malformations of the cervical vertebrae (the Klippel-Feil syndrome). In general, movement at the shoulder joint is only slightly limited and the principal problem is that of deformity.

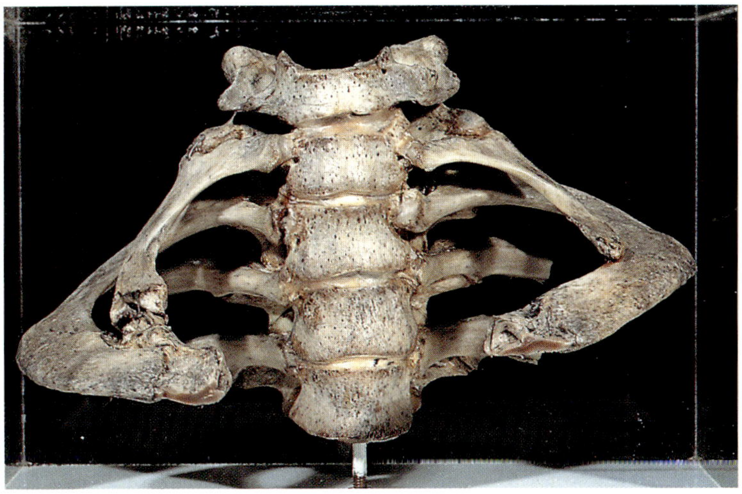

10.7 Spine: Bilateral Cervical Ribs

No clinical details are available.

The lower cervical and upper thoracic vertebrae are shown with the normal first ribs. There is also a well-developed cervical rib on each side.

The congenitally anomalous presence of a cervical rib (which is most often unilateral) is not uncommon and is more frequent in females. It may remain asymptomatic, being an incidental X-ray finding, or it may give rise to features resulting from compression of the lower brachial plexus, particularly in patients with drooping shoulders. In this latter circumstance, symptoms typically develop in the 4th and 5th decades.

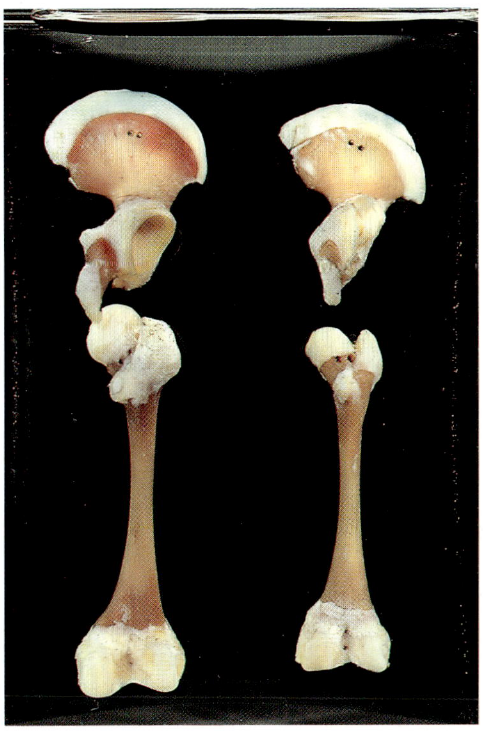

10.8 Hip: Congenital Dislocation

This is a post-mortem specimen from a male neonate. No other clinical details are available.

Mounted on the right, the femur has an abnormally small and conical head, associated with a shallow acetabulum which is also diminished in size. The corresponding bones from a normal child are mounted on the left for comparison.

Congenital dislocation of the hip is a common malformation which is predominant in females, occurs most often in first-born children and is often bilateral. There is a recognised familial tendency. Aetiological factors include inherited joint laxity and acetabular dysplasia, the effects of which may be exaggerated by intra-uterine breech position, oligohydramnios and tight swaddling with the hips extended in the neonatal period. Complications include delayed walking and, later in life, lumbar lordosis and/or osteoarthrosis of the hip.

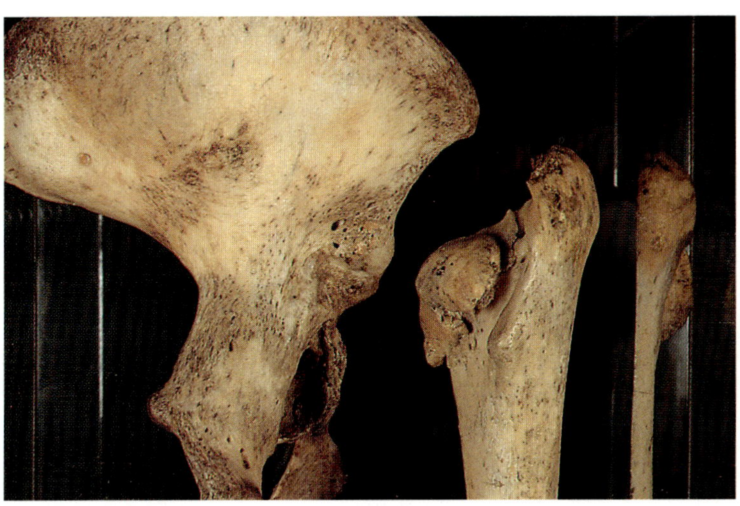

10.9 Hip: Congenital Dislocation

No clinical details are available.

The right femur and the hip bone have been mounted to show a congenital posterior dislocation of the femoral head onto the dorsum ilii, where a false articular depression has formed just above the sciatic notch. The acetabulum is very small and deformed, as is the femoral head, which also appears to be dysplastic.

Congenital hip dislocation almost always occurs anterosuperiorly. There is usually associated acetabular hypoplasia.

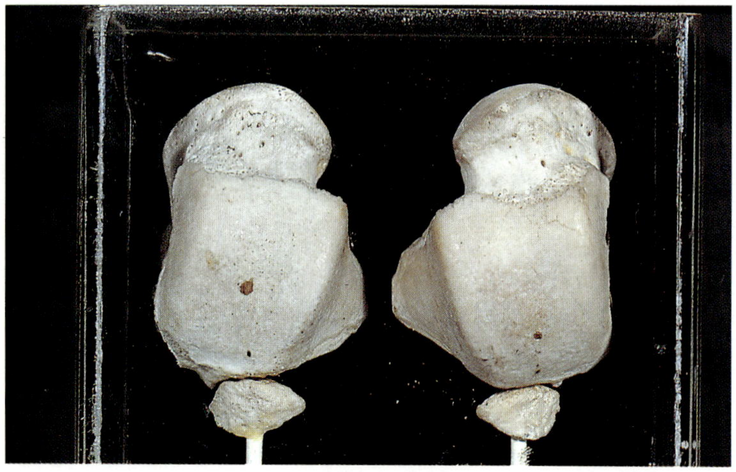

10.10 Ankle: Os Trigonum

No clinical details are available.

A pair of talus bones are mounted, each of which shows a separate os trigonum posteriorly.

This accessory ossicle simply represents the posterior process of the talus which sometimes ossifies separately and may or may not become joined to the main bone. It is a common minor congenital malformation of no pathological significance.

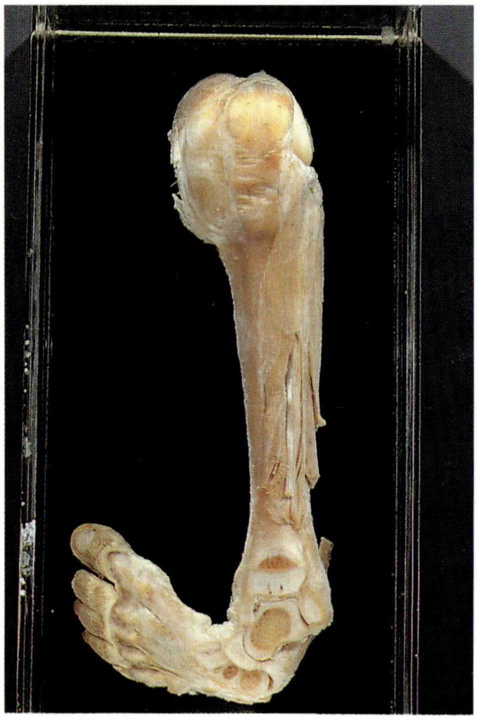

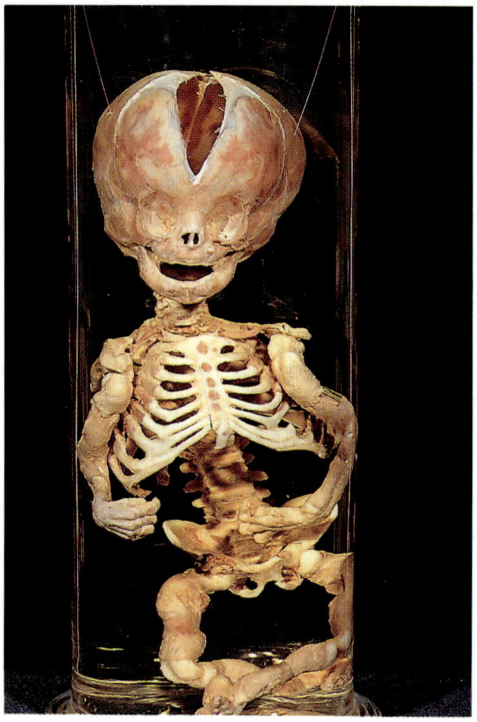

10.11 Ankle: Talipes Equinovarus

No clinical details are available.

The left lower leg and foot of a child, coronally sectioned through the tarsus, shows marked adduction of the forefoot, the latter being smaller than normal. The calcaneum and navicular bone are displaced medially and the hind foot is held in a varus position.

Talipes equinovarus (synonym: club foot) is a relatively common congenital malformation of the osteoarticular system which is most often idiopathic. It may result from intra-uterine malposition and was a recognised feature of thalidomide babies. Males are more often affected than females and the malformation is sometimes bilateral. This deformity may also be associated with spina bifida (see Chapter 11) or congenital hip dislocation.

10.12 Skeleton: Osteogenesis Imperfecta

This is the skeleton of a 5-month-old baby girl. No other clinical details are available.

There is prominent hydrocephalus with wide separation of the sutures. The bones of the arms and legs are markedly deformed and the feet are held in a position of equinovarus. There are numerous recent and healed fractures. Note also the deformed pelvis.

Osteogenesis imperfecta may be divided clinically into two main types: congenital, manifest from birth and usually fatal, and tarda, which is less severe and usually presents in early infancy or later in childhood. The congenital variant is thought to represent a sporadic mutation, while the tarda variant shows autosomal dominant inheritance. This disease usually comprises widespread bony deformities, a tendency to multiple fractures, ligamentous laxity, poorly formed teeth, otosclerosis and blue sclerae. It is thought that the underlying abnormality is a variable quantitative and qualitative alteration in collagen synthesis.

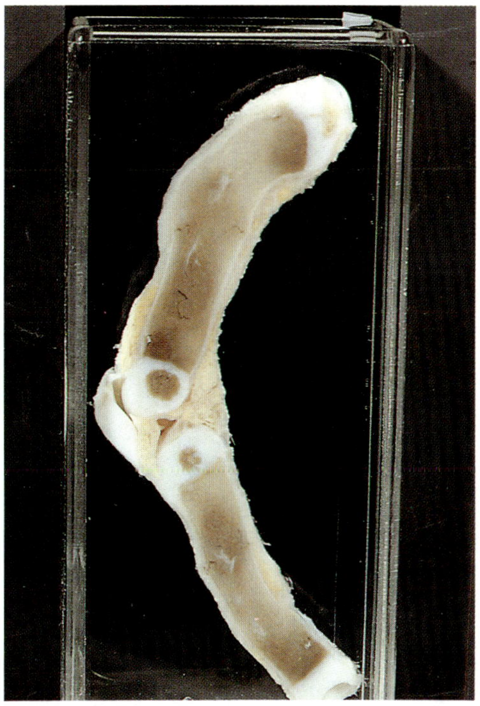

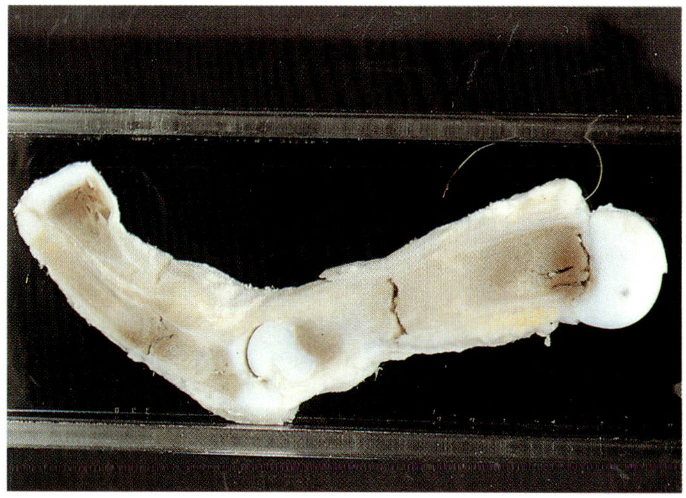

10.13 Limb Bones: Osteogenesis Imperfecta

These are post-mortem specimens from a 16-day-old baby girl, who was noticed to be very short and who cried when her limbs were handled. X-rays revealed fractures of both femora and all the long bones of the right arm. She became gradually cyanotic and died.

The bones of the right arm (10.13a), seen in vertical section, show regular epiphyses with diminished adjacent bone formation. The cortex is abnormally thin and there are fractures in the mid-humerus and ulna. The left femur, tibia and patella from the same infant (10.13b) show normal growth plates and indistinct bony trabeculae. Both long bones are deformed by multiple irregular fractures.

This infant had no positive family history of a skeletal disorder or of blue sclerae and therefore represents either an autosomal recessive case or a spontaneous mutation.

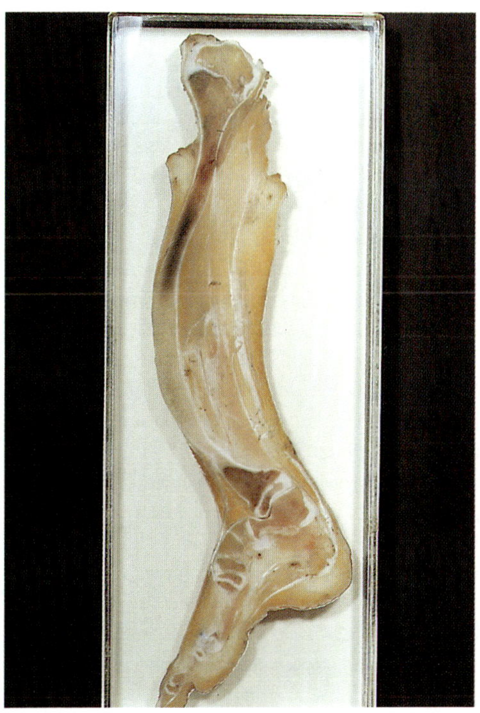

10.14 Left Lower Leg: Osteogenesis Imperfecta

This is an amputation specimen from a 13-year-old boy who had suffered repeated fractures of the left leg. The limb was deformed and measured 10cm less than the right leg; a through-knee amputation was performed.

A vertical section through the left lower leg shows very marked anterior bowing of the tibia and extreme thinning of all the bony cortices. Very little cancellous bone is evident, despite the presence of normal endochondral ossification centres.

This is an example of osteogenesis imperfecta tarda, in which the deformity has resulted from multiple fractures, associated with extreme disuse osteoporosis. In delayed cases such as this, the disease is usually limited to the lower limbs and sometimes may only give rise to minimal deformity.

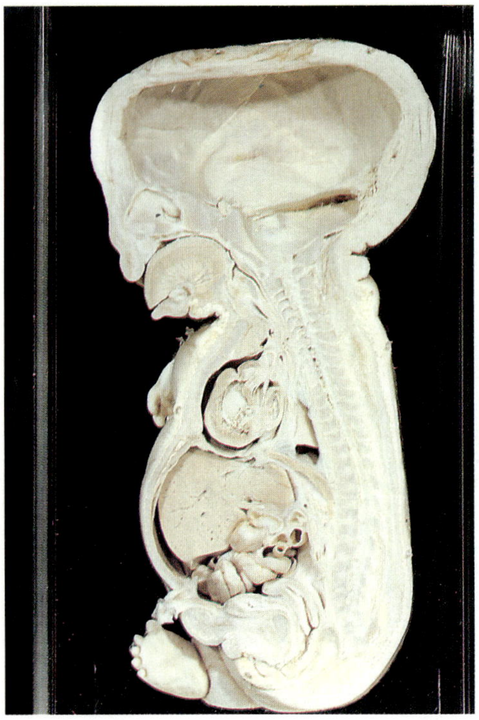

10.15 Fetus: Achondroplasia

No clinical details are available.

This is the right half of a female achondroplastic fetus. The limbs are stunted owing to defective growth of the long bones and the base of the skull is shortened in the basisphenoid region.

Achondroplasia may be an autosomal dominantly inherited condition or may rarely occur as a spontaneous mutation. The majority of affected infants are either stillborn (as here) or die in the neonatal period. The disease is characterised by diminished endochondral ossification, particularly in the long bones and at the base of the skull which leads to diminished growth at the epiphyses. This is the commonest cause of dwarfism and typically, the trunk is fairly normal.

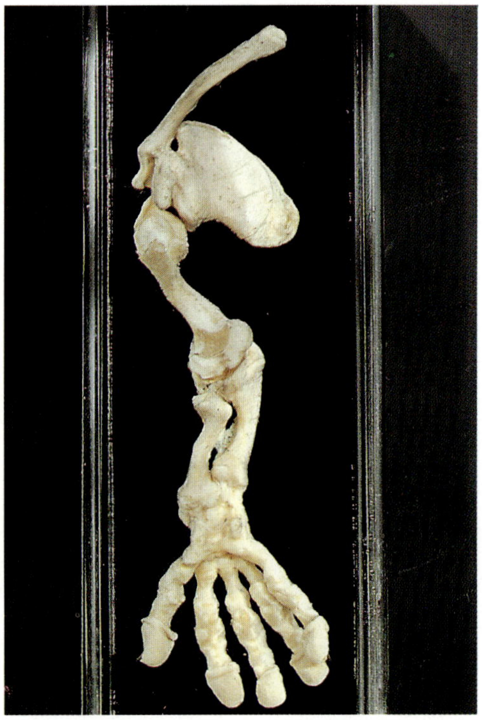

10.16 Fetal Arm Bones: Achondroplasia

This specimen is from a full-term stillborn fetus.

All the arm bones are stunted and deformed, particularly if compared to the normal clavicle. The epiphyses appear widened and the shaft of each bone appears abnormally thick and dense: these latter phenomena are illusions consequent upon the marked shortening.

These are the typical features of an achondroplastic limb.

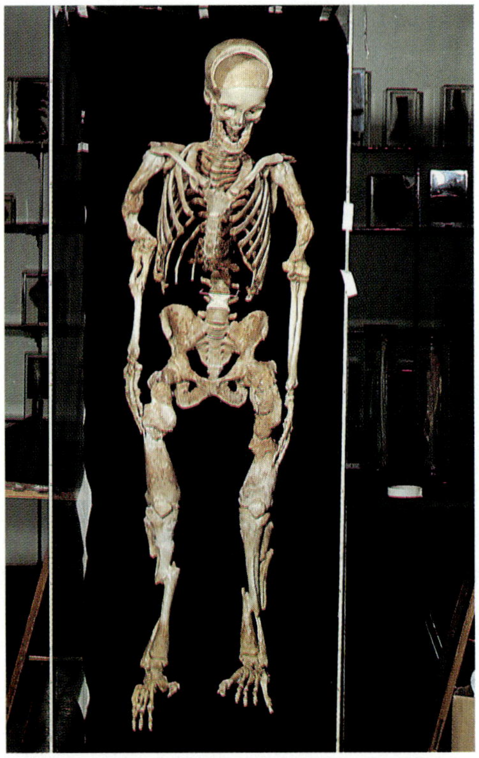

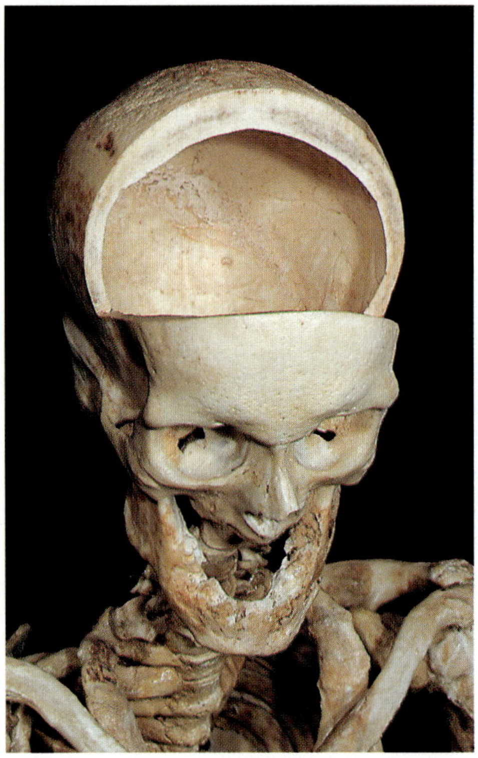

10.17 Skeleton: Osteopetrosis

This is the skeleton of a 43-year-old male, who died of pneumococcal meningitis with a cerebral abscess. He had sustained his first fracture in early infancy when his mother had rubbed his arm. By the time of his death, he had suffered over 80 fractures, including an unpleasant series following a road traffic accident. From the age of 22, his vision had gradually deteriorated such that he was almost completely blind by the time of his death.

Features to be noted in the skeleton (10.17a) are: thickening of the skull and femora; gross deformity of both femora, tibiae, fibulae, humeri and the left radius and ulna due to malunited fractures; severe kyphoscoliosis, and irregularity of many of the ribs due to malunited fractures. A close-up view of the skull (10.17b) shows extensive replacement by dense, compact bone which has obliterated the medullary cavity. Note also the mandibular irregularity, probably secondary to osteomyelitis.

Osteopetrosis (synonym: Albers-Schöenberg disease, marble bone disease) is a rare genetic disorder of variable autosomal inheritance, which is characterised by greatly increased bony density with a failure of remodelling at the metaphyses. The skeleton is composed of irregular, disorganised compact bone which retains a cartilaginous core, due to a failure of primary spongiosa remodelling; hence the tendency to multiple fractures. Anaemia and pancytopenia commonly result from obliteration of the medullary cavity, leading to susceptibility to infection. In addition, thickening of the calvaria commonly gives rise to cranial nerve compression with consequent optic atrophy or deafness.

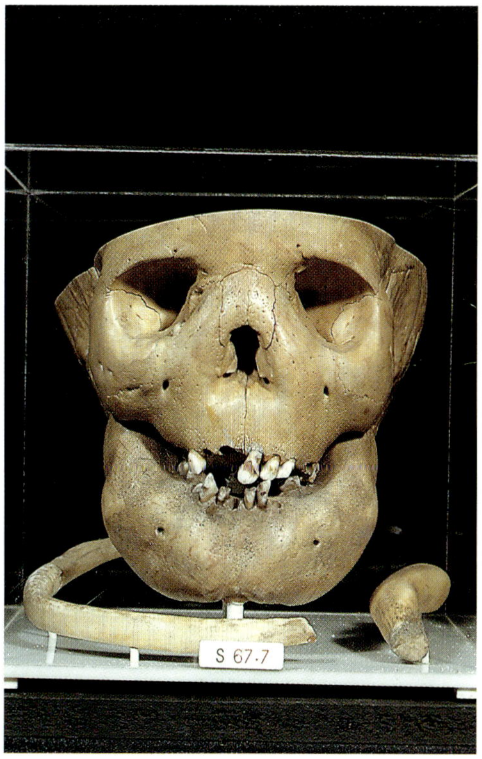

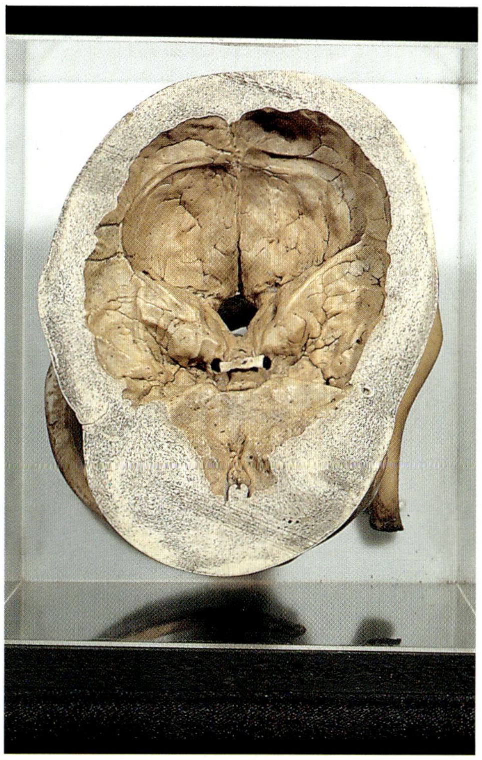

10.18 Skull, Clavicle and Rib: Hyperostosis Corticalis Generalisata

These are post-mortem specimens from a 10-year-old girl, who died suddenly for no apparent reason. Since the age of 3 she had developed progressive enlargement and deformity of the skull. X-rays revealed extreme thickening and sclerosis of the calvaria, mandibles, clavicles and ribs. For 3 years prior to death the patient had suffered from severe occipital headaches, progressive bilateral optic atrophy and episodes of unconsciousness.

The skull, clavicle and rib (10.18a) are greatly enlarged and thickened. The process is particularly well marked in the nasal region, zygomatic arches and mandible and it is noteworthy that the bones have retained a smooth surface. A horizontal section through the skull (10.18b) demonstrates clearly the gross thickening of compact lamellar bone.

Hyperostosis corticalis generalisata is a rare condition of young children, which shows a variable autosomal inheritance and may take several different clinical forms. The best known variant (Camurati-Engelmann disease) predominantly affects the long bones of the limbs (particularly the legs), while this case falls into the group which shows prominent skull involvement. A similar appearance may be seen in hyperphosphatasaemia (juvenile Paget's disease).

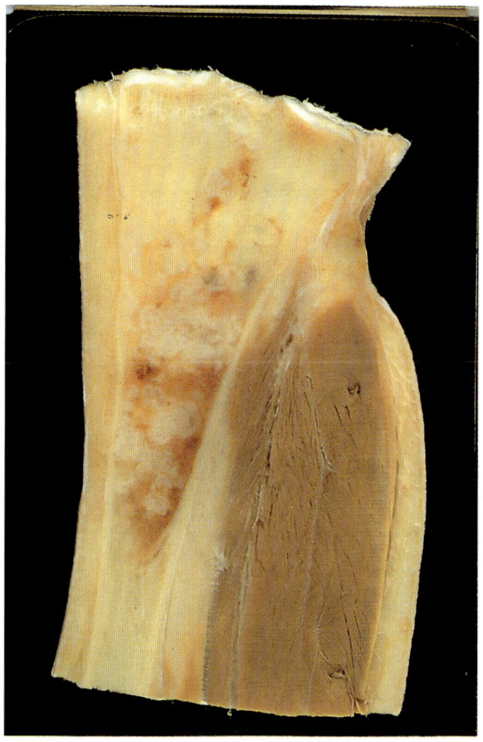

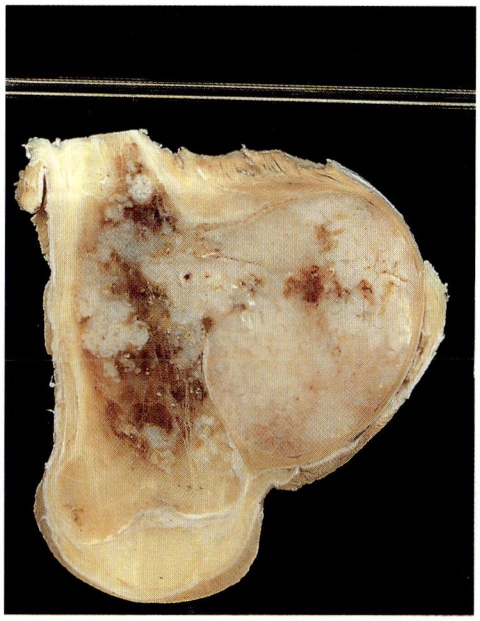

10.19 Leg Bones: Enchondromatosis

These are amputation specimens from a 29-year-old woman, who had been known to suffer from enchondromatosis of the right leg since childhood. She subsequently developed a large mass on the medial aspect of the lower thigh and, since limb function was poor, amputation was performed.

A section through the upper third of the tibia and adjacent soft tissues (10.19a) shows multiple, bluish cartilaginous nodules in the medullary cavity. A section through the lower third of the femur (10.19b) shows similar features but, in addition, a separate large cartilaginous mass has developed in the cortex and is extending into adjacent soft tissues. Histologically, this latter lesion is a chondrosarcoma.

Enchondromatosis (synonyms: Ollier's disease, dyschondroplasia) is an uncommon developmental anomaly, characterised by the development of multiple cartilaginous nodules (of varying size) usually in several bones. This condition is most often unilateral and is commonest in the hands, feet and long limb bones. It may be associated with multiple haemangiomas of skin, soft tissue or viscera (Maffucci's syndrome). Patients with enchondromatosis have a significantly increased risk of developing chondrosarcoma, as here.

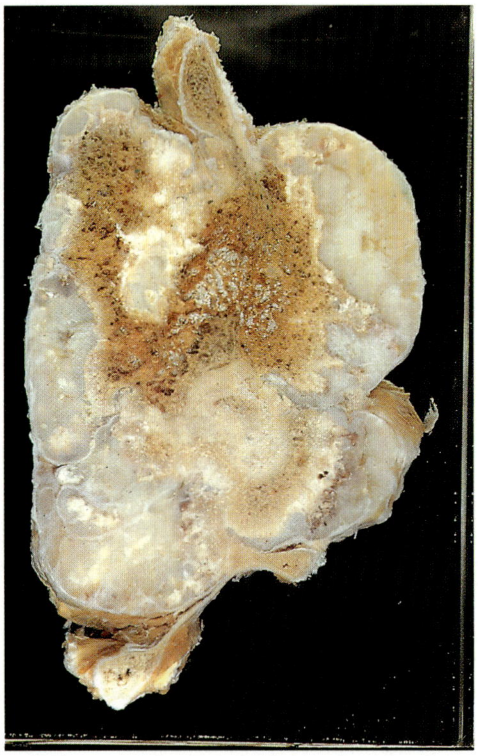

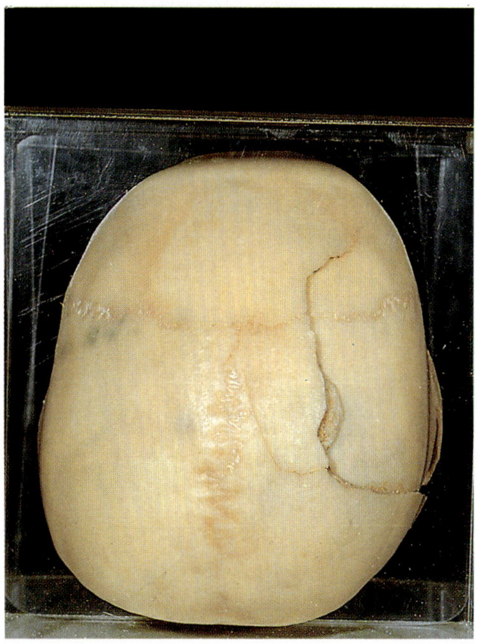

10.20 Scapula: Enchondromatosis

This specimen was excised from a 19-year-old man, who had first noticed a painless swelling of the right scapula 9 months previously. X-rays revealed further enchondromata in both tibiae and the right femur. The body of the scapula was excised.

A vertical section through the scapula shows a multinodular cartilaginous mass arising from the body of the bone below the spine. Centrally the lesion has undergone extensive ossification.

Enchondromatosis is most often manifest in the limb bones but may, on occasion, affect any part of the skeleton.

10.21 Skull: Fracture

This is a post-mortem specimen from a soldier who sustained a severe head injury in the course of a manic-depressive illness while a prisoner-of-war. He died of massive extradural haemorrhage associated with an underlying cerebral laceration.

The calvaria, viewed from above, shows a fracture commencing in the right frontal region which has extended posteriorly over a distance of about 20cm, crossing both the right fronto-parietal and coronal sutures.

Closed linear fractures such as this are the commonest type seen in the skull. While they themselves do little harm, there is often associated cerebral injury and/or damage to one of the meningeal arteries resulting from displacement of the brain within the skull on impact.

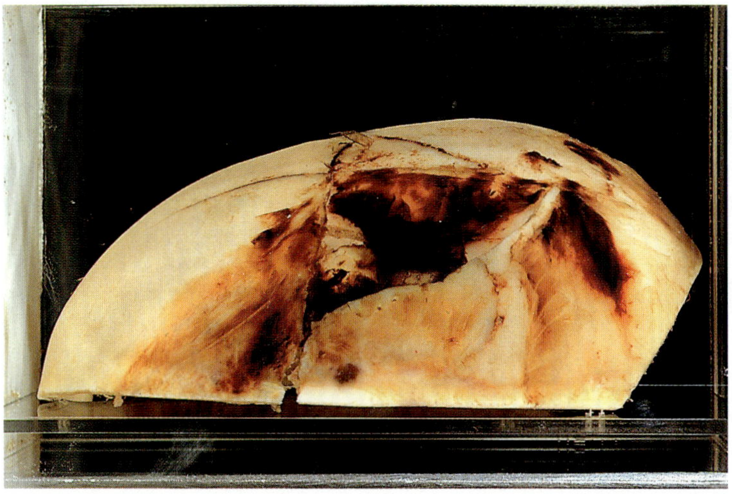

10.22 Skull: Comminuted Fracture

This is a post-mortem specimen from a 70-year-old woman, who threw herself from a window 6m above the ground while being treated for depression.

There is an extensive depressed and comminuted fracture of the left parietal and squamous temporal bones. Note the surrounding haemorrhage. In the fresh state there were extensive lacerations of the left cerebral hemisphere.

The term comminuted implies that the fractured bone has been broken into multiple fragments of varying size.

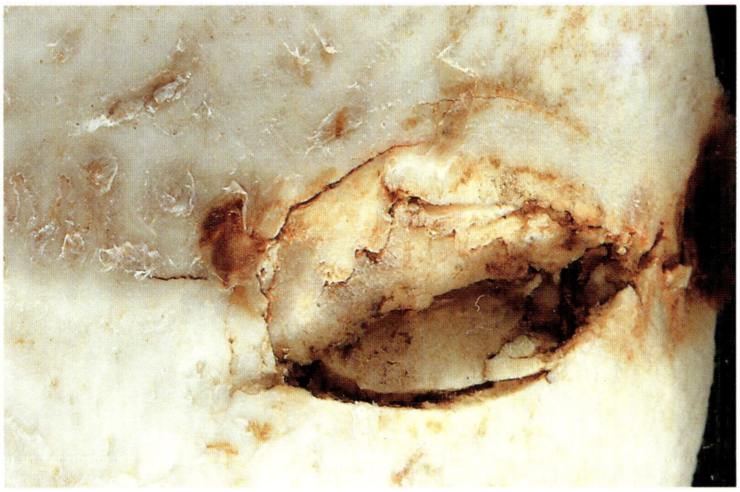

10.23 Skull: Depressed Compound Comminuted Fracture

This is a post-mortem specimen from a 22-year-old man who sustained fatal injuries in a road traffic accident.

A close-up view of the parietal bone shows a depressed fracture, measuring 5cm in maximum diameter and 1.5cm in depth. The fragments of bone are comminuted and in the fresh state the fracture was in continuity with the external surface of the scalp. The underlying brain was compressed and showed contusions.

Depressed skull fractures are common and are the result of localised indentation of the skull, often by rounded objects. They may remain closed (i.e. the scalp and usually the dura remains intact), in which case they are known as pond fractures, and typically heal. Compound fractures have a poorer prognosis.

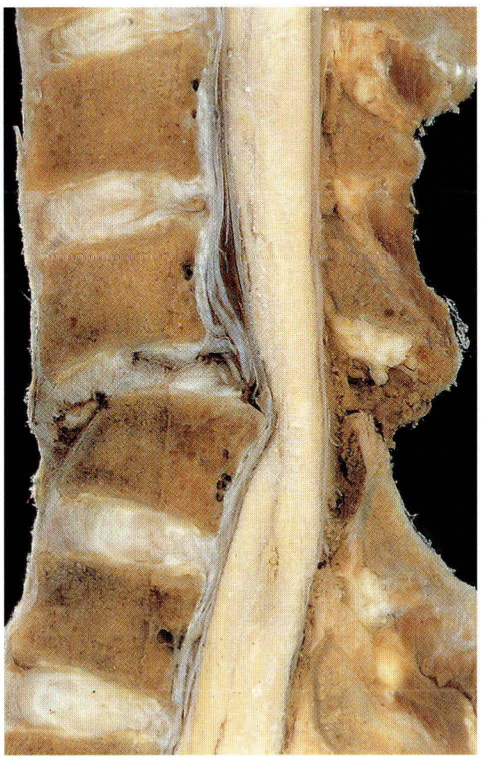

10.24 Cervical Spine: Fracture Dislocation

This is a post-mortem specimen from a 50-year-old man who fell down some stairs. He died 2 hours later, having become quadriplegic and having developed increasing respiratory difficulties.

A sagittal section through the cervical part of the vertebral column shows a fracture dislocation between C4 and C5. The 5th cervical vertebral body is displaced posteriorly and has caused severe cord compression.

Spinal fractures are of clinical significance because of the secondary damage to the cord which frequently occurs. Those injuries which tear the posterior ligaments render the cord most liable to damage because of the consequent instability of the vertebral column. Fracture dislocations most often follow a rotational shearing injury, particularly if the spine is flexed.

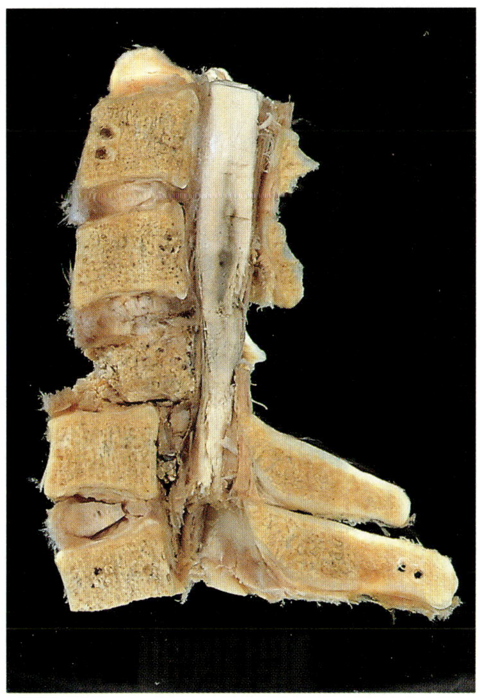

10.25 Cervical Spine: Fracture Dislocation

This is a post-mortem specimen from a young man who sustained a forceful blow to the head while swimming, when hit by another man diving into the water. He suffered immediate quadriplegia and died 2 days later in respiratory failure.

A sagittal section through the cervical spine shows crushing and posterior displacement of C5, associated with compression and bleeding into the cord.

This case is remarkably similar to Legend 10.24. The injury here probably represents a 'burst' fracture in which compressive force has been applied from above, driving the intervertebral disc into the vertebral body beneath. It should be noted that vertebral dislocation with cord damage may occur in the absence of a fracture solely as a result of ligamentous injury.

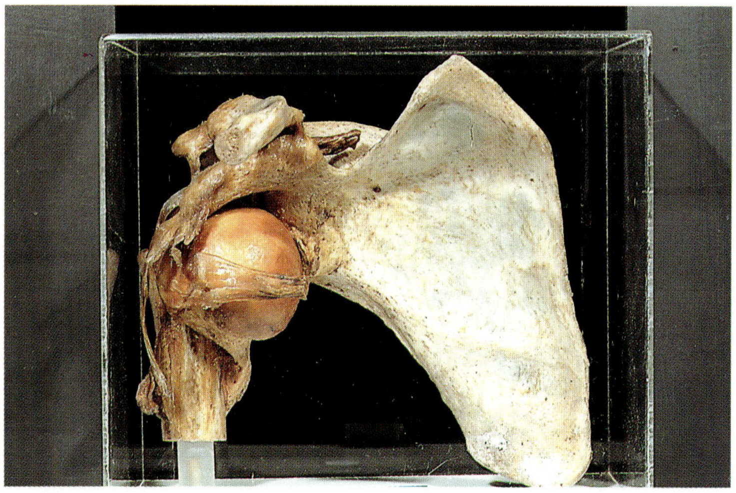

10.26 Shoulder: Fracture Dislocation

No clinical details are available, other than that the causative injury occurred 3 months before death.

The right shoulder joint, viewed anteriorly, shows an oblique fracture of the neck of the humerus associated with anterior subcoracoid dislocation of the humerus head. New bone formation has provided a false articular surface just below the anterior margin of the glenoid fossa.

Acquired dislocation of the shoulder is a common injury, usually caused by a fall on an outstretched hand, and is almost always anterior in direction. There may be an associated fracture of the greater humeral tuberosity or the neck of the humerus and neurovascular damage is not infrequent. It should be noted that, if the glenoid labrum is severely damaged, recurrent dislocation may occur.

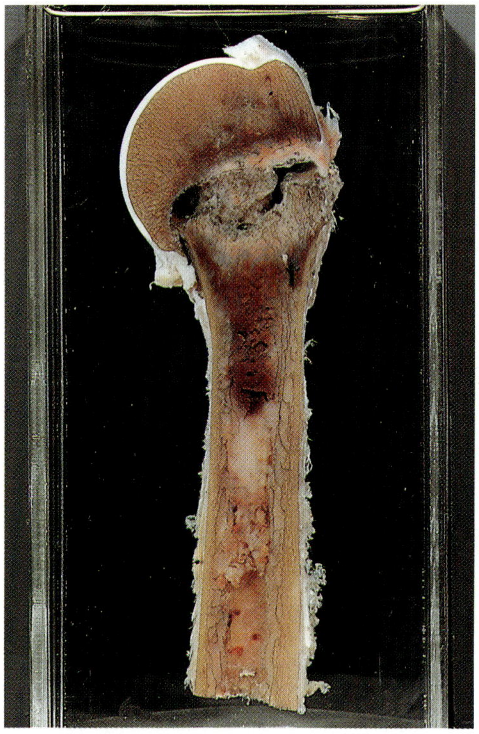

10.27 Humerus: Fracture

No clinical details are available.

A vertical section through the upper end of this humerus shows a recent transverse fracture through the neck with extensive intramedullary haemorrhage.

Fractures of the neck of the humerus are commonest in the elderly and usually follow a fall on an outstretched hand. There is often associated damage to the greater tuberosity and the humeral shaft may be impacted in the head, often leading to malunion.

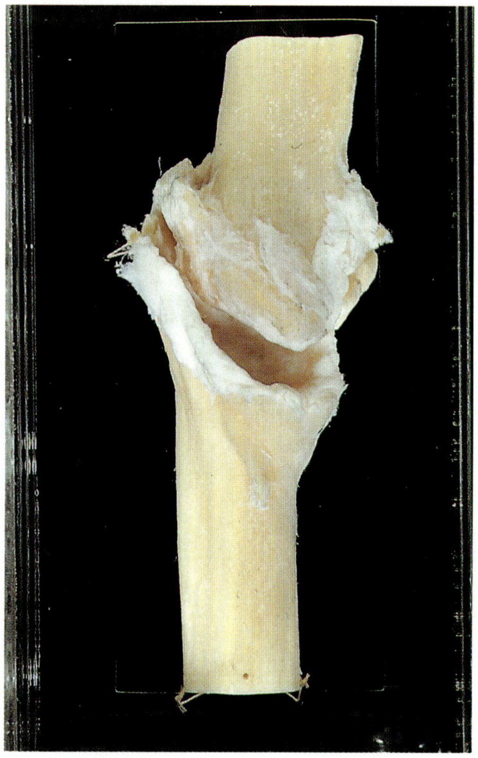

10.28 Humerus: Fracture with False Joint (Pseudarthrosis)

No clinical details are available.

Part of the shaft of the humerus shows an oblique fracture. A false joint with a surrounding fibrous capsule has formed between the bone ends.

Transverse or oblique fractures of the humeral shaft typically follow a severe direct blow or a fall on the elbow. Delayed or non-union, as here, is a well recognised complication if too much traction is employed following the injury. Important general causes of non-union include ischaemia, local infection, malnutrition, excessive mobility at the fracture site and interposition of extraneous tissue between the bone ends.

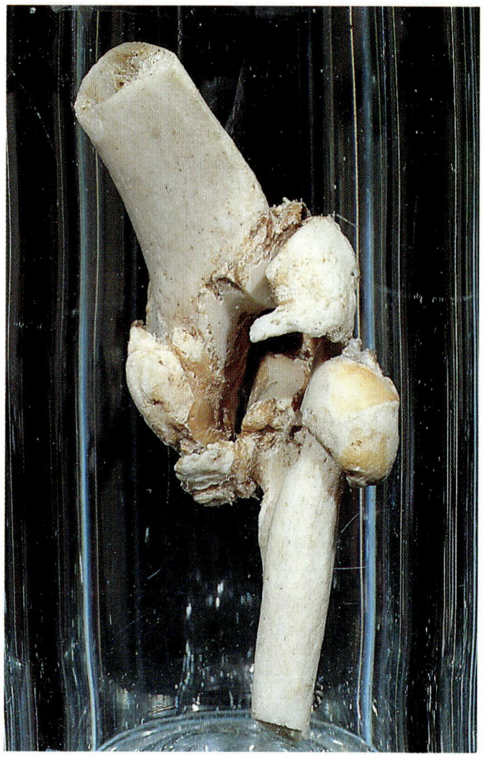

10.29 Elbow: Fracture Dislocation

No clinical details are available.

The bones of the left elbow joint show a comminuted fracture of the distal humerus, associated with detachment of the capitulum and lateral humeral condyle. The radius was dislocated in the fresh state. There is extensive secondary osteoarthrosis with new bone formation, particularly around the new articular surface formed between the ulna and the fractured aspect of the distal humerus.

Dislocation of the elbow may be associated with fractures of any of the bones around the joint. Such an injury typically follows a fall on the hand and may be followed by neurovascular damage or severe joint stiffness.

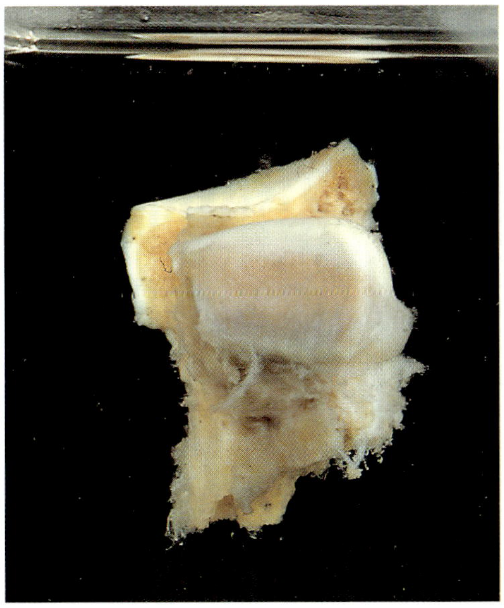

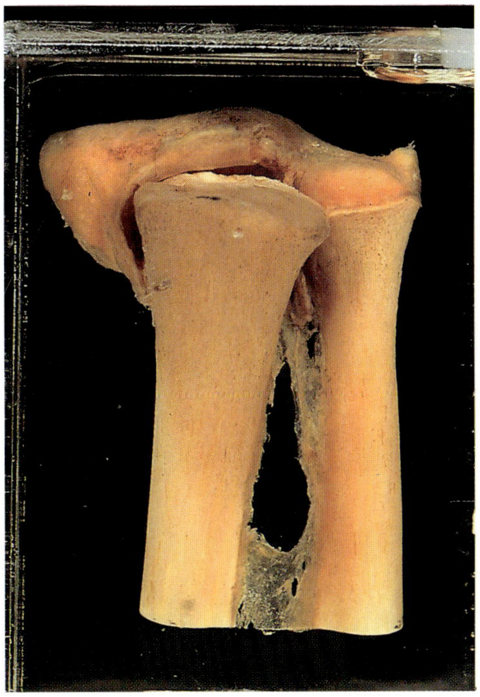

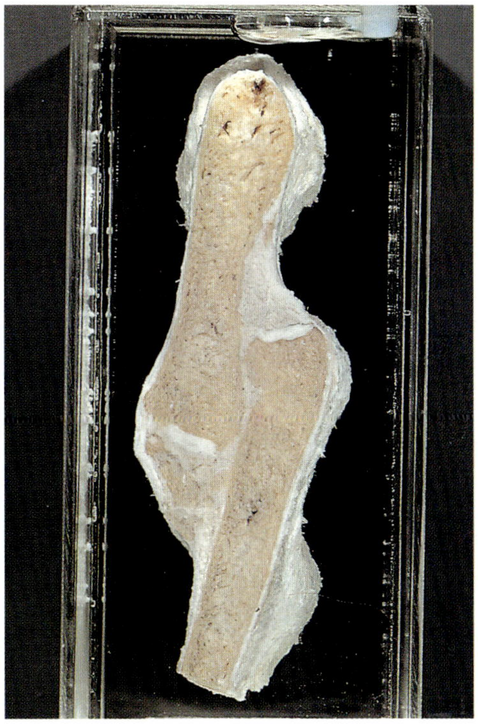

10.30 Head of Radius: Fracture

This specimen was excised from a 50-year-old woman who had fallen and injured her left elbow and presented with swelling and limited flexion. Despite conservative treatment with splinting, symptoms persisted and, at operation, a fragment of bone was found wedged between the articular surfaces, and the head of the radius was excised.

The excised left radial head shows a fracture through the articular surface with considerable displacement of the main fragments.

Fractures of the radial head are virtually confined to adults who have fallen on an outstretched hand. Similar injuries in childhood cause fractures of the radial neck. Fragmentation of the bone or overlying articular cartilage is quite common and is an important cause of joint stiffness.

10.31 Wrist: Detached Lower Radial Epiphysis

This specimen is from an adolescent boy who fell on his outstretched hand.

The bones of the lower arm at the wrist joint show backward displacement of the lower radial epiphysis, which has occurred through the epiphyseal growth plate.

Fracture-separation of the lower radial epiphysis is the rare childhood equivalent of a Colles' fracture and typically follows a fall on a dorsiflexed hand. While, most often, growth of the radius and later epiphyseal fusion are not affected, any degree of crushing damage to the epiphysis itself may be followed by premature fusion such that the ulna outgrows the radius.

10.32 Sternum: Fracture Dislocation

This is a post-mortem specimen from a 60-year-old man who, 5 months previously, had fallen from a tree and sustained severe injuries to the head and chest. At autopsy part of the pericardium and adjacent left lung were adherent to the internal aspect of the sternal injury.

The left half of the upper sternum, viewed from the mid-line, shows a 1.5cm postero-inferior displacement of the manubrium behind the body of the sternum. The bones are firmly united in their new position.

This is clearly a rather unusual site for a fracture dislocation but was probably the result of a severe anterior crushing force, as may also be sustained by road traffic accident victims.

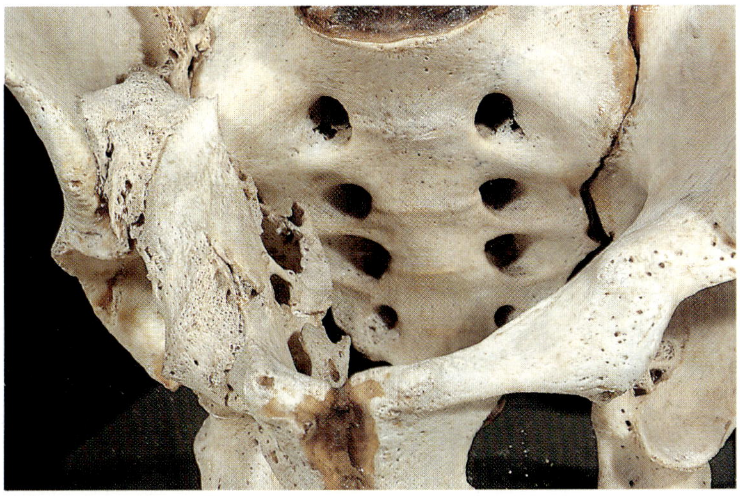

10.33 Pelvis: Extensive Healed Fracture

This is a post-mortem specimen from a 61-year-old man who died of typhus fever. Four months previously he had fallen from a height on to some stones but had gradually recovered, being left with a limp and apparent shortening of the right leg.

The pelvis (viewed anteriorly) shows extensive right-sided fractures of the ilium, pubic ramus and ischium which have healed with considerable displacement. The head of the femur had been forcibly driven inwards and upwards, grossly distorting the acetabulum.

Multiple pelvic fractures, leading to disruption of the pelvic ring of bones, typically follows either a severe crush injury or a severe vertical force in which the patient falls on to one leg (as here). Commonly there is extensive bony and soft tissue damage with massive haemorrhage and often injury to the genito-urinary tract. Affected patients are therefore treated as a surgical emergency. In contrast, solitary fractures of one of the pelvic bones, which do not compromise pelvic stability, often have little ill effect and may not require active treatment.

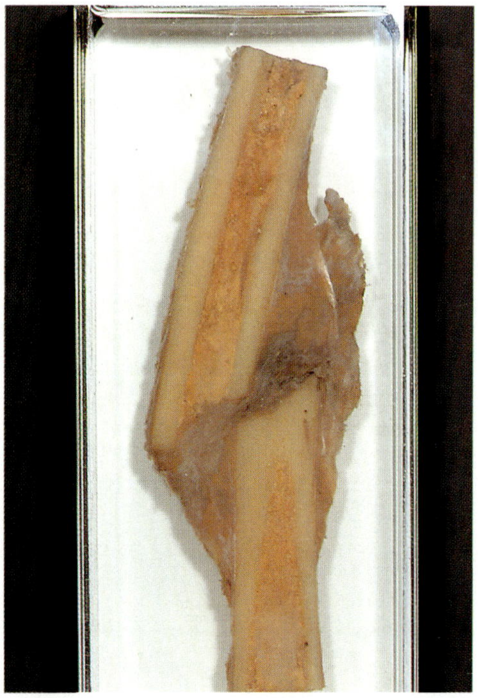

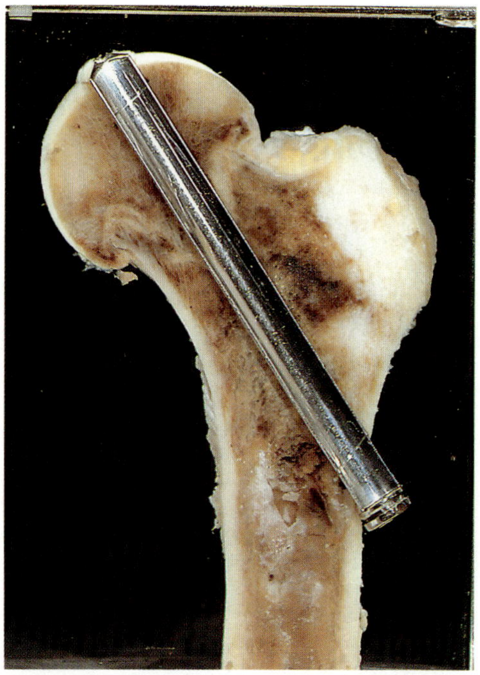

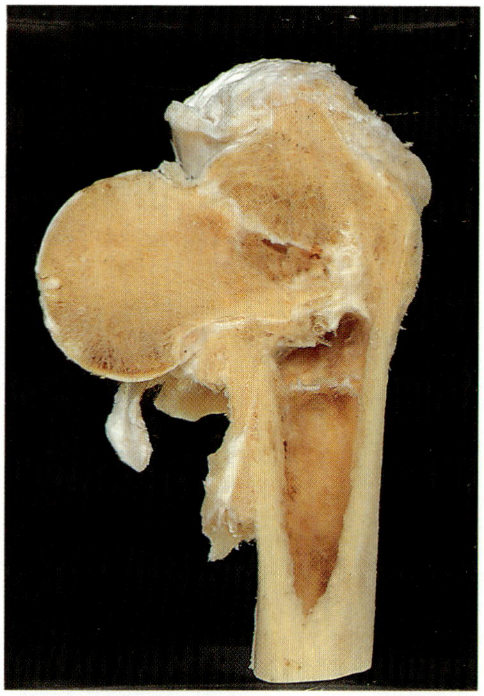

10.34 Femur: Healing Fracture

This is a post-mortem specimen from a 56-year-old man who had fractured his femur 3 months previously. Initial treatment over the first month had been unsuccessful, but then the fracture was reduced by traction and started to heal. The patient died of pneumonia.

Part of the shaft of the femur, viewed in vertical section, shows an oblique fracture in the course of repair. The callus which has formed on either side of the lateral displacement is undergoing ossification.

Healing of an uncomplicated fracture is achieved by the formation of provisional callus, derived from the periosteum and medulla. Thereafter, complete ossification and gradual remodelling of the bone to adapt to incident stress occurs. Factors which impair bone healing include instability or wide separation of the bone fragments, local infection, ischaemia or extensive bony necrosis, comminution, and the presence of massive periosteal damage. Important systemic factors include malnutrition, particularly deficiencies of vitamins D or C, and coincident steroid treatment.

10.35 Femur: Fracture of Neck

No clinical details are available.

The upper end of the femur has been sectioned to show a recent, transverse subcapital fracture, which is slightly impacted. The fracture has been fixed with a Trifin nail.

Fractures of the femoral neck are extremely common and almost invariably occur in the elderly, particularly females. While a fall is the most frequent precipitating injury, quite trivial trauma may be responsible, largely because most cases are attributable to underlying osteoporosis. Less often, such fractures are pathological, occurring through a metastatic tumour deposit. Currently the majority of patients are treated surgically, either by internal fixation or occasionally hip replacement, so as to prevent long periods of immobilisation. Important local complications include avascular necrosis of the femoral head or non-union. More significantly, however, the associated risk of deep venous thrombosis, pulmonary embolism, myocardial infarction or bronchopneumonia is particularly high in the elderly.

10.36 Femur: Intracapsular Fracture of Neck with Severe Varus Deformity

No clinical details are available.

A vertical section through the upper femur shows a healed, intertrochanteric fracture showing partial fibrous union. The head and neck show extreme displacement, lying at a right angle to the shaft.

Gross displacement such as this would clearly be corrected surgically nowadays, perhaps by hip replacement if the fracture is irreducible.

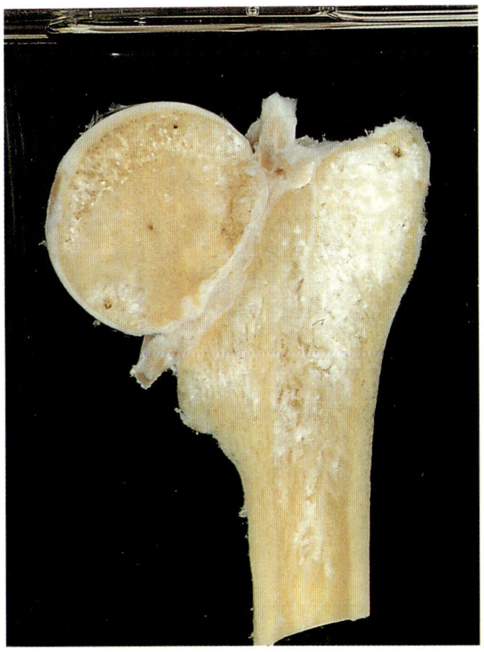

10.37 Femur: Fracture of Neck with Fibrous Union

This is a post-mortem specimen from a 66-year-old woman, who died 5 months after sustaining a fracture of the right hip following a fall.

A vertical section through the upper end of the femur shows a clearly delineated subcapital fracture, which has been followed by almost total resorption of the femoral neck and fibrous union.

Fibrous union of any fracture most often follows delayed union (see Legend 10.34), wide separation of the bone ends or the interposition of either dead bone or adjacent soft tissue between the bone ends.

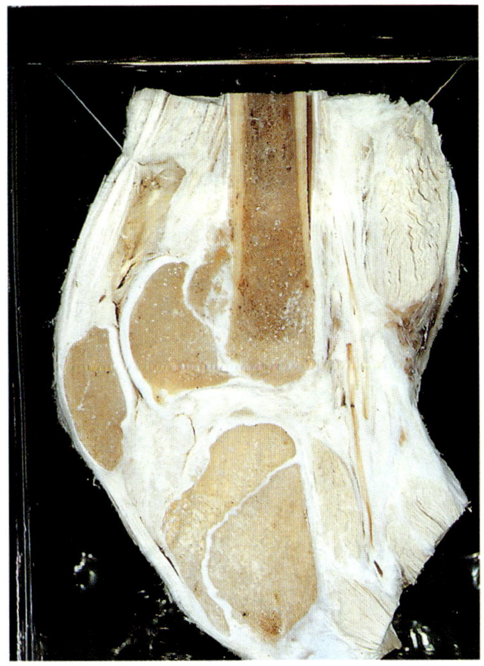

10.38 Femur: Detachment of Lower Epiphysis

This is a post-mortem specimen from a young boy who died 5 weeks after sustaining a severe blow to the front of the knee from the handle of a grocer's cart. He died during the course of an operation to replace the epiphysis.

A vertical section through the bones and soft tissues of the left knee joint shows marked antero-superior displacement of the distal femoral epiphysis, which is also slightly rotated. Between the epiphysis and shaft there is a mass of callus, with a fragment of bone torn from the metaphysis at the time of injury embedded within it.

Fracture-separation of the lower femoral epiphysis is an injury seen in adolescence, usually following excessive abduction or extension forces at the knee. While vascular damage is not uncommon, interference with femoral growth is rarely a complication since reduction of the displacement by conservative means is usually possible.

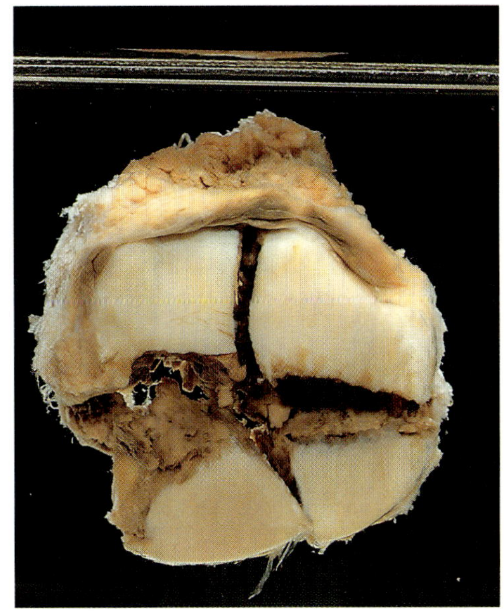

10.39 Patella: Stellate Fracture

No clinical details are available.

The patella is shattered in both the vertical and transverse planes, the intervening central space being occupied by recent blood clot.

Stellate patellar fractures result from a direct blow or fall, which usually smashes the patella on the femur. In the absence of any significant displacement or comminution, such fractures are usually amenable to conservative treatment.

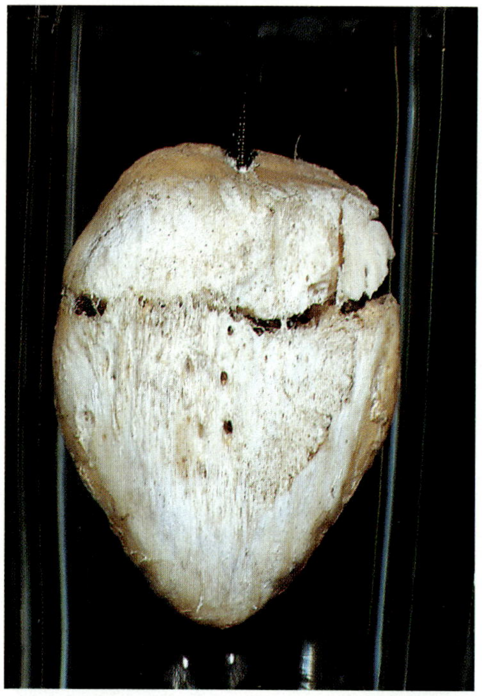

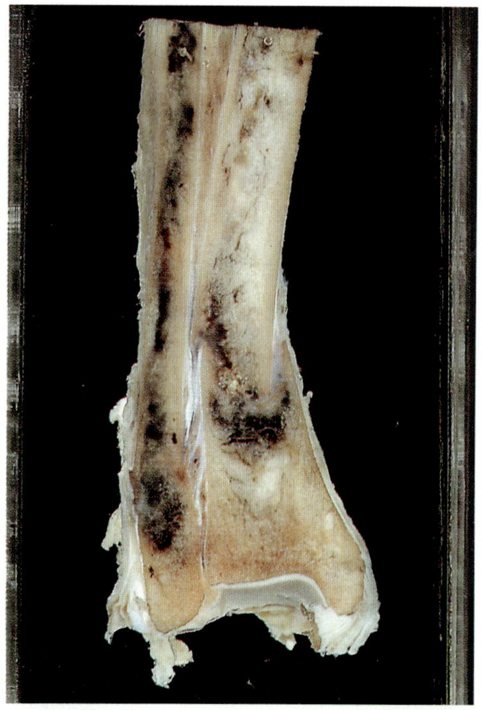

10.41 Tibia and Fibula: Transverse Fractures

This is a post-mortem specimen from a 90-year-old woman, who died of bronchopneumonia 6 weeks after falling out of bed and severely twisting her ankle. The fractures had been fixed in plaster.

A coronal section through the lower ends of the tibia and fibula show recent transverse fractures of both bones, associated with slight lateral displacement and extensive intramedullary haemorrhage. Note the marked cortical atrophy of both bones, indicative of senile osteoporosis.

It is more usual for both distal leg bones to be fractured at the same time than for one to be broken in isolation. While direct trauma may be responsible, a twisting injury (particularly in the elderly) is more common. There is frequently coexistent injury to the skin and soft tissues, so wound infection and, later, non-union are important complications.

10.40 Patella: Transverse Fracture

This is a post-mortem specimen from a 24-year-old man, who fell from a considerable height on to his knee. He died 7 weeks later of fulminant suppurative osteomyelitis.

The patella shows a well demarcated transverse fracture, across which foci of bony union have taken place.

Transverse patellar fractures result from rupture of the knee extensor mechanism, usually as a result of a fall in which the knee cannot be straightened. Fractures such as this, if displaced, require prompt surgical repair, otherwise knee extension is permanently impaired and the joint becomes unstable.

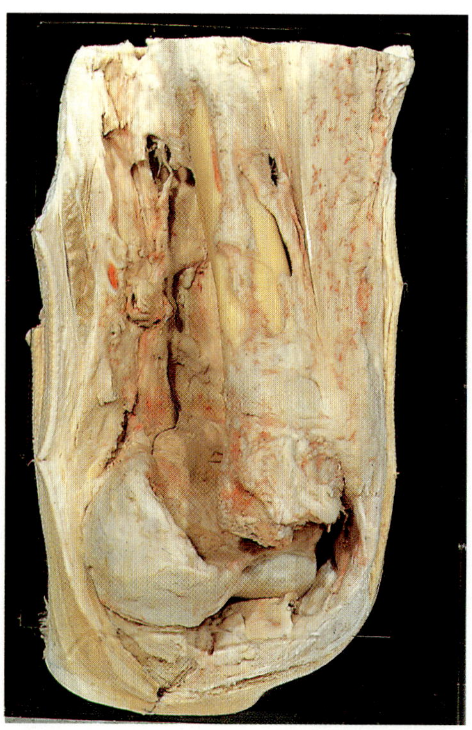

10.42 Femur: Acute Osteomyelitis

This is an amputation specimen from a 16-year-old boy, who had presented with a 3 week history of fever and pain in the right thigh. A large fluctuant swelling developed in the lower thigh musculature which, when drained, contained copious pus. Symptoms persisted and, since antibiotics were not available, amputation became necessary.

The lower end of the femur, with the knee joint, is shown. The periosteum is separated from the femoral shaft, which is almost completely necrotic. The intervening gap, in the fresh state, was filled with pus and represents an extensive abscess cavity. The lower epiphysis has become separated and the suppurative process communicates with the joint space.

Pyogenic osteomyelitis is typically a disease of children and adolescents and most often commences in the metaphysis of a long bone, more frequently in the leg than the arm. The majority of cases represent the result of haematogenous dissemination of an often asymptomatic bacteraemic illness but other causes include trauma (particularly compound fractures) and spread from some other local source of infection. The most frequently implicated organism is *Staphylococcus aureus*; less frequently, streptococci and various coliforms may be responsible. Patients with sickle cell anaemia or Gaucher's disease may also be prone to Salmonella infection.

Infection typically commences in the highly vascular medullary cavity of the metaphysis from whence it spreads both within the marrow but also through the cortical bone to the subperiosteum. The periosteum is then stripped off and, with time, begins to form new bone (the involucrum) while the central necrotic bone is known as the sequestrum. Complications include the development of a localised bone abscess, soft tissue sinuses or an abscess, suppurative arthritis and septicaemia. Given time, chronic infection, secondary amyloidosis and disrupted growth of the affected bone may also occur.

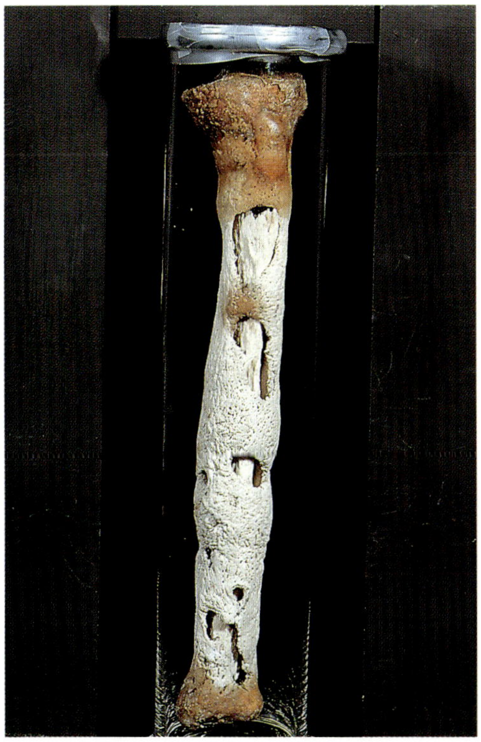

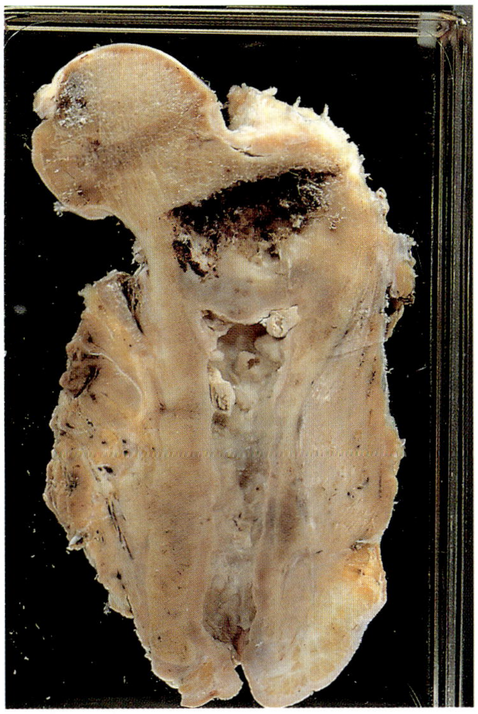

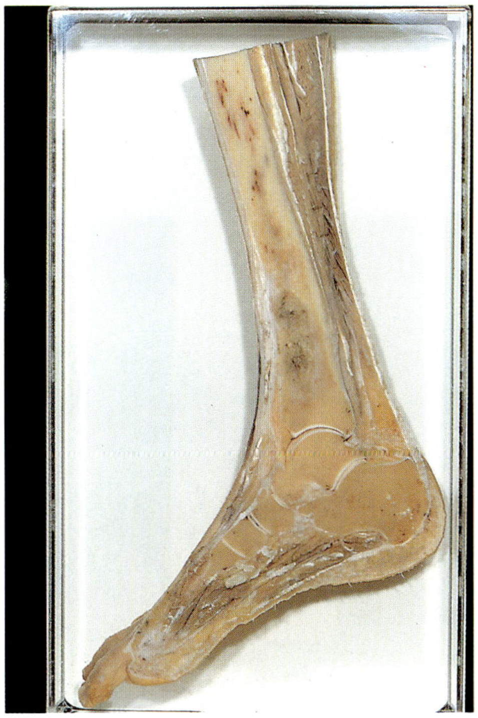

10.43 Tibia: Chronic Osteomyelitis

No clinical details are available.

The left tibia shows complete necrosis of the shaft (sequestrum) which is separated from the periosteum. The latter is thickened and shows extensive new bone formation (the involucrum). Numerous sinuses, known as cloacae, penetrating through the involucrum are apparent.

The tibia is the second commonest site of origin of an osteomyelitic process, the femur being most frequently affected. This is a typical case of chronic infection, as indicated by the presence of a well-developed involucrum.

10.44 Femur: Chronic Osteomyelitis

This is a disarticulation specimen through the left hip joint from a 45-year-old man who had sustained a severe gunshot wound to the left leg 20 years previously. This had necessitated an above-knee amputation for unremitting osteomyelitis; thereafter the proximal femur had remained infected with the formation of a cutaneous sinus and further surgery became inevitable.

The upper half of the left femur, with adjacent soft tissues, shows that the medullary cavity is filled with necrotic, purulent material. The cortex is markedly thickened and congested. At the distal end of the specimen, a sinus tract extending from the infected sequestrum can be seen opening on to the skin of the amputation stump.

Sinuses between the infected bone and the skin surface often develop in long-standing osteomyelitis. Such sinuses may occasionally be complicated by the development of squamous cell carcinoma, a phenomenon known as Marjolin's ulcer (see Chapter 8).

10.45 Tibia: Osteomyelitis with Brodie's Abscess

This is an amputation specimen from a 32-year-old man who had developed a tumour at the lower end of the right tibia sometime previously. Biopsy revealed a non-Hodgkin's lymphoma which was treated by radiotherapy. Thereafter, the patient developed osteomyelitis at the same site which, despite antibiotic treatment, threatened to cause a pathological fracture so amputation was performed.

A sagittal section through the right lower leg shows a well-delineated abscess cavity in the lower tibia, which measures 5 × 2 × 2cm and contains greenish pus. The abscess is surrounded by a layer of pale, sclerotic bone.

It is well-recognised that a focus of osteomyelitis, particularly if partially treated, may become localised and 'walled-off', a phenomenon known as Brodie's abscess. This case also demonstrates that immunocompromised individuals are at particular risk of developing osteomyelitis.

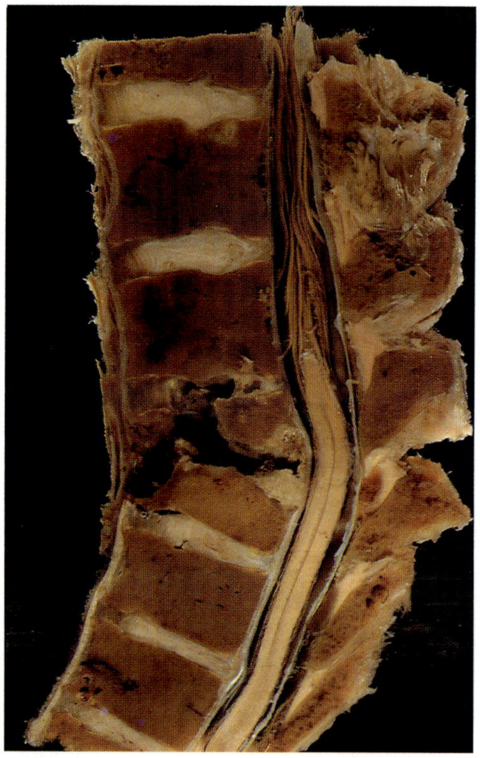

10.46 Spine: Tuberculous Osteomyelitis

This is a post-mortem specimen from a 52-year-old man, who died of heart failure. He was known to have had pulmonary tuberculosis for the preceding 4 years. During the last 6 months of his life, he had developed back pain associated with gradual loss of power and sensation in the legs. Latterly he was completely paraplegic with loss of excretory sphincter control.

A sagittal section through the lower thoracic and lumbar vertebrae shows extensive destruction of two of the vertebral bodies by cavitating caseous necrosis. The damaged bone bulges posteriorly into the spinal canal, compressing the cord.

Tuberculous osteomyelitis is usually a complication of mycobacterial infections elsewhere in the body, most often the lungs. Haematogenous spread of organisms to bones and joints may give rise to multifocal osteomyelitis but, in general, the thoracolumbar spine is most often involved, followed by the long bones of the leg. Children and young adults are usually affected. Spinal involvement, which nearly always leads to vertebral collapse and a gibbous deformity (kyphoscoliosis), is known as Pott's disease and may be complicated by cord compression, tuberculous meningitis or a psoas 'abscess'. (Courtesy of St. Thomas's Hospital Medical School Museum)

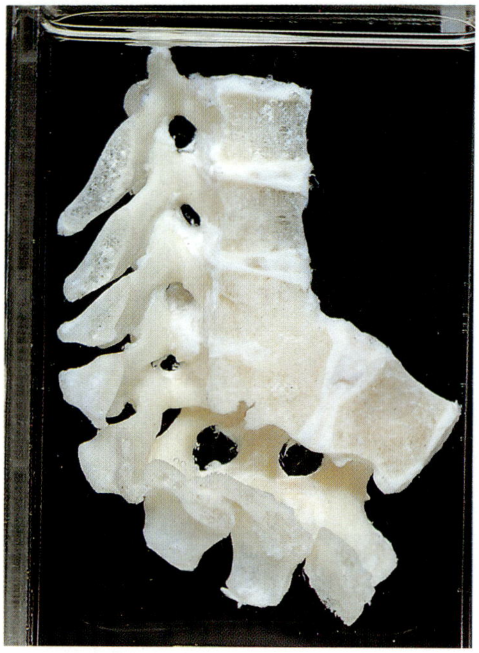

10.47 Spine: Tuberculous Osteomyelitis

No clinical details are available other than that the patient was a child.

This macerated specimen shows a sharp angular curvature due to tuberculous destruction of the 3 lower thoracic and first lumbar vertebrae. The caseous process has healed, resulting in bony ankylosis. The vertebral canal appears normal.

Spinal angulation following tuberculous destruction is characteristic of Pott's disease, which is now only rarely seen in the Western world. Modern surgical techniques in combination with antituberculous chemotherapy may prevent the development of kyphosis.

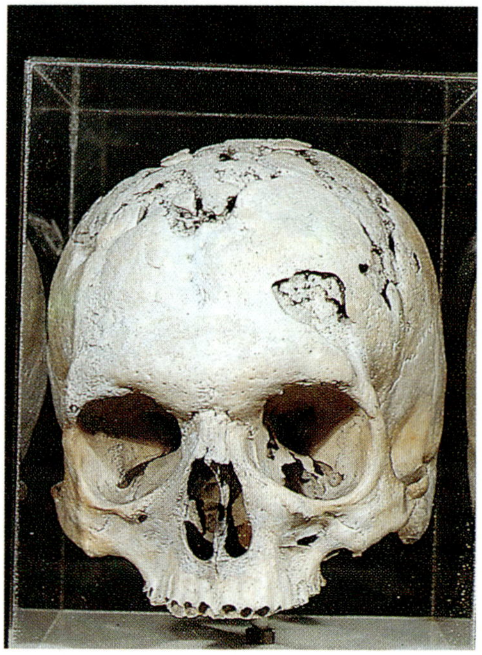

10.48 Skull: Acquired Syphilis

No clinical details are available.

This adult's skull shows extensive, irregular destruction of the frontal and parietal bones with occasional areas of complete perforation.

The skeleton is typically affected in the tertiary stage of syphilitic infection, the tibia, skull or clavicle being most often involved. The principal features are those of gummatous bone destruction, associated with florid periostitis and new bone formation. Multiple superficial erosions of the skull, as here, are known as *caries sicca*; perforation of the inner table is an infrequent feature.

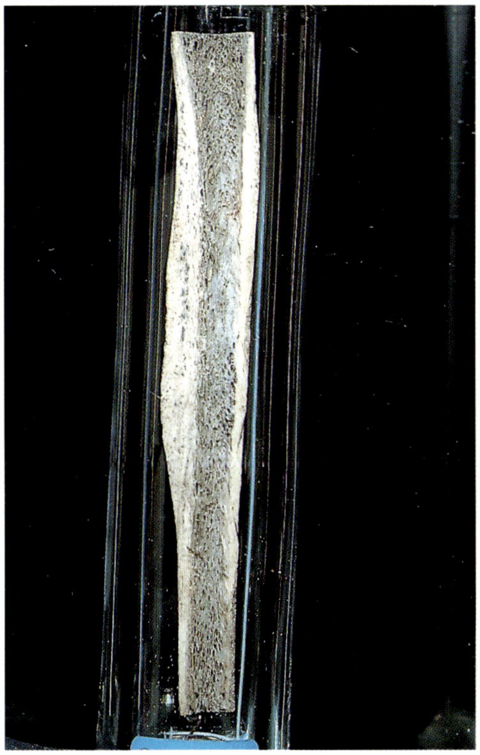

10.49 Tibia: Acquired Syphilis

No clinical details are available.

A section through the tibia shows very marked cortical thickening due to periosteal new bone formation.

As already stated, the tibia is one of the most frequently affected bones in tertiary syphilis. As shown in this case, florid periostitis is much more often seen than gummatous destruction.

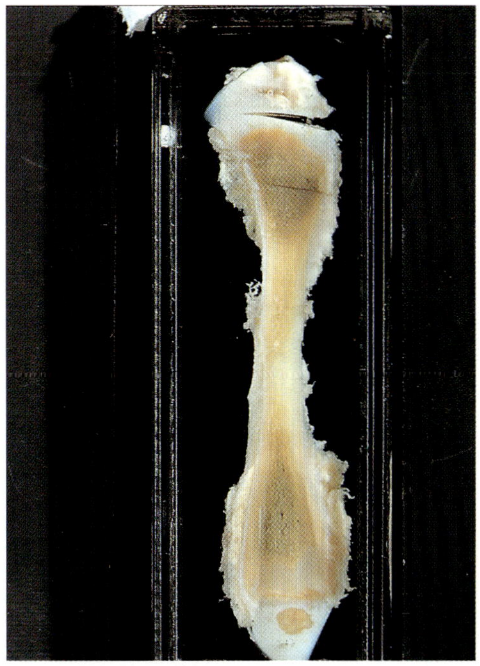

10.50 Femur: Congenital Syphilis

This is a post-mortem specimen from a 6-week-old baby girl who had been unable to move her limbs since the age of 2 weeks. Examination revealed a flaccid paresis and X-rays showed florid syphilitic osteochondritis. The mother's Wassermann reaction was positive. The child became pyrexial and died of bronchopneumonia.

A vertical section through the femur shows that the epiphyses are thickened, opaque and yellowish. Note also that the ends of the diaphysis are replaced by greyish granulation tissue. There is minimal periosteal thickening.

The features of congenital syphilis and tertiary acquired syphilis are very similar although in the former granulomatous osteochondritis, particularly at the ends of long bones, is usually a predominant feature. Epiphyseal destruction, often with separation, may lead to disrupted growth.

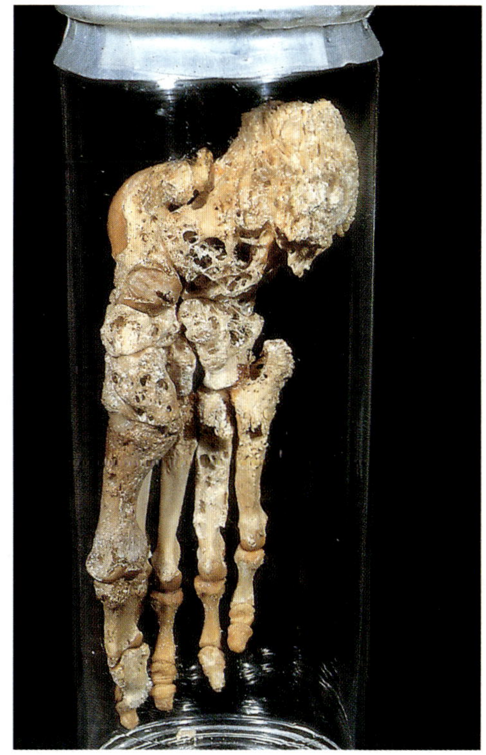

10.51 Foot: Maduromycosis

No clinical details are available, other than the patient was a native of India.

The bones of this right foot show very extensive necrosis and destruction at multiple sites.

Maduromycosis (also known as mycetoma) is almost exclusively a tropical disease, resulting from infection by either fungi or actinomycetes which are acquired through a penetrating injury. The condition is characterised by an extensive, ramifying suppurative process, which destroys soft tissues, tendosynovial structures and bone alike. The clinical course tends to be indolent and chronic.

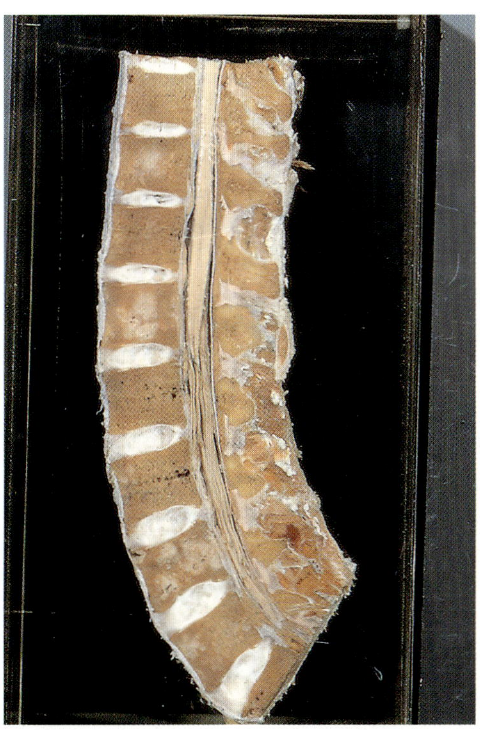

10.52 Spine: Melioidosis

This is a post-mortem specimen from a soldier, who had served for many years in the Far East. He had suffered from melioidosis for the previous 5 years with recurrent septicaemic episodes. The culpable organism was isolated from a subcutaneous abscess. Because, at the time, antibiotics were unavailable, the patient's condition deteriorated and he died with extensive foci of infection in the lungs, liver, kidneys and spine.

A sagittal section through the spine shows multiple, pale rounded abscesses in several of the vertebral bodies.

Melioidosis is very uncommon in the Western world but is endemic in the Far East and South East Asia. It is caused by the bacterium *Pseudomonas pseudomallei*, which is found in the soil or water in endemic areas and is thought to be transmitted in rodent faeces. Infection may follow either contamination of an infected wound, ingestion or inhalation. The clinical course is variable but systemic dissemination is common.

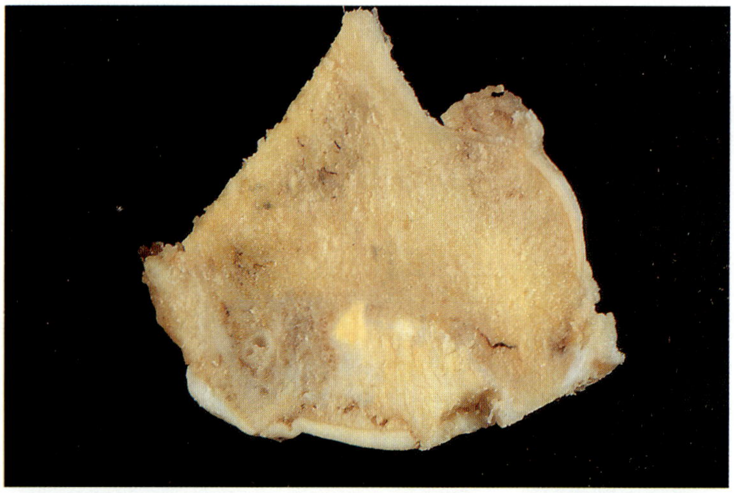

10.53 Femoral Head: Avascular Necrosis

No clinical details are available.

This femoral head has been sectioned to show a vaguely wedge-shaped area of greyish-yellow infarction beneath the articular surface. Note the small area of collapse above the infarct, with flattening of the articular surface.

Avascular necrosis of the femoral head is not uncommon and represents an important predisposing cause of osteoarthrosis. The condition is characterised by infarction of bone and bone marrow due to ischaemia, resulting from vascular occlusion or compression. Common predisposing causes include a subcapital femoral fracture, systemic steroid therapy (e.g. in rheumatoid arthritis or transplant recipients) or alcoholism. Less common causes include sickle cell anaemia and Gaucher's disease. Microfractures of the necrotic bone may lead to collapse of the articular surface and hence to secondary osteoarthrosis. (Courtesy of Drs. C.D.M. Fletcher and P.H. McKee, St. Thomas's Hospital Medical School)

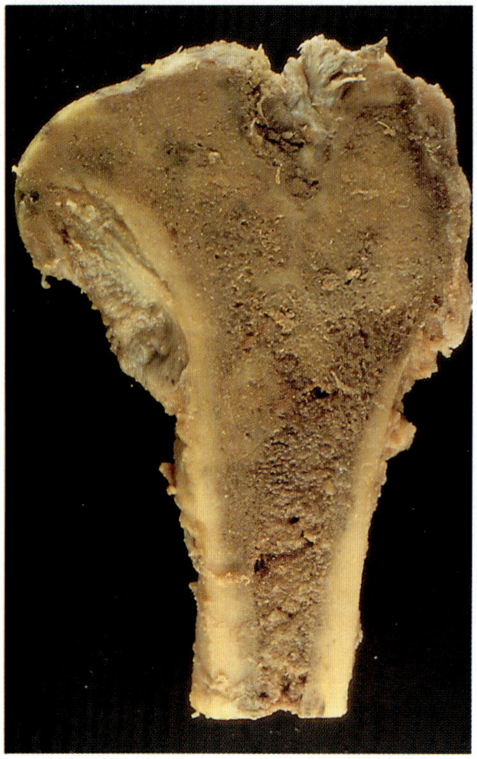

10.54 Femoral Head: Avascular Necrosis

No clinical details are available.

The proximal femur has been sectioned to show an extensive area of pale infarction, affecting the head, neck and greater trochanter. In this case, there has been very marked collapse of the femoral head such that the articular surface is severely flattened and shows degenerative changes.

This is a good example of the joint destruction that may follow avascular necrosis. Some authorities claim that up to 20 per cent of hip joints requiring prosthetic replacement (other than those fractured) show evidence of avascular necrosis. (Courtesy of Drs. C.D.M. Fletcher and P.H. Mckee, St. Thomas's Hospital Medical School)

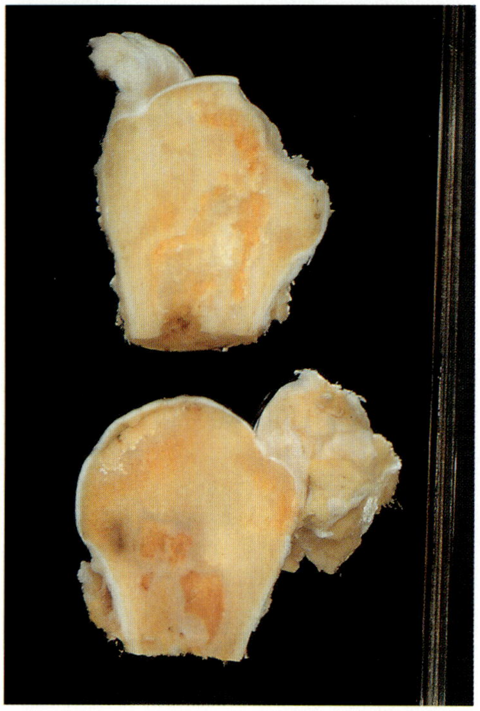

10.55 Humerus: Decompression Sickness

These are post-mortem specimens from a 37-year-old man who died of a coronary thrombosis. Two months previously he had presented with a 9 month history of intermittent pains in the shoulders and right hips, having spent the previous 4 years engaged in tunnelling work at high atmospheric pressure under compressed air. X-rays of the shoulders revealed irregular erosion of the central articular surfaces of both humeri, with fragmentation and condensation of the underlying bone.

Vertical sections through the heads of both humeri show collapse of the articular surfaces (particularly above), while the underlying cancellous bone has an opaque, yellowish necrotic appearance which extends down the shaft bilaterally.

Decompression sickness (synonym: Caisson disease) results from the formation of nitrogen bubbles in the bloodstream, which are derived from the increased soluble nitrogen produced by working at high atmospheric pressure if gradual decompression is not undertaken. These bubbles act as emboli and hence lead to infarction, particularly of subchondral bone and cerebral tissue. Some authorities currently believe that these bone infarcts result from the dissolution of nitrogen in medullary fat, leading to swelling and venous compression.

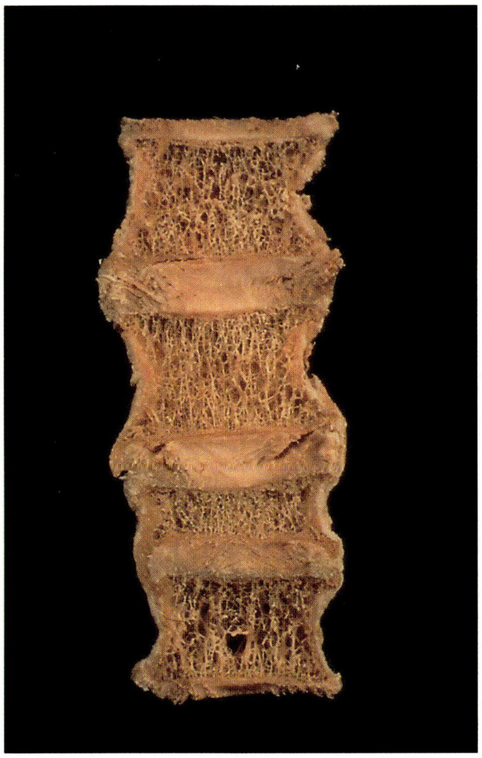

10.56 Spine: Senile Osteoporosis

No clinical details are available.

This coronal section of the lower thoracic and upper lumbar vertebrae shows a marked diminution in the amount of cortical and trabecular bone, associated with a characteristic compression fracture.

Osteoporosis represents a diminution in total bone mass, which is otherwise normal in its relative mineralised and organic components. This condition, which affects the whole skeleton, is seen most often in the elderly, particularly females. It may be secondary to immobility, postmenopausal diminished oestrogen levels, malnutrition, various endocrine disorders (e.g. Cushing's syndrome and thyrotoxicosis), drugs (e.g. alcohol) and a variety of inherited conditions, including osteogenesis imperfecta. Many cases, however, remain idiopathic. Because of the resultant cortical thinning and resorption of cancellous bone, affected patients are rendered very susceptible to vertebral compression fractures and fractures of the limb bones (particularly the femoral neck and the wrist) following negligible trauma. (Courtesy of Dr. P.G. Bullough, Hospital for Special Surgery, New York)

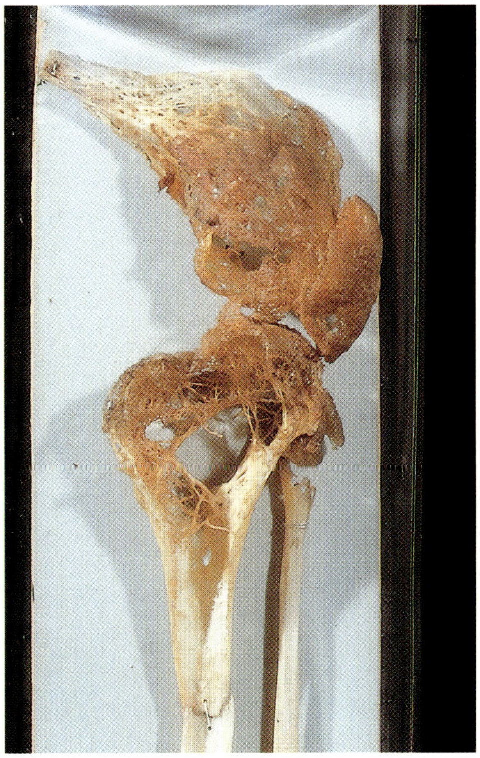

10.57 Leg Bones: Disuse Atrophy

This is an amputation specimen from a young man with a 10 year history of tuberculous osteomyelitis of both ankles. He had been bedridden for the past 3 years.

The right tibia, fibula, patella and the lower end of the femur show extreme atrophy. There is very little remaining cancellous bone and the cortices are severely thinned being virtually absent in some places.

Osseous atrophy such as this is typically seen as a consequence either of prolonged disuse (e.g. in neuromuscular paralytic disorders), malnutrition, severe ischaemia or various endocrine disorders. Basically it represents a subgroup of osteoporosis (see Legend 10.56).

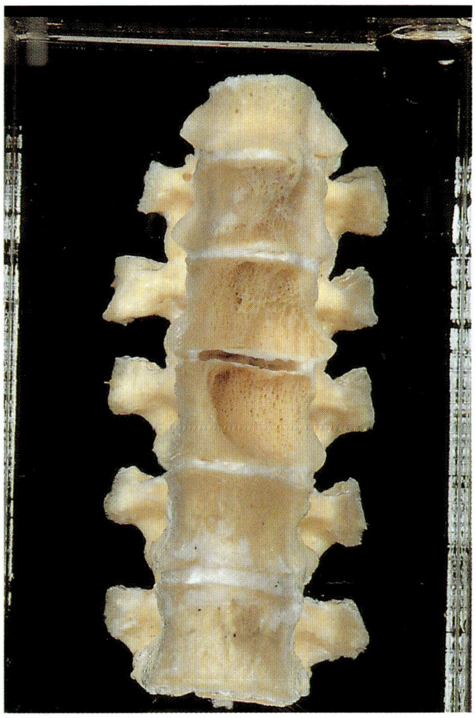

10.58 Spinal Column: Pressure Atrophy

This is a post-mortem specimen from a 37-year-old man who died of left-sided bronchopneumonia. At autopsy there was a large, probably syphilitic, aneurysm of the ascending aorta which had compressed the left main bronchus and which was also impinging on the vertebrae.

Three of these thoracic vertebral bodies show smooth bony erosion on the left side at the site of pressure from the aneurysm.

Pressure exerted for any length of time on bone typically leads to increased local osteoclastic resorption.

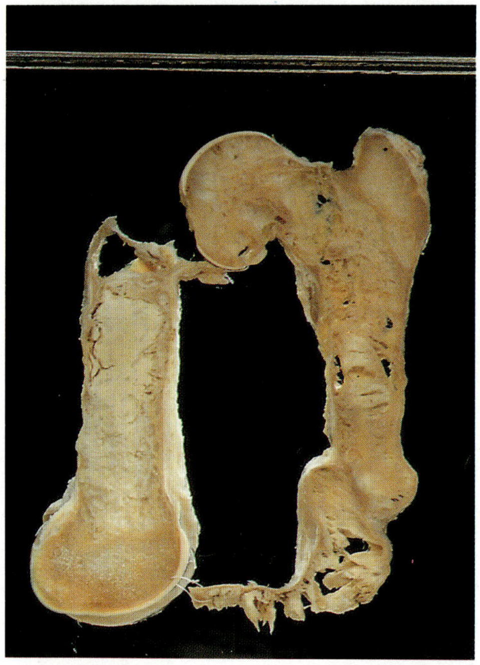

10.59 Femur: Osteomalacia

This is a post-mortem specimen from a 35-year-old woman, who had suffered from a 'softening of the bones' for 5½ years. She had developed a rolling, stooping gait with curvature of the spine and severe pain in the hips. She had suffered bilateral femoral fractures prior to death.

This fractured left femur was so soft at post-mortem that it could be longitudinally sectioned with a knife. Almost the entire diaphysis is replaced by soft, pale osteoid, leaving in some places only an outer layer of periosteum. A thin layer of cancellous bone remains at either end. Note the partially united old fracture beneath the greater trochanter.

Osteomalacia is the adult equivalent of rickets and is characterised by inadequate bony mineralisation leading to a relative increase in the amount of osteoid. It may result from vitamin D deficiency (of whatever cause), impaired vitamin D metabolism (due usually to renal or hepatic disease), and renal phosphaturia, or it may form part of a uraemic renal osteodystrophy. The failure of mineralisation leads to softening and fragility of bones with stress deformities and fractures. Epiphyseal pseudofractures, known as Looser's zones, may be seen. Recognition of this condition is vital since many cases, particularly those due to dietary, malabsorptive or environmental vitamin D deficiency, are eminently treatable.

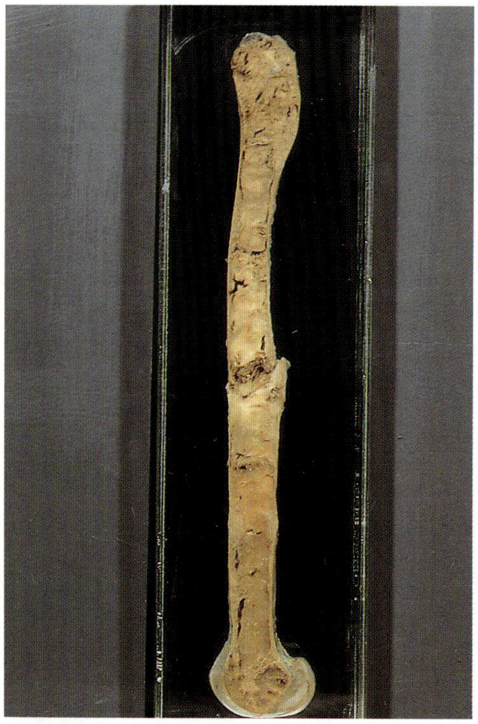

10.60 Femur: Osteomalacia

This is a post-mortem specimen from a 72-year-old woman who had been bedridden for 4 years. Previously she had developed severe pain in both legs, associated with gradual bending. Shortly before death she had suffered fractures of the left femur and right humerus while being moved in bed.

A vertical section of the femur, which was easily cut with an ordinary knife, shows a marked reduction in cortical thickness and the cancellous bone is replaced by yellowish-red fatty tissue. There is a recent transverse fracture of the mid-shaft.

This case is also typical of very severe osteomalacia. This degree of disease is very rarely seen in modern practice.

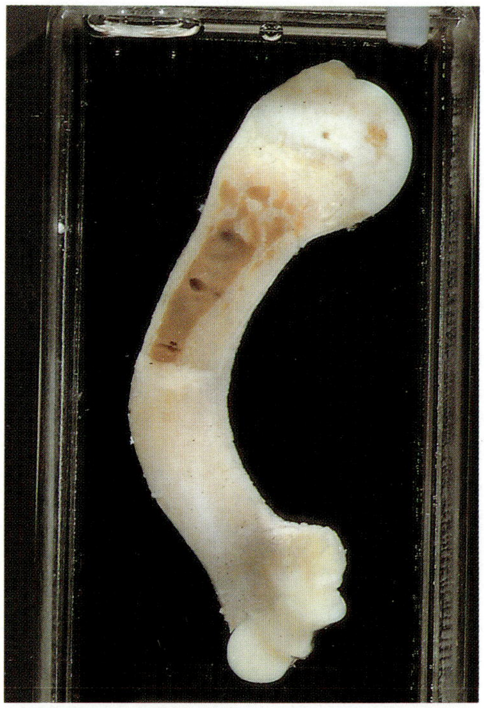

10.61 Humerus: Rickets

This is a post-mortem specimen from a 16-month-old girl who died of bronchopneumonia and marasmus. She had been noted to suffer from rickets since birth and her long limb bones could be bent like rubber.

This infantile right humerus shows a prominent zone of cartilage at the upper epiphysis and the advancing calcification front (which is more opaque and darker in colour) is very irregular. The cortex of the diaphysis is thickened and consists almost entirely of soft cancellous bone. Note the marked lateral curvature of the bone.

Rickets represents the effects of defective mineralisation, entirely comparable to osteomalacia, occurring in childhood (prior to epiphyseal fusion). In the Western world rickets is now most often due to renal tubular disease (e.g. renal tubular acidosis) or severe coeliac disease, but vitamin D deficiency remains the most important cause on a world-wide scale. The accumulation of large amounts of unmineralised epiphyseal cartilage and cortical osteoid leads to softening of bones, marked curvature (particularly in the limbs and spine) and a pigeon-breast deformity of the chest.

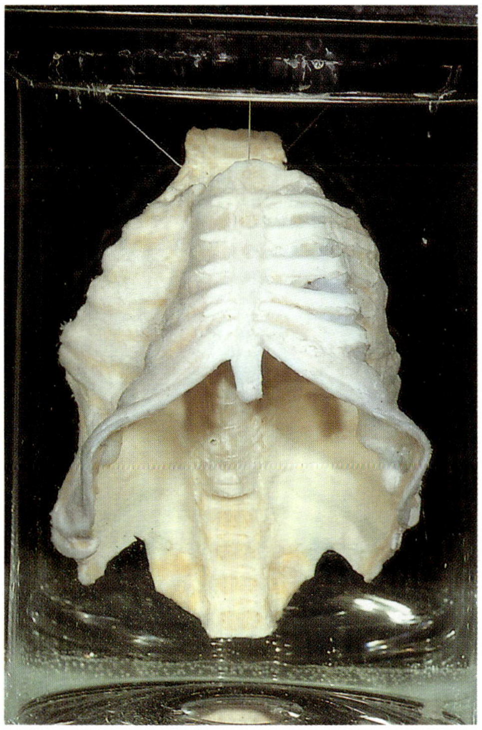

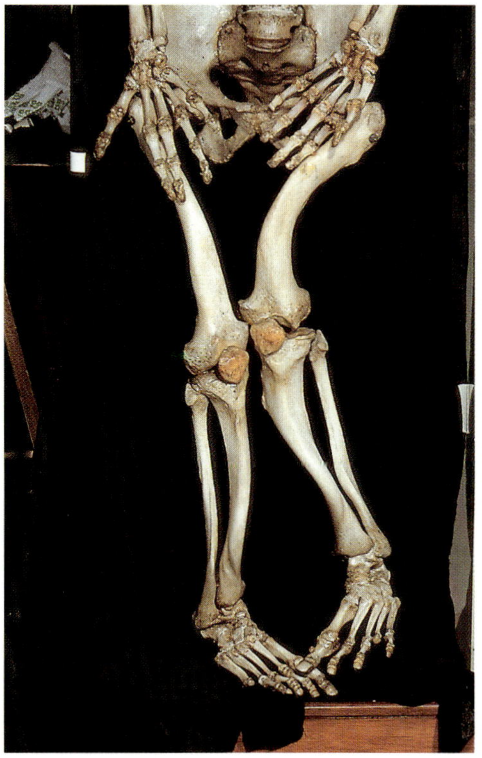

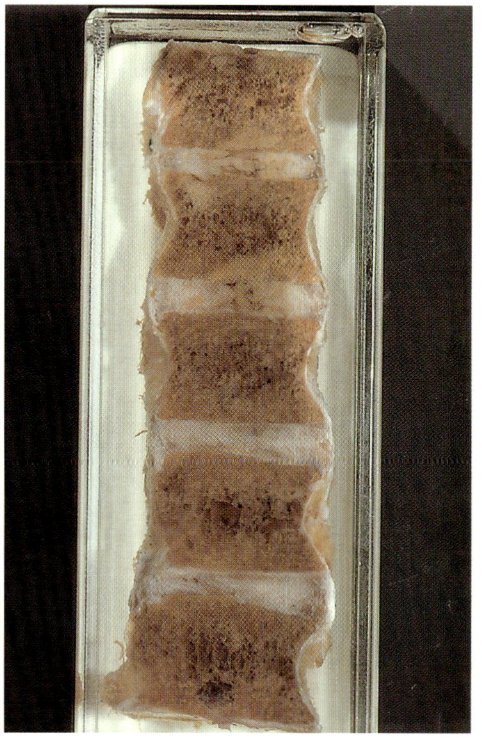

10.62 Thorax: Rickets

This is a post-mortem specimen from a 12-month-old infant known to suffer from rickets.

The thoracic skeleton, viewed anteriorly, shows a gross pigeonbreast deformity of the rib cage. There is prominence of the sternum and costochondral cartilages ('rickety rosary') and, posteriorly, the ribs are bent anteromedially behind the costal cartilages.

These are the characteristic appearances of the rib cage deformities seen in rickets.

10.63 Lower Limb Bones: Rickets Deformity

This is a post-mortem specimen from an adult female who had suffered from rickets in childhood. She measured 1.38m in height, the stunting being largely attributable to shortening and bending of the lower limbs.

Both femurs show marked antero-medial bowing, as does the tibia on each side. The leg bones thus form a sigmoid curve, the total length of each limb being only 0.55m.

These are the typical fixed deformities seen in adults, following rickets in childhood.

10.64 Vertebrae: Renal Osteodystrophy

This is a post-mortem specimen from a 57-year-old woman who died of chronic renal failure, thought to be due to chronic pyelonephritis. She had been noted to have proteinuria with hypertension and grade III retinopathy for the preceding 13 years. At autopsy the parathyroid glands were noted to be hyperplastic.

The bodies of these five vertebrae show central softening with loss of the normal trabecular pattern and, adjacent to the intervertebral discs, there is marked sclerosis. This is an example of the so-called 'rugger jersey' spine.

Renal osteodystrophy is a complex process, owing to the kidney's role in calcium and phosphate excretion, hydroxylation of vitamin D and the secondary hyperparathyroidism which results from chronic renal disease. In essence the features are those of osteomalacia combined with a degree of osteitis fibrosa cystica. A degree of osteosclerosis, most often evident in the spine or pelvis, may also be seen due to the increased deposition of immature woven bone.

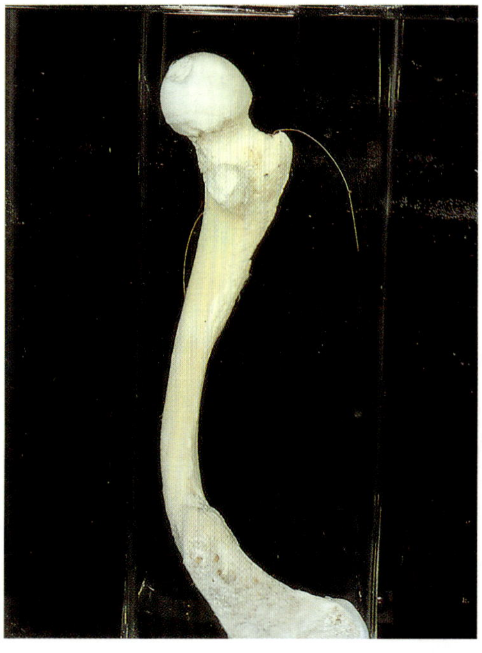

10.65 Femur: 'Renal Rickets'

This is a post-mortem specimen from a 17-year-old girl who, from the age of 5, had developed marked bowing of the legs. She died following an attack of vomiting and convulsions, the cause of which is unknown. At autopsy the kidneys were noted to be shrunken and showed granular cortical scarring. However, no histological material or biochemical data are available.

The right femur, viewed posteriorly, shows considerable bowing.

It is probable, although not proven, that this child had rickets due to renal disease; possible causes include renal tubular damage, Fanconi's syndrome or familial hypophosphataemia.

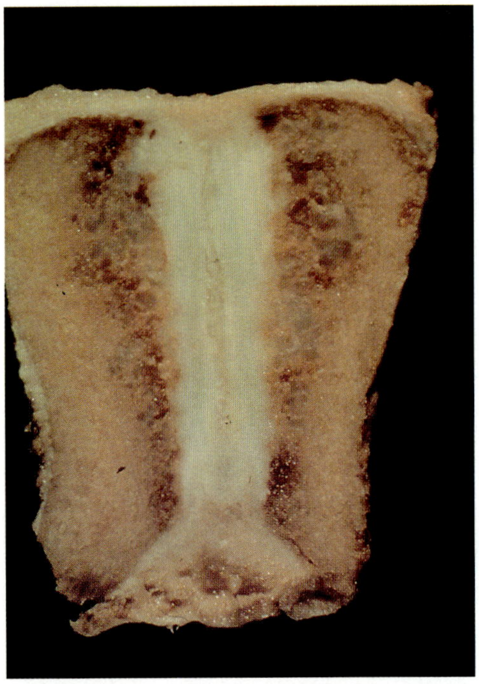

10.66 Symphysis Pubis: Osteitis Fibrosa Cystica

No clinical details are available.

This portion of the pelvis has been sectioned to show extensive resorption of bone on either side of the symphysis, producing a rather cystic appearance. Note the adjacent hyperaemia.

Osteitis fibrosa cystica (synonym: von Recklinghausen's disease of bone) is the term used to describe the bony changes seen in hyperparathyroidism, a condition which is fully discussed in the Endocrine System volume. These changes are typically more severe in primary than in secondary hyperparathyroidism but, in general, reflect increased resorption and demineralisation of bone. These lead both to osteomalacia-like features, associated with cortical and cancellous thinning, medullary fibrosis and cystic changes at the sites of marked resorption. Classically the bone destruction is greatest in the subperiosteal region of the phalanges. Occasionally a so-called 'brown tumour' or reparative granuloma may be seen which is a localised mass, typically located in a long bone or the jaw, of organised haemorrhage associated with a focus of resorption. (Courtesy of Dr. P.G. Bullough, Hospital for Special Surgery, New York)

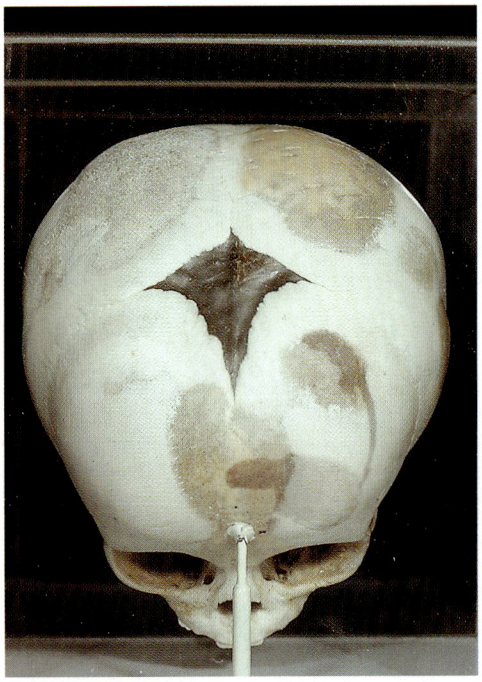

10.67 Skull: Infantile Scurvy

No clinical details are available.

This infantile skull, viewed from above, shows nearly symmetrical, rounded deposits of cancellous new bone in both frontal and parietal regions. These represent organised foci of subperiosteal haemorrhage.

The skeletal lesions of scurvy (vitamin C deficiency) are extremely rare nowadays and are only usually seen in young infants. The typical features are subperiosteal haemorrhages, diminished growth, impaired osteoid synthesis and deficient endochondral ossification. All these features are attributable to a disruption of collagen synthesis and increased capillary fragility.

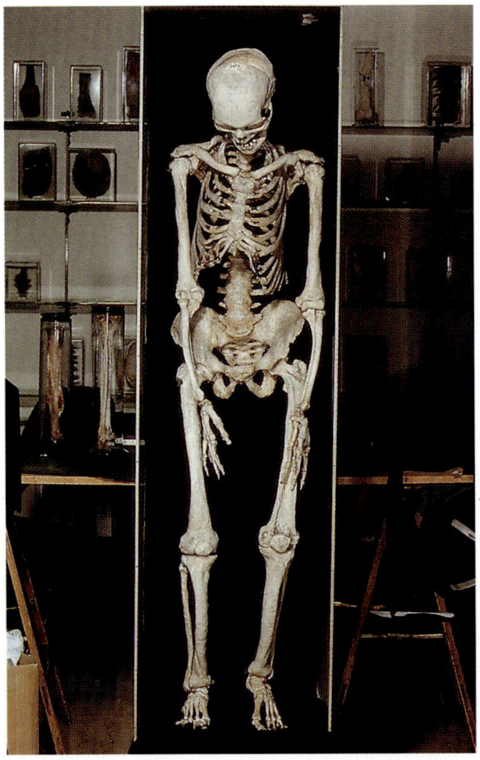

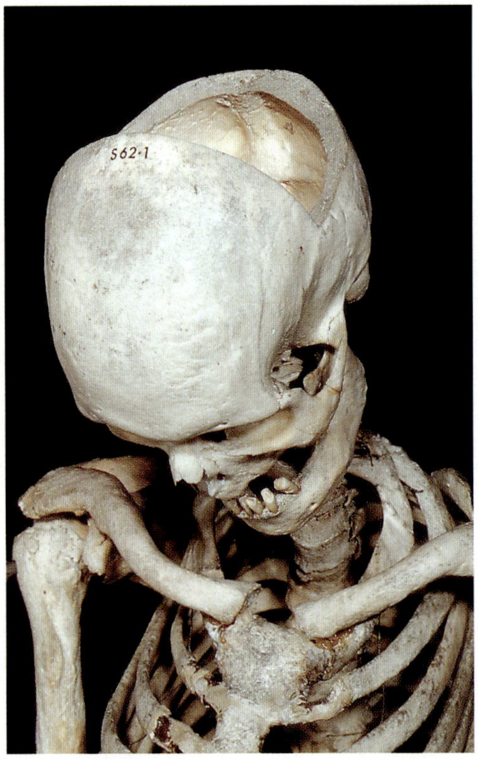

10.68 Skeleton: Paget's Disease

This is the skeleton of a 75-year-old man who, in life, walked with a stooping gait, with his shoulders raised and thrown forward and his chin almost resting on his sternum. His head measured 60cm in maximum circumference.

The skeleton (10.68a) shows enlargement of the skull, with the neck held in flexion. The spinal column shows marked kyphosis and the rib cage is flattened laterally. All the long bones of the limbs are markedly thickened and the femora and tibiae are slightly curved anteriorly. A closer view of the skull (10.68b) shows gross thickening of the bones of the vault.

Paget's disease (synonym: osteitis deformans) is a condition of late adulthood, which shows a predilection for males. A slow viral infective aetiology is postulated. It is characterised initially by increased bony resorption, later associated with new bone formation and finally by marked irregular osteosclerosis. It is most often asymptomatic and monostotic (particularly affecting the axial skeleton) or, less commonly, polyostotic, most frequently involving the spine, pelvis and long bones of the leg. The incidence in elderly Caucasians is said to be between 2-4 per cent. At all stages of the disease, the affected bones are fragile and hypervascular. Complications include pathological fractures, high output cardiac failure, secondary osteoarthrosis and a significantly increased risk of developing a sarcoma in bone.

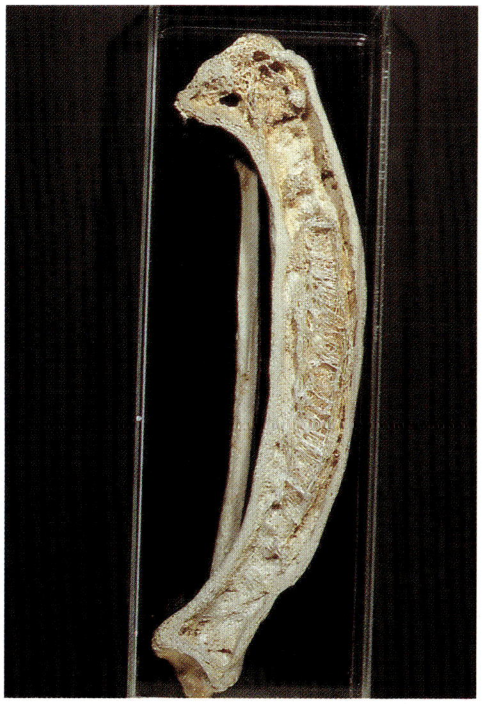

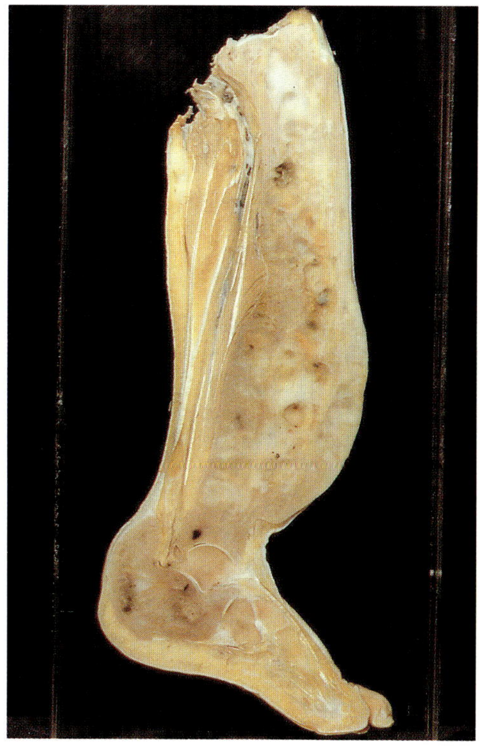

10.70 Tibia: Paget's Disease

This is an amputation specimen from a 74-year-old woman, who had first been noted to have Paget's disease of the left tibia 30 years previously. Recently the left leg had become hot and tender and the patient had developed dyspnoea and ankle oedema. On admission to hospital she was found to be in gross congestive cardiac failure; there was radiological evidence of widespread Paget's disease and the serum alkaline phosphatase was markedly elevated. The left leg was amputated through the knee joint and, within 36 hours, all features of her hyperkinetic circulatory state had disappeared.

A sagittal section through the left lower leg and foot shows marked anterior curvature. The cortex of the tibia is grossly expanded by soft, woven bone and the medullary cavity shows cystic and haemorrhagic degenerative features (as does the calcaneus). Histologically this latter feature was attributed to multiple small intramedullary fractures of the softened, disorganised bone. There was no evidence of a sarcoma.

High output cardiac failure is probably the commonest significant complication of Paget's disease. It is a consequence of the greatly increased vascular bed which develops in the expanded soft medullary fibrous tissue, seen particularly in the active osteolytic stage of the disease. This latter acts effectively as a large, often multifocal, arteriovenous shunt.

10.69 Tibia: Paget's Disease

This is a post-mortem specimen from a 73-year-old woman, who had first noticed bowing of her lower legs 30 years previously. Latterly she had been bedridden.

The tibia is grossly thickened and is bowed anteriorly. The normal cancellous bone is replaced by irregular, coarse trabeculae. The fibula, visible on the left, is normal.

Anterior bowing of the tibia or femur is a characteristic clinical feature of Paget's disease.

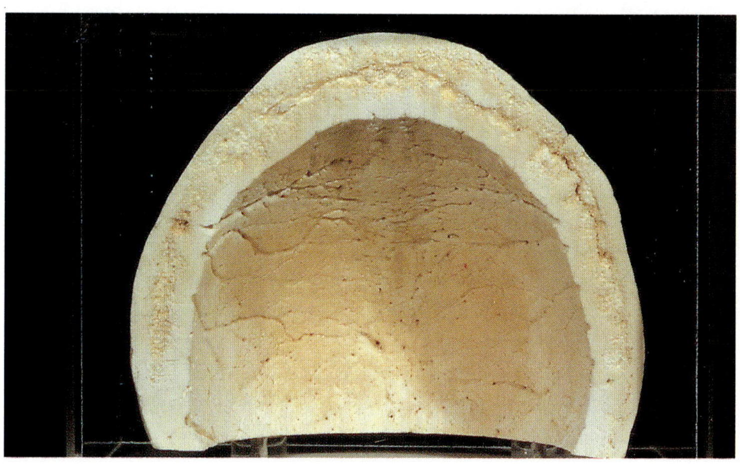

10.71 Skull: Paget's Disease

This is a post-mortem specimen from a 76-year-old woman, who had noticed a gradual increase in the size of her head for about 2 years, more recently associated with severe headaches.

The anterior part of the calvaria shows gross thickening of the frontal bones, which measure 2.5cm in cross-section. The sutures are obliterated and the normal structure is replaced by very dense cancellous bone. At autopsy no changes were observed in any other bone.

The skull is very commonly involved in Paget's disease and sometimes patients present with the complaint that their hat size has increased for no apparent reason. Thickening of the base of the skull may lead to cranial nerve compression, most often resulting in deafness.

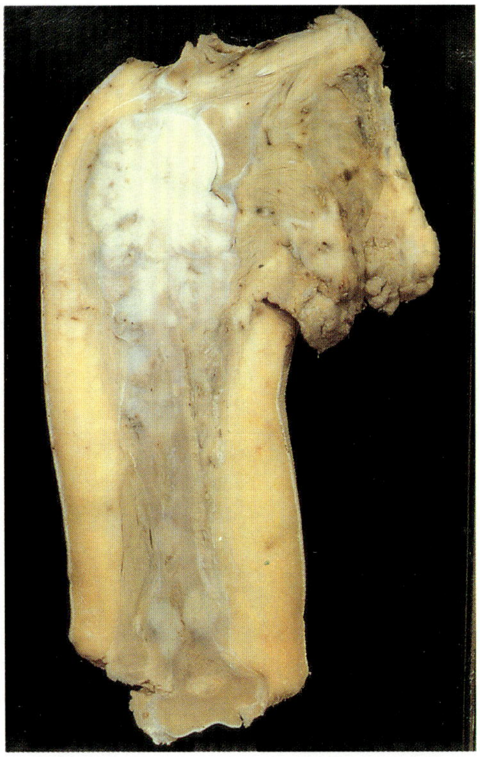

10.72 Humerus: Paget's Disease complicated by Osteosarcoma

This is a forequarter amputation specimen from a 59-year-old woman, who had been found to have Paget's disease when she fractured her right lower humerus 3 years previously. She presented with a 4 month history of a painful ache in the right shoulder region and examination revealed diffuse swelling of the proximal humerus. X-rays revealed an undoubted osteolytic sarcoma complicating Paget's disease.

A longitudinal section through the right upper arm and shoulder joint shows an extensive, pale neoplasm destroying the head and upper shaft of the humerus over a distance of 5cm. The tumour has spread distally down the shaft (note the discrete nodules), is invading adjacent soft tissue and has metastasised to the axillary lymph nodes (top right).

Up to 1 per cent of patients with monostotic or polyostotic Paget's disease are said to develop a primary osseous sarcoma, most often in the femur or humerus. While histologically this may be a typical osteosarcoma or chondrosarcoma, very often such tumours show a mixed or anaplastic pattern. The prognosis of these neoplasms is extremely poor.

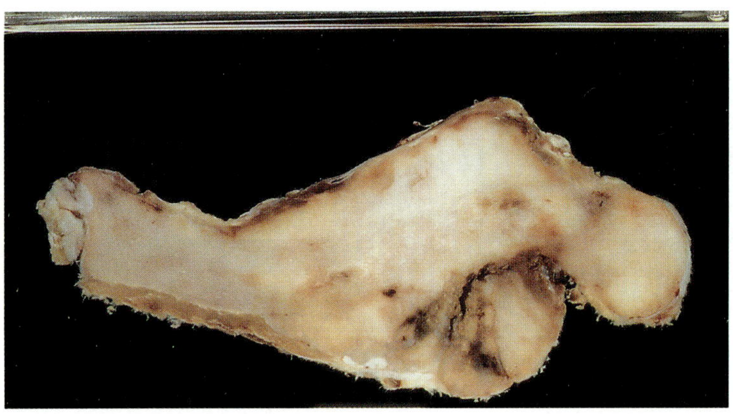

10.73 Clavicle: Paget's Disease complicated by Anaplastic Sarcoma

This specimen was excised from a 62-year-old man, who was known to suffer from Paget's disease. Eighteen months previously he had undergone amputation of the right arm for a sarcoma of the humerus. On this occasion, he presented with a one month history of enlargement of the left clavicle. In the absence of demonstrable metastases elsewhere, this was thought to represent a second sarcoma and the clavicle was excised.

The left clavicle has been sectioned in its long axis to show typical Pagetic changes in its medial third (left) and expansion by a pale, fusiform neoplasm in its outer two-thirds.

The independent development of more than one sarcoma in Paget's disease is extremely rare but well documented.

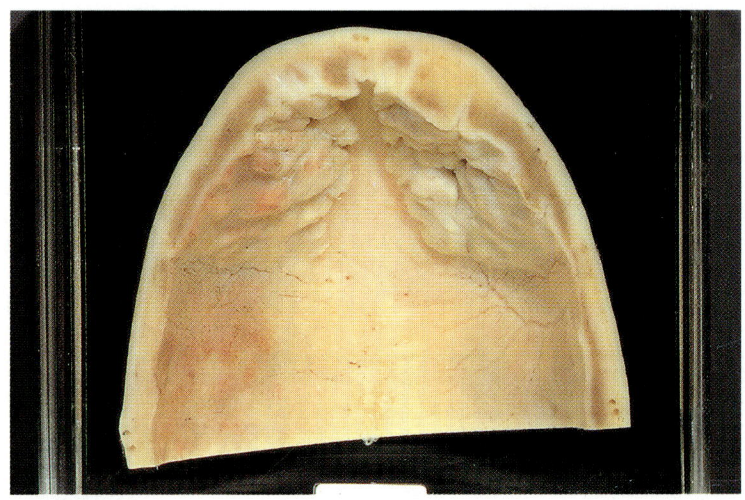

10.74 Skull: Hyperostosis Frontalis Interna

No clinical details are available.

The anterior half of the calvaria shows symmetrical areas of nodular bony thickening on either side of the mid-line. Where the bone has been sectioned it is apparent that this represents deposition of dense bone on the inner table.

Hyperostosis frontalis interna is an idiopathic condition which very rarely has any clinical effects. It is quite a common incidental finding at post-mortem, most often being seen in elderly adults (particularly females).

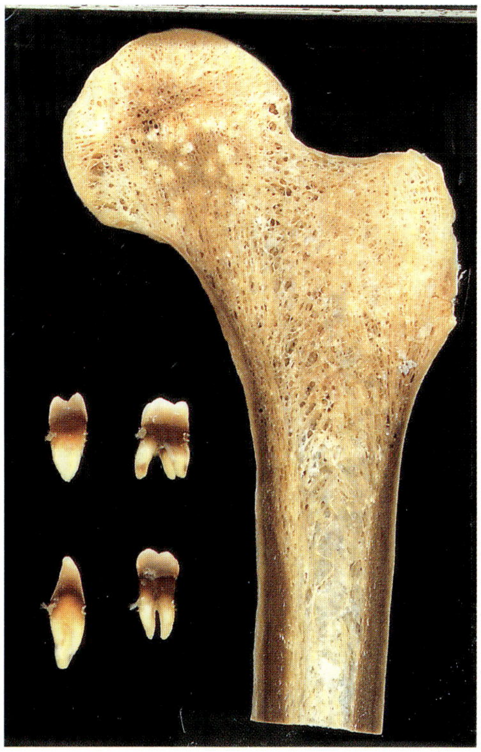

10.75 Femur and Teeth: Congenital Erythropoietic Porphyria

These are post-mortem specimens from a known case of erythropoietic porphyria.

Both the compact bone of the femoral shaft and the cementum of the 4 teeth, show purplish, so-called 'burgundy-coloured' staining. When examined under ultraviolet light, these areas show characteristic red fluorescence.

Congenital erythropoietic porphyria is a rare inherited disorder of porphyrin metabolism characterised by abnormal haem synthesis. Typical clinical features include photosensitivity, a bullous dermatosis and, less often, haemolytic anaemia. Deposition of excess porphyrins in bones and teeth is typical.

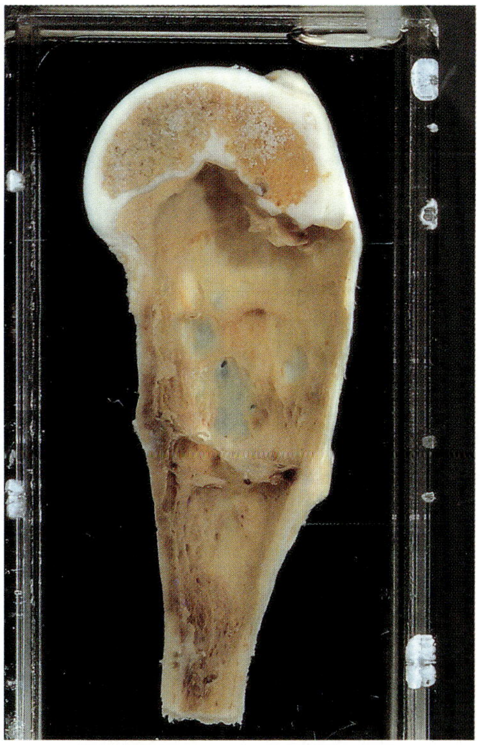

10.76 Humerus: Unicameral Bone Cyst

This is an amputation specimen from a 7-year-old boy who had noticed painful swelling of his left upper arm following two recent falls.

A vertical section through the proximal humerus shows that the upper 7cm of the shaft are expanded by a thin-walled, rather pseudoloculated cyst, which characteristically extends right up to the growth plate. In the fresh state, the cyst contained yellowish fluid.

Unicameral bone cysts (synonym: simple or solitary bone cysts) are unusual idiopathic lesions, most often detected in childhood or adolescence, which are typically located in the metaphysis of a long bone, particularly the proximal humerus. These lesions are entirely benign (hence amputation would not be performed nowadays) but, by attenuating the overlying cortex, are commonly complicated by a pathological fracture. Recurrence after excision is common because of their juxta-epiphyseal location, since the surgeon wishes to avoid damaging the growth plate.

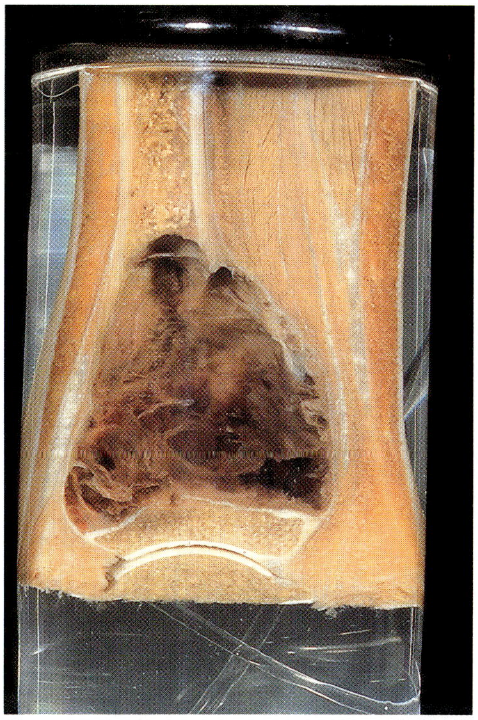

10.77 Tibia: Unicameral Bone Cyst

This is an amputation specimen from a 14-year-old girl, who presented with a gradually increasing swelling of the left lower leg which was painful on walking.

A vertical section through the distal end of the left tibia shows that the metaphysis and distal diaphysis are markedly expanded by a loculated, blood-filled cyst, measuring 7.5cm in maximum diameter. The cortex is grossly thinned and, focally, the tumour has eroded the cortex and has elevated the periosteum (right).

While the proximal end of the humerus is by far the commonest site of these lesions, they may occur in the metaphysis of any long bone. In this case, because of the lateral 'blow-out', the differential diagnosis should include aneurysmal bone cyst and telangiectatic osteosarcoma. The latter can only be ruled out by extensive tissue sampling.

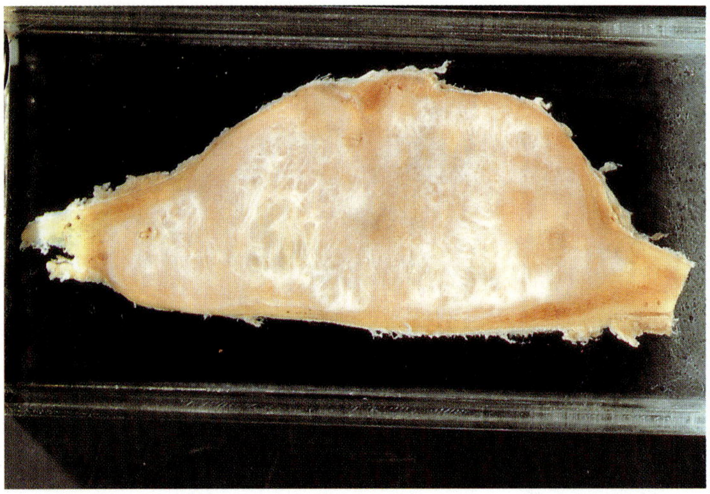

10.78 Rib: Monostotic Fibrous Dysplasia

This specimen was excised from a young adult male, who had developed a painless swelling along the line of the 9th rib in the left posterior axillary line. The mass gradually increased in size and the affected segment of rib was excised.

A section through the 9th rib shows a fusiform mass, measuring 10 × 5 × 5cm, which is well-circumscribed and has expanded the bone. The cut surface has a pale, fibrous appearance with a thin rim of normal cortical bone remaining on its outer aspect. Note the small foci of cystic change.

Fibrous dysplasia is a fairly common hamartomatous malformation which, in the vast majority of cases, affects only one bone. It typically presents in childhood or adolescence and is commonest in the ribs, jaw or long bones of the leg. The lesion arises in the marrow or endosteal region and is composed of mature fibrous tissue with a variable amount of woven bone, sometimes associated with cartilage formation and xanthomatous degeneration. Complications include a pathological fracture and, extremely rarely, sarcomatous change. Note that the wide range of histological appearances that may be present in fibrous dyplasia may be readily confused with a malignant tumour without adequate tissue sampling. Fibrous dysplasia is very occasionally polyostotic (see Figure and Legend 10.79) or may give rise to diffuse facial asymmetry.

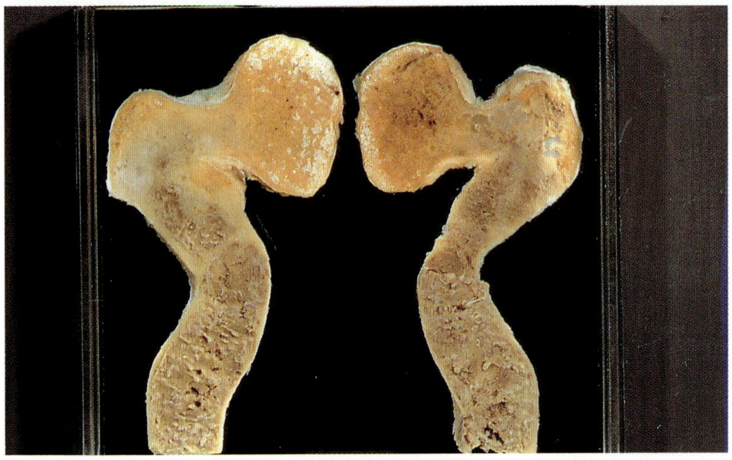

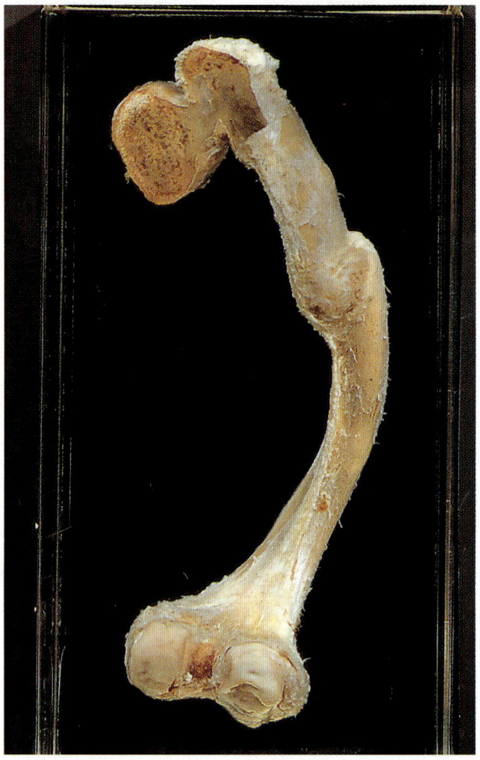

10.79 Femora: Polyostotic Fibrous Dysplasia

These are post-mortem specimens from a 19-year-old girl who died of acute appendicitis. Since the age of 15 she had developed swelling of both knees followed by increasing deformity of all the long bones, the pelvis and spine. She had also recently suffered a spontaneous fracture of the right tibia.

The upper end of the left femur (10.79a) has been bisected to show that the upper shaft and neck are expanded by a greyish, microcystic mass. The femoral head is composed largely of cancellous bone. There is gross deformity, probably due to repeated subclinical fractures through the lesion. The right femur (10.79b) also shows marked varus deformity (so-called 'shepherd's crook' deformity) with an obvious oblique fracture in the upper third of the shaft.

The polyostotic variant of fibrous dysplasia is extremely rare and is not typically as extensive as this case. It may be associated with café-au-lait skin macules, endocrine disorders and precocious puberty in females (Albright's syndrome).

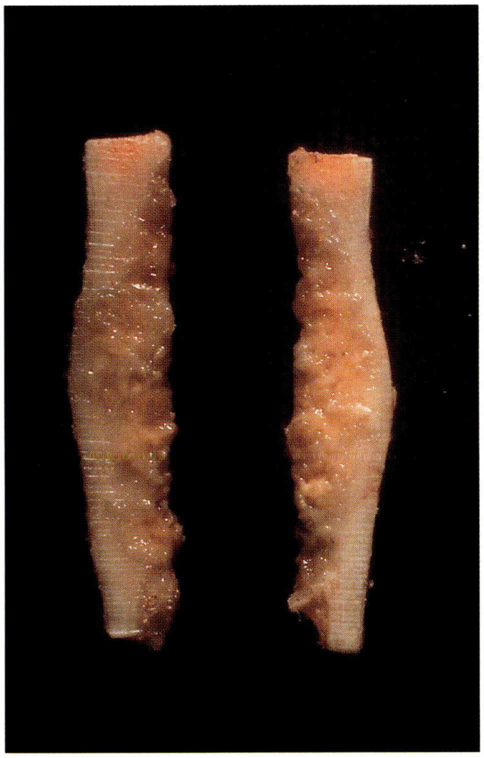

10.80 Fibula: Non-Ossifying Fibroma

No clinical details are available.

This specimen has been removed intact from the distal fibula and bisected to reveal a reasonably defined tumour, which has a soft, yellowish-orange, cut surface. Note the focal erosion of the overlying cortical bone.

Non-ossifying fibroma (synonym: fibrous cortical defect) is probably one of the most common benign bone tumours and shows a predilection for the long limb bones of children. It is thought that up to 50 per cent of all children develop this lesion at some time. However, very many non-ossifying fibromas remain asymptomatic and it is probable that a large proportion regress spontaneously suggesting that they are not true neoplasms. These lesions may sometimes arise in adulthood, when they are known as benign fibrous histiocytomas, and bone pain may be a presenting feature. (Courtesy of Dr. P.G. Bullough, Hospital for Special Surgery, New York)

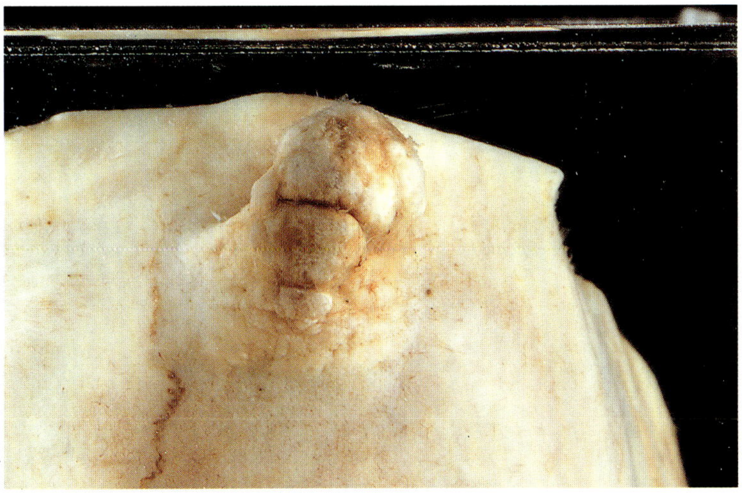

10.81 Skull: Ivory Osteoma

This was an incidental finding at post-mortem in a 60-year-old man, who died of chronic obstructive airways disease.

Projecting from the outer surface of the right frontal bone is a rather nodular, well-circumscribed bony tumour, measuring 3 × 2 × 1.5cm.

Ivory osteomas are common benign lesions, composed of dense sclerotic bone, which classically arise from the skull or facial bones. While they most often develop in childhood or early adulthood, they are nearly always asymptomatic and only present clinically for cosmetic reasons. They have no capacity to undergo malignant change.

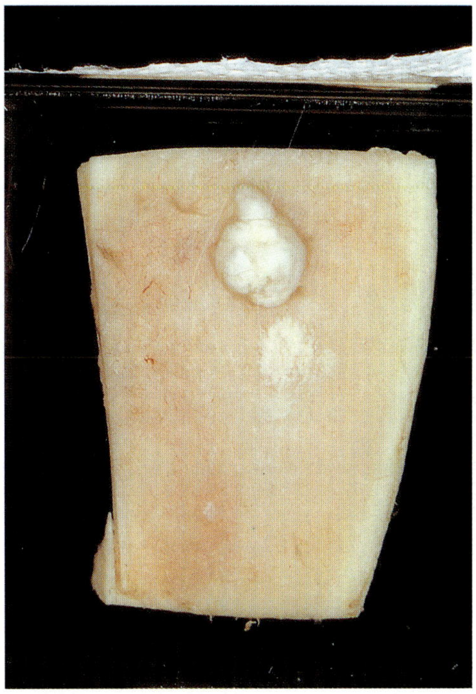

10.82 Skull: Ivory Osteoma

This was an incidental finding at post-mortem in an 80-year-old woman, who died of unrelated intercurrent disease.

Projecting from the outer surface of this portion of one of the frontal bones is a rounded, rather nodular pale osteoma, measuring 1.5cm in maximum diameter.

This is another typical ivory osteoma. It is worth remembering that similar lesions, usually situated in the nasal sinuses, are occasionally associated with familial polyposis coli (Gardner's syndrome).

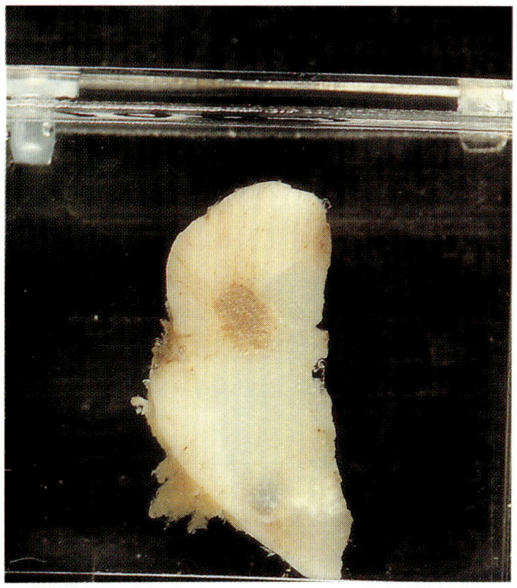

10.83 Femur: Osteoid Osteoma

This specimen was excised from a 46-year-old man, who presented with pain in the thigh. At operation, a small tumour was excised from the medial aspect of the proximal femoral shaft, just below the level of the greater trochanter. No further clinical details are available.

The specimen consists of a rounded, rather lobulated mass of pale tissue, measuring 3 × 1.5 × 1cm. Note the central, reddish 'nidus', which constitutes the tumour, and the surrounding rim of active sclerosis.

Osteoid osteomas are not uncommon benign tumours, which present most often in childhood or adolescence and show a predilection for the diaphysis of the long bones in the leg. Characteristically, the affected patient complains of localised pain, which is worse at night and is relieved by aspirin. These tumours are usually cortical in location and show a central nidus of immature bone surrounded by radiolucent, hyperaemic fibrous tissue and an outer rim of sclerotic bone. There is no potential for malignant change. (Courtesy of the Royal National Orthopaedic Hospital, Stanmore)

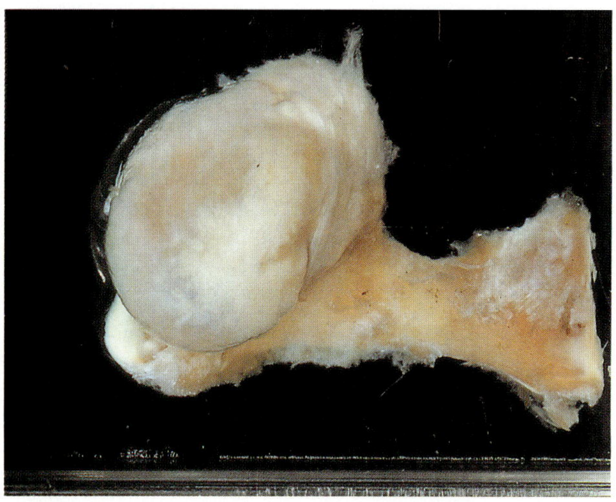

10.84 Metatarsal Bone: Osteochondroma

This specimen was excised from a 12-year-old boy, who had noticed a swelling in the sole of his left foot for 2 weeks. X-rays revealed an exostosis arising from the neck of the second metatarsal bone.

A section through the long axis of the metatarsal bone shows a lobulated mass arising from the under-surface of the distal half of the shaft. The surface of the lesion has a glassy cartilaginous appearance.

Osteochondroma (synonym: cartilage-capped exostosis, ecchondroma) is the commonest benign tumour of bone and is, in fact, regarded by some as a developmental abnormality. It is thought to develop by lateral herniation of the growth plate through the perichondrial ring. This cartilage then gradually becomes ossified, remaining only as a rim over the surface. The vast majority of these lesions present in childhood or adolescence and arise in the juxta-epiphyseal region of long bones, particularly the lower femur or upper tibia. These lesions are occasionally multiple, an inherited phenomenon known as diaphyseal aclasis. Very rarely they may be complicated by the development of a chondrosarcoma, especially in inherited cases.

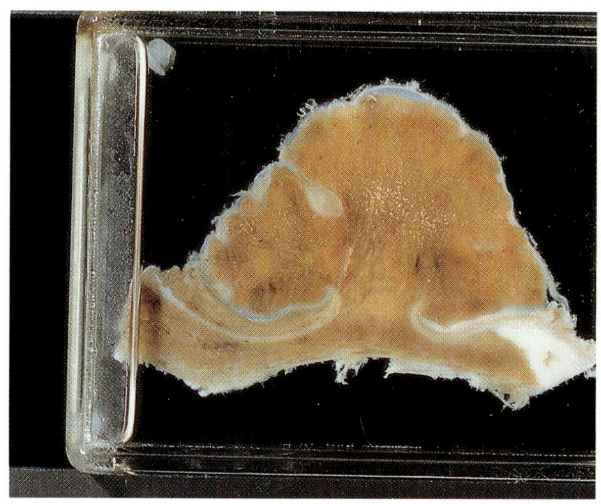

10.85 Iliac Crest: Osteochondroma

This specimen was excised from a 14-year-old boy. No further clinical details are available.

A section through the iliac crest shows a mushroom-shaped neoplasm, projecting from its surface. The 'stalk' of the lesion is contiguous with the underlying cancellous bone. Most of the tumour is ossified but the surface is covered by a thin layer of cartilage.

These are the classical macroscopical appearances of an osteochondroma.

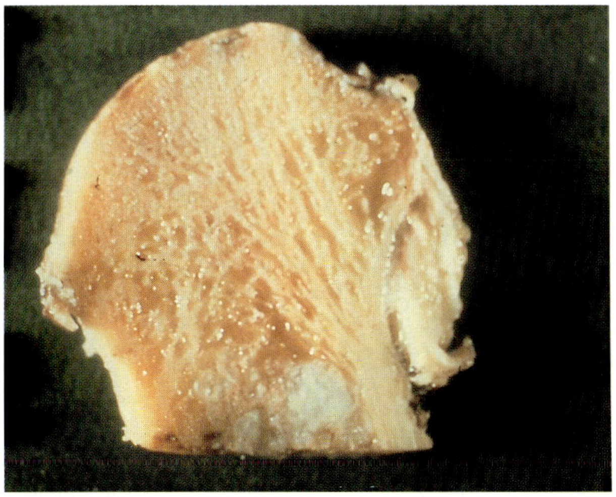

10.86 Femur: Enchondroma

This was an incidental finding in a specimen resected during the course of a prosthetic hip replacement for osteoarthrosis.

Within the medulla of the neck of the femur is a small lobulated neoplasm, showing the typical glistening bluish-white appearance of a cartilaginous lesion.

Solitary enchondromas are benign lesions which originate most often in the small bones of the hand or foot, usually in adults. They may also arise in the metaphysis of long tubular bones. While they often remain asymptomatic, weakening of the affected bone may predispose to a fracture and hence to clinical presentation. Extension of the tumour from the medulla through the cortex may occur following a fracture. The majority of these tumours have no malignant potential; however occasional cases, usually arising in long limb bones, may be complicated by the development of a chondrosarcoma. (Courtesy of Dr P.G. Bullough, Hospital for Special Surgery, New York)

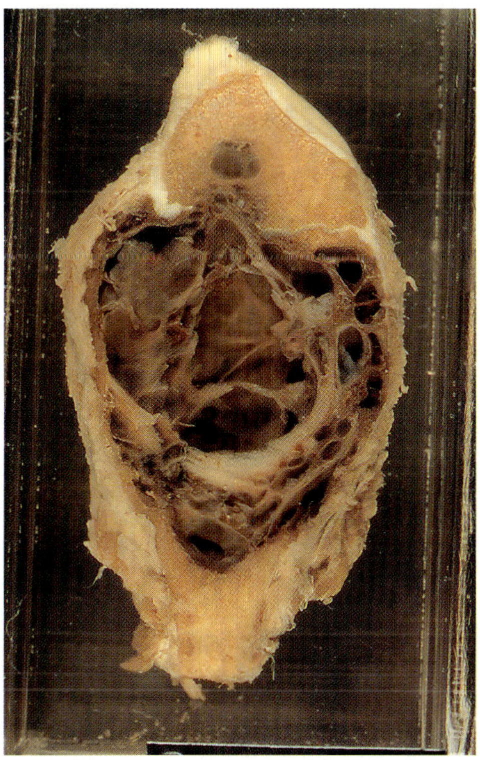

10.87 Fibula: Aneurysmal Bone Cyst

No clinical details are available in this case.

The medulla of the proximal fibula is expanded by a well-demarcated, multilocular haemorrhagic mass, measuring 8cm in maximum diameter. In the fresh state the cystic spaces were filled with blood. Note the adjacent periosteal elevation and focal erosion of the growth plate.

Aneurysmal bone cysts are uncommon benign lesions of uncertain nature, which typically arise in the long bones or spine of adolescents or young adults of either sex. Some cases appear to represent degenerative change in a chondroblastoma, osteoblastoma, non-ossifying fibroma or simple bone cyst. Local recurrence, which may be repeated, is a feature in up to half of the affected patients. There is no potential for malignant change. Care should be taken to differentiate these lesions histologically from telangiectatic osteosarcoma. (Courtesy of the Royal National Orthopaedic Hospital, Stanmore)

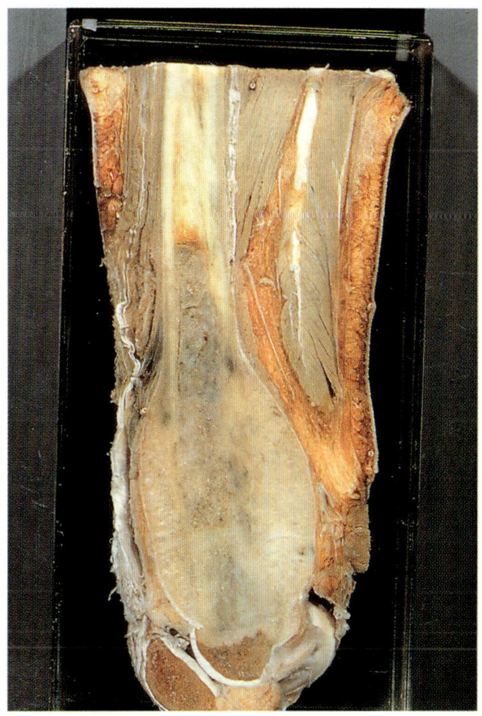

10.88 Femur: Osteosarcoma

This is an amputation specimen from a 14-year-old boy who presented with a 4 month history of swelling in the lower thigh, associated with an effusion into the knee joint. The patient died with pulmonary metastases 2 years later.

A vertical section through the lower thigh shows a fusiform, greyish tumour arising in the metaphyseal region of the lower femur. The tumour has invaded the epiphysis and diaphysis and the periosteum is very markedly elevated.

Osteosarcoma is the commonest primary malignant neoplasm of bone, if haemopoietic tumours (such as multiple myeloma) are excluded. The majority arise in the metaphysis of long limb bones (particularly the femur, tibia and humerus) of children, adolescents or young adults, predominantly males. A very small proportion of osteosarcomas, however, develop either secondary to Paget's disease, previous irradiation or chronic osteomyelitis.

While osteosarcomas, by definition, show formation of malignant bone or osteoid, up to half of these tumours may show extensive chondroblastic or fibroblastic differentiation. Hence small biopsies may be histologically misleading. In general, irrespective of histological type, these tumours tend to rapid haematogenous dissemination and metastases are often present at the time of presentation. The overall 5-year-survival is about 50 per cent using modern multimodal treatment.

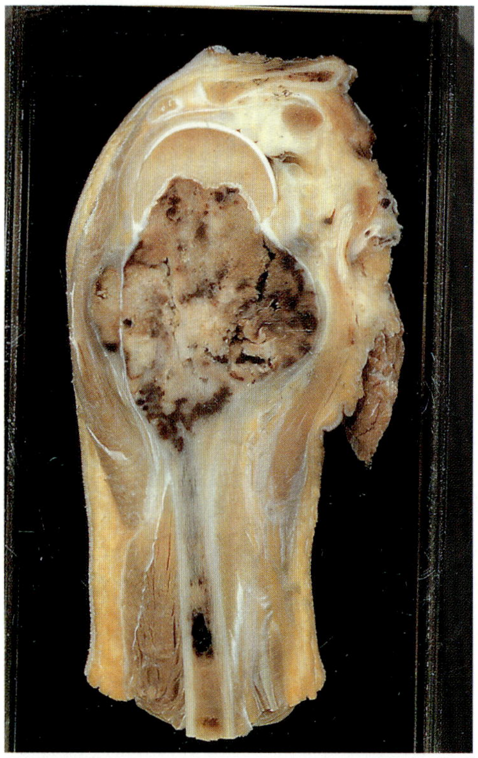

10.89 Humerus: Osteosarcoma

This is an amputation specimen from a 14-year-old boy, who presented with a one month history of pain in the left upper arm. Following a course of radiotherapy, the limb was amputated. However the patient died one year later with pulmonary metastases.

Arising in the upper metaphysis of the humerus is a haemorrhagic neoplasm, measuring 7.5cm in diameter. There is extensive periosteal elevation and the tumour has spread down the medullary cavity. Although the epiphyseal cartilage is distorted, it has remained intact.

The upper end of the humerus is the third most common primary site of osteosarcoma (after the lower femur and upper tibia).

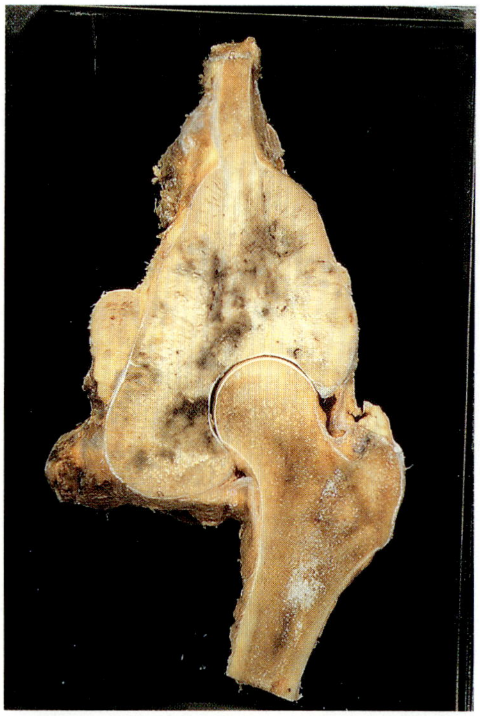

10.90 Pelvis: Osteosarcoma

This is a hindquarter amputation specimen from a young adult male, who presented with pain in the left hip. X-rays revealed a bony mass arising in the acetabular region.

A vertical section through the hip joint shows that much of the ilium and pubic ramus are infiltrated by a haemorrhagic neoplasm, which is surrounding the acetabulum. The femur is completely uninvolved.

Osteosarcoma arising primarily in the axial skeleton is uncommon.

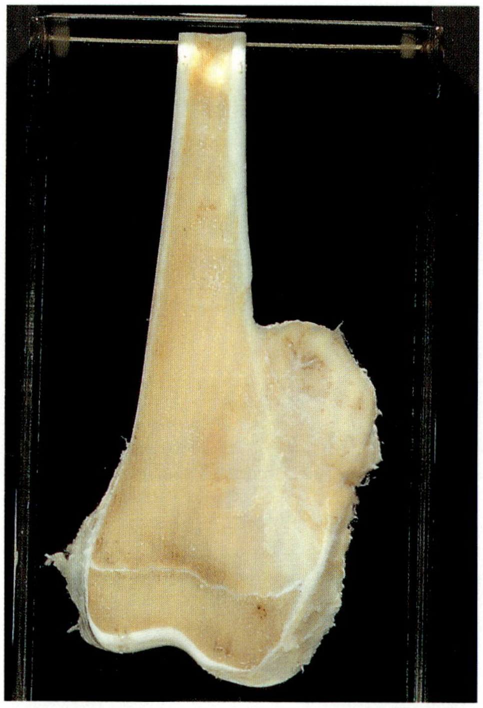

10.91 Femur: Juxtacortical Osteosarcoma

This is an amputation specimen from a 14-year-old boy, who presented with a 3 month history of a painful swelling above the right knee.

The lower end of the femur has been sectioned to show a pale tumour, measuring 8cm in maximum diameter, arising from the external aspect of the cortex; the tumour has spread into the diaphysis and is invading adjacent soft tissues widely.

Juxtacortical (parosteal) osteosarcoma is a rare neoplasm, which typically presents in young or middle-aged adults and always arises from the external surface of the bone, where it is attached to the cortex. Medullary invasion is an occasional feature and is important to detect pre-operatively so as to avoid incomplete excision. Histologically, this variant of osteosarcoma is usually well-differentiated and, in this circumstance, the 5-year-survival is about 90 per cent (i.e. very significantly better than most osteosarcomas). However if the tumour is histologically of high grade, the prognosis is poor. These lesions should be distinguished from periosteal osteosarcoma, an even rarer variant, which is commonest in adolescence and carries an intermediate prognosis.

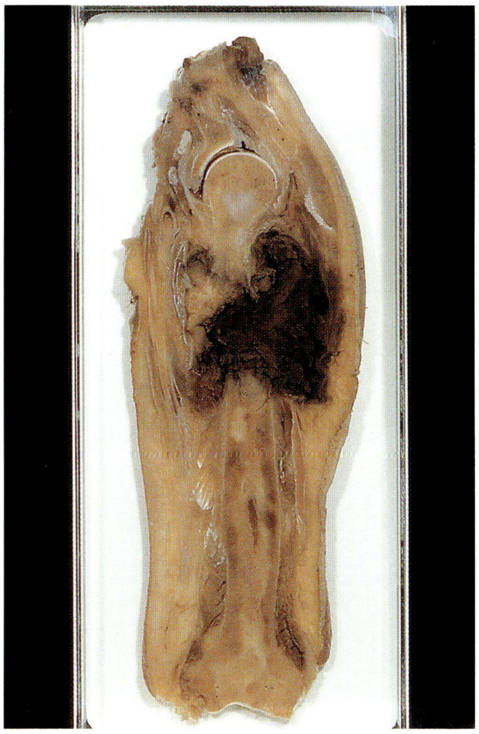

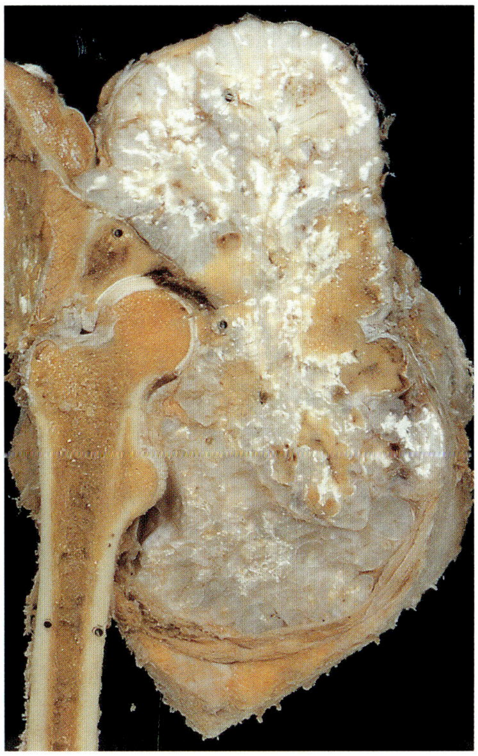

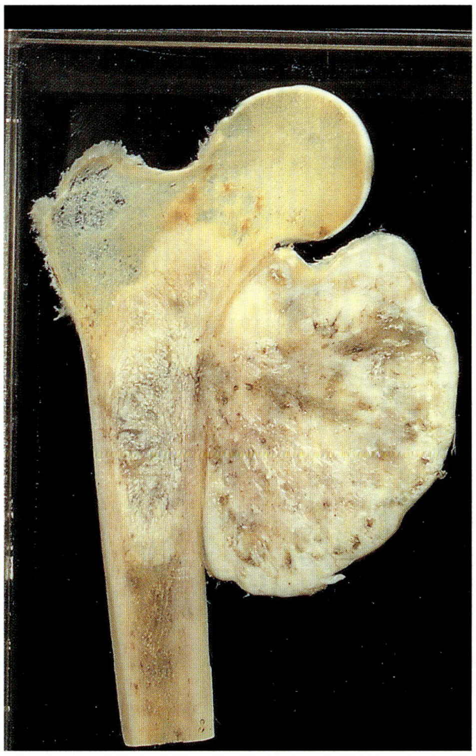

10.92 Humerus: Osteosarcoma complicating Paget's Disease

This is an amputation specimen from a 54-year-old woman, known to have Paget's disease, who suffered a pathological fracture of the upper humerus following a fall.

A section through the right humerus and adjacent soft tissues shows a fracture through the upper shaft. The fracture has occurred at the site of a large, haemorrhagic tumour which is invading adjacent soft tissues. The lower humerus shows the typical features of Paget's disease (see Figure and Legend 10.68 et seq.).

Sarcomas complicating Paget's disease of bone have already been discussed (see Figure and Legend 10.72 et seq.).

10.93 Pelvis: Well Differentiated Chondrosarcoma

This is a hindquarter amputation specimen from a 27-year-old man, who presented with a 6 year history of pain in the left groin and a gradually increasing swelling in the inguinal region. Following a course of radiotherapy, amputation was performed.

A vertical section through the left hip shows a bulky, lobulated tumour arising from the inner aspect of the pelvis near the acetabulum. The cut surface of the tumour has a characteristic bluish, glassy appearance and shows foci of calcification. The lesion has extended far down into the thigh, but does not actually involve the femur.

Chondrosarcoma accounts for about 20 per cent of primary malignant osseous neoplasms. It is commonest in late adulthood and shows a slight predilection for males. Up to 10 per cent of cases arise in a pre-existing lesion, particularly enchondromatosis. By far the commonest sites are the pelvis, femur and humerus but almost any bone may be affected. These tumours are significantly less malignant than osteosarcoma, in general being histologically low grade, and the overall 5-year-survival is about 70 per cent. However, high grade tumours and the dedifferentiated variant in which foci of a relatively low grade lesion adopt a variably anaplastic appearance, carry a poor prognosis.

10.94 Femur: Chondrosarcoma with Extensive Calcification

This is an amputation specimen from a 61-year-old man, who presented with a one year history of a gradually increasing swelling of the upper inner thigh. X-rays revealed a neoplasm arising in the proximal femoral diaphysis. Nine months post-operatively he remained alive and free from tumour.

A section through the upper half of the femur shows a rounded tumour, measuring 12cm in maximum diameter. It has invaded through the cortex, extending widely into soft tissues, and shows extensive white calcification.

The majority of chondrosarcomas of long bones arise in the medullary cavity, as here. While calcification is a common finding, it is important to determine, on histological grounds, that the lesion is not a true osteosarcoma showing chondroblastic differentiation, as the prognosis is much worse in this event.

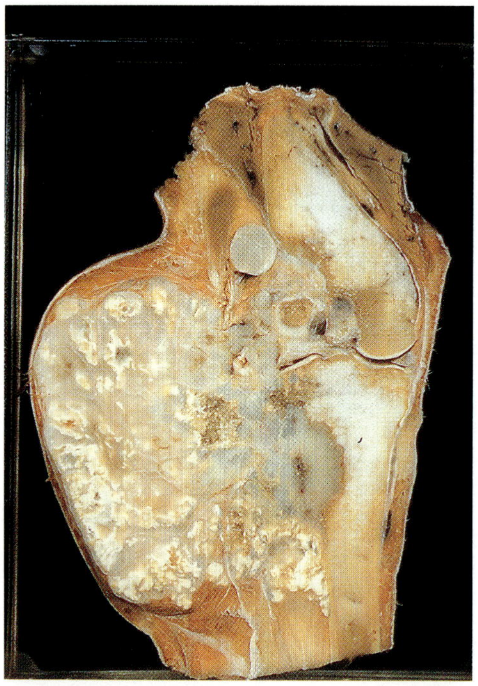

10.95 Tibia: Chondrosarcoma

This is an amputation specimen from a 66-year-old woman, who had noticed a gradually increasing swelling below the left knee for 8 years. She only presented to her doctor when the lesion ulcerated through the skin.

A vertical section through the left knee joint shows a lobulated cartilaginous tumour, measuring 14cm in maximum diameter, arising in the tibia. The tumour shows extensive invasion of the joint space and popliteal fossa. The upper end of the fibula was not included in this section. Note the coexistence of apparent enchondromatosis in the upper tibia and lower femur.

Well-differentiated chondrosarcomas are often very slow-growing, as here, and haematogenous dissemination is only a late feature.

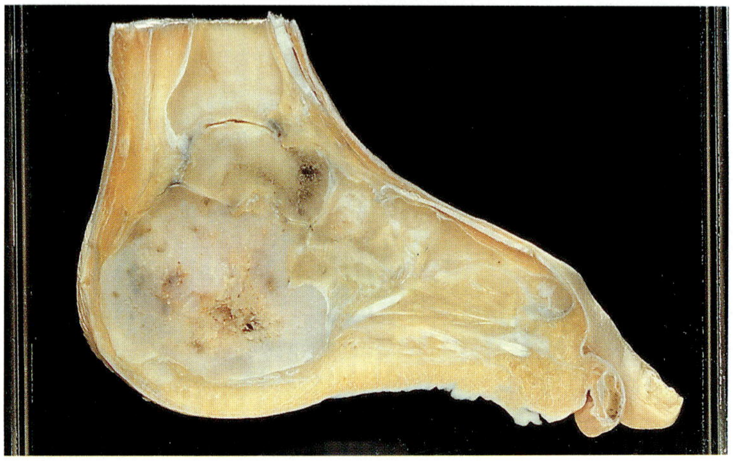

10.96 Calcaneus: Well Differentiated Chondrosarcoma

This is an amputation specimen from a 60-year-old woman, who presented with an 18 month history of a painful swelling in the right heel.

A sagittal section through the right foot shows almost complete replacement of the calcaneus by a glassy, pale cartilaginous neoplasm, which is invading adjacent soft tissues.

Chondrosarcoma arising in the bones of the hands or feet is fairly unusual but well recognised.

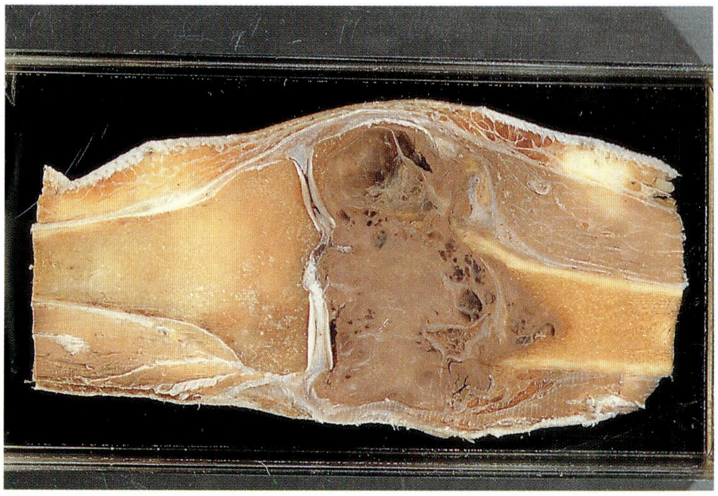

10.97 Femur: Giant Cell Tumour

This is an amputation specimen from a 59-year-old man, who presented with a 4 month history of a painful right knee. X-rays showed a radiolucent lesion in the epiphysis and metaphysis of the lower femur.

A vertical section through the right knee joint, viewed posteriorly, shows virtual replacement of the epiphysis and metaphysis of the lower femur by a brown, focally haemorrhagic and necrotic neoplasm. The tumour has extended through the cortex on both sides. Note the characteristic extension to the articular surface.

Giant cell tumour of bone (synonym: osteoclastoma) presents most often between the ages of 20 and 50 and typically arises in the epiphysis of a long bone, most often in the lower femur, upper tibia or fibula. Whether this tumour is derived from osteoclasts or tissue histiocytes remains uncertain. Giant cell tumours are the only primary osseous neoplasms that are more common in females than males. Their clinical behaviour is notoriously hard to predict, but is largely dependent upon the histological degree of anaplasia in the neoplastic stroma. Approximately 90 per cent of cases showing a conventional pattern pursue a benign course, although local recurrence is common.

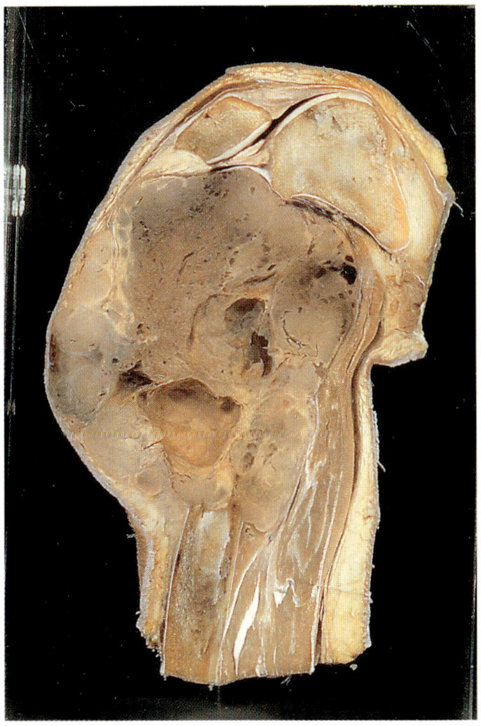

10.98 Tibia: Giant Cell Tumour

This is an amputation specimen from a 31-year-old woman, who presented with a 14 month history of pain in the right knee. The upper end of the tibia was palpably enlarged.

The lateral aspect of the right knee joint has been sectioned to show a reasonably circumscribed tan-coloured tumour, measuring 10cm in diameter, arising in the upper tibial epiphysis. The lesion has undergone extensive cystic degeneration and is invading adjacent soft tissues.

Haemorrhage, necrosis and cystic degeneration are common features of giant cell tumours, but do not, of themselves, imply malignancy. Many tumours labelled as malignant giant cell tumour in the past would probably nowadays be reclassified as malignant fibrous histiocytoma (see Figure and Legend 10.100).

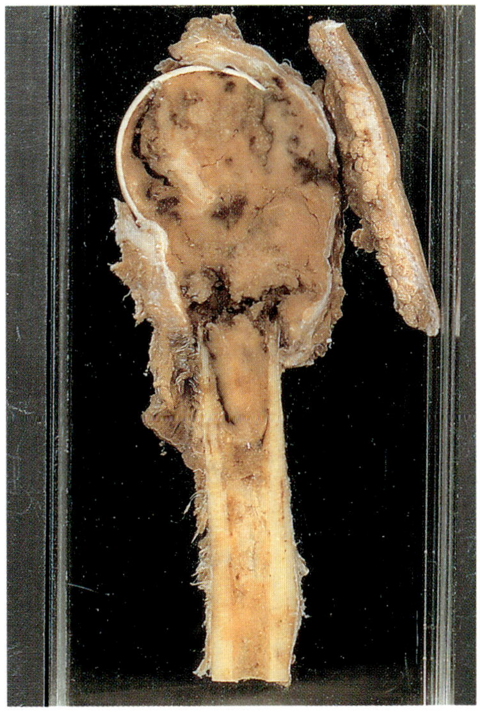

10.99 Humerus: Giant Cell Tumour

This specimen was excised from a 46-year-old man, who presented with a few months' history of pain in the left shoulder associated with limitation of movement. X-rays revealed an osteolytic lesion in the head of the humerus, associated with a pathological fracture.

A section through the upper humerus and adjacent skin shows a focally haemorrhagic and necrotic, tan-coloured neoplasm arising in the head of the humerus and extending distally into the shaft. A pathological transverse fracture is apparent just below the humeral neck.

A pathological fracture is a fairly common mode of presentation for giant cell tumours.

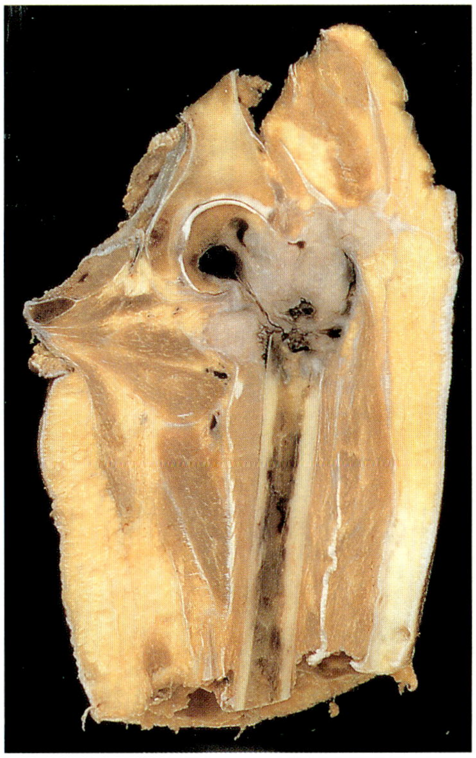

10.100 Femur: Malignant Fibrous Histiocytoma

This is an amputation specimen from a 50-year-old woman, who presented with a 4 month history of pain in the left thigh. Radiologically and pathologically, a simple bone cyst was diagnosed but, 4 months later, the patient suffered a pathological fracture and biopsy revealed a sarcoma.

A vertical section through the left hip and adjacent soft tissues shows a pale, focally haemorrhagic neoplasm arising in the intertrochanteric region of the femur. The tumour has invaded the femoral head and neck and is extending into soft tissues.

Primary malignant fibrous histiocytoma of bone is now a well-recognised and not uncommon tumour. It shows a wide age distribution and arises most often in the femoral and tibial metaphyses. Up to a quarter of cases are associated with a pre-existent bony lesion, most often Paget's disease or a bone infarct. The 5-year-survival is of the order of 35 per cent.

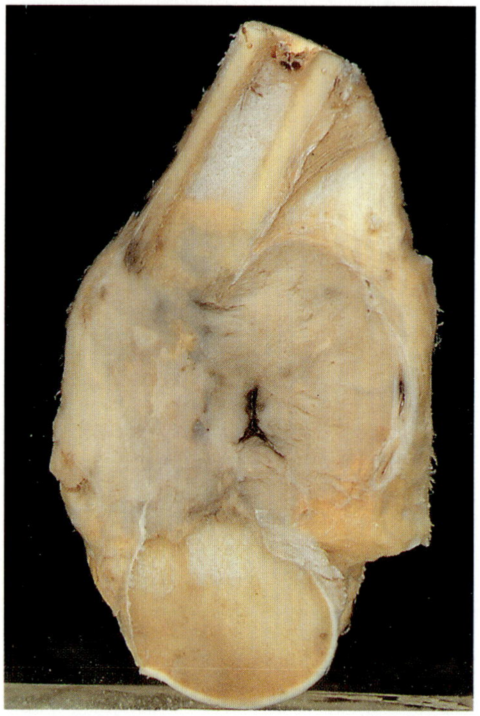

10.101 Femur: Fibrosarcoma

This is an amputation specimen from a 69-year-old man, who presented with a 9 month history of a painful leg. X-rays revealed a pathological fracture through a tumour in the lower femur.

A vertical section through the lower femur shows a pale, rather fibrous neoplasm, measuring 10cm in diameter, arising in the metaphyseal region and invading both the shaft and the epiphysis. The periosteum appears intact over the surface of the tumour.

Primary fibrosarcoma of bone is a rare neoplasm, which most often arises in the metaphysis of a long limb bone (particularly around the knee) and typically presents in adulthood. The prognosis is directly related to the histological grade of the tumour.

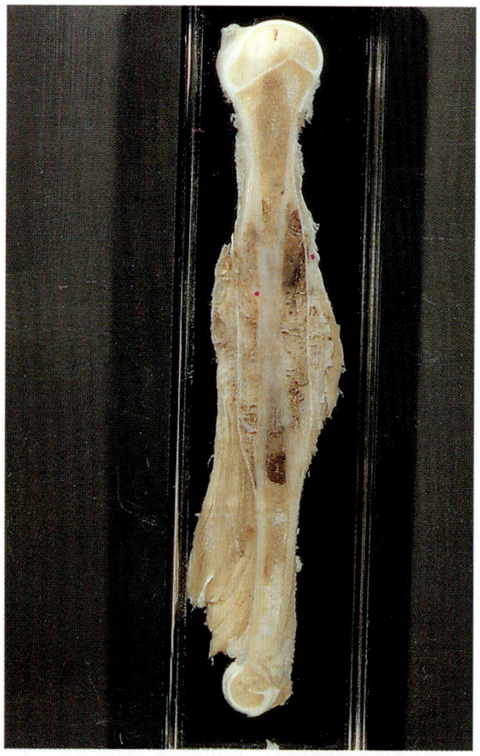

10.102 Humerus: Ewing's Sarcoma

This is an amputation specimen from a 10-year-old girl, who presented with a 3 week history of pain in the right arm. Examination revealed a tender, ill-defined swelling of the postero-lateral aspect of the upper arm and X-rays showed an extensive neoplasm in the humeral shaft.

A vertical section through the right humerus shows a haemorrhagic neoplasm, measuring 12 × 2.5 × 2cm, arising in the shaft and spreading extensively beneath the elevated periosteum. The tumour has invaded adjacent soft tissue.

Ewing's sarcoma is a relatively uncommon neoplasm of uncertain histogenesis, which typically arises in the long bones or ilium in childhood; however, almost any bone may be affected. The prognosis is generally poor.

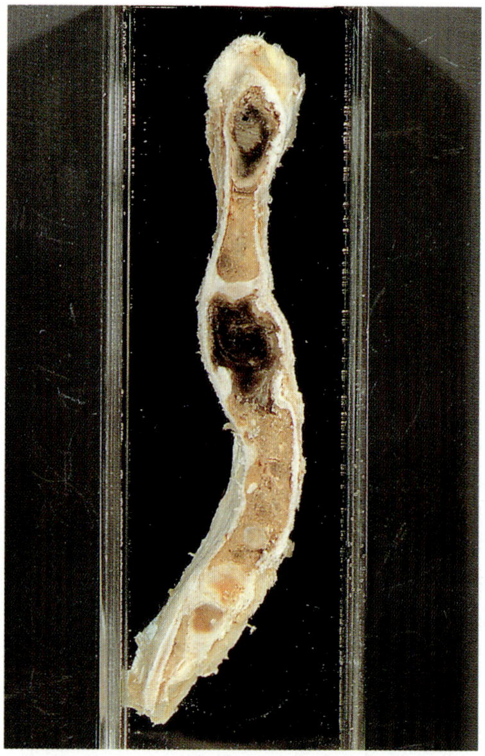

10.103 Sternum: Multiple Myeloma

This is a post-mortem specimen from a 72-year-old woman, who had been treated for multiple myeloma. At autopsy there was also extensive myelomatous infiltration of the vertebral column.

A vertical section through the sternum shows patchy, multifocal replacement of the cancellous bone by greyish neoplastic tissue, some areas of which are haemorrhagic. The residual bone marrow is pale and rather yellow, reflecting a degree of aplastic change following cytotoxic chemotherapy.

Multiple myeloma is the commonest primary malignant neoplasm that arises in bone and is derived from medullary plasma cells. Patients in late adulthood, particularly males, are most often affected. The disease is characterised by multifocal osteolytic lesions, which show a predilection for the axial marrow-containing bones (especially the skull and spine). Rarely, the tumour deposits may be osteoblastic, in which circumstance distinction from metastatic carcinoma may be difficult. The diagnostic *sine qua non* is the production (by tumour cells) of abnormal, circulating monoclonal immunoglobulins, the light chains of which are classically detected in the urine (Bence-Jones protein). Complications include renal damage (see Chapter 4), a predisposition to infection, vertebral collapse and neuropathy. The prognosis is generally poor.

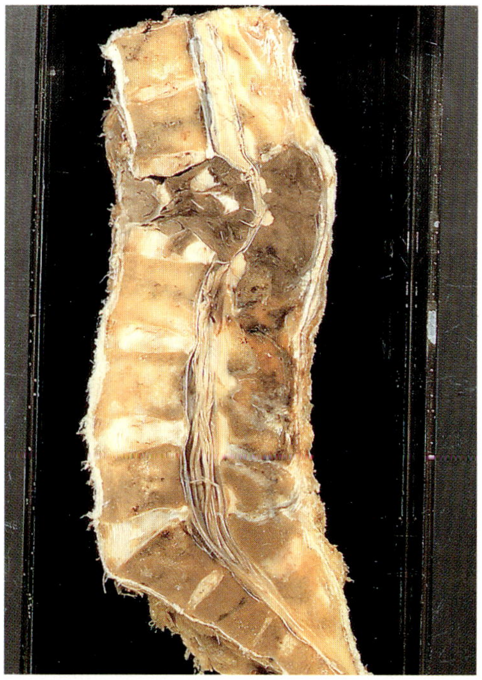

10.104 Spine: Multiple Myeloma

This is a post-mortem specimen from a 59-year-old man, who presented with a 9 month history of lumbar back pain. Examination revealed a soft tissue swelling over the upper lumbar vertebrae and X-rays revealed an osteolytic neoplasm of L1 and L2. The serum immunoglobulin concentration was increased and Bence-Jones protein was detected in the urine. The patient was treated with repeated courses of radiotherapy over the succeeding 5 years but he eventually returned with intractable bone pain and died of bronchopneumonia.

A sagittal section through the lower spine reveals a mass of haemorrhagic tumour destroying the bodies of T12, L1 and L2. The neoplasm has extended into the extradural space, compressing the spinal cord, and is invading adjacent soft tissues. Note the radiation-induced fibrosis in adjacent vertebral bodies.

While the myelomatous process appears to be characterised by a single tumour mass in this specimen, the diagnosis of solitary plasmacytoma can be excluded by this patient's abnormal immunoglobulins. Solitary plasmacytoma is typically a localised lesion of young adults, unassociated with any protein abnormality, which carries a much better prognosis than multiple myeloma.

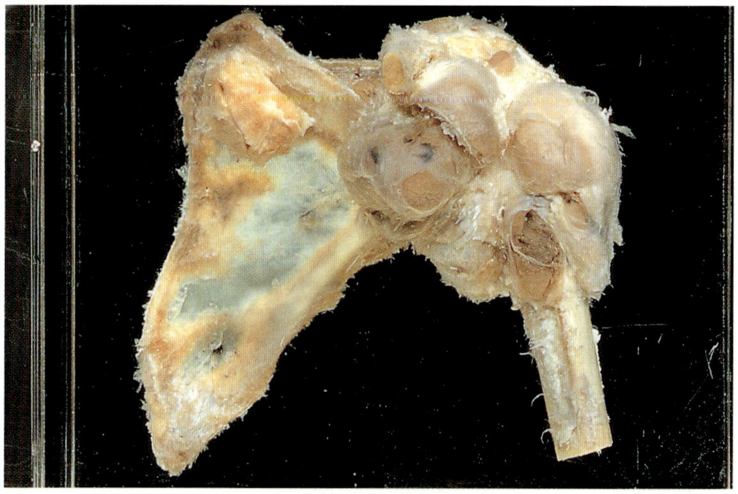

10.105 Shoulder: Amyloidosis complicating Multiple Myeloma

This is a post-mortem specimen from a 52-year-old woman, who presented with multifocal bone pain. Four years previously she had suffered a seemingly 'spontaneous' rib fracture and more recently, had been treated for 'nephritis' on the basis of proteinuria. On this admission, however, multiple osteolytic lesions were found on X-ray and Bence-Jones protein was detected in the urine. The patient died 11 months later of bronchopneumonia. At autopsy, in addition to multiple neoplastic bone lesions, large, yellowish translucent nodules were found in the shoulder and hip joints and adjacent bursae.

The left shoulder has been dissected to show gross distension of the joint capsule and bursae by rounded masses which, in section, are seen to be composed of yellowish material. Histologically this proved to be amyloid.

Amyloidosis is a well-recognised complication in about 20 per cent of cases of multiple myeloma, in which circumstance the characteristic ß-pleated sheets of fibrillary protein are composed of abnormal immunoglobulin light chains. Most often there is diffuse deposition in the kidneys, heart vessels and gastrointestinal tract: nodular, tumour-like deposition, as seen here, is extremely unusual.

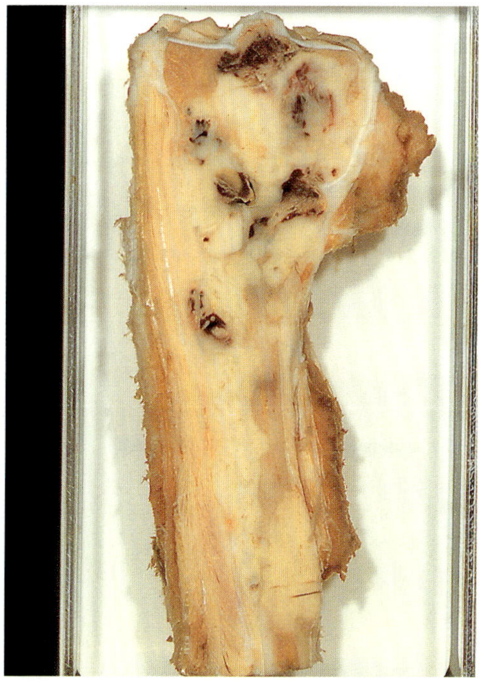

10.106 Tibia: Adamantinoma

This is an amputation specimen from an 11-year-old girl, who presented with a 7 year history of pain in the left leg which had been attributed in the past to a bone cyst. Surgical exploration revealed numerous fluid-filled cysts and, one year later following a spontaneous fracture, a biopsy revealed an adamantinoma. Radiotherapy was given but 2 years later a further fracture occurred. Local excision with bone-grafting was performed, but subsequent local recurrence led to amputation being performed. One year after the latter operation the patient died with pulmonary metastases.

The proximal half of the tibia has been sectioned to reveal extensive replacement of the bone by a pale, haemorrhagic neoplasm.

Adamantinoma arising in a long bone is histologically very similar to the more common ameloblastoma seen in the jaw. It is a rare, slow-growing neoplasm, which typically presents in adolescence or early adulthood and is virtually confined to the tibial diaphysis. Local recurrence is a common feature but only approximately 30 per cent of tumours eventually metastasise.

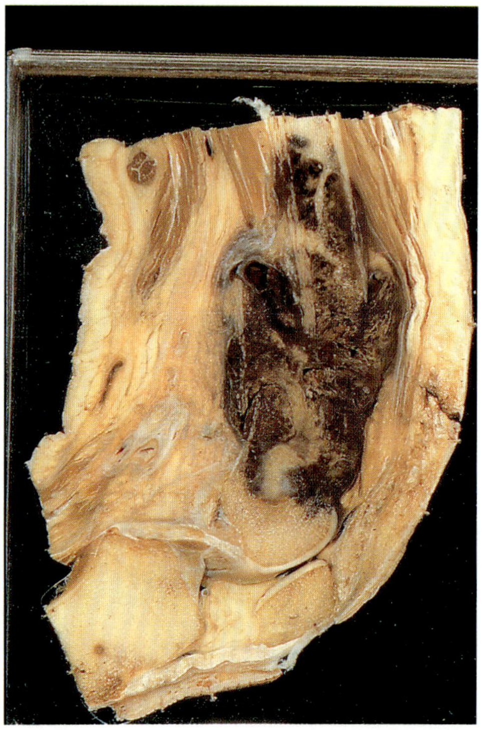

10.107 Femur: Haemangioendothelioma

This is an amputation specimen from an 80-year-old woman, whose right leg suddenly gave way when she was walking. She was found to have a pathological fracture of the lower femoral shaft, associated with an osteolytic neoplasm.

A sagittal section through the knee joint and adjacent soft tissues shows an extensive haemorrhagic mass arising in the lower femur, through which a fracture has occurred. The cut surface of the tumour has a rather 'honeycomb' appearance owing to the presence of numerous vascular channels.

Primary vascular endothelial tumours of bone are rare; they typically arise in the long limb bones in adulthood. Primary multifocality within one limb is not uncommon. Their behaviour is directly related to the degree of histological atypia and pleomorphism present: well differentiated lesions, as here, tend to be locally aggressive but only rarely metastasise, while full-blown angiosarcomas carry a poor prognosis.

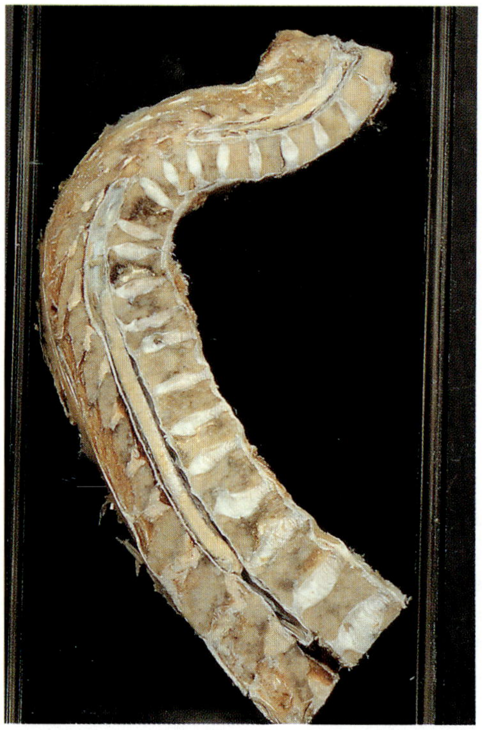

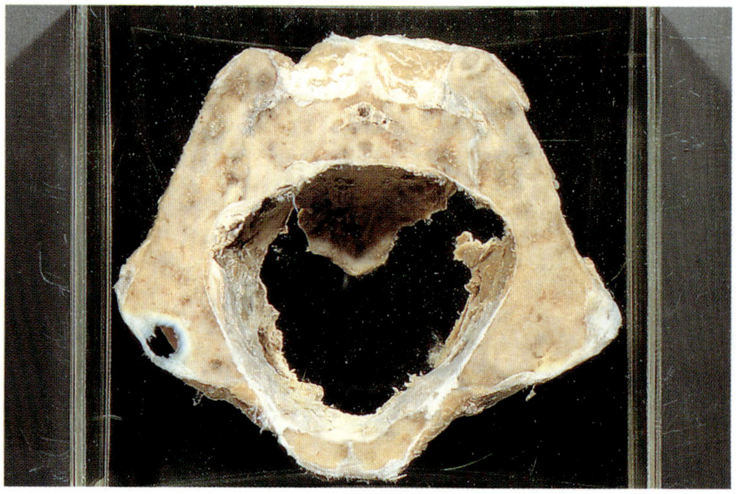

10.108 Spine and Pelvis: Metastatic Breast Carcinoma

These are post-mortem specimens from a 37-year-old woman, who died of carcinomatosis one year after undergoing radical mastectomy.

A vertical section through the spine (10.108a) shows diffuse infiltration of nearly all the vertebral bodies by pale, focally haemorrhagic tumour. Several of the vertebrae have collapsed. The pelvis of the same patient (10.108b), sectioned at the level of the acetabula, shows diffuse infiltration by pale neoplastic tissue.

Metastases in bone are far more common than primary osseous malignant tumours. The commonest primary sites of origin are carcinomas of the breast, prostate, bronchus, kidney and thyroid. The majority of such metastases are osteolytic, but prostatic cancer, and sometimes breast cancer, tend to produce sclerotic, osteoblastic deposits. The axial skeleton, i.e. the major marrow-containing bones, are most often involved. The frequency with which metastatic tumours involve bone probably reflects the very marked vascularity of the medullary cavity.

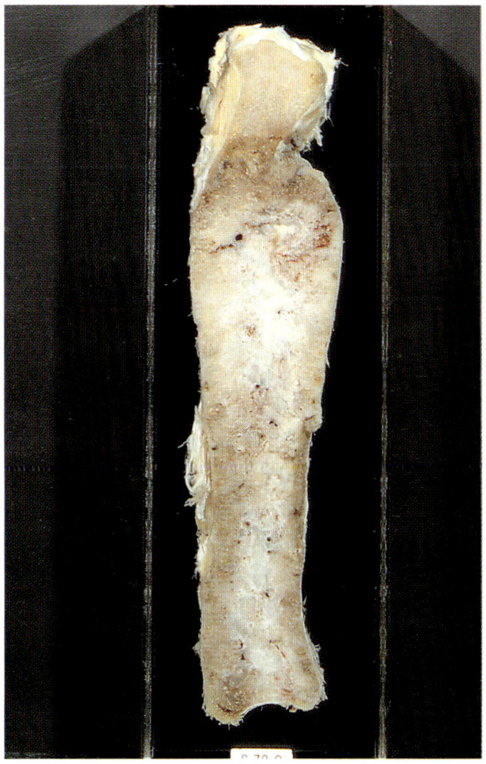

10.109 Tibia: Metastatic Prostatic Carcinoma

This is an amputation specimen from a 73-year-old man who, 10 years previously, had undergone prostatectomy for carcinoma. He then developed pain in the left shin, followed by a pathological fracture of the tibia and, in the absence of demonstrable metastatic disease elsewhere, amputation was performed. He died of bronchopneumonia one month post-operatively and, at autopsy, there was no local recurrence or metastasis elsewhere.

The left tibia has been sectioned to show extensive bony replacement by a dense, pale neoplasm within which there are foci of calcification and necrosis.

Osteosclerotic tumour deposits such as this are characterised by new bone formation in the tumour stroma. This is thought to be an effect of an osteoblastic-stimulating substance secreted by the metastatic tumour cells.

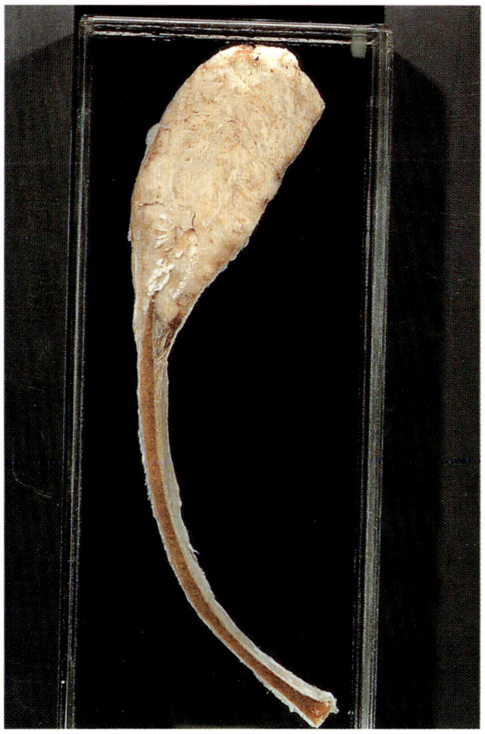

10.110 Rib: Metastatic Renal Carcinoma

This is a post-mortem specimen from a 68-year-old man, who presented with a one month history of pain in the left side of his chest. A mass was palpable posteriorly and X-rays showed a predominantly intrathoracic mass destroying the left 6th rib. A presumptive diagnosis of lung cancer was made and the patient soon died. Autopsy revealed a large carcinoma of the left kidney with metastases in the lungs, adrenals, ribs, skin, contra-lateral kidney and thyroid.

A section through the left 6th rib shows expansion of its posterior end by a large, yellowish deposit of tumour, measuring 10 × 4.5 × 4cm.

Carcinomas of the kidney and thyroid are particularly prone to present with bony metastases in association with an occult primary neoplasm.

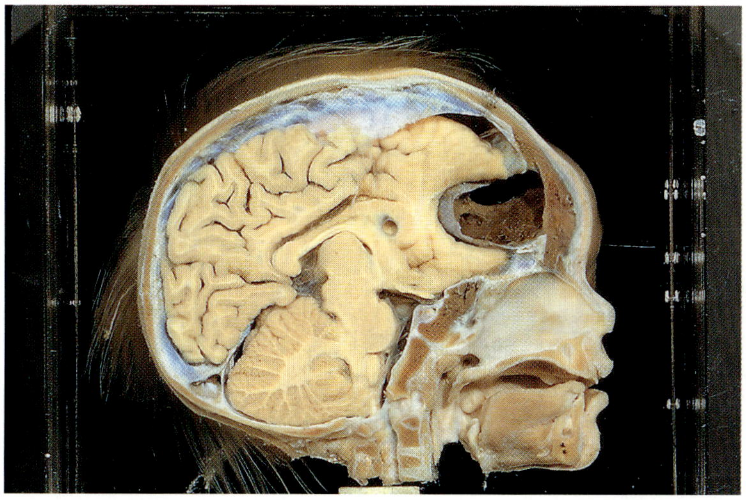

10.111 Orbit: Metastatic Adrenal Neuroblastoma

This is a post-mortem specimen from a 17-month-old girl, whose mother had noticed a mass in the patient's right loin. Laparotomy revealed a cystic neoplasm arising in the right adrenal gland, which was excised along with the kidney. Within a matter of days, metastases were found in the left orbit, right humerus and left femur. The child died 4 months after the onset of symptoms.

A section through the skull shows a deposit of haemorrhagic tumour extending backwards from the orbit and compressing the frontal lobe.

In childhood, neuroblastoma is by far the commonest neoplasm to metastasise to bone. In the absence of careful clinical examination and estimation of urinary catecholamines, such metastases may be histologically misinterpreted as primary Ewing's sarcoma (see Figure and Legend 10.102). The orbit is a particularly common site for such spread, a phenomenon known in the past as Hutchison's syndrome.

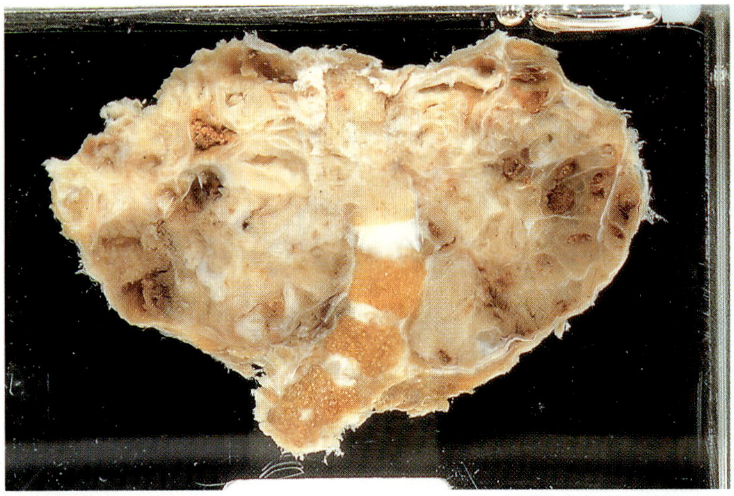

10.112 Sacrococcyx: Chordoma

This specimen was excised from a 49-year-old man, who presented with a slow-growing mass at the base of his spine which he had first noticed 2 years previously. Examination revealed a sacrococcygeal neoplasm with diffuse extension into the right sacro-iliac region. Complete excision was not technically feasible.

A sagittal section through the sacrococcygeal region shows a very large, lobulated, gelatinous tumour extensively infiltrating the sacrum and showing foci of haemorrhage. The coccyx is largely spared.

Chordomas are rare neoplasms, thought to be derived from notochordal remnants, which most often arise in the sacrococcygeal region but may also be seen in the spheno-occipital area. These tumours usually arise in middle or late adulthood, and show a predilection for males. While they tend to be relentlessly locally aggressive, only about 35 per cent actually metastasise. The majority of cases do, however, pursue a fatal course owing to infiltration of adjacent vital structures.

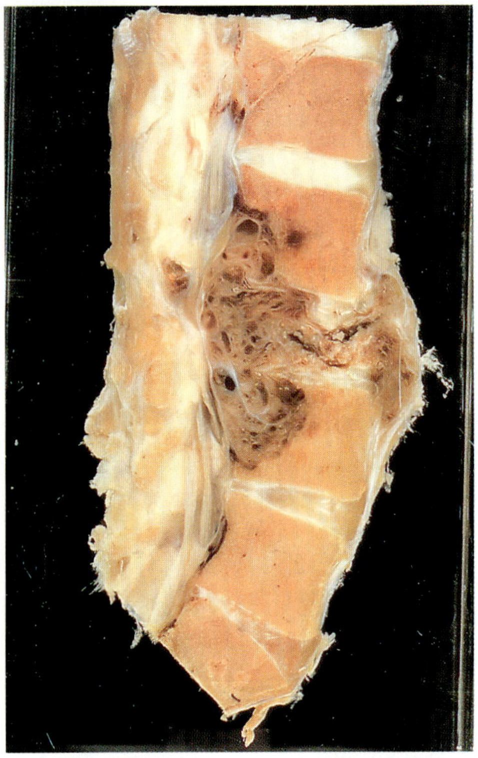

10.113 Lumbar Vertebra: Chordoma

This is a post-mortem specimen from a 70-year-old man, who was found to have an osteolytic lesion in his 3rd lumbar vertebra. This was assumed to represent metastasis from an occult prostatic cancer, despite lack of histological evidence and normal serum acid phosphatase levels. Biopsy revealed only necrotic material. The patient died one year later having become paraplegic with intractable urinary infection.

A sagittal section through the lumbar spine shows destruction of the 3rd lumbar vertebra by an extensive haemorrhagic neoplasm, which has invaded the bodies of adjacent vertebrae and is compressing the cauda equina. Histology revealed the classical features of a chordoma.

Chordomas arising in the vertebral column other than at the most proximal and distal ends are extremely rare.

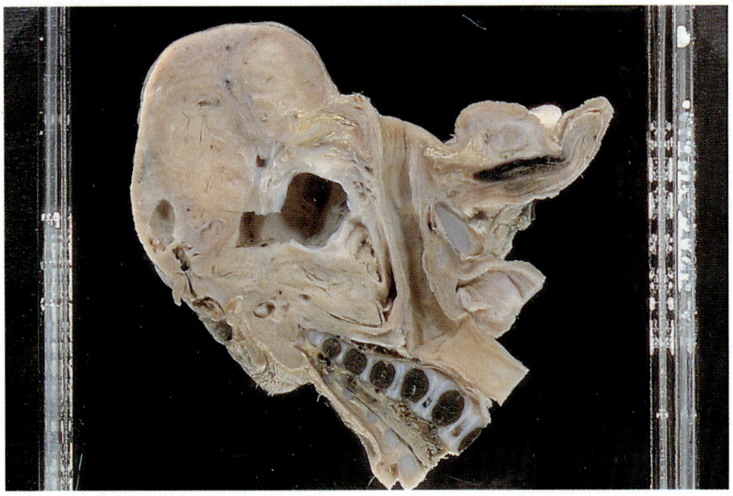

10.114 Sacrococcyx: Benign (Mature) Teratoma

This is a post-mortem specimen from a premature infant who lived for only a short time.

A sagittal section through this infant's lower trunk shows a rounded neoplasm, measuring 8cm in maximum diameter, arising between the sacrum and the rectum. The tumour is focally cystic and has compressed and distorted the overlying perineal skin.

Benign (mature) teratomas may classically arise anywhere in the mid-line, probably at the site of anomalous totipotential cell rests. Such sites include the sacrococcygeal region, retroperitoneum, mediastinum and pineal gland: histologically identical tumours are seen in the testis and ovary. They are commonly cystic lesions and rupture of these cysts may lead to inflammatory adhesions to adjacent structures, giving a mistaken clinical impression of malignancy.

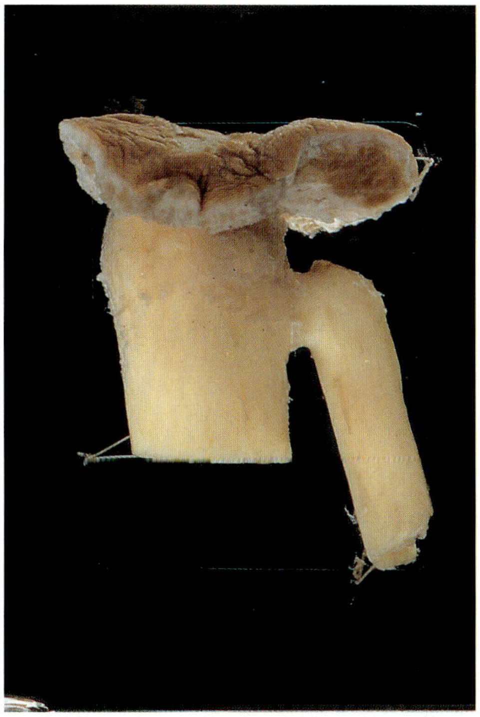

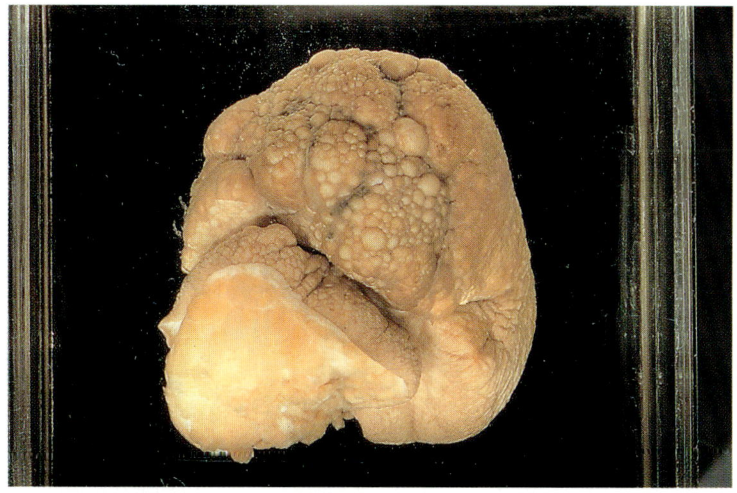

10.116 Amputation Stump: Viral Warts

No clinical details are available.

These pendulous folds of skin, which were excised from an above-knee amputation stump, are covered by multiple, pale warty lesions.

Redundant folds of skin over an amputation stump are prone to chronic eczematous irritation and to infection. The occasional development of viral warts in a moist area such as this is not surprising.

10.115 Amputation Stump: Bony Cross Union

No clinical details are available.

This below-knee amputation stump shows cross union between the tibia and fibula. The overlying skin is firmly adherent to the tibia and, in the fresh state, was extensively ulcerated.

Bony cross union in an amputation stump is unsatisfactory because it reduces the resilience of the stump, particularly if a prosthesis is to be fitted. It typically follows post-operative wound infection, which also gives rise to cutaneous complications.

JOINTS AND TENDONS

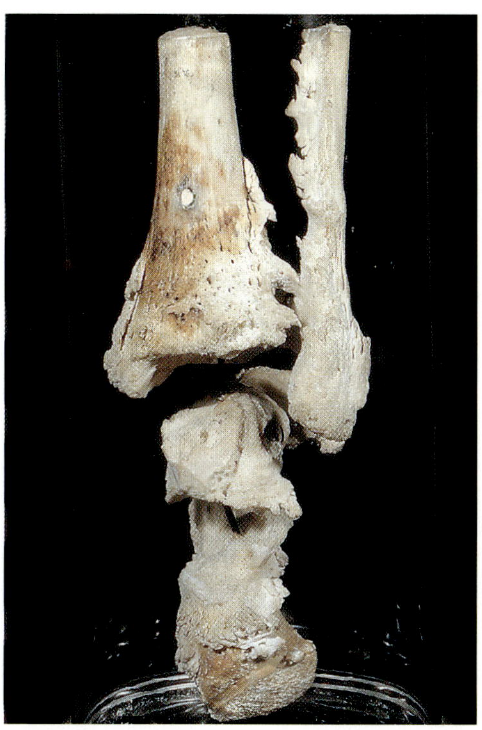

10.117 Ankle Joint: Chronic Suppurative Arthritis

No clinical details are available.

The bones of this macerated ankle joint show erosion of the cancellous bone. There is adjacent subperiosteal new bone formation, which has extended to form a bridge at the site of the obliterated inferior tibio-fibular ligament.

Suppurative (septic) arthritis is most often a consequence of trauma, haematogenously spread infection or local spread from an osteomyelitic process. Young children are most often affected and the joints of the lower limb are usually involved. Since articular cartilage is rapidly destroyed, prompt surgical intervention and antibiotic treatment is imperative to avoid changes such as those seen in this case.

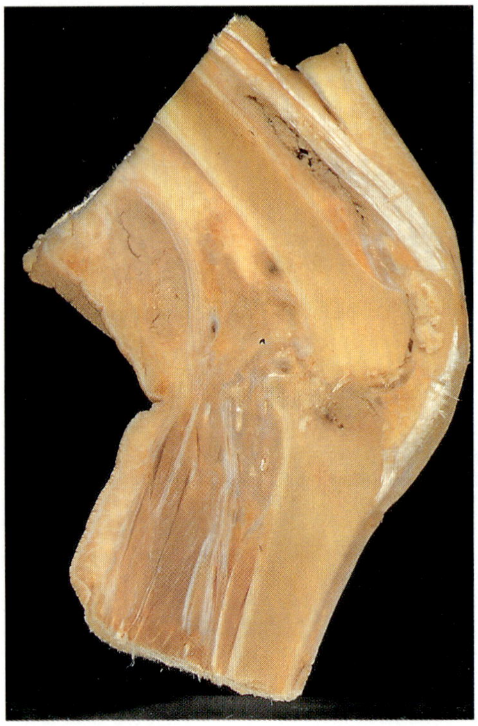

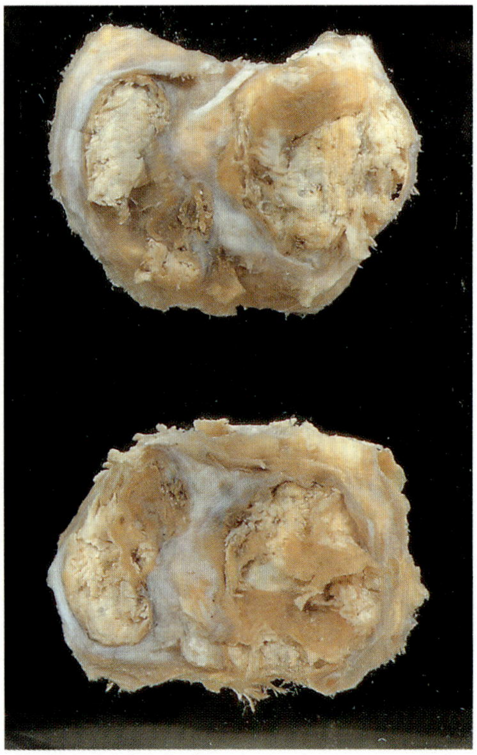

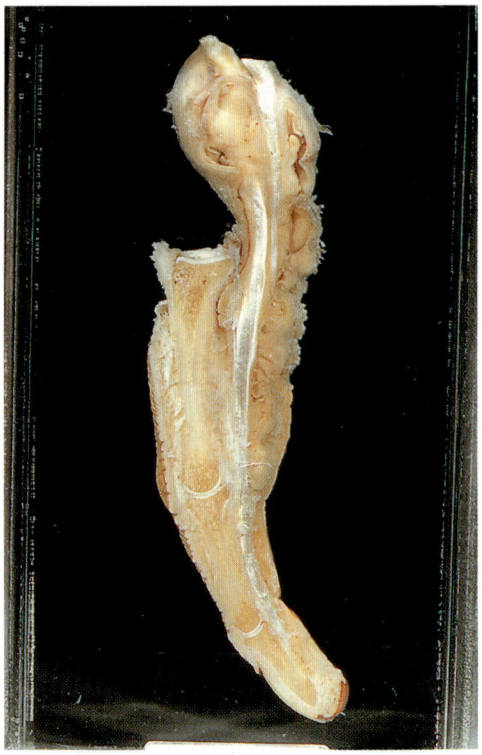

10.118 Knee Joint: Tuberculous Arthritis

This is an amputation specimen from a 59-year-old woman, who presented with pain in her left knee which had been deformed from birth. X-rays showed gross joint destruction but the patient refused further investigation. However, a fluctuant swelling with a sinus developed around the head of the fibula and eventually amputation became necessary.

A vertical section through the left knee joint shows complete disorganisation and destruction of the articular surfaces. There is extensive fibrosis with joint adhesions and multiple small foci of yellowish caseous necrosis are evident, particularly in the partly dislocated patella.

Tuberculous arthritis, like tuberculous osteomyelitis (see Figure and Legend 10.46 et seq.), most often results from haematogenous spread of infection, usually from the lungs. The hip and knee are most often affected in patients of almost any age. Commonly, synovitis and osteomyelitis develop at the same site. Spontaneous bony ankylosis may occur. Complications include the formation of a 'cold abscess', joint destruction with deformity and reactivation of infection at a later date.

10.119 Knee Joint: Tuberculous Arthritis

This specimen was excised from a 27-year-old man, who presented with a one month history of pain in the right knee. He had been successfully treated for pulmonary tuberculosis 12 years previously. Examination revealed swelling of the knee joint with an effusion and thickening of the synovium in the suprapatellar pouch. X-rays showed erosion of the femoral condyles and the head of the tibia so the joint was excised.

The excised articular surfaces of the knee joint show extensive destruction of the cartilage and superficial bone. The damaged areas are filled with yellow, caseous material with adjacent haemorrhage.

This case demonstrates well the damage caused by tuberculosis to the articular surfaces of a joint.

10.120 Finger: Tuberculous Tenosynovitis

This is an amputation specimen from a 25-year-old woman, who presented with a 3 year history of progressive swelling of the right middle finger. A chest X-ray revealed evidence of quiescent tuberculosis.

The middle finger of the right hand has been divided in the long axis to show multinodular thickening and fibrosis along the flexor tendon sheath. There is no evidence of active caseation.

Involvement of tendons and their sheaths is uncommon nowadays but most frequently affects the hands, particularly the wrist.

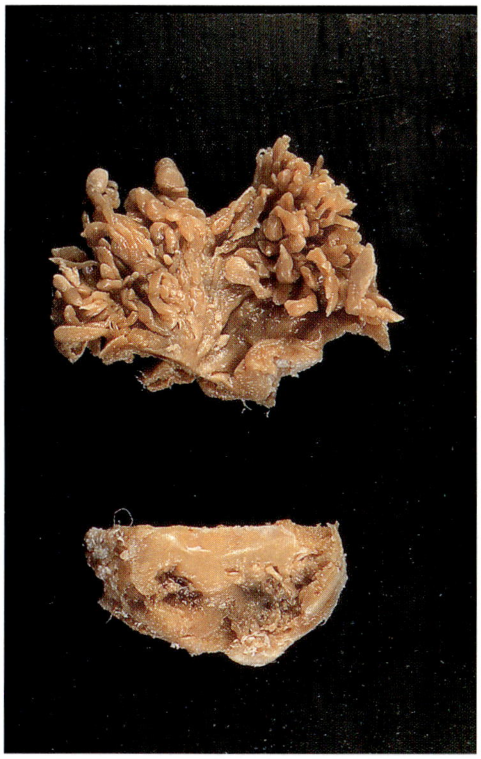

10.121 Knee Joint: Rheumatoid Arthritis

These specimens were excised from the knee joint of an adult female. No other clinical details are available.

The synovium (above) shows numerous hyperplastic papillary excrescences which are brownish in colour due to haemosiderin deposition. The articular surface of the tibia (below) shows irregular peripheral erosion and destruction of the cartilage.

Rheumatoid arthritis is a multisystem chronic inflammatory disorder, the precise aetiology of which is unknown. It has been suggested that an unknown infective agent initiates cell damage, most especially in synovial tissue, which is succeeded by a vigorous host autoimmune response. The disease is commonest in the 4th and 5th decades, shows a predilection for females and has an overall incidence in the adult population of about 2 per cent. The majority of patients demonstrate a circulating antibody to IgG, known as the rheumatoid factor.

Joint involvement is usually symmetrical and is most often seen in the metacarpophalangeal joints, wrists, elbows and knees. The proliferating inflamed synovial tissue (pannus) erodes articular cartilage and the joint capsule and may eventually destroy ligaments and underlying bone. Systemic manifestations include the development of rheumatoid nodules, particularly in the skin, heart or lungs, splenomegaly, vasculitis, myositis and sometimes, Sjögren's syndrome. (Courtesy of St. Thomas's Hospital Medical School Museum)

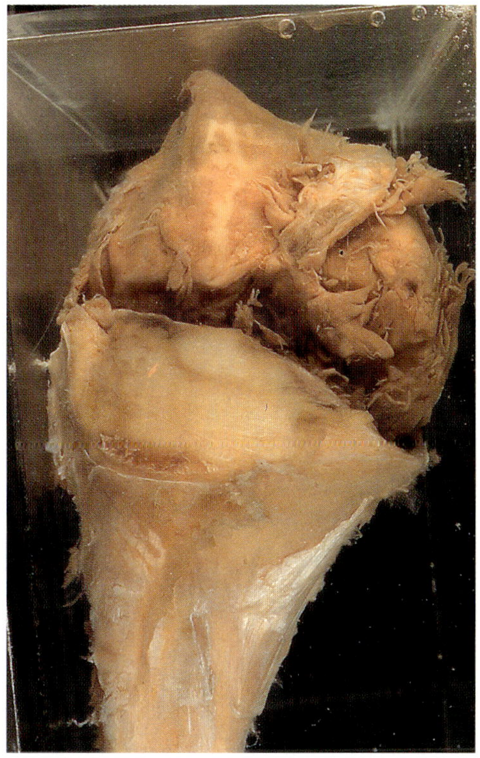

10.122 Knee Joint: Rheumatoid Arthritis

This is a post-mortem specimen from a 35-year-old woman, who had first presented with the features of rheumatoid arthritis at the age of 20. She had been treated with high-dose steroids, leading to osteoporosis and vertebral collapse. Latterly she presented with renal failure, found to be due to secondary amyloidosis, and she died.

This flexed knee joint, viewed anteriorly, shows synovial pannus formation, which is eroding the articular cartilage of the femur and tibia. Note also the pale, fibrinous exudate and the area of bony necrosis in the proximal tibia. The latter may be accounted for by this patient's high dose steroid treatment.

Secondary amyloidosis, as in this case, is a well-recognised complication of chronic rheumatoid arthritis. There are a variety of inflammatory joint disorders thought to be related variants of rheumatoid arthritis, but which usually lack circulating rheumatoid factor. The most important of these are ankylosing spondylitis, Still's disease (seen in childhood) and the arthritides associated with inflammatory bowel disease or psoriasis. (Courtesy of St. Thomas's Hospital Medical School Museum)

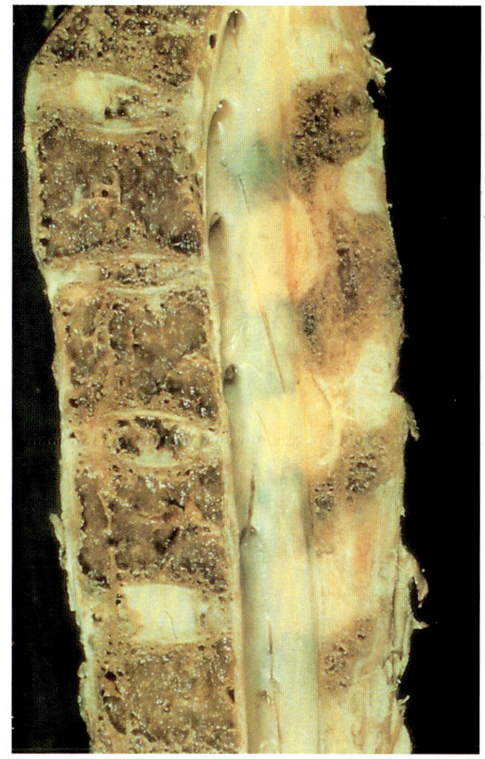

10.123 Spine: Ankylosing Spondylitis

No clinical details are available.

This close-up view of the lumbar spine shows that the bulk of each intervertebral disc has been replaced by bony tissue, leading to osseous fusion of the vertebrae.

Ankylosing spondylitis is a fairly uncommon disorder, which typically affects young adults (predominantly males) and is characterised by bony ankylosis of the sacro-iliac joints, facet joints of the spine and across the intervertebral discs. The vast majority of affected patients have the HLA type B27 and this condition may be associated with psoriasis, inflammatory bowel disease and Reiter's syndrome. While the histological features are said to be similar to those of rheumatoid arthritis, inflammation is by no means so severe. (Courtesy of Dr. P.G. Bullough, Hospital for Special Surgery, New York)

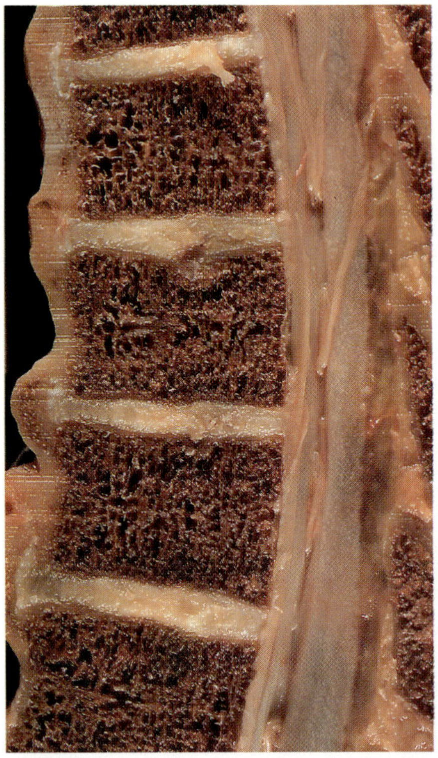

10.124 Spine: Diffuse Idiopathic Skeletal Hyperostosis

No clinical details are available.

This sagittal section through the thoracic spine shows pale ossification of the anterior longitudinal ligament. Note that the intervertebral discs are well preserved.

Diffuse idiopathic skeletal hyperostosis is a fairly common disorder, which is being increasingly recognised and typically is seen in the elderly (predominantly males). Up to 30 per cent of older patients may show evidence of this condition at autopsy. It is characterised by ossification of the anterior and/or posterior ligaments, particularly in the thoracic spine, but may also affect tendons or ligaments around any of the major joints. Stiffness is the principal presenting complaint. (Courtesy of Dr. P.G. Bullough, Hospital for Special Surgery, New York)

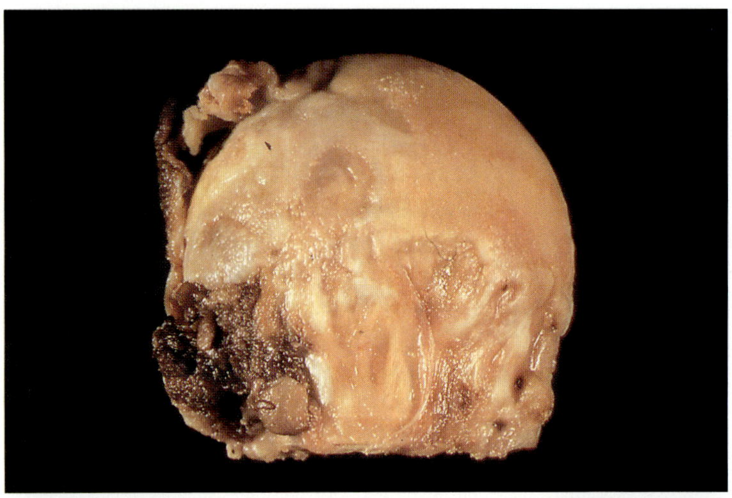

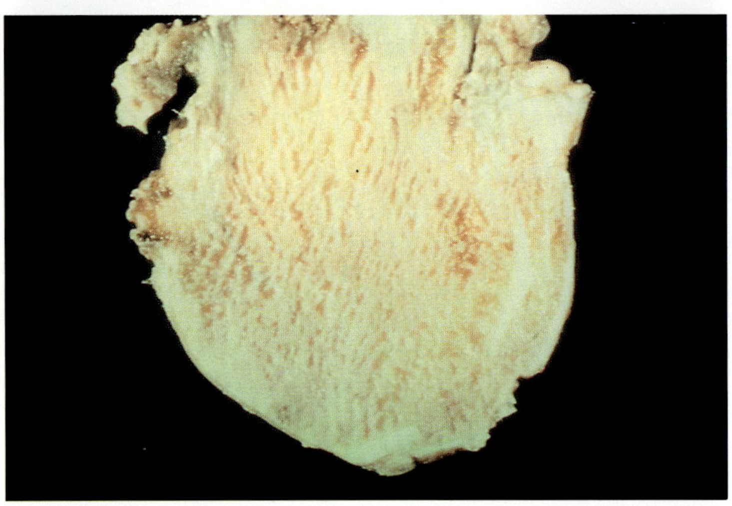

10.125 Femoral Head: Osteoarthrosis

No clinical details are available in either case.

This resected femoral head (10.125a) shows gross irregularity with extensive erosion of articular cartilage, eburnation of bone (top) and focal damage to subchondral bone with cyst formation. A separate case (10.125b), seen in cross-section, shows supero-lateral cartilage destruction and a large, flat medial osteophyte (right).

These are the characteristic appearances of the articular surface of a joint affected by this condition. Osteoarthrosis (more often known as osteoarthritis, despite the lack of an inflammatory pathogenesis) is a ubiquitous disorder, particularly in the elderly, and tends to affect the major weight-bearing joints (hips and knees) or joints that are used a great deal. Most often this process is idiopathic, probably representing the result of abnormal mechanical forces and ageing phenomena, but some cases may complicate pre-existent disease, such as congenital hip dislocation or a slipped epiphysis. The basic cause in all cases is probably repeated trauma to articular cartilage, which becomes eroded and splits. Characteristically, affected joints become stiff and painful (particularly in the early morning) and movement becomes limited.
(10.125a courtesy of Drs. C.D.M. Fletcher and P.H. McKee, St. Thomas's Hospital Medical School; 10.125b courtesy of Dr. P.G. Bullough, Hospital for Special Surgery, New York)

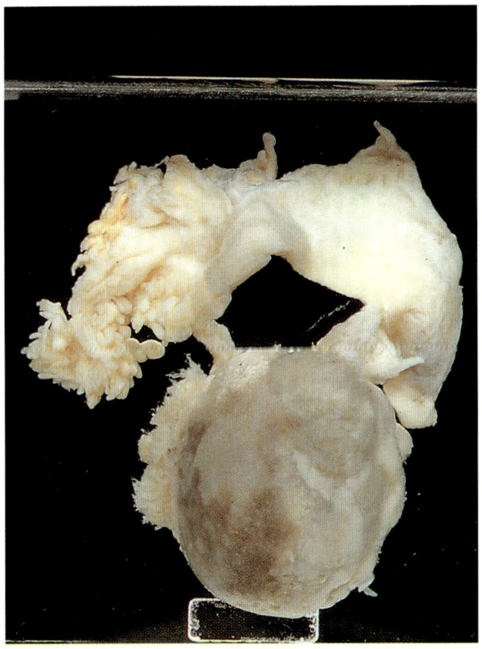

10.126 Shoulder Joint: Osteoarthrosis

This specimen was excised from a soldier, who had suffered repeated severe trauma to the right shoulder which had led to intractable stiffness, pain and swelling.

The head of the humerus with part of the adjacent joint capsule is mounted. The articular surface is completely denuded of cartilage, leading to eburnation of the underlying bone. Projecting from the lateral aspect (right) are many irregular spicules of new bone (osteophytes). The capsular synovium shows villous hyperplasia.

Osteoarthrosis of the shoulder is rare and most often affects the acromioclavicular joint.

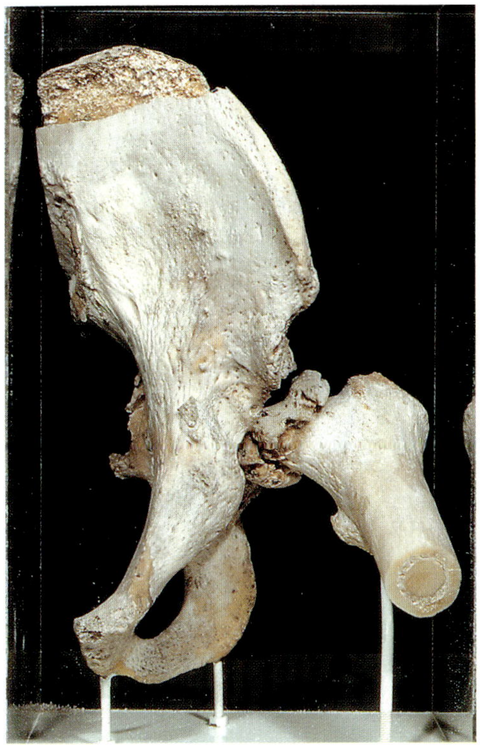

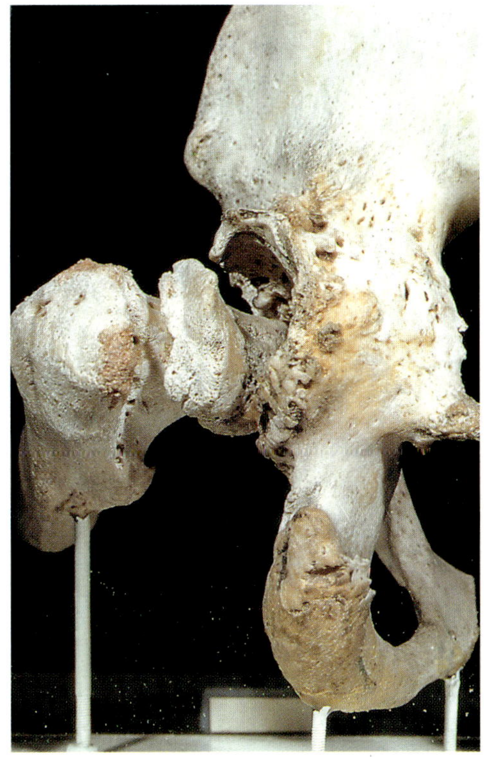

10.127 Hip Joint: Osteoarthrosis

No clinical details are available.

The left hip joint, with the upper femur, (10.127a) shows great distortion and destruction of the femoral head and neck. Large osteophytes project from the medial aspect of the articular surface ('lipping'). Seen in close-up from behind (10.127b), irregular osteophytes are also visible at the margin of the acetabulum.

Osteoarthrosis of the hip is probably the single commonest indication for hip replacement (arthroplasty). In this case, the lesion appears to be secondary to an old slipped epiphysis.

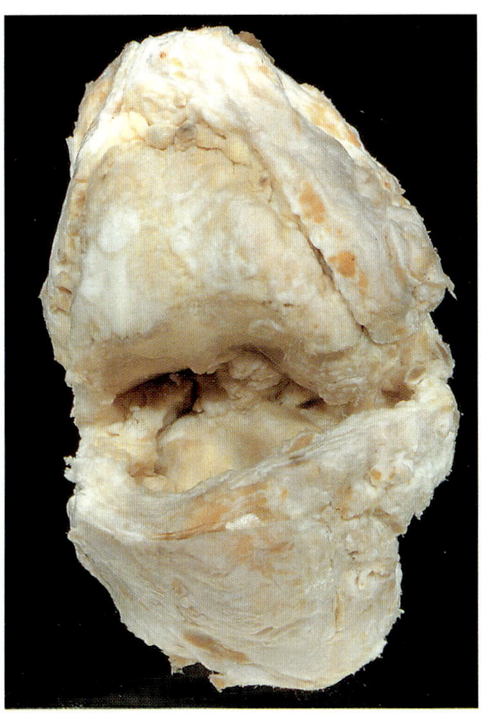

10.128 Knee Joint: Osteoarthrosis

No clinical details are available.

The knee joint has been opened anteriorly to show erosion and eburnation of the articular surfaces, marked capsular thickening and nodularity of the semilunar cartilages. Note also the opaque, chalky deposits on both sides of the joint, indicative of chondrocalcinosis.

It should be remembered that a proportion of patients with osteoarthrosis show an ill-understood genetic predisposition to this condition. This is particularly true of those cases affecting the distal interphalangeal joints of the hand (Heberden's nodes), in which there is a strong familial tendency and a predilection for postmenopausal women.

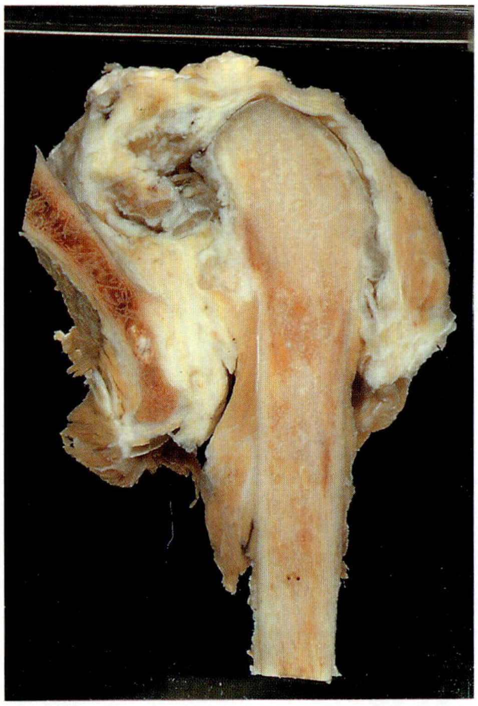

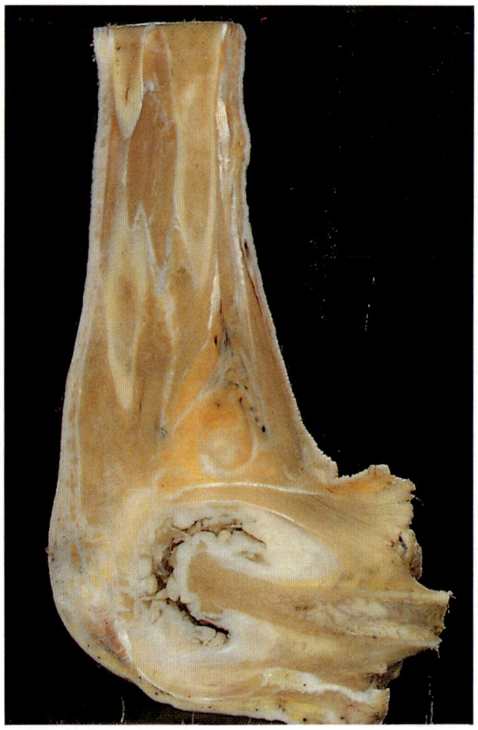

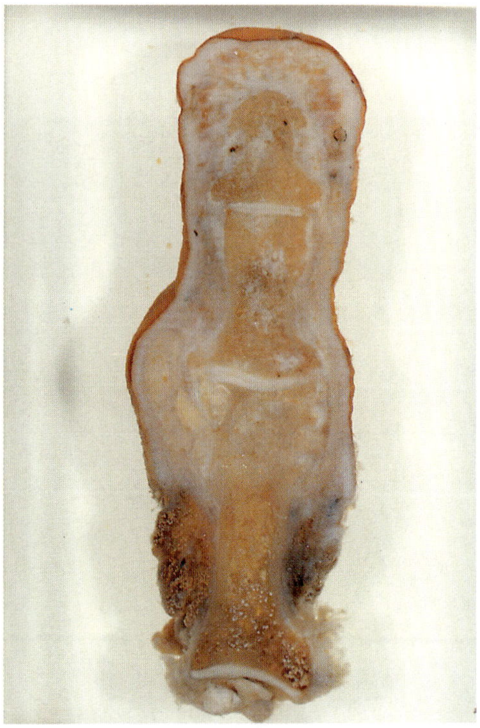

10.129 Hip Joint: Charcot's Osteoarthropathy

This is a post-mortem specimen from a 58-year-old man, who died of a pulmonary embolism. He was known to have long-standing tabes dorsalis, with advanced damage to the right hip and left knee. At autopsy there was also a syphilitic aneurysm of the aortic arch.

A section through the right hip shows complete disorganisation and dislocation of the joint. The femoral head and the acetabulum have been completely destroyed and the bones are joined by a grossly thickened fibrous capsule.

Charcot's osteoarthropathy is characterised by extreme osteoarthrosis and joint destruction secondary to an underlying neurological deficit (classically with anaesthesia and loss of proprioception). While the classical preceding cause is always regarded as neurosyphilis, currently more common causes include subacute combined degeneration of the cord (in pernicious anaemia), diabetic neuropathy and syringomyelia. The presence of loose bodies or bony detritus in the affected joint is a common feature.

10.130 Elbow Joint: Charcot's Osteoarthropathy

This is an amputation specimen from a 74-year-old woman, who presented with progressive painless swelling of the right elbow. She had dislocated her right shoulder 15 years previously. Examination revealed a completely flail, disorganised elbow and evidence of a neurological deficit in the median, radial and ulnar nerves. There was no evidence of syringomyelia and serological tests for syphilis were negative.

A vertical section through the elbow joint shows complete disorganisation with destruction of the proximal ends of both the ulna and radius. The joint capsule is swollen, extensively scarred and is lined by hyperplastic synovium.

It must be assumed that this patient's joint destruction was attributable to unnoticed local nerve damage proximally at the time of the shoulder dislocation.

10.131 Toe: Gouty Arthritis

This is an amputation specimen from a 64-year-old man, who had developed gout 2 years previously. There were multiple tophi in the heels, ears and elbows and the right second toe became extremely painful.

A section through the right second toe shows erosion and replacement of the head of the proximal phalanx by opaque, yellowish material. There is erosion of the cartilage at the articular margins and further deposits of tophaceous material are apparent in the adjacent subcutaneous tissue.

Gout is characterised by hyperuricaemia and the deposition of urate crystals in joints and the kidneys. It may be due to a primary inherited disorder of purine metabolism, which is more common in males, or secondary to disorders in which there is an increased turnover of nucleic acids e.g. psoriasis, malignant disease (particularly multiple myeloma) and cytotoxic treatment. The disease is initially manifest as acute episodes of crystal-induced inflammation in joints but gradually progresses to extensive crystal deposition with the formation of tophi. The development of coexistent urate stones in the urinary tract is an important complication.

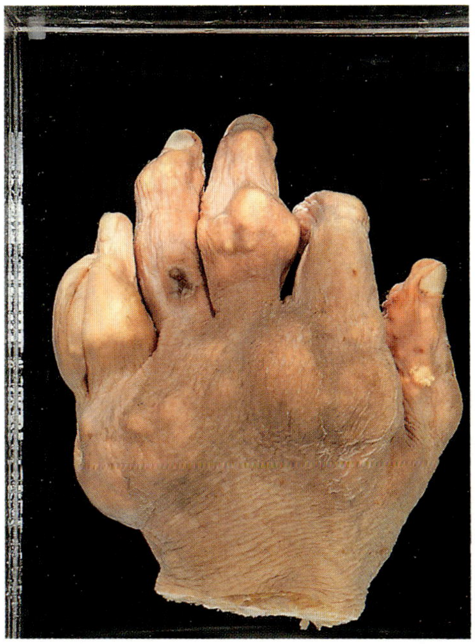

10.132 Hand: Gouty Arthritis

No clinical details are available.

The left hand shows multiple, yellowish irregular swellings over the metacarpophalangeal and interphalangeal joints.

Acute gout is most often monoarticular but polyarticular involvement occurs in chronic disease. Joints in the distal portions of the limbs, most especially the metatarsophalangeal joints, are usually affected.

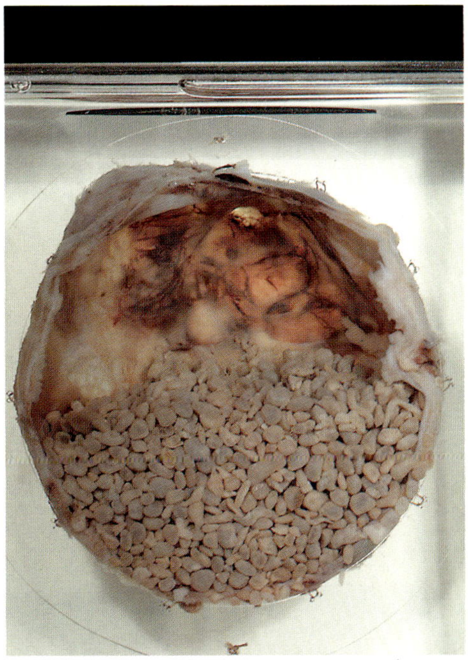

10.133 Olecranon Bursa: Gout

This specimen was excised from a 66-year-old man, who had suffered from gouty tophi in the hands and elbows for 20 years. Latterly he presented with a grossly enlarged olecranon bursa.

The bursa is greatly increased in size, now measuring 10cm in diameter, and is almost completely filled with fibrinous 'melon-seed' loose bodies. The wall is thickened and congested and, histologically, contained numerous amorphous masses of urate crystals with associated inflammatory changes.

Chronic gout may affect tendosynovial structures throughout the body. Fibrinous loose bodies such as these are more often a feature of rheumatoid arthritis.

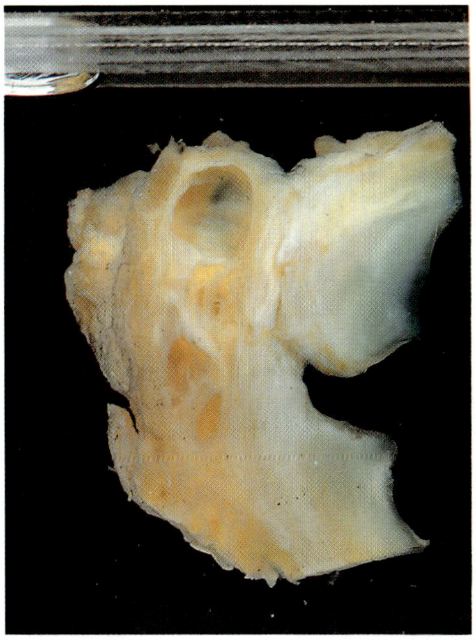

10.134 Lateral Meniscus: Tear and Cysts

This specimen was excised from a 25-year-old man, who fell and twisted his left knee violently. There was pain and a joint effusion for about one week, which resolved spontaneously. Five months later he presented with a swelling on the outer aspect of the knee.

Part of the lateral meniscus shows a smoothly healed cartilaginous tear and, on its lateral aspect there is a mass of fibrous tissue containing several smooth-walled cysts.

The medial meniscus is more often torn than its lateral counterpart but, in either event, this lesion is commonest in young men who have applied a severe twisting force to the knee (usually in the course of sport). The later development of small mucoid cysts is quite common and, in fact, is more frequent on the lateral side.

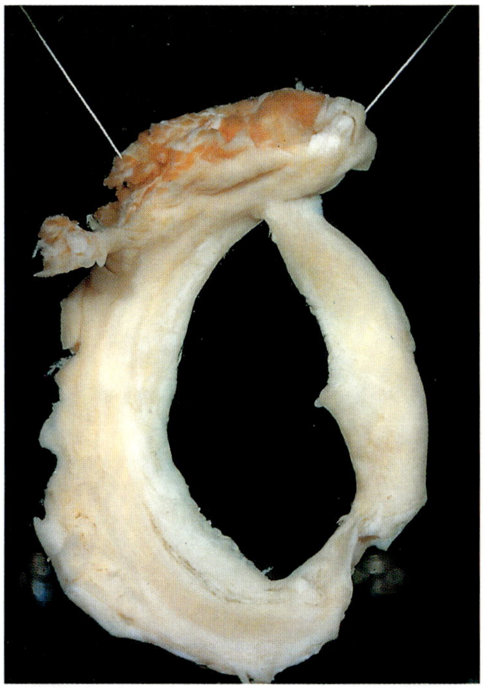

10.135 Medial Meniscus: Tear

This specimen was excised from a 27-year-old man, who had suffered a severe twisting injury of the right knee 2 years previously. Since then he had suffered frequent episodes of pain and swelling of the knee associated with a feeling of 'giving way'.

The medial meniscus shows an almost complete longitudinal split.

This is a typical example of the so-called 'bucket-handle' tear of the medial meniscus, in which there is a split in both the anterior and posterior horns.

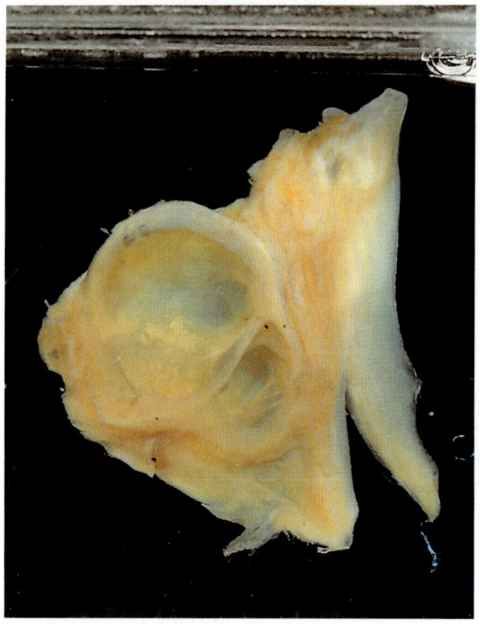

10.136 Medial Meniscus: Cysts

This specimen was excised from a 36-year-old man, who presented with a 5 year history of pain in the right knee. Examination revealed a soft swelling on the medial aspect of the joint.

Attached to the medial meniscus are a collection of small cysts, measuring up to 2cm in diameter. The adjacent cartilage has a rather mucoid appearance and is scarred at one end, suggesting a healed tear.

Tearing of the medial meniscus is the commonest cause of locking at the knee joint. Cysts such as these may lead to juxta-articular erosion of bone.

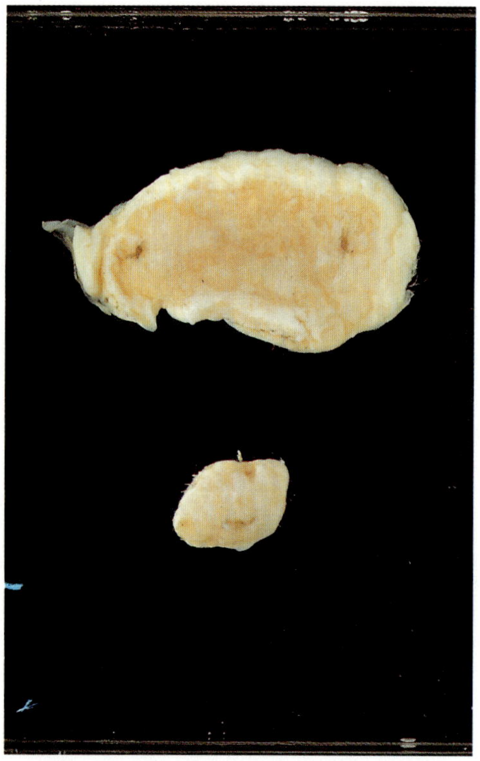

10.137 Knee Joint: Loose Bodies

These specimens were removed from a 24-year-old man, who presented with a 2 year history of pain and locking of the left knee joint following a fall. X-rays showed two loose bodies and a defect in the medial condyle of the femur.

The larger specimen (above), measuring $4 \times 2 \times 1$cm, is composed principally of bone, covered on one surface by articular cartilage. This fragment corresponds closely in size and shape to the femoral defect. The smaller specimen is composed solely of a rounded nodule of cartilage.

Loose bodies, which are commonest in the knee joint, have a variable aetiology. In young patients, as here, they are most often the result of a single, fairly severe injury. In older patients, they may represent fragmented osteophytes (in osteoarthrosis) or may be fibrinous in nature (in rheumatoid arthritis). A primary disorder, known as synovial chondromatosis, in which multiple cartilaginous loose bodies are formed is discussed in Legend 10.146.

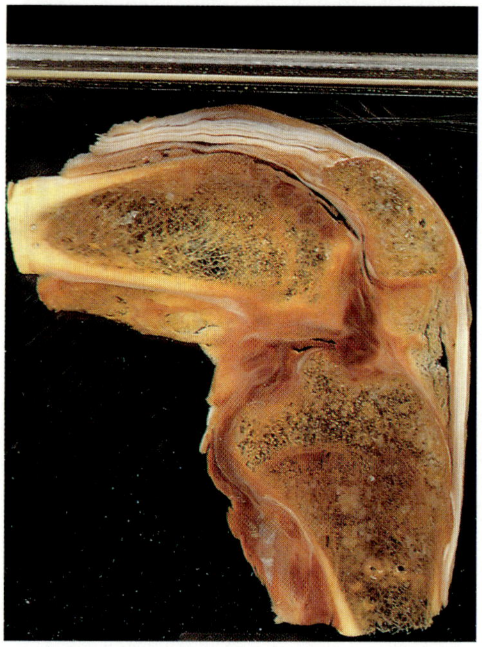

10.138 Knee Joint: Haemophilia

This is a post-mortem specimen from a 17-year-old boy, known to suffer from haemophilia, who had a long history of nose bleeds and haemorrhage into various joints. He died following a massive retroperitoneal haemorrhage.

A vertical section through the knee joint shows the results of repeated haemorrhage into the synovium and joint cavity. The synovial membrane is markedly thickened and discoloured by haemosiderin deposition. Small collections of partly organised blood clot are also visible. Note the characteristic, prominent juxta-articular osteoporosis, which is confined to the epiphysis.

Bleeding into joints, often following insignificant trauma, is a very frequent complication of haemophilia and most often affects the knees, ankles and elbows. The consequent chronic haemorrhagic effusions that may develop are associated with progressive destruction of adjacent osteocartilaginous structures.

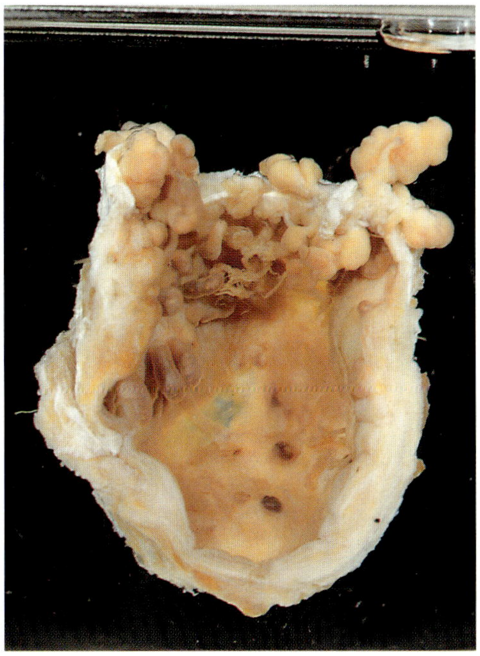

10.139 Prepatellar Bursa: Chronic Bursitis

This specimen was excised from a 50-year-old woman, whose job entailed a great deal of kneeling.

The prepatellar bursa has been opened to show gross fibrous thickening of its wall, which is roughened and covered in a thick, shaggy fibrinous exudate.

Chronic inflammation of any bursa results from repeated trauma and leads to painful swelling around the adjacent joint, most commonly the knee. When affecting the prepatellar bursa it is known as 'housemaid's knee' and when the infrapatellar bursa is involved, 'clergyman's knee': the difference lies in the fact that those with religious inclinations tend to kneel in a more upright position than those who are scrubbing the floor.

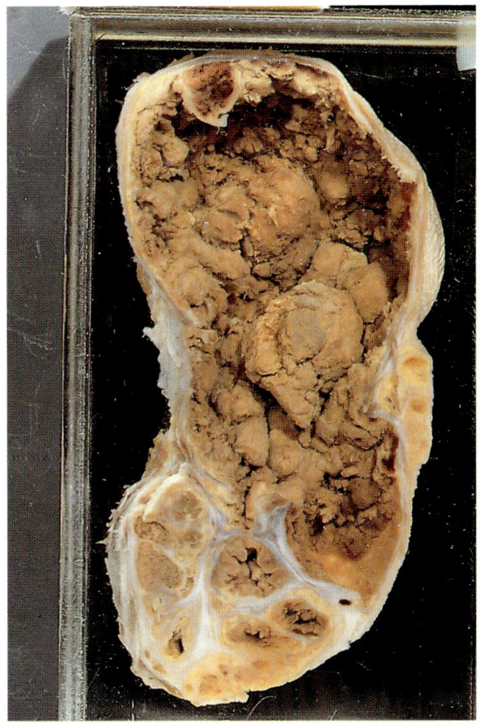

10.140 Olecranon Bursa: Chronic Bursitis

This specimen was excised from an elderly trawler fisherman, who had noticed a slow-growing lump over his elbow for many years.

The bursa, which now measures 18 × 8 × 8cm, has been bisected to show gross fibrous thickening, loculation and large quantities of organised blood clot within its cavity.

Olecranon bursitis is relatively uncommon but is usually associated with repeated pressure or friction, as here. The trauma in this case clearly led to episodic haemorrhage.

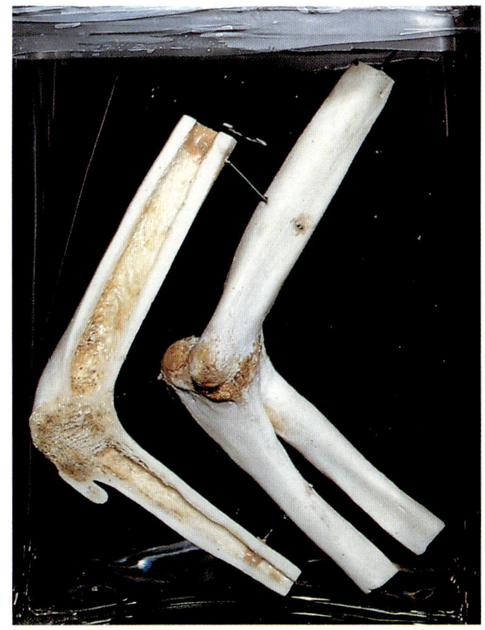

10.141 Elbow Joint: Bony Ankylosis

No clinical details are available.

The bones of the left elbow joint show complete bony ankylosis. The joint is held in fixed flexion with the radius semi-pronated.

Bony ankylosis is a non-specific sequela of complete destruction of the articular cartilage of a joint, which leads to total loss of movement at the joint. Predisposing causes include chronic rheumatoid arthritis, suppurative or tuberculous arthritis.

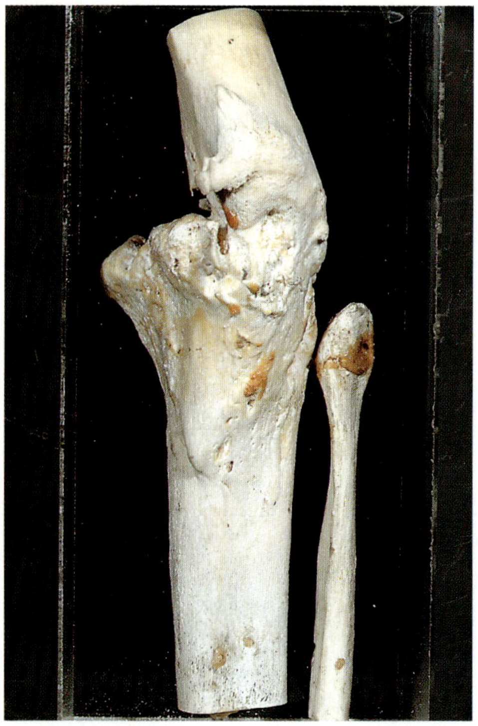

10.142 Knee Joint: Bony Ankylosis

This is an amputation specimen from a soldier, who suffered a severe gunshot injury to the right knee with comminution of the lower femur and upper tibia. The wound was complicated by prolonged suppurative arthritis and amputation eventually became necessary.

The bones of the right knee joint show fixed osseous ankylosis between the femur and tibia. The medial femoral and tibial condyles have been largely destroyed.

The clinical history in this case is a typical example of disease leading to bony ankylosis. When such a joint is created surgically, as a therapeutic measure, it is known as an arthrodesis.

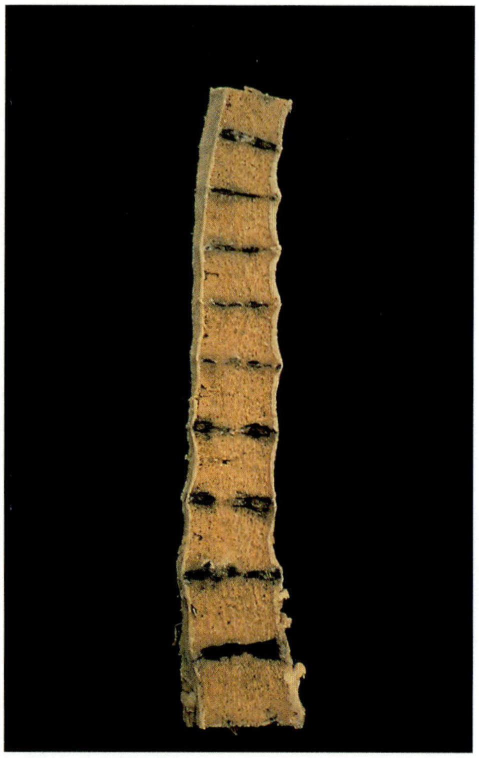

10.143 Spine: Ochronosis

No clinical details are available.

A coronal section through this vertebral column shows dense black pigmentation of the intervertebral discs. Note the associated narrowing of the disc spaces.

Ochronosis results from the deposition of homogentisic acid and its metabolites in soft tissues and is nearly always associated with the inherited disorder alkaptonuria. Cartilage tends to be particularly affected with collagenous disorganisation, often becoming brittle and fragmented which leads to changes similar to osteoarthrosis. (Courtesy of Dr. P.G. Bullough, Hospital for Special Surgery, New York)

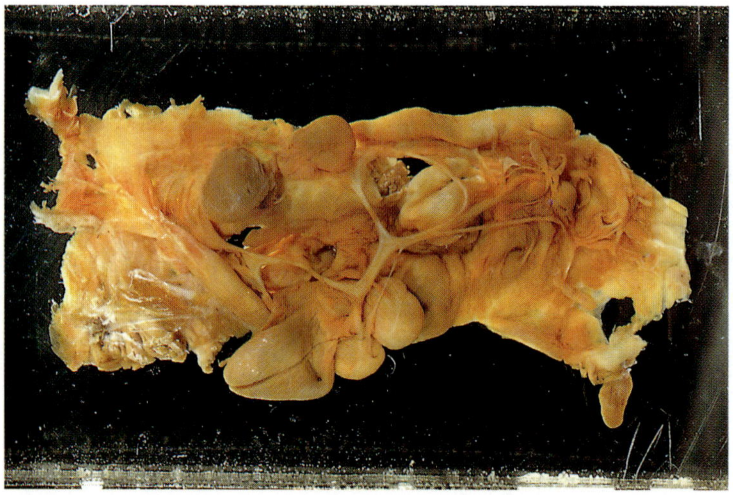

10.144 Knee Joint: Pigmented Villonodular Tenosynovitis

This specimen was excised from a 32-year-old man, who presented with a 3 year history of swelling just above the knee.

Part of the suprapatellar pouch has been opened to show a number of smooth, rounded nodules projecting from the synovial surface. The tissue has a diffuse rust-coloured pigmentation.

Pigmented villonodular tenosynovitis is a fairly common benign tumour, which typically presents in young or middle-aged adults, particularly males, and is most frequent in the knee joint. It is a locally aggressive lesion, which may erode bone, and recurs in up to a third of cases following excision. It is thought to be derived from fibrohistiocytic cells in the synovial stroma and may adopt a diffuse or localised appearance. Localised lesions arising in a tendon are known as giant cell tumours of tendon sheath: these are commonest in the fingers and show a predilection for females. The pigmentation, which is characteristic, represents extensive haemosiderin deposition which results from haemorrhage into the lesion.

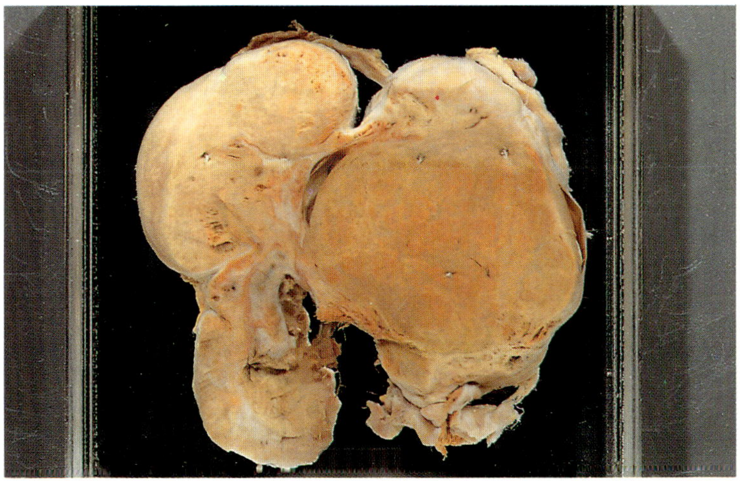

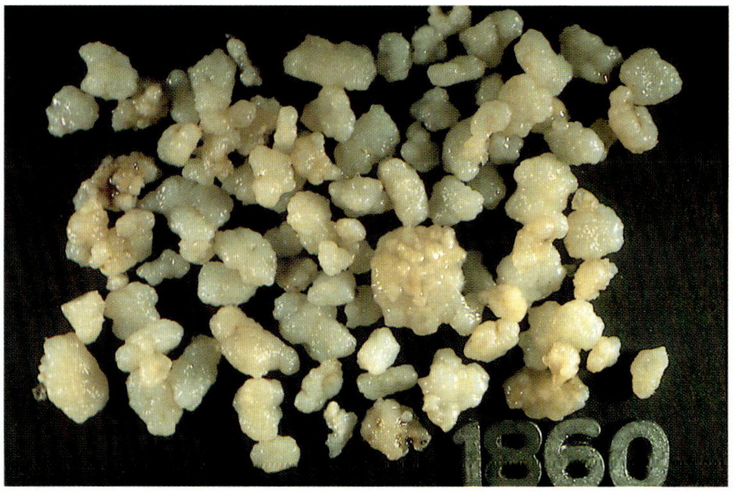

10.145 Knee Joint: Pigmented Villonodular Tenosynovitis

This specimen was excised from a 25-year-old man, who presented with a 2 year history of swelling of the right knee. Examination revealed a blood-stained joint effusion and a mass in the suprapatellar pouch, which was adherent to the quadriceps tendon anteriorly.

The specimen consists of a large lobulated mass, measuring 12 × 12 × 5cm, over which part of the quadriceps tendon is attached (top right). The cut surface of the mass shows multiple foci of brownish pigmentation, cystic degeneration and fibrosis. At the lower aspect, several villous synovial processes, which projected into the knee joint, are apparent.

This is an example of a very large localised lesion in this disease. Macroscopically it bears a close resemblance to a giant cell tumour of tendon sheath, which is rarely seen at this site, thus demonstrating that the two entities are closely related variants of one spectrum.

10.146 Joint: Synovial Chondromatosis

No clinical details are available.

The specimen consists of innumerable, glassy cartilaginous loose bodies that have been removed from a joint space.

Synovial chondromatosis is a fairly uncommon disorder, which typically presents in adulthood and is commonest in the knee or hip: it is usually monoarticular. This condition is characterised by multifocal proliferation of rather immature cartilage in the synovium or tendon sheath of a joint. The cartilaginous nodules which develop commonly fragment, giving rise to numerous loose bodies in the joint. Local recurrence following excision is common, but malignant change, for all practical purposes, does not occur. However, histological distinction from well differentiated chondrosarcoma can be extremely difficult. (Courtesy of Dr. P.G. Bullough, Hospital for Special Surgery, New York)

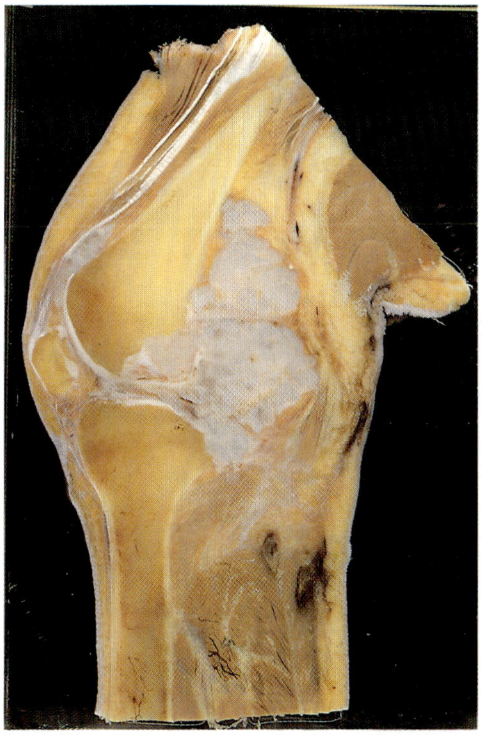

10.147 Knee Joint: Synovial Chondrosarcoma

This is an amputation specimen from a 40-year-old male, who presented with a 2 year history of swelling of the left knee. A tumour measuring 8cm in diameter, was excised from the suprapatellar pouch and was thought to represent synovial chondromatosis. However the lesion rapidly recurred and extended into the popliteal fossa, necessitating a further excision. Four years after the original onset, the mass had recurred again and now involved the entire knee joint and a biopsy was reported as chondrosarcoma.

A sagittal section through the knee joint shows a large, multinodular, bluish translucent tumour in the popliteal fossa. Neoplastic tissue is also visible in the suprapatellar pouch (top left) and the lesion has invaded both the lower end of the femur and the head of the tibia.

Primary synovial chondrosarcoma is a very rare neoplasm which has only been reported to arise in the knee joint of middle-aged males. It is generally a fairly low grade neoplasm, biopsies of which may be easily confused with synovial chondromatosis. It is considered unlikely that these lesions arise in a pre-existent benign tumour. However, histological distinction between the two is exceedingly difficult.

11. NERVOUS SYSTEM

CRANIAL MENINGES

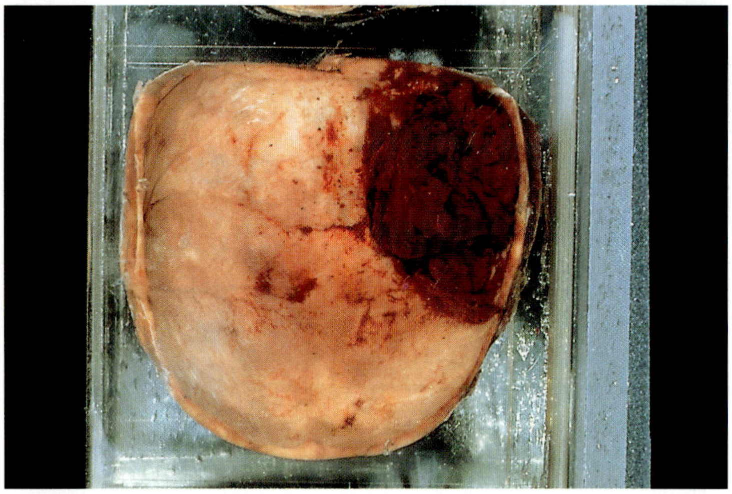

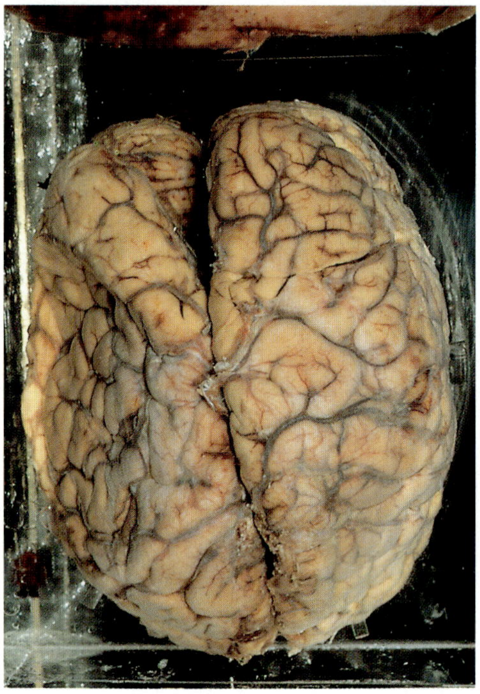

11.1 Calvaria and Brain: Extradural Haematoma

This is a post-mortem specimen from an 80-year-old man who fell in the street and knocked his head. He was detained in hospital for 3 days and then returned home. Three weeks later he fell again and died following a quite separate subdural haemorrhage.

The calvaria (11.1a) has been stripped of the dura to reveal an extensive, dark red organising haematoma occupying much of the right side. In the fresh state, there was a fracture of the temporal bone which extended into the parietal bone. The brain (11.1b) shows marked compression of the right cerebral hemisphere, particularly in the parietal area, corresponding to the overlying haematoma. The separate, more recent subdural haemorrhage is not shown.

Extradural haemorrhages are relatively uncommon, but typically result from trauma to one of the meningeal arteries (most often the middle one) commonly associated with an overlying skull fracture. The prognosis is generally poor, since there is often coexistent damage to the cerebral cortex, but symptoms of raised intracranial pressure may be delayed or absent in the elderly where the brain is relatively atrophic.

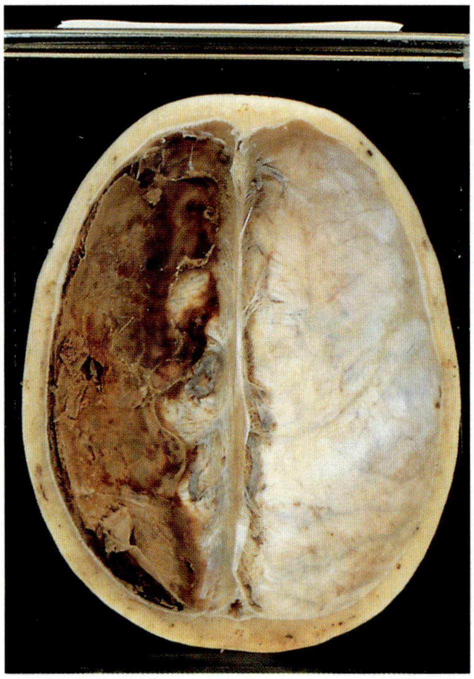

11.2 Skull: Chronic Subdural Haematoma

This is a post-mortem specimen from an 86-year-old man who died following a recent history of weakness and several falls.

The vault of the skull shows extensive haemorrhage beneath the dura on the right side, which has organised to form an irregular layer of blood clot. Note also the false subdural membrane on the internal aspect of the haematoma.

Subdural haemorrhages are fairly common, particularly in association with head injuries even if the latter are seemingly minor. They usually result from a shearing tear in one of the cerebral veins at its junction with a venous sinus. While brisk haemorrhage may lead to a rapid rise in intracranial pressure, bleeding may be gradual (but progressive) over a period of weeks. This gives rise to a chronic haematoma, the symptoms of which may not be related by the patient or clinician to the original injury and hence this treatable lesion may go undetected.

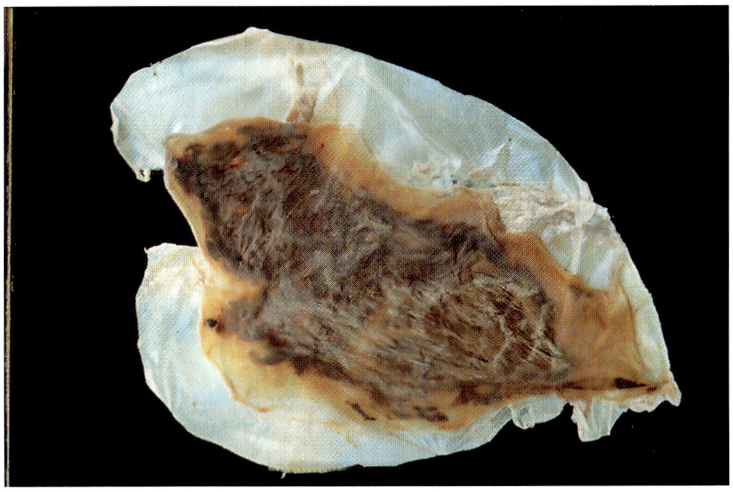

11.3 Dura Mater: Organised Chronic Subdural Haematoma

This is a post-mortem specimen from an 82-year-old woman who died of unrelated causes, having been bedridden for the last 12 months.

This portion of dura mater, which has been stripped from the skull vault shows a rust-coloured area of fibrous tissue adherent to its inner surface, which represents a completely organised small subdural haemorrhage.

This case serves to demonstrate that subdural haemorrhages may not only be delayed in presentation but on occasion may remain completely undetected and asymptomatic.

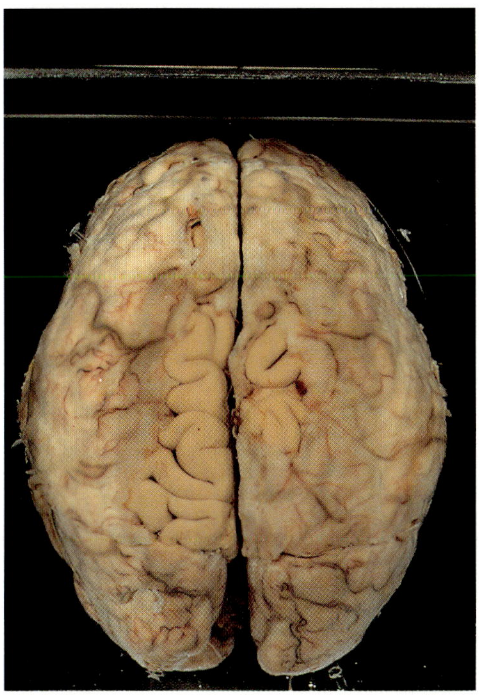

11.4 Brain: Pneumococcal Meningitis

This is a post-mortem specimen from a 77-year-old man who was found in a severely confused state and died shortly after admission to hospital.

The cerebral hemispheres, viewed from above, show a florid, greenish purulent exudate particularly over the frontal lobes. The superficial blood vessels are engorged and there is obvious gyral flattening, a consequence of the patient's cerebral oedema.

Suppurative leptomeningitis is commonest in the young or the very old and may complicate a septicaemic illness or local infection (e.g. sinusitis or otitis media). Direct spread from inhaled organisms in the nasopharynx is also pathogenetically important. Children and young adults most often develop meningococcal or *Haemophilus influenzae* infection, while pneumococci are most often isolated in infants and the elderly. Neonates may acquire infection (usually streptococci or coliforms) from the maternal genital tract, particularly after a prolonged or traumatic delivery. It should be remembered that, in the immunocompromised individual, almost any organism may be responsible.

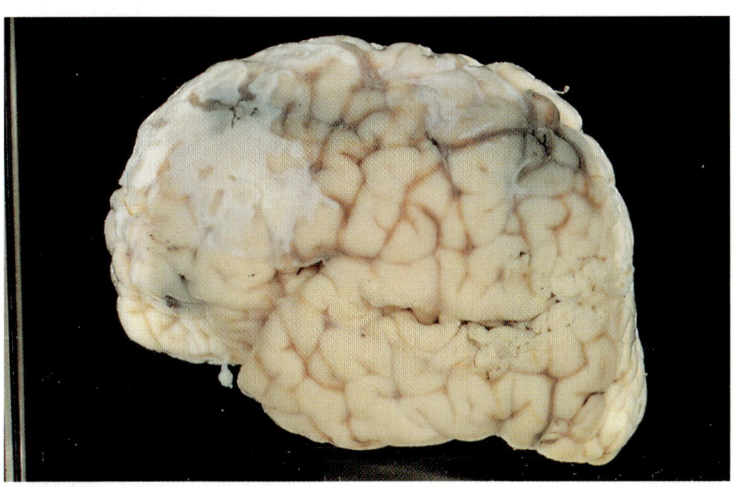

11.5 Brain: Pneumococcal Meningitis

This is a post-mortem specimen from an 8-month-old girl, who was born with a congenital heart defect and was mentally handicapped. She suffered recurrent episodes of pneumonia, the last of which was complicated by the development of meningitis.

The left cerebral hemisphere, viewed from the lateral aspect, shows a thick, pale inflammatory exudate over the frontal and parietal lobes. Note also the gyral flattening due to cerebral oedema.

Meningitis due to *Streptococcus pneumoniae*, which is commonest in young children and the very old, is most often a complication of pulmonary or middle ear infection. Despite modern antimicrobial chemotherapy it still carries a significant mortality.

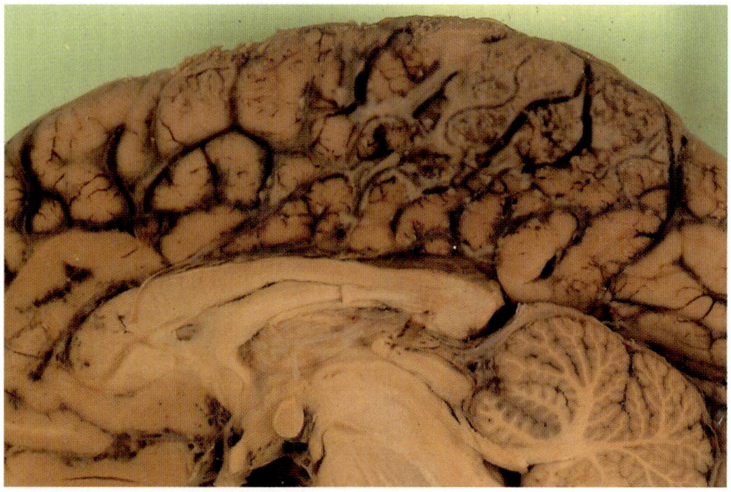

11.6 Tuberculous Meningitis

No clinical details are available.

Over the parietal lobe of this cerebral hemisphere, viewed from the medial aspect, there is a dense, greyish-white inflammatory exudate associated with numerous discrete tubercles. Note that the exudate is most marked along the course of adjacent blood vessels.

Tuberculous meningitis, in the vast majority of cases, represents a complication of miliary infection associated with primary pulmonary disease (see Chapter 2). In this circumstance, children are typically affected. A small proportion of cases result from rupture of a Rich focus (a solitary cerebral tuberculous lesion) into the subarachnoid space. The meningitic process is usually most marked over the base of the brain. Despite modern antituberculous chemotherapy, tuberculous meningitis is still a life-threatening disease. (Courtesy of St. Thomas's Hospital Medical School Museum)

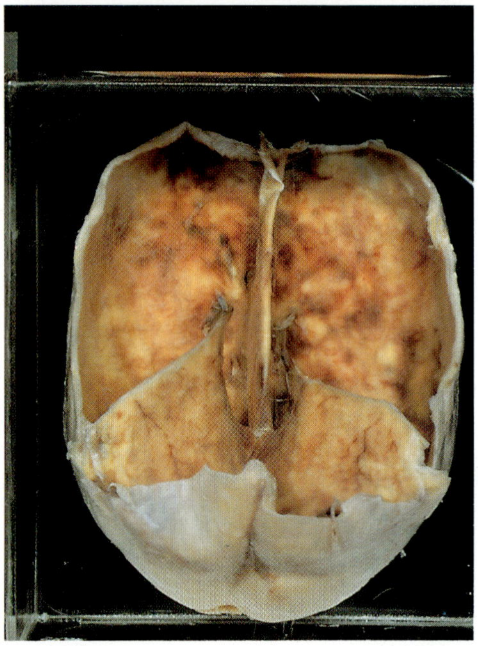

11.7 Dura Mater: Chronic Pachymeningitis

This is a post-mortem specimen from a 72-year-old woman who was found dead. Eight years previously she had undergone a surgical operation on the nasal antrum and recently had begun to complain of repeated attacks of giddiness and severe headaches. At autopsy, in addition to the meningeal lesion, inflammatory exudate was present in the left middle ear.

The dura mater, falx cerebri and tentorium cerebelli are all grossly thickened measuring up to 0.5cm in cross section. Their internal surfaces are congested and have a granular appearance.

Pachymeningitis (inflammation of the dura) is far less common than suppurative leptomeningitis (inflammation of the arachnoid and pia), but is most often associated with trauma to the skull or spinal osteomyelitis. However, spread of infection from the nasal sinuses, middle ear or mastoid air cells may lead to subdural infection, as appears to be the case here. Pachymeningitis may be complicated by the development of an extra- or subdural abscess but chronic infection, as in this case, is very unusual.

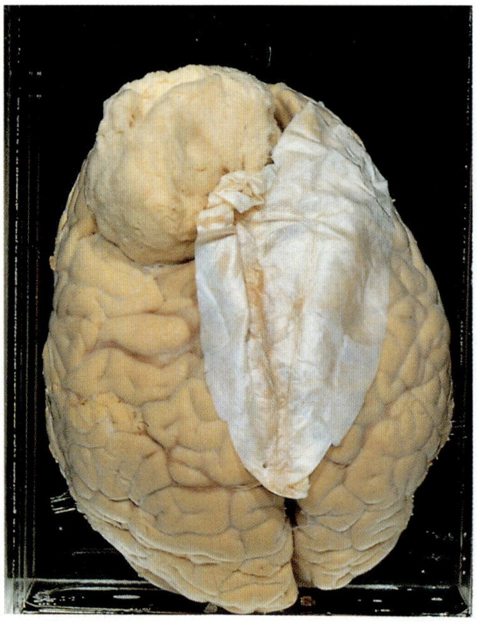

11.8 Brain: Meningioma

This is a post-mortem specimen from a 47-year-old woman who died suddenly; she had recently complained of severe headaches and bouts of depression.

The brain, with a piece of attached dura, is viewed from above to show a large, parasagittal tumour on the left, which measures 7 × 5 × 5cm. The tumour, which is pale in colour, has produced a deep hollow in the left frontal lobe (due to compression atrophy), the full extent of which is not readily apparent in this picture.

Meningiomas are the commonest primary neoplasm of the central nervous system and arise from arachnoid endothelium, often close to the dural venous sinuses. They are slow-growing lesions which typically present in late adulthood, affecting females rather more than males. Frequently, they remain asymptomatic and are found incidentally at autopsy. Their most common site of origin is adjacent to the superior sagittal sinus, but they may arise wherever arachnoid endothelium is present. The vast majority run an entirely benign course although local invasion of the adjacent cranial bone is a well-recognised feature. Recurrence may complicate incomplete primary excision.

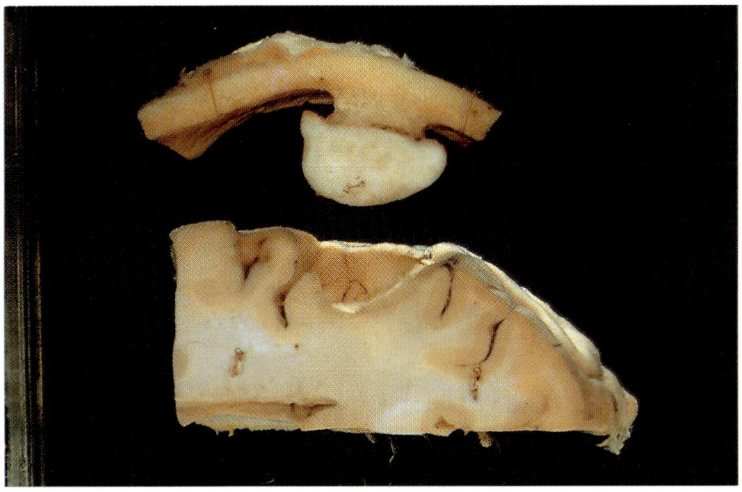

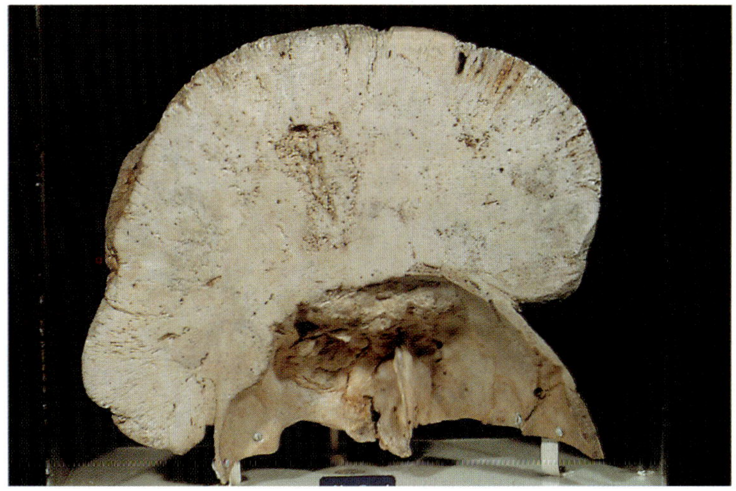

11.9 Dura Mater: Meningioma

This was an incidental finding at post-mortem in an 86-year-old woman who died of cerebral infarction.

A portion of the left parietal lobe with the corresponding segment of overlying skull and dura are shown. Projecting from the inner aspect of the dura is a rounded, pale tumour, measuring 2cm in maximum diameter. Note that the adjacent bone shows reactive hyperostosis. The underlying cerebral cortex shows a corresponding depression.

The frequency with which these tumours remain asymptomatic is surprisingly high. Reactive hyperostosis of the adjacent skull, at the site of local invasion, is a common feature and may provide a radiological pointer to the underlying tumour.

11.10 Skull: Meningioma

This is a post-mortem specimen from a 40-year-old man who had noticed a gradually enlarging swelling over his occiput for about 10 years. Recently the mass had become so large that he had needed to lie down owing to the weight of the tumour; he had also developed headaches and diplopia. Latterly he suffered severe respiratory problems, for which no cause could be found, and he died.

The left side of the base of the skull shows a dural meningioma (below) which has extensively infiltrated the occipital, temporal and parietal lobes. Massive reactive hyperostosis has accompanied this invasion of bone: the new bone shows a typical radial trabecular pattern at its periphery.

It is well recognised that, on occasion, meningiomas (benign or malignant) may penetrate the full thickness of the skull and this is particularly true of tumours located at the base of the brain. A more common circumstance in which these tumours may become apparent in the scalp is when they recur locally, following craniotomy when the skull flap has not been completely closed.

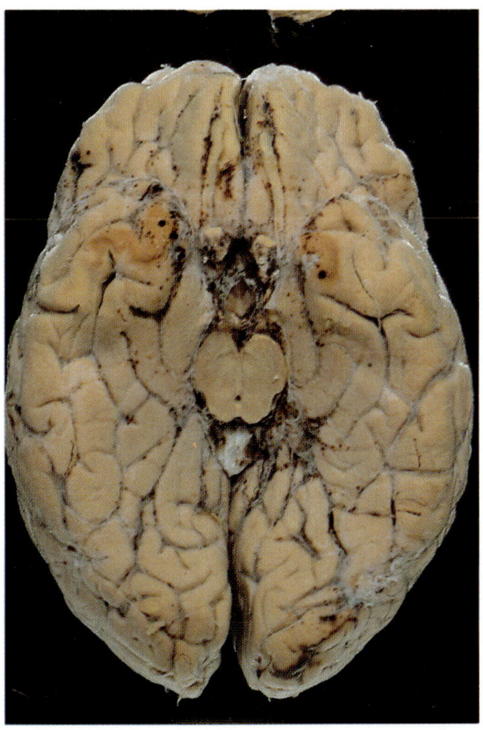

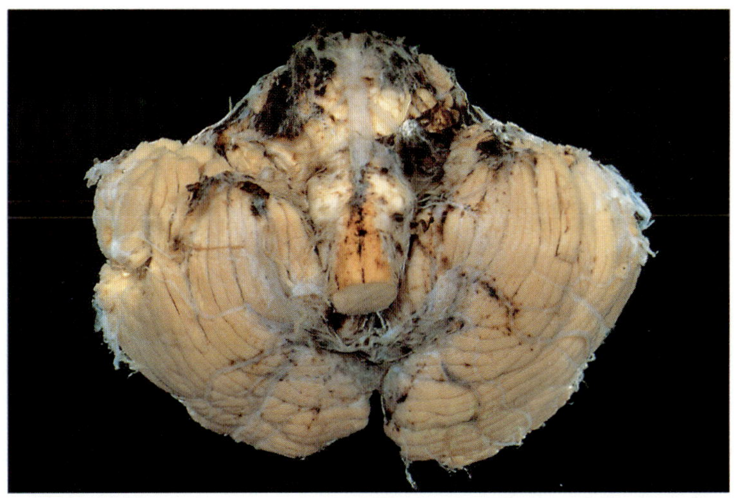

11.11 Meninges: Metastatic Malignant Melanoma

This is a post-mortem specimen from a 60-year-old man who presented with severe dyspnoea and chest pain; he rapidly developed multifocal bone pain, became anorexic and died 10 weeks later. Autopsy revealed metastatic melanomatous deposits in the lungs, liver, skeleton, lymph nodes, serous cavities and meninges. The primary tumour was found to be an inconspicuous ulcerated cutaneous lesion on the chest wall.

Scattered in the pia-arachnoid over the base of the brain (11.11a) are small pigmented nodules which form larger, confluent masses about the pons and brain stem (11.11b). Note that these metastases are largely situated near small blood vessels.

Meningeal involvement by metastatic cutaneous malignant melanoma is a common finding in fatal cases. It should also be remembered that, more rarely, primary meningeal melanomas may arise from the scattered melanocytes which normally exist in the leptomeninges (see Figure and Legend 11.12).

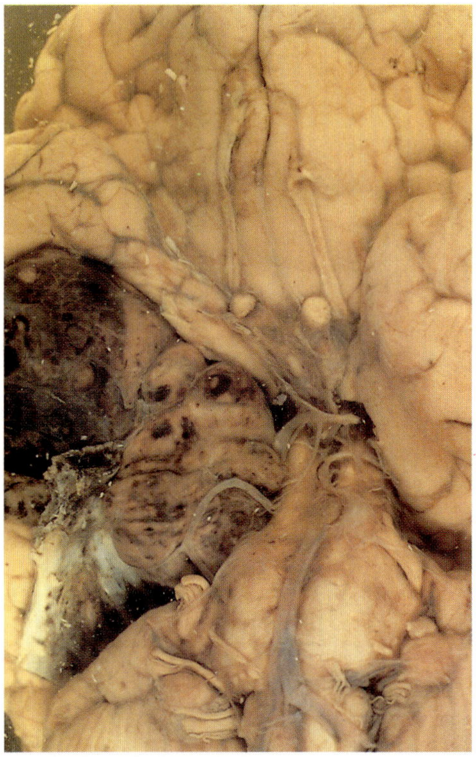

11.12 Meninges: Primary Malignant Melanoma

This is a post-mortem specimen from a 28-year-old man, who presented with a 6 week history of weakness in the legs and left arm, associated with difficulty in swallowing. More recently he had developed severe headaches and vomiting. An intracranial tumour was diagnosed and treated with radiotherapy, but his symptoms recurred and, despite further treatment, the patient died 22 months later.

Arising from the leptomeninges over the right temporal lobe (viewed inferiorly) is a multinodular, heavily pigmented mass which is compressing the mid-brain. There was also invasion of the brain substance and dissemination throughout the ventricular system (not seen in this view).

As already stated, primary meningeal malignant melanoma is much rarer than metastatic spread from a cutaneous melanoma. However, young or middle-aged adults are typically affected and the prognosis is uniformly poor. (Courtesy of St. Thomas's Hospital Medical School Museum)

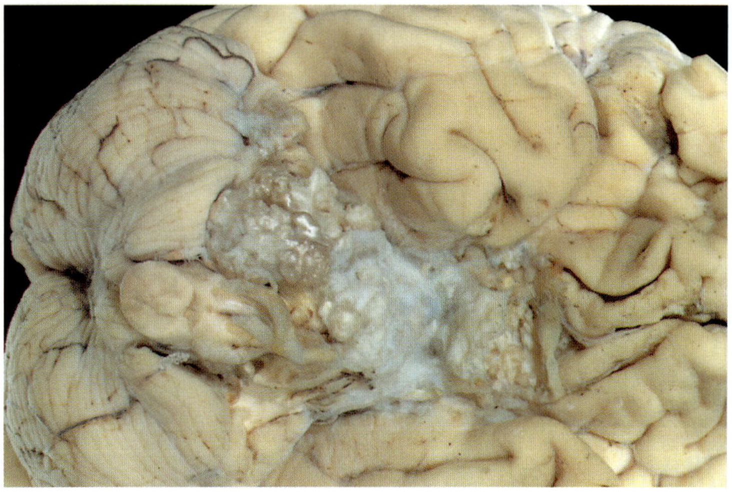

11.13 Meninges: Epidermoid Cyst

This was an incidental finding at post-mortem in a 61-year-old man who died of a myocardial infarct.

At the base of the brain, an irregular pearly-white and yellowish multilocular mass can be seen extending from the region of the pituitary stalk to the right lateral aspect of the brain stem.

Intracranial epidermoid cysts (or so-called cholesteatomata) are relatively rare lesions derived from ectopic squamous epithelium. They are most often located in the region of the pituitary or the cerebellopontine angle and, if symptomatic, typically present in adulthood. The macroscopic appearances in this case are characteristic.

BRAIN

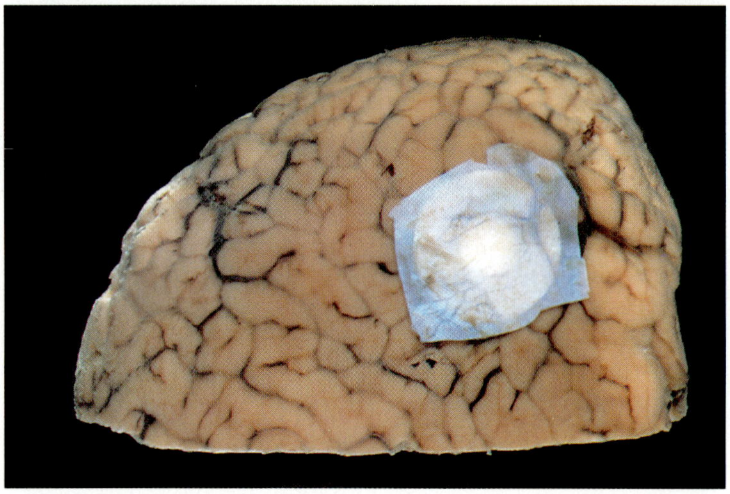

11.14 Microgyria

This is a post-mortem specimen from a 7-month-old child, who was born with an Arnold-Chiari malformation and a lumbar myelocele. The infant died of an upper respiratory tract infection, having undergone two surgical attempts to treat the hydrocephalus.

The posterior portion of the left cerebral hemisphere shows an abnormal gyral pattern, the majority being small with shallow sulci. A Forest disc with adherent dura (remaining from the first attempt to treat the hydrocephalus) is embedded in the brain surface.

When abnormally small gyri are present, they are usually increased in number (micropolygyria), but this may only be apparent histologically. This is a congenital anomaly, which tends to affect the cerebral cortex rather than the cerebellum, and may represent either a failure of neuroblastic development or migration, or the effects of intrauterine hypoxia or ischaemia. Congenital infection with cytomegalovirus or toxoplasmosis may produce a similar appearance. The clinical features are very variable.

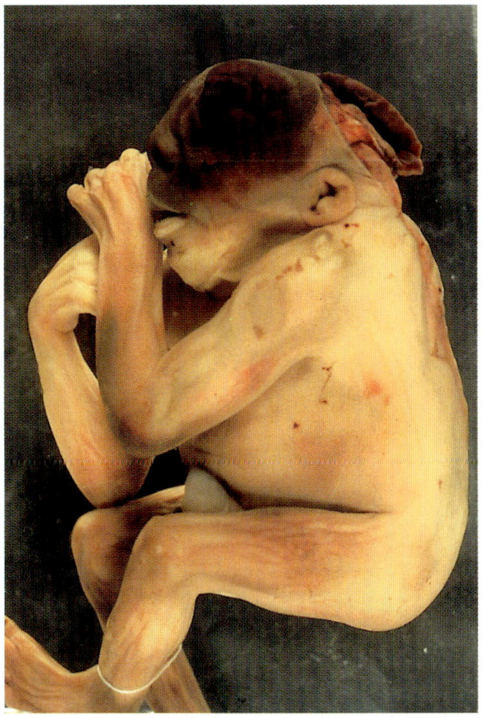

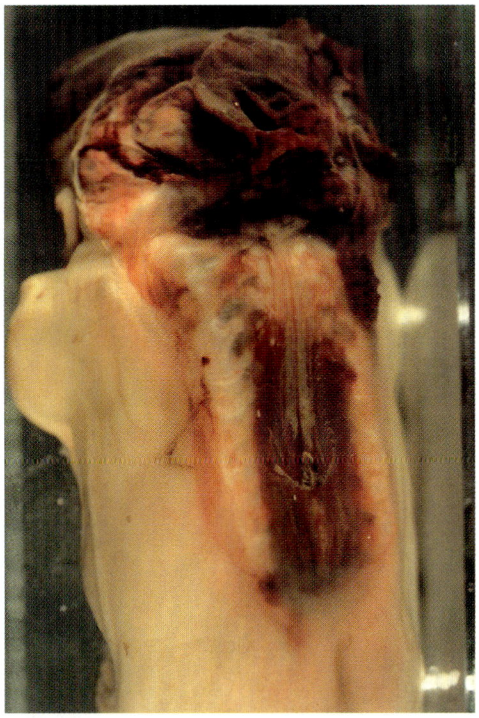

11.15 Anencephaly

No clinical details regarding this stillborn infant are available.

The lateral view of this fetus (11.15a) shows complete absence of the calvaria, associated with shallow orbits, leading to exophthalmos. The ear is also abnormally shaped and located. A posterior view (11.15b) shows the cerebrum to be replaced by a red, friable mass of vascular tissue. In addition there is complete craniorrhachischisis.

Anencephaly is a not uncommon congenital malformation, which shows a predilection for female fetuses and often leads to spontaneous abortion or stillbirth. While its pathogenesis is unknown, the same factors regarded as important in spina bifida (see Legend 11.61) may be implicated. There is frequently coexistent pulmonary hypoplasia or spina bifida and the mother may present with polyhydramnios. (Courtesy of St. Thomas's Hospital Medical School Museum)

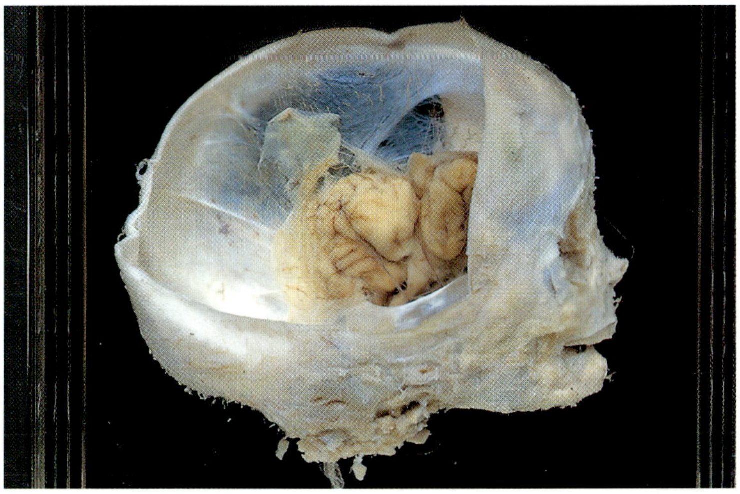

11.16 Hydranencephaly

No clinical details are available.

The head of a small infant has been dissected to show that much of the cranial cavity is filled by a large, thin-walled sac, which in the fresh state was filled with cerebrospinal fluid. All that remains of the brain are very small, cystic cerebral hemispheres and a relatively normal cerebellum and brain stem.

Hydranencephaly is an uncommon malformation which results from an impaired blood supply from the internal carotid arteries *in utero*, due either to spasm, occlusion or atresia. Hence massive cerebral infarction occurs. While the majority of infants die shortly after birth, a few survive for some time in a severely underdeveloped and quadriparetic state.

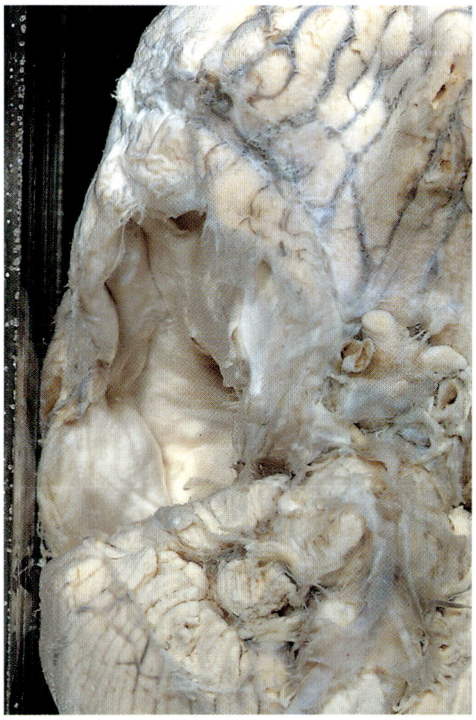

11.17 Porencephaly

This is a post-mortem specimen from a 28-year-old man who died following an operation for a perforated gastric ulcer. He had been severely mentally handicapped and suffered from epilepsy.

At the base of the brain, a large cavity lined by pia-arachnoid replaces much of the right temporal lobe and communicates directly with the subjacent lateral ventricle.

Porencephaly, characterised by a cystic defect in the brain substance, may result from a localised intra-uterine vascular lesion (as in hydranencephaly see Legend 11.16) or may represent a developmental abnormality in cerebral cleavage and migration. In the latter group the defect is most often bilateral and symmetrical.

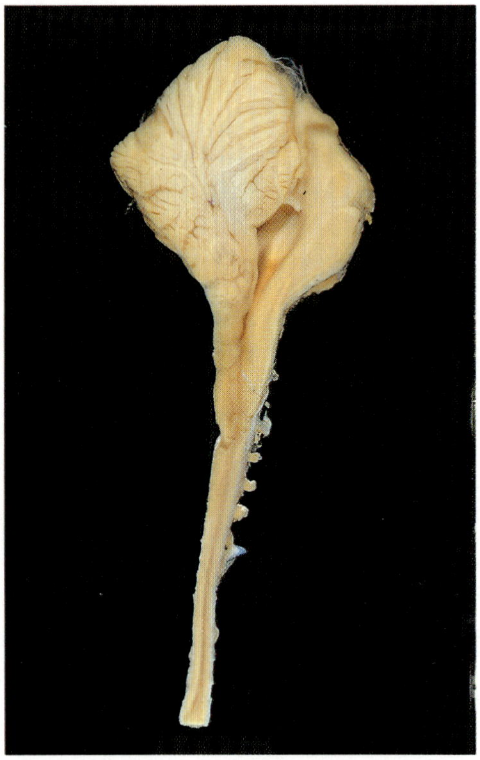

11.18 Brain: Hydrocephalus with Arnold-Chiari Malformation

This is a post-mortem specimen from a 9-month-old baby girl who was born with spina bifida and a mild degree of hydrocephalus, which rapidly increased. There was also bilateral talipes equinovarus. Eventually the lumbothoracic myelocele ulcerated and ruptured and a week later she died.

This is a sagittal section through the hind-brain and upper spinal cord. The cerebellum, which is poorly lobulated, extends as a mid-line process down the spinal canal over a distance of 2cm. The pons is elongated, but entirely intracranial, while the majority of the medulla is located intraspinally. The cerebral aqueduct (above) is dilated and the 4th ventricle is narrow and grossly elongated, measuring 3cm in length; the latter terminates in the substance of the medulla, well below the foramen magnum. Note that the upper spinal nerve roots have deviated upwards to reach their intervertebral exit foramina.

The Arnold-Chiari malformation is the commonest cause of congenital hydrocephalus. The intraspinal location of part of the cerebellum and the medulla blocks the foramen magnum so that cerebrospinal fluid cannot leave the 4th ventricle and cerebral aqueduct. This form of non-communicating, internal hydrocephalus leads to a rapid rise in intraventricular pressure with associated separation of the skull bones and cerebral atrophy. The coexistence of a meningomyelocele is almost invariable.

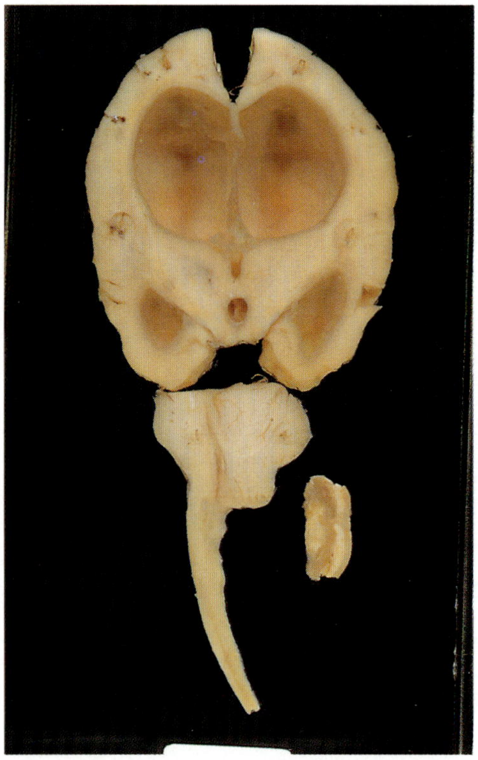

11.19 Hydrocephalus with Arnold-Chiari Malformation

This is a post-mortem specimen from a 1-month-old baby boy who was born with a lumbosacral myelocele. The child was noted to have an increasing head circumference and he died following an episode of respiratory stridor.

This is a coronal section through the cerebral hemispheres and a sagittal section of the hind-brain. The gyral pattern is completely obliterated and the lateral ventricles are grossly dilated with associated cerebral atrophy. The cerebellum is grooved and a narrow cerebellar tongue and the majority of the medulla are intraspinal.

The finding of a meningomyelocele at birth should always raise the possibility of a coexistent Arnold-Chiari malformation. This case demonstrates well the effects of internal hydrocephalus.

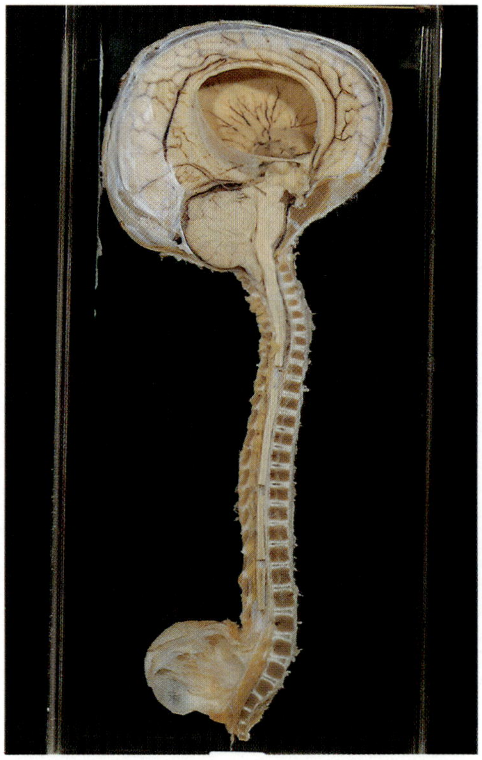

11.20 Hydrocephalus with Arnold-Chiari Malformation and Meningomyelocele

This is a post-mortem specimen from a 6-month-old baby girl, who was born with hydrocephalus and a large lumbar meningomyelocele. Ventriculography revealed an Arnold-Chiari malformation and, at 5 months of age, a Spitz-Holter valve was inserted. The surgical wound became infected and she died one month later with florid osteomyelitis of the sternum and ribs.

This is a sagittal section through the skull and vertebral column to show the left side of the brain and cord. There is gross dilatation of the lateral and 3rd ventricles with marked cerebral atrophy. The cerebellum shows a long spinal process and the medulla is markedly elongated (being largely intraspinal). There is hydromyelia of the spinal cord, which terminates in a meningomyelocele at the level of the lumbar vertebrae.

This is a classical example, showing both malformations which commonly coexist.

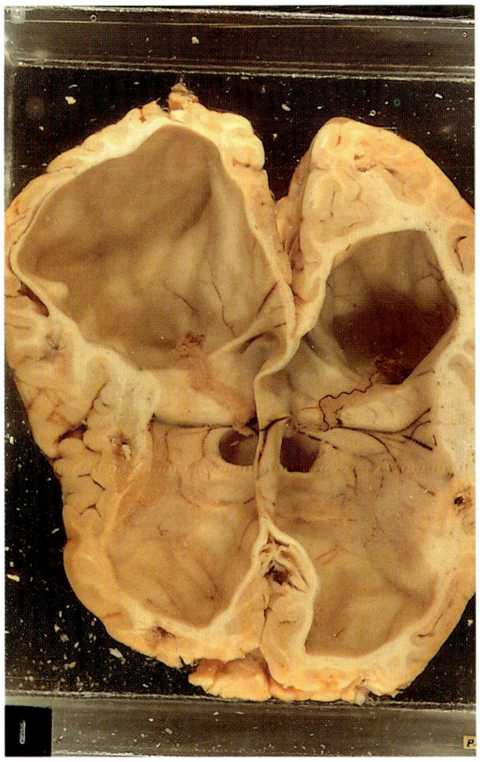

11.21 Communicating Hydrocephalus

This is a post-mortem specimen from 1-year-old boy, who had developed progressive enlargement of the skull over the previous 4 months. He had become increasingly irritable, constipated and was noticed to have staring eyes and a squint. An air encephalogram demonstrated internal hydrocephalus which was relieved by insertion of a Spitz-Holter valve. The latter, however, became occluded and he died shortly afterwards.

A horizontal section through the child's brain shows massive dilatation of the lateral ventricles and foramina of Monro, associated with gross cortical atrophy. Not apparent in this view are dense leptomeningeal adhesions which were found over much of the base of the brain.

Communicating hydrocephalus is usually a post-infective (most often meningitic) phenomenon, which results from the development of adhesions in the region of the subarachnoid cisterns, thus preventing the upward flow of cerebrospinal fluid to the arachnoid villi in the sagittal sinus. No preceding episode of meningitis or any other relevant illness could be identified in this case. (Courtesy of St. Thomas's Hospital Medical School Museum)

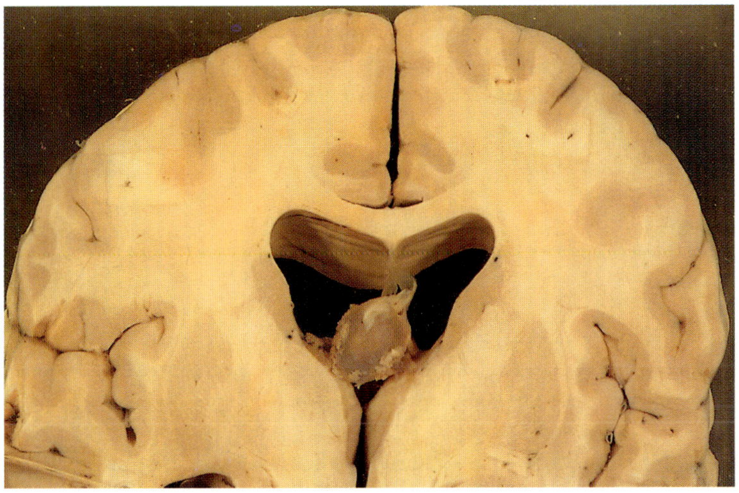

11.22 Colloid Cyst of the Third Ventricle

This is a post-mortem specimen from an adult male who presented with a 12 year history of intermittent headaches, associated with vomiting. Examination revealed papilloedema, but the day before the patient was due for operation, he had a series of fits and died.

Arising from the septum pellucidum is a small, smooth cyst, measuring 1.5cm in diameter. Note the marked dilatation of the lateral ventricles but a normally sized third ventricle. This suggests that the cyst, which was mobile, intermittently obstructed the foramina of Monro leading to hydrocephalus.

Colloid cysts of the third ventricle are very uncommon developmental anomalies, derived either from the diencephalon or the roof of the third ventricle. They are typically solitary lesions which are well known to cause intermittent hydrocephalus (usually in adulthood) as a consequence of their anatomical location. (Courtesy of St. Thomas's Hospital Medical School Museum)

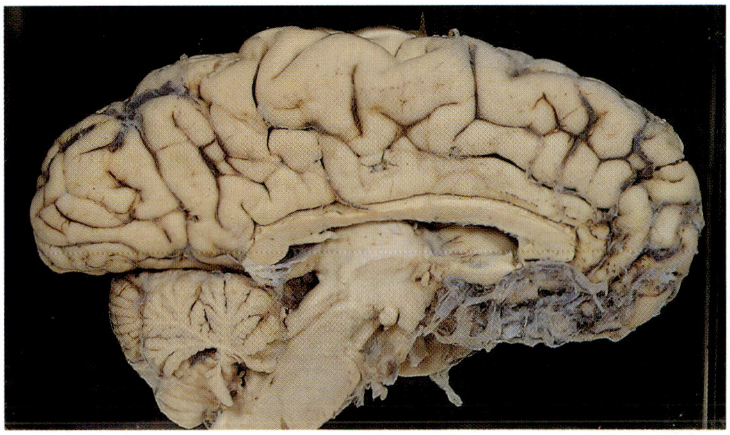

11.23 Arteriovenous Malformation

No clinical details are available.

A medial sagittal section of the brain shows a tangled mass of tortuous vessels in the leptomeninges over the subcallosal area. Histologically these proved to be a mixture of arteries and veins.

Intracranial arteriovenous malformations are relatively uncommon congenital lesions, which are most often posteriorly located (involving the great vein of Galen and one of the posterior cerebral arteries). The development of similar anomalies anteriorly is, however, well recognised. Important complications include the development of high-output cardiac failure and cerebral symptoms (dependent upon the site and extent of the malformation).

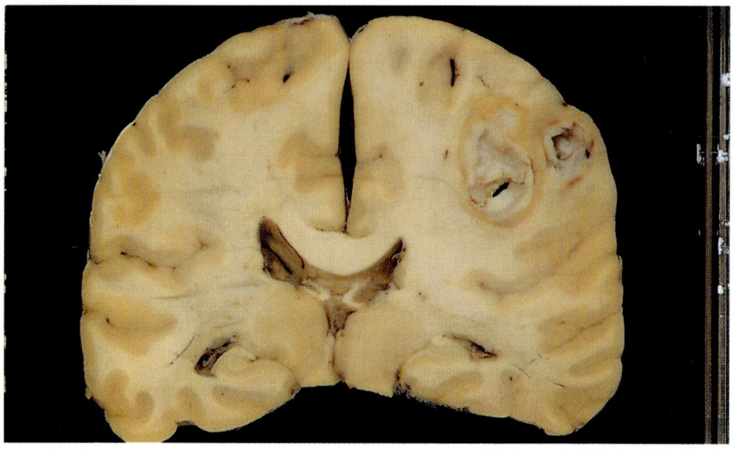

11.24 Cerebral Abscess

This is a post-mortem specimen from a 60-year-old man, who had developed multiple staphylococcal carbuncles following an operation for a perforated gastric ulcer. One month later he represented with right-sided pneumonia and shortly afterwards, suffered a series of epileptiform fits. His condition improved temporarily with antibiotic treatment but 2 months later he died.

A coronal section through the brain shows a multilocular abscess cavity, measuring 2cm in diameter, located in the left parietal lobe. The cavity contains purulent debris. Note that persistent cerebral oedema (due to this inflammatory process) has resulted in marked gyral flattening.

Cerebral abscesses are most often a consequence of haematogenous spread of infection from a site elsewhere in the body, particularly the lungs or heart. However, local spread of organisms may occur from otitis media, sinusitis or mastoiditis. Those lesions of septicaemic origin are not infrequently multiple and almost any organism may be responsible. Complications include rupture onto the brain's surface (hence meningitis) or into the ventricular system.

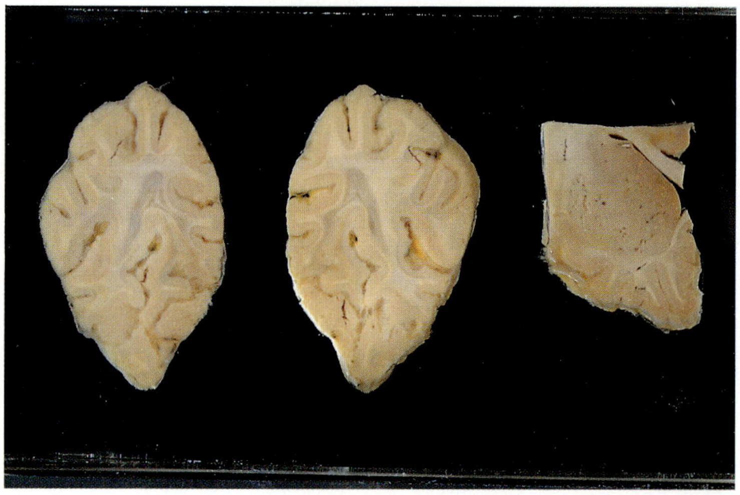

11.25 Cryptococcosis

This is a post-mortem specimen from a 7-year-old boy, who presented with a 4½ month history of progressively severe headaches and drowsiness. Examination revealed marked papilloedema and culture of the cerebrospinal fluid revealed cryptococci. He died soon afterwards.

Three separate sections of the brain show that the sulci are distended by pale, gelatinous material and there are multiple small cystic cavities throughout the cortex and in the region of the basal ganglia.

Cerebral infection with *Cryptococcus neoformans* is most often seen in patients who are immunocompromised (for whatever reason), particularly in those with lymphomas or in individuals receiving cytotoxic treatment. The organism, which is typically transmitted in bird faeces, is usually inhaled and there is often a coexistent focus of pulmonary infection. Despite modern antimicrobial chemotherapy, there is still a significant fatality rate.

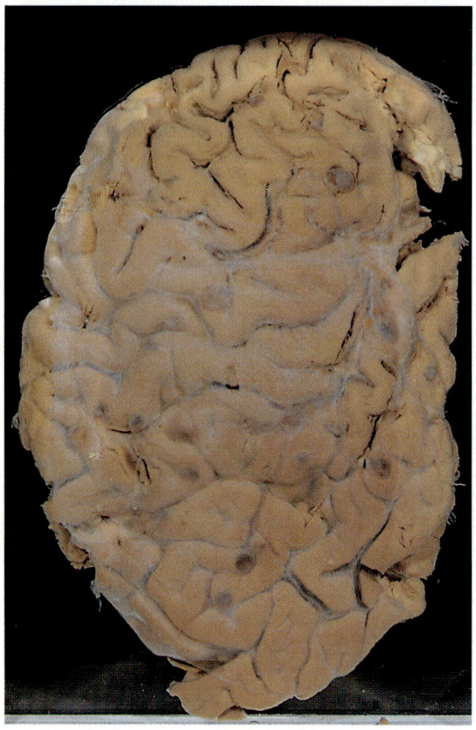

11.26 Cysticercosis

This is a post-mortem specimen from a 30-year-old Indian man who presented with a 2 week history of being unable to walk. Tender nodules were palpable in many of the leg muscles, particularly the calf, and biopsy revealed cysticerci. The patient died 3 months later of lobar pneumonia. At autopsy, cysts were present in many of the skeletal muscles, the heart, pancreas and brain.

The right cerebral hemisphere, which is rather poorly preserved, shows numerous small greyish cysts scattered within the cortex.

Cysticercus cellulosae represents the larval form of the tapeworm *Taenia solium*; the latter, which infests the bowel, is typically derived from pork and is endemic in the Indian subcontinent and South America. The larvae reach other somatic tissues by oro-faecal spread and entry into the portal venous system. Cerebral involvement may either be asymptomatic (as in this case) or may give rise to hydrocephalus or epilepsy.

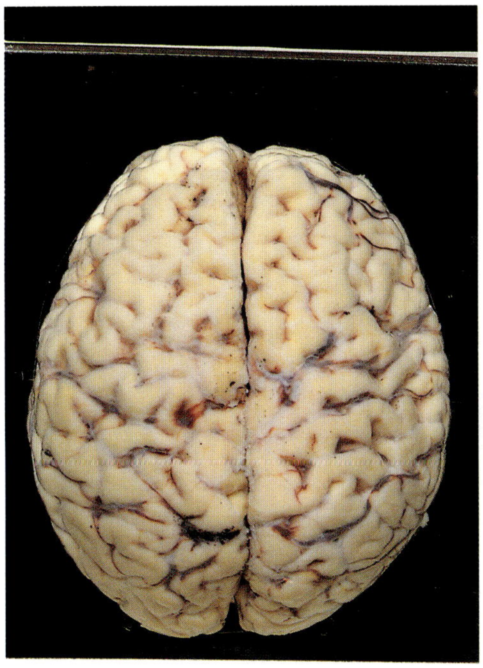

11.27 General Paresis of the Insane

This is a post-mortem specimen from a 49-year-old man who had recently been certified insane and thereafter developed general paralysis. After a euphoric period, he became demented and died of bronchopneumonia.

The superior surface of the brain shows marked gyral atrophy and widening of the sulci particularly over the frontal and parietal lobes. The pia-arachnoid membrane shows multifocal thickening, most marked in the right precentral area.

Syphilitic involvement of the central nervous system may take 3 principal forms (which are not mutually exclusive). In the tertiary stage chronic leptomeningitis and arteritis (with or without gumma formation) may occur; the former was probably responsible for the meningeal thickening in this case. Much later, general paresis (characterised by a florid encephalitis and cerebral atrophy) or tabes dorsalis (typified by dorsal root degeneration and localised atrophy within the cord) may develop. In general, these latter manifestations are commonest in males and tend to present up to 50 years after the primary infection.

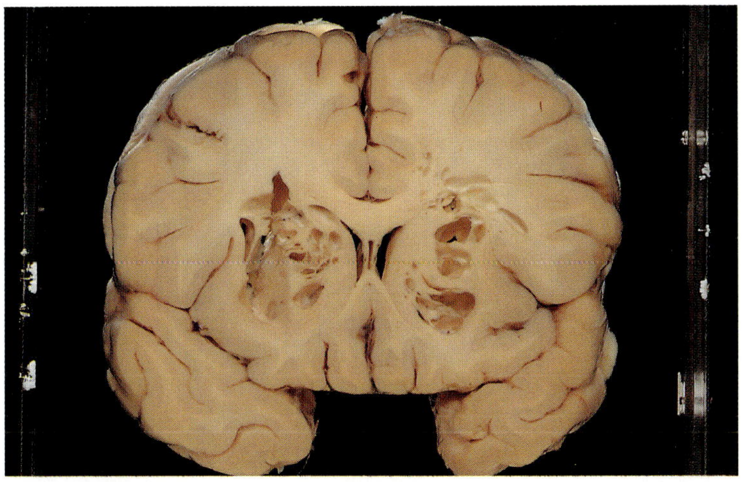

11.28 Post-Mortem Cystic Decomposition

This was an incidental finding in a dissecting room cadaver.

A coronal section through the brain shows a number of small, smooth-walled cysts located mainly around the thalamus on either side. Histological examination of these areas reveals numerous Gram-positive bacilli and no sign whatever of a vital tissue reaction.

This appearance, which may be seen in almost any organ, but which is commonest in the liver, is a frequent post-mortem finding of no actual significance. It simply reflects the spread and activity of gas-forming organisms [most often *Clostridium perfringens (welchii)*] in the devitalised tissues after death.

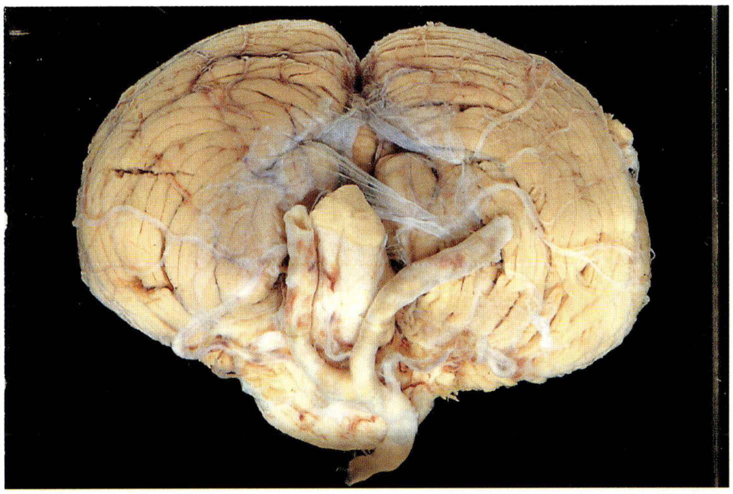

11.29 Hind-Brain: Vertebrobasilar Atheroma

This is a post-mortem specimen from a 67-year-old myxoedematous woman, who died of myocardial infarction.

Over the hind-brain, both vertebral arteries and the proximal portion of the basilar artery show numerous, yellowish atheromatous plaques (clearly visible through the vessel walls); note also the marked vascular tortuosity.

Atheroma is a common finding in the vertebral and basilar arteries particularly with advancing age (see Chapter 1). The clinical significance of this occurrence lies in the fact that associated intraluminal thrombosis may lead to local occlusion or intracerebral embolisation, and that plaque fragments may also enter and obstruct the cerebral circulation: hence vertebrobasilar atheroma is an important cause of cerebral infarction.

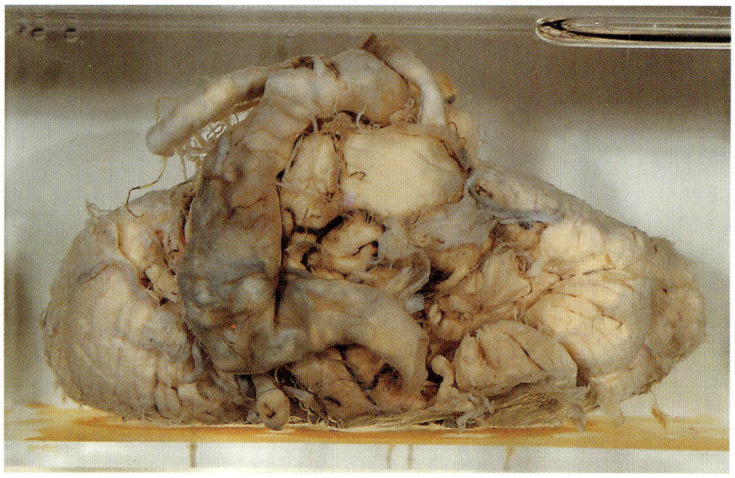

11.30 Hind-Brain: Atheromatous Fusiform Aneurysm of the Basilar Artery

This is a post-mortem specimen from an 88-year-old woman, who had suffered a number of cerebrovascular accidents in the preceding 3 years; she finally collapsed unconscious and died.

At the base of the hind-brain, the basilar and left vertebral arteries show fusiform dilatation and are severely atheromatous. The left vertebral artery is largely occluded by thrombus (upper right).

Aneurysmal dilatation of the vertebrobasilar arteries is a fairly common complication of severe atheroma and develops in the same way as in the systemic arteries elsewhere (see Chapter 1).

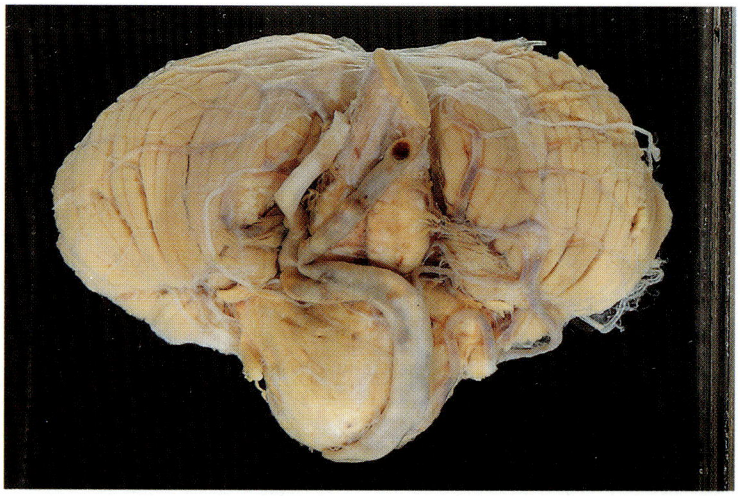

11.31 Hind-Brain: Thrombosis of Right Vertebral Artery

This is a post-mortem specimen from a 73-year-old woman, known to be diabetic and hypertensive, who presented with a 6 week history of dizziness, ataxia, blurred vision and slurred speech. She developed a left-sided hemiplegia and died.

Over the hind-brain, both the basilar and vertebral arteries are extremely tortuous and show severe atheroma. The right vertebral artery is completely occluded by recent dark thrombus over a distance of 2cm, which is well seen at the proximal cut end of the vessel.

This case, which demonstrates a typical thrombosis complicating vertebrobasilar atheroma, testifies to the importance of this condition as a cause of cerebrovascular accidents (see Figure and Legend 11.33 et seq.).

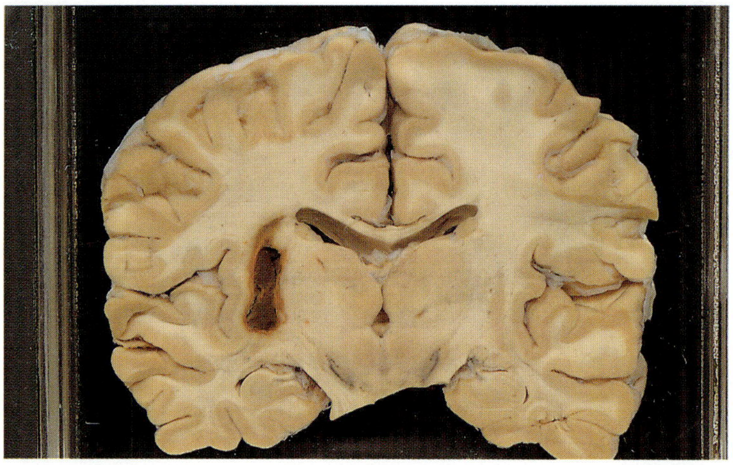

11.32 Old Intracerebral Haemorrhage

This is a post-mortem specimen from a 73-year-old hypertensive woman, who had suffered a cerebrovascular accident with left-sided hemiparesis 5 years previously.

A coronal section through the brain shows an organised, partly cystic area of haemorrhage, which is golden-brown in colour, located in the region of the basal ganglia on the right side. The lesion abuts onto the ipsilateral internal capsule.

Cerebral haemorrhage is less frequent than cerebral infarction as a cause of cerebrovascular accidents ('strokes') at the present time: this is thought to be a result of generally improved control of essential hypertension in most populations. Intracerebral haemorrhage is most often the consequence of rupture of a small atheromatous artery, usually in a hypertensive patient, and is therefore more common with advancing age. The lentiform nucleus, mid-brain or cerebellum are most often affected. It should be noted that vascular rupture is said to occur at the site of Charcot-Bouchard micro-aneurysms, which are a classical feature of hypertensive cerebrovascular disease. Clearly the clinical consequences are very variable, depending largely upon the site and extent of bleeding.

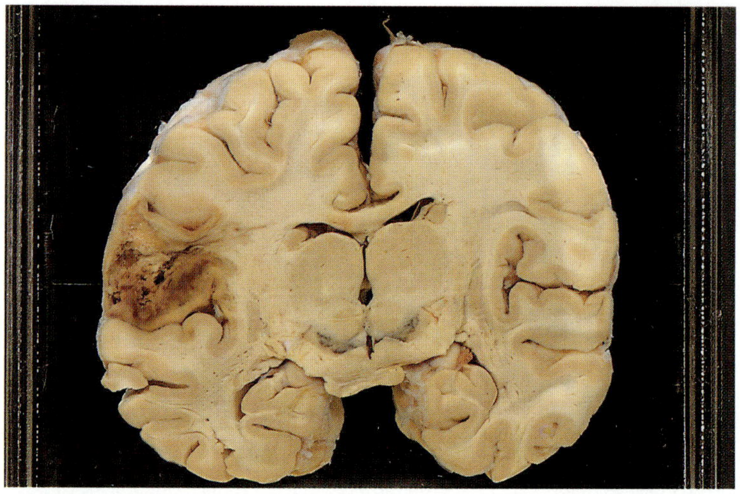

11.33 Recent Cerebral Infarct

This is a post-mortem specimen from a 57-year-old man, who was known to have rheumatic heart disease and atrial fibrillation. He presented with an acute right-sided hemiplegia and died one month later.

A coronal section through the brain at the rear of the frontal lobes, viewed posteriorly, shows a reasonably circumscribed infarct, measuring 2.5cm in diameter, situated in the lower lateral cortex of the left hemisphere. There is central softening and necrosis, with adjacent oedema and congestion.

Cerebral infarction, the commonest cause of cerebrovascular accidents in the Western world, is most often due either to local thrombosis in an atheromatous vessel or to an embolus (composed of thrombus or fragmented plaque), usually derived from the internal carotid or vertebrobasilar arteries or the heart. Other causes of thrombosis such as polycythaemia, hypercoagulability and the oral contraceptive pill are important in some cases. Generally, the elderly tend to be affected and the clinical outcome is very variable. In the case here, endocardial mural thrombus due to the patient's atrial fibrillation was probably the root cause.

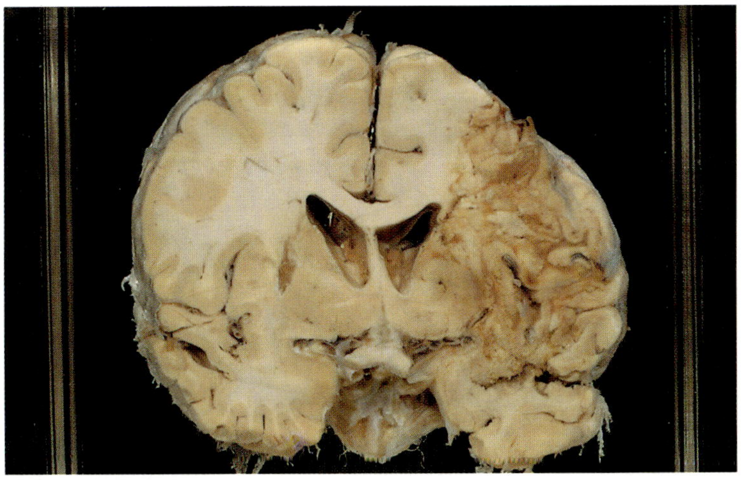

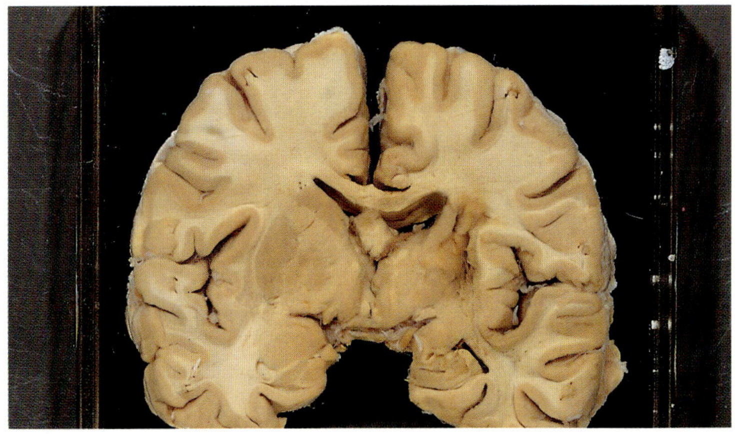

11.34 Extensive Recent Cerebral Infarct

This is a post-mortem specimen from a 75-year-old woman, who had suffered a cerebrovascular accident about one month previously which had resulted in marked mental deterioration.

A coronal section through the brain, at the level of the optic chiasma, shows massive infarction of the left cerebral hemisphere. Note the loss of brain substance, yellowish-red discoloration and extensive softening.

This is a very large cerebral infarct, which clearly resulted from occlusion of a major vessel. Note that the early yellowish liquefaction, seen in this specimen, reflects the start of gradual breakdown of the necrotic cerebral tissue, which is typically seen within a few weeks of infarction.

11.35 Old Cerebral Infarct

This is a post-mortem specimen from a 62-year-old man, who died of a myocardial infarct. Two years before death he had developed a right-sided hemiplegia and was found to have suffered thrombotic occlusion of the left internal carotid artery.

A coronal section through the brain, viewed anteriorly, shows a cystic, shrunken area in the region of the left basal ganglia. The edges of the infarct have a yellowish-brown appearance.

These are the typical appearances of an old, organised cerebral infarct; the discoloured edges are attributable to the accumulation of haemosiderin and lipid within microglial cells (macrophages).

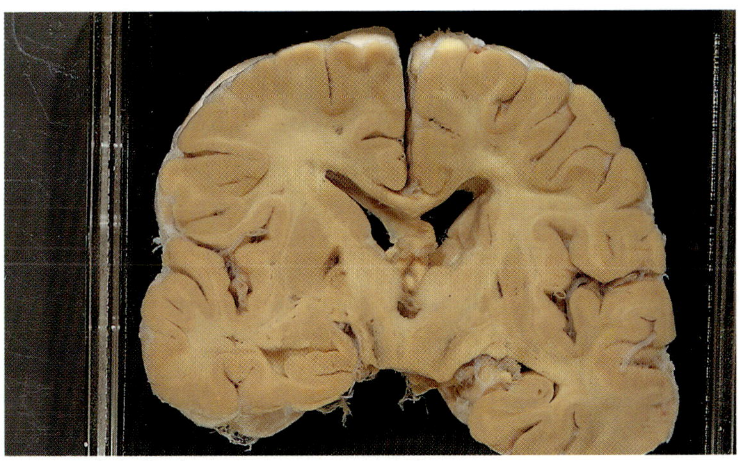

11.36 Multifocal Infarction

This is a post-mortem specimen from a 70-year-old woman, who had developed a left-sided hemiplegia 3 years previously. Latterly she had presented with rapidly progressive Parkinson's disease. At autopsy there was severe atheroma of the anterior and middle cerebral arteries.

A coronal section through the brain shows several small areas of cystic softening in the basal ganglia, most marked in the globus pallidus of the left lentiform nucleus, but also apparent in the right lentiform and caudate nuclei and the left claustrum.

Multiple small infarcts are a fairly uncommon finding but are a well recognised cause of dementia, in addition to the more usual sensorimotor features of a stroke. Occasionally, as here, features of Parkinsonism may develop.

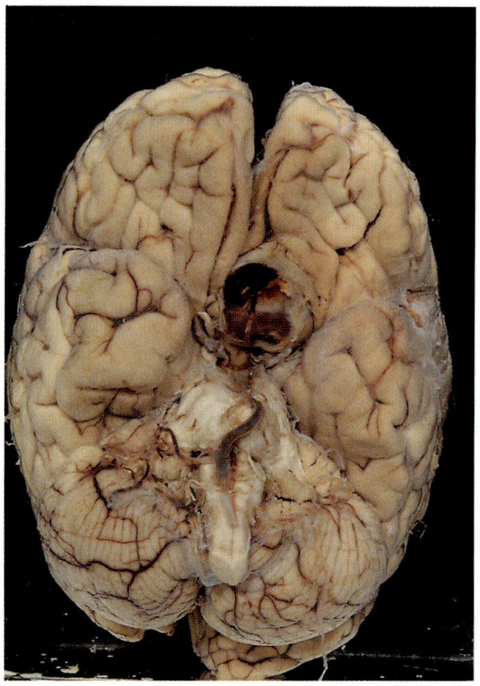

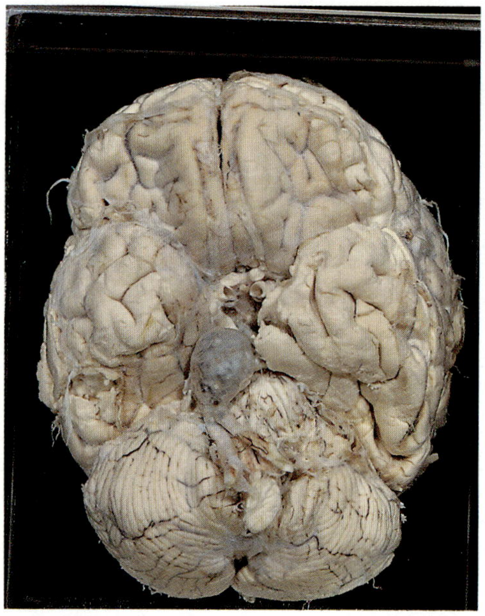

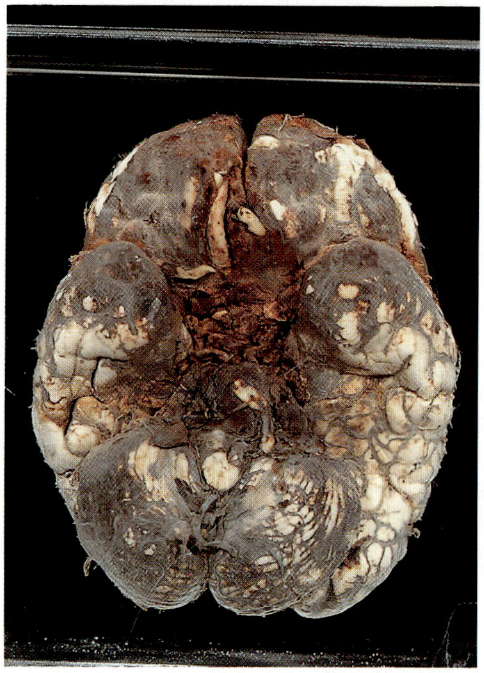

11.37 Berry Aneurysm of the Anterior Communicating Cerebral Artery

This is a post-mortem specimen from a 56-year-old hypertensive woman, who was found dead at her home. Autopsy revealed death to be due to a dissecting aneurysm of the aortic arch which had ruptured into the pleural cavity.

This view of the base of the brain shows an unruptured, saccular aneurysm of the left anterior communicating cerebral artery, which measures 1.5cm in diameter. The aneurysm has been bisected to show the laminated thrombus with which it is filled.

Berry aneurysms are fairly common lesions of the cerebral arterial system, which are said to develop at the site of a congenital defect or weakness in the media. The later development of atheroma may further weaken the vessel wall. These aneurysms, which may be multiple, are more common with increasing age and are seen most frequently around the bifurcations of the circle of Willis, particularly in the middle cerebral artery. They frequently rupture, especially in a hypertensive patient, and as such berry aneurysms are the commonest cause of subarachnoid haemorrhage (see Legend 11.39). As in this case, very many berry aneurysms go undetected in life and are an incidental finding at post-mortem. It is said that the true incidence may be about 2 per cent the adult population.

11.38 Berry Aneurysm of the Bifurcation of the Basilar Artery

This is a post-mortem specimen from a 62-year-old hypertensive man, known to have ischaemic heart disease, who suddenly collapsed and died.

At the junction of the basilar artery with the posterior cerebral and posterior communicating arteries is arising a large saccular aneurysm, which measures 2.5cm in diameter. The bluish colour of the aneurysm reflects discoloration of extensive intraluminal thrombus.

Berry aneurysms of the posterior cerebral vessels are much less common than those situated anteriorly. At whatever site, this example is unusually large, the vast majority of these lesions being less than 2cm in diameter.

11.39 Subarachnoid Haemorrhage

This is a post-mortem specimen from a 77-year-old man. He was thought to have Marfan's syndrome but no further clinical details are available.

Almost the whole base of the brain is covered by extensive haemorrhage, which is located in the subarachnoid space. The vertex (not seen in this view) had a similar appearance. The interpeduncular fossa is completely filled with thick blood clot, beneath which there was thought to be a small berry aneurysm of the circle of Willis.

Subarachnoid haemorrhage is a common cause of sudden death and, in the vast majority of cases, results from rupture of a cerebral berry aneurysm (see Legends 11.37 et seq.), often in a hypertensive patient. Adults in the 5th and 7th decades of either sex, are typically affected and the principal sites of bleeding reflect the topographical incidence of the underlying aneurysm. Trauma is an infrequent cause in adulthood but is probably the principal aetiological factor in neonatal cases (premature infants or those requiring an instrumental delivery being most often affected).

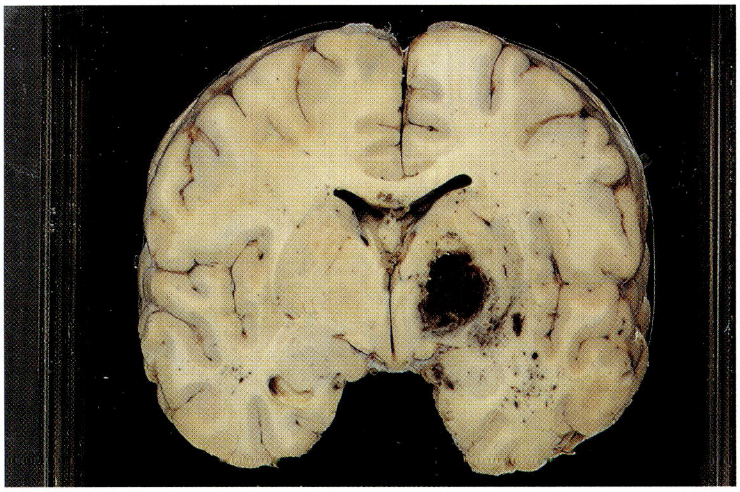

11.40 Traumatic Intracerebral Haemorrhage

This is a post-mortem specimen from a 34-year-old man, who was admitted to hospital in an unconscious state following an accident in a motorcycle race. Bleeding from the left ear was noted and following a series of tonic fits, he died shortly afterwards.

A coronal section through the brain shows extensive haemorrhage in the region of the internal capsule on the left side. Note the adjacent smaller punctate haemorrhages.

These appearances are typical of a severe non-penetrating head injury, of which the commonest cause is a road traffic accident of some kind. The frontal and temporal lobes are most often affected; the two principal pathogenetic factors are shearing of small blood vessels and forcible contact with sharp or irregular portions of the internal aspect of the cranium.

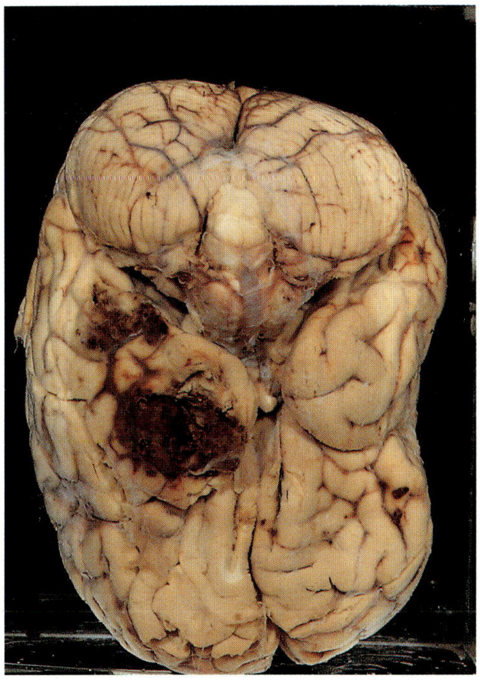

11.41 Traumatic Cerebral Haemorrhage

This is a post-mortem specimen from a 46-year-old man who was a known epileptic and also an alcoholic. He suffered a grand mal fit, fell, injured the right side of his head and died shortly thereafter. At autopsy there was also a right-sided extradural haemorrhage.

The base of the brain shows extensive laceration of the inferior surface of the left temporal lobe with associated haemorrhage.

Since the primary injury was to the right side of the head, the features here are those of a contrecoup injury: in other words, as the head was propelled laterally and then decelerated, the opposite cortex was torn from the small arachnoid vessels and perhaps damaged on the sphenoid ridge. It should be remembered that the contrecoup injury is often more extensive or severe than that of the coup (i.e. the primary impact) in cases of head injury.

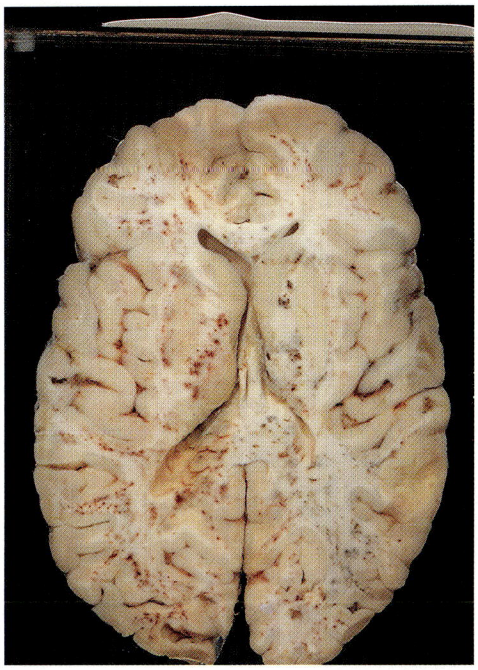

11.42 Fat Embolism

This is a post-mortem specimen from a 45-year-old man, who had been admitted to hospital 5 days previously with multiple injuries (including fractures) following a road traffic accident. He became comatose, jaundiced and died. At autopsy, in addition to the cerebral findings, there were petechial haemorrhages in the lungs and peritoneum.

A coronal section through the brain shows numerous, small petechial haemorrhages scattered throughout the white matter. Note the relative sparing of the grey matter.

Cerebral fat embolism results from the entry of marrow fat into damaged vessels at the site of trauma to a long bone, in the vast majority of cases. While most of this fat is held up in the lungs, some often passes into the systemic circulation. Consequent occlusion of small cerebral vessels results in vascular damage and local haemorrhages, as seen here; these classically lead to coma or delirium. It should be remembered that pituitary fat emboli may induce endocrine dysfunction in those patients who survive.

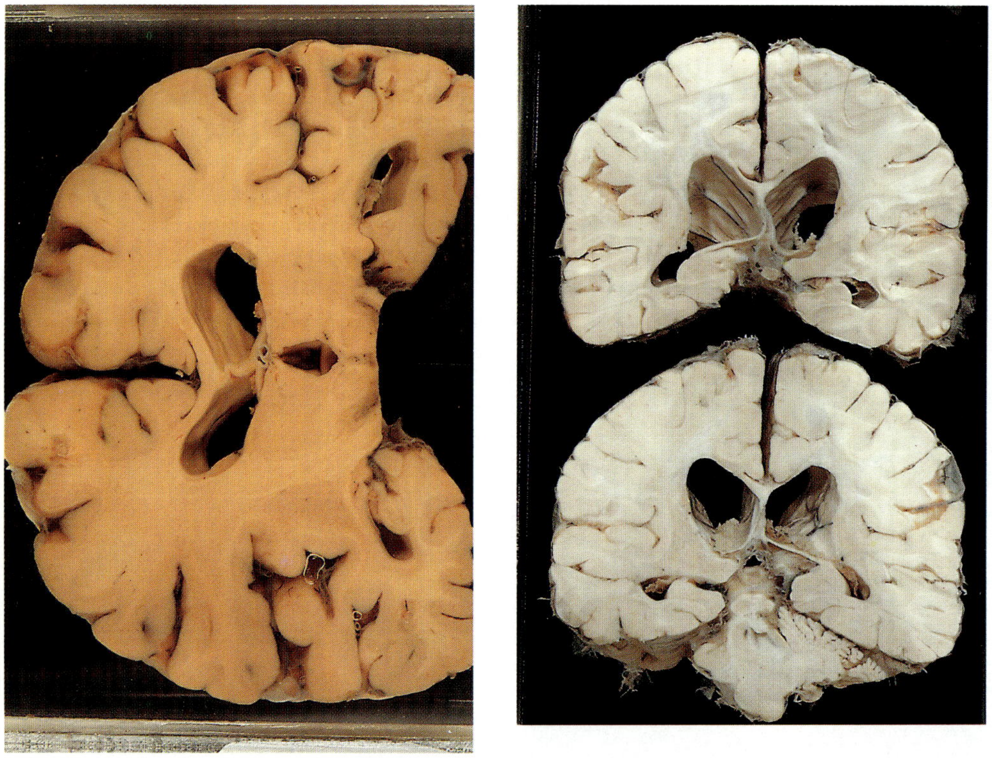

11.43 Multiple Sclerosis

This is a post-mortem specimen from a 44-year-old woman, who had been diagnosed as suffering from multiple sclerosis 8 years previously. Her condition had been gradually deteriorating but she eventually died of endometrial adenocarcinoma.

Coronal sections through the frontal lobes and one cerebral hemisphere (11.43a) show numerous, reasonably defined greyish plaques of demyelination, most obviously seen above the lateral ventricle in the lower section. Two further coronal sections through both cerebral hemispheres (11.43b) show numerous additional greyish lesions, classically situated in the periventricular white matter.

Multiple (synonym: disseminated) sclerosis is a common condition, which typically affects young adults, particularly females. It is a chronic progressive condition, characterised by a remitting and relapsing course, which is due to multifocal demyelination and gliosis. It is commonest in Caucasians, particularly Northern Europeans, and, while the aetiology remains uncertain, a slow or persistent viral infection is thought to be responsible. A small proportion of cases are familial. The neurological symptoms and clinical features are variable but the development of plaques in the mid-brain or loss of excretory sphincter control are often poor prognostic signs.

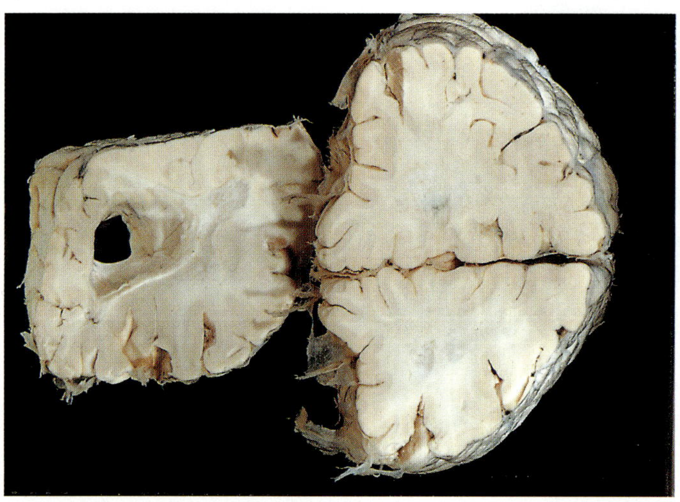

11.44 Idiopathic Senile Dementia

This is a post-mortem specimen from an 82-year-old woman, who had required admission to a psychiatric hospital because of increasing dementia, associated with totally inappropriate behaviour.

The cerebral cortex is atrophied and there is symmetrical dilatation of the ventricles. Note also the shallow sulci. The cerebral arteries showed minimal atheroma and histology revealed the classical features of senile dementia. In persons below 60 years of age these features are to be found in Alzheimer's disease, which is characterised by dementia associated with apraxia, aphasia and epilepsy.

In the elderly, care should be taken to distinguish this condition from dementia due either to senile arteriosclerosis or to multiple infarcts (see Figure and Legend 11.36). The aetiology is unknown but current possible causative agents include a slow viral infection (or other transmissible agent) or chemical toxicity (perhaps due to aluminium). Gradual mental, and then physical deterioration, typically leads to death within 5 years. (Courtesy of St. Thomas's Hospital Medical School Museum).

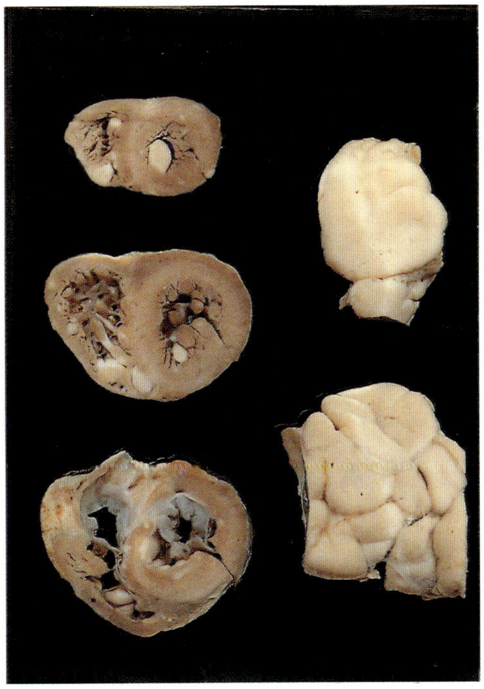

11.45 Brain and Heart: Tuberous Sclerosis

These are post-mortem specimens from a young infant, who was thought to have died of tuberculous meningitis.

On the right, two portions of cerebral cortical tissue show irregular, rounded, rather protuberant areas which, in the fresh state, were palpable as hard lumps. On the left, a series of transverse sections through the heart shows multiple, discrete pale nodules located in the myocardium.

Tuberous sclerosis (synonym: epiloia, Bournville's disease) is an autosomal dominantly inherited condition of variable penetrance which is characterised by the development of multiple hamartomatous lesions in almost any organ system. Patients, who are most often female, typically present with neurological symptoms in childhood, due to the development of cortical and subependymal tubers: these latter are composed of aberrant astrocytes. Other typical findings include various skin lesions, angiomyolipomas or adenomas of the kidney and so-called 'rhabdomyomas' of the heart (as seen in this case, see Chapter 1).

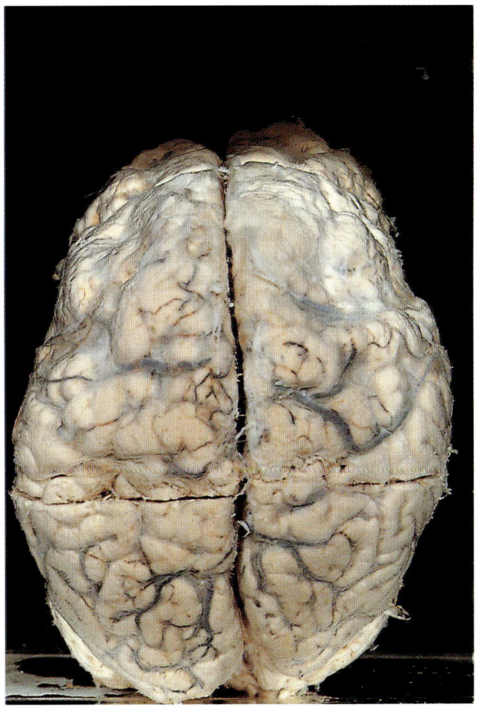

11.46 Cerebral Atrophy

This is a post-mortem specimen from a 72-year-old woman, who died of colonic carcinoma. She had been mentally subnormal and temperamentally volatile for several years, necessitating confinement to a psychiatric hospital.

The brain shows generalised atrophy, which is most marked in the frontal lobes (above). Note the flattened, rather simplified gyral pattern.

It was not possible to ascertain whether the lesion was congenital or acquired in this case, hence the precise nature of the atrophy is uncertain. Generalised (or diffuse) cerebral atrophy reflects gradual neuronal loss and is seen to some extent as part of the ageing process. Important causes of clinically significant atrophy include senile dementia, Alzheimer's disease, severe ischaemia, Pick's disease and some of the encephalitides.

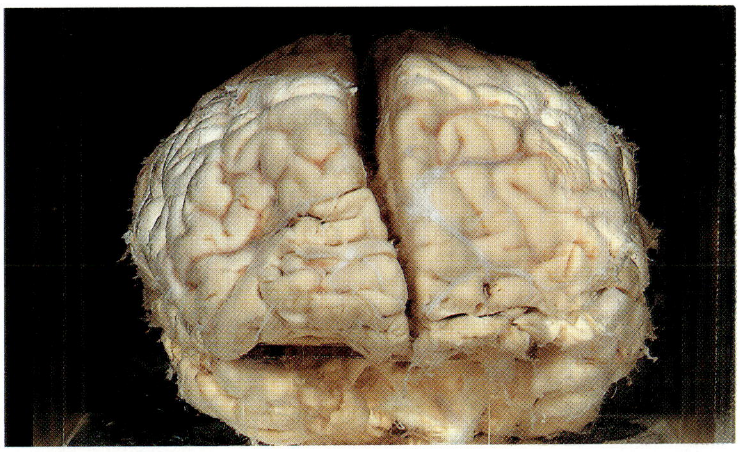

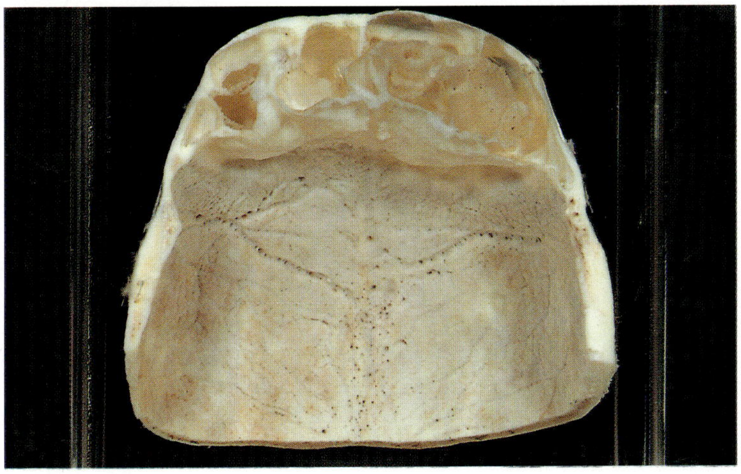

11.47 Pressure Atrophy

This was an incidental finding at post-mortem in a 76-year-old woman who died of a coronary thrombosis. There had been no clinical symptoms attributable to the loss of cerebral tissue.

The anterior portions of the frontal lobes (11.47a) show marked symmetrical atrophy and flattening, which corresponds in distribution to the greatly enlarged and dilated frontal sinuses seen in the calvaria (11.47b).

Chronic localised lesions, located outside the cerebrum but within the skull, commonly give rise to pressure atrophy of the underlying cortex, often with surprisingly few, if any, symptoms. Other good examples include the chronic subdural haematoma and meningioma (Legend 11.8). The appearance of the frontal sinuses in this case may reflect a congenital malformation or perhaps the effects of chronic sinusitis.

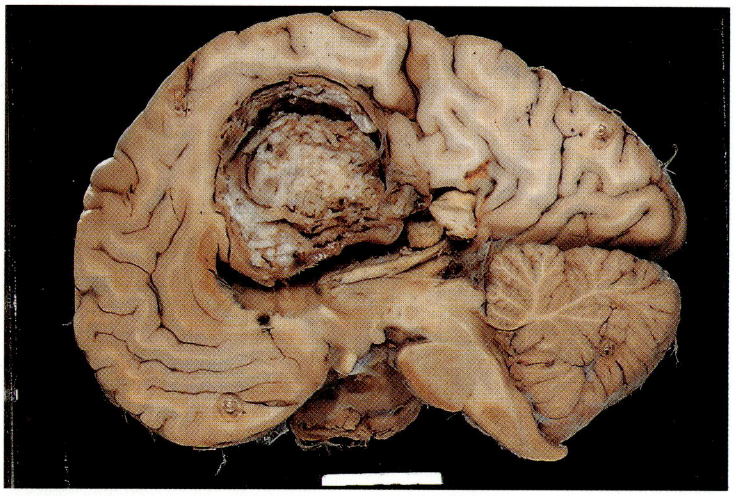

11.48 Epidermoid Cyst

This is a post-mortem specimen from a 27-year-old man, who had collapsed unconscious 2 years previously and on recovering had suffered a transient left hemiparesis. He had 2 further similar attacks over the next 9 months and the hemiparesis became permanent. He developed headaches and failing vision and was found to have a tumour in the left lateral ventricle. This was removed, seemingly completely, but the patient died suddenly on the 7th post-operative day.

The right half of the brain, viewed from the medial aspect, shows a rounded, encapsulated mass, measuring 5cm in diameter, arising in the centre of the hemisphere. The tumour, which is composed of pale, friable material, has replaced much of the corpus callosum and projects into the lateral ventricle. Note the flattened gyral pattern due to raised intracranial pressure.

This case demonstrates well that these histologically innocuous lesions may extend into the cerebral cortex to a significant degree (see Legend 11.13).

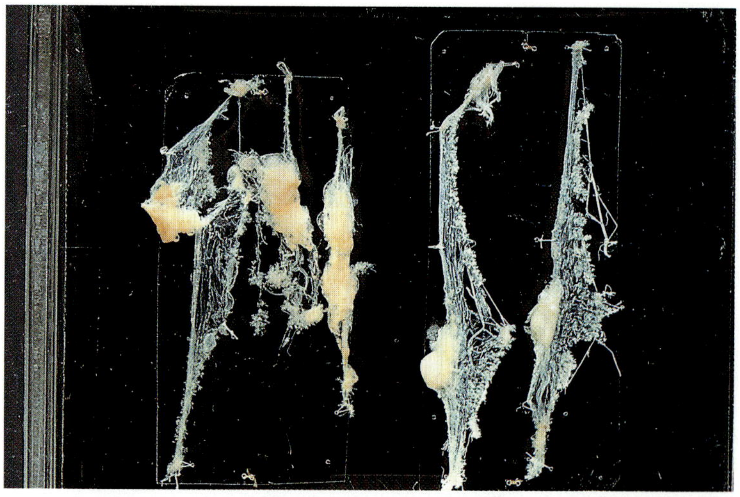

11.49 Choroid Plexus: Xanthogranuloma

No clinical details are available.

Arising in these fragments of choroid plexus are several yellowish, well-circumscribed nodules.

Xanthogranulomas of the choroid plexus are not uncommon incidental findings at post-mortem, being typically seen in the lateral ventricles (often bilaterally). They tend to be small lesions, usually measuring less than 1cm in diameter, and are regarded by most as a reactive (rather than neoplastic) entity which are most often associated with hypercholesterolaemia.

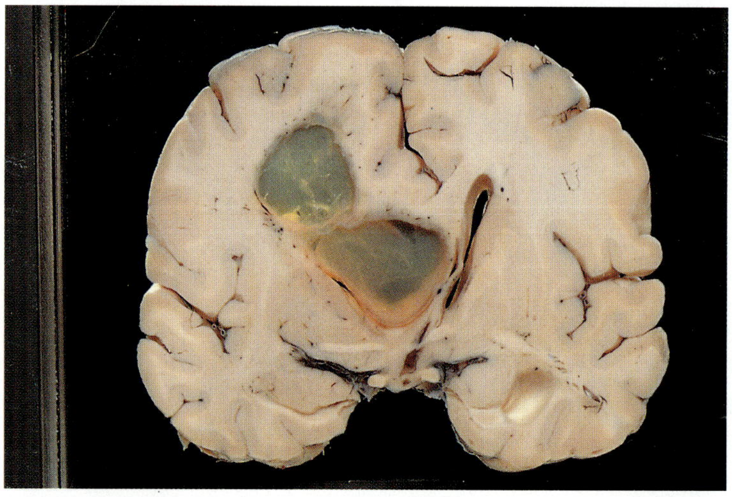

11.50 Cystic Glioma

This is a post-mortem specimen from a 52-year-old man, who had presented 7 weeks previously with severe bitemporal headaches and a tendency to fall to the right. Investigations revealed a left frontal tumour, biopsy of which was interpreted as a glioma of uncertain type. The lesion was aspirated and radiotherapy was given, but the patient died shortly afterwards of bronchopneumonia.

A coronal section through the frontal lobes shows a large, bilocular cystic lesion on the left side. The cyst is filled with greenish, thick material and is lined by a yellowish layer of neoplastic tissue. Note the marked compression and lateral displacement of the lateral ventricles to the right.

Gliomas are the commonest primary intracerebral tumours and are derived from neuroglial cells, hence they may be divided into astrocytomas, oligodendrogliomas, ependymomas, mixed types and choroid plexus papillomas. In general, gliomas are commonest in adulthood and arise most often in the cerebral hemispheres (particularly the frontal lobe). They are all locally invasive and therefore should always be regarded as malignant. However, they do not spread outside the central nervous system, except on very rare occasions following craniotomy. The prognosis is largely dependent upon the tumour's anatomical location, the stage at which it causes symptoms, and its rate of growth.

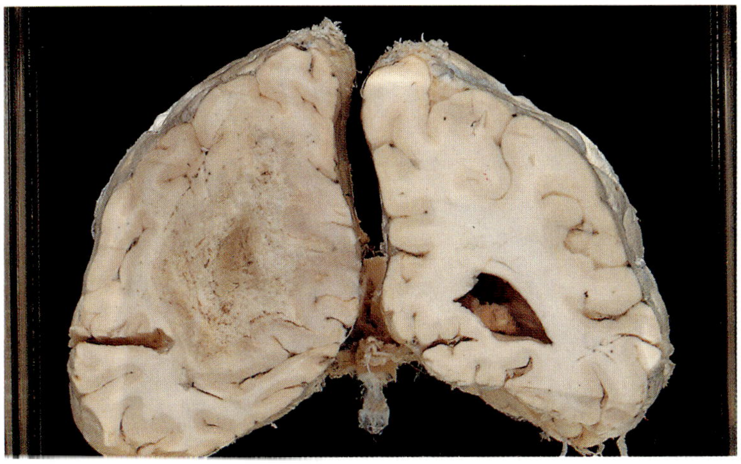

11.51 Glioblastoma Multiforme

This is a post-mortem specimen from a 74-year-old man, who had presented 6 months previously with acute weakness of the right arm. A brain scan suggested a left-sided cerebral tumour and, after a period of progressive right-sided weakness, the patient died.

A coronal section through the parietal lobes shows an ill-defined, large mass, which measures 6cm in maximum diameter, on the left side. The tumour, which shows extensive necrosis, has completely obliterated the left lateral ventricle.

Glioblastoma multiforme is the single commonest type of glioma and represents an anaplastic neoplasm which may be derived from any of the types of neuroglial cell; the designation of Grade III or IV astrocytoma may sometimes therefore be histogenetically inaccurate. This tumour arises most often in middle-aged adults and is typically located in the frontal lobes, basal ganglia or septum pellucidum. It is a rapidly growing lesion and carries a poor prognosis.

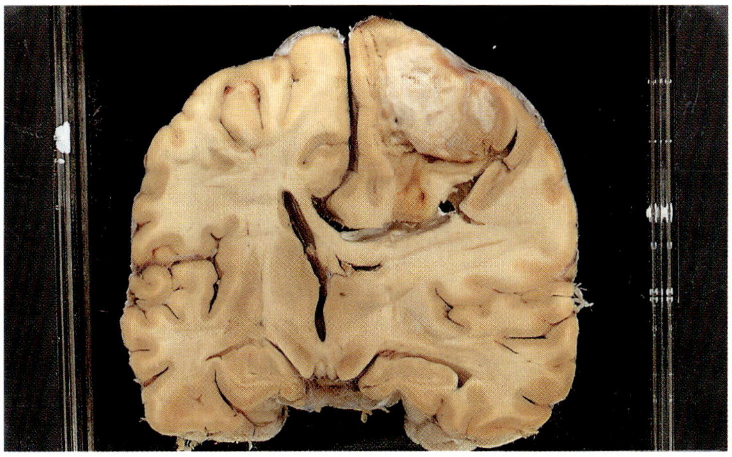

11.52 Grade III Astrocytoma

This is a post-mortem specimen from a 66-year-old man, who had undergone exploratory craniotomy for a cerebral tumour 5 months previously. No further clinical details are available.

A coronal section through the brain at the level of the mammillary bodies shows a pale, largely necrotic neoplasm, which measures 4cm in maximum diameter, situated in the upper part of the right parietal lobe. Note the compression and distortion of the corresponding lateral ventricle.

Astrocytomas are the second commonest type of glioma; while they may present at any age, children and young adults are most often affected and the most frequent sites of origin are the frontal or parietal lobes. They are graded histologically from I to IV, higher grade lesions being poorly differentiated, rapid growing, and carrying the poorest prognosis. In general these tumours behave more aggressively the older the age of the patient.

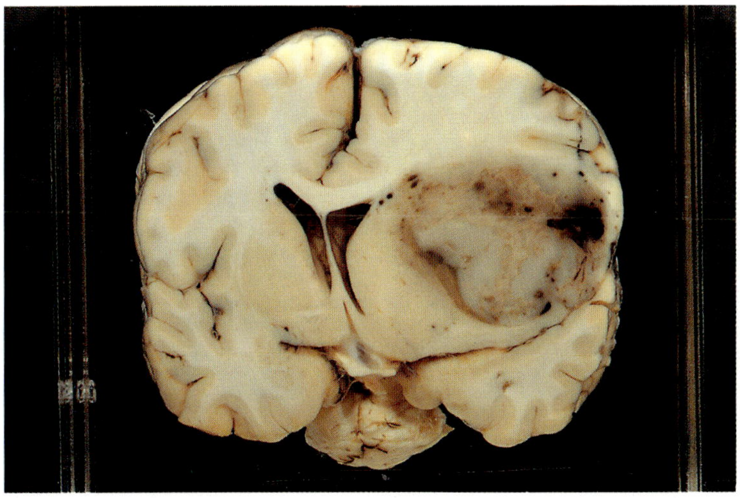

11.53 Grade I Astrocytoma

This is a post-mortem specimen from a 55-year-old man, who had presented one year previously with headaches for which no cause could be found. A fortnight before death he developed signs of increasing intracranial pressure and a left-sided intracerebral lesion. Biopsy through a burrhole revealed an astrocytoma. He died shortly thereafter of bronchopneumonia.

A coronal section through the brain at the level of the optic chiasma shows an ill-defined, haemorrhagic mass, measuring 5cm in diameter, located in the left frontal lobe. Note the marked displacement of mid-line structures to the right and the gyral flattening due to raised intracranial pressure.

This case demonstrates that even histologically well-differentiated gliomas can induce extensive cerebral destruction and pursue a fatal course.

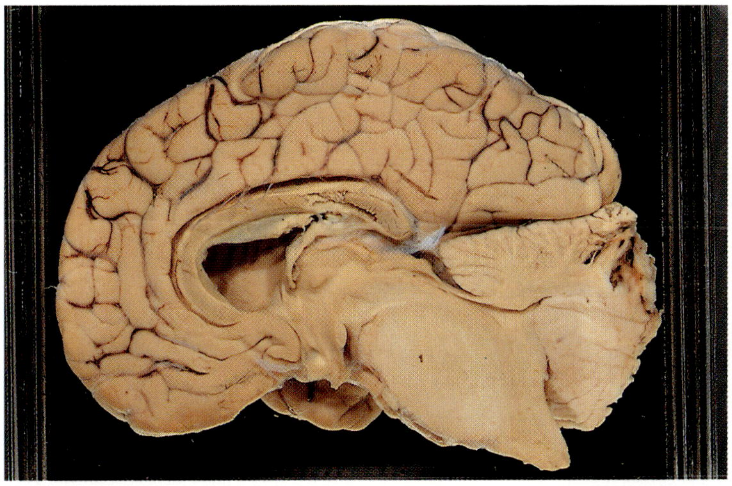

11.54 Grade I Fibrillary Astrocytoma

This is a post-mortem specimen from a 9-year-old boy, who presented with headaches and an unsteady gait. Air encephalography revealed a tumour in the posterior fossa. Following biopsy, radiotherapy was given but 6 months later he returned with nausea, headache, diplopia and dysarthria; soon after, he died.

The right half of the brain, viewed from the medial aspect, shows an ovoid, pale neoplasm, measuring 4.5cm in maximum diameter, located within the pons and extending into the cerebellum. The term fibrillary denotes a common histological variant of astrocytoma which by producing copious astroglial fibrils, tends to adopt a pale, firm appearance. Astrocytomas in childhood, while less common, frequently arise in the brainstem, around the 3rd ventricle or in the optic nerve. These tumours have a rather better prognosis in children than in adults.

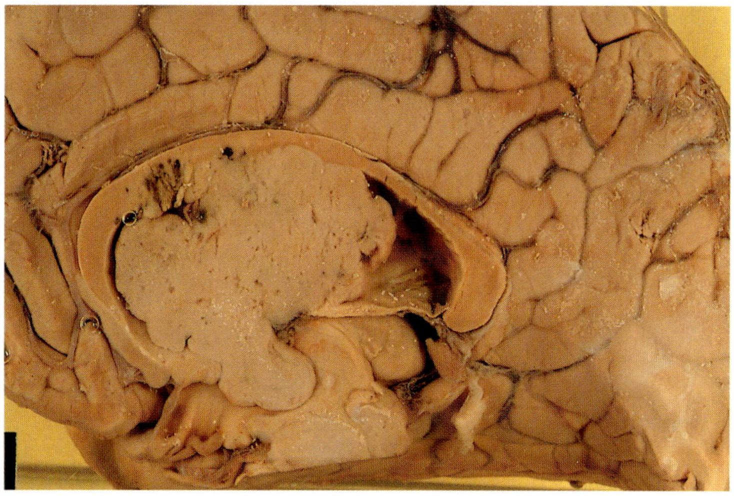

11.55 Oligodendroglioma

This is a post-mortem specimen from a 43-year-old man who presented with a 6 month history of gradually deteriorating vision and periodic loss of consciousness. A skull X-ray revealed almost complete destruction of the sella turcica and at craniotomy, an inoperable tumour was found and biopsied. The patient died soon afterward.

The right cerebral hemisphere, viewed from the midline, shows a large infiltrative mass which has extended to fill much of the 3rd ventricle.

Oligodendrogliomas are relatively uncommon tumours, which typically present in middle age and most often arise in the frontal lobes. These lesions tend to be fairly slow growing, often retaining a reasonable circumscribed appearance, and frequently undergo dystrophic calcification. (Courtesy of St. Thomas's Hospital Medical School Museum)

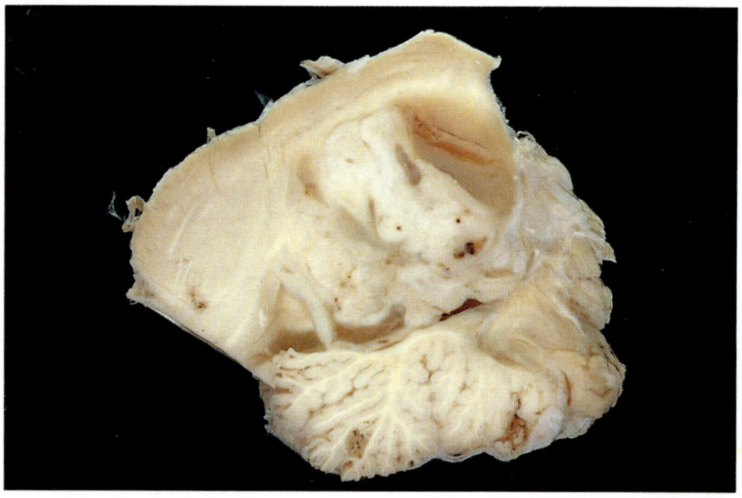

11.56 Ependymoma

This is a post-mortem specimen from a 38-year-old man, who had first presented 17 years previously complaining of occipital headaches and vomiting. Examination revealed papilloedema and nystagmus. At that time, an ependymoma was removed from the floor of the 4th ventricle and radiotherapy was given. Six years later he developed vomiting and blurred vision; no recurrent tumour was found and ventriculocisternostomy was performed to relieve fibrous obstruction of the foramen of Magendie. He later died of bronchopneumonia.

A sagittal section through the brainstem and cerebellum shows a pale, cystic tumour, measuring 4cm in diameter, distending the lower part of the 4th ventricle and infiltrating the superior surface of the medulla.

Ependymomas are an uncommon type of glioma but are the most frequent to arise primarily in the spinal cord (see Figure and Legend 11.67). They typically present in young adults and are, overall, most often seen in the 4th ventricle, although they may develop from the ventricular lining at any site. Classically they are slowly growing tumours (as demonstrated by the long history in this case), but their anatomical location, by rendering surgery difficult, often confers a poor prognosis.

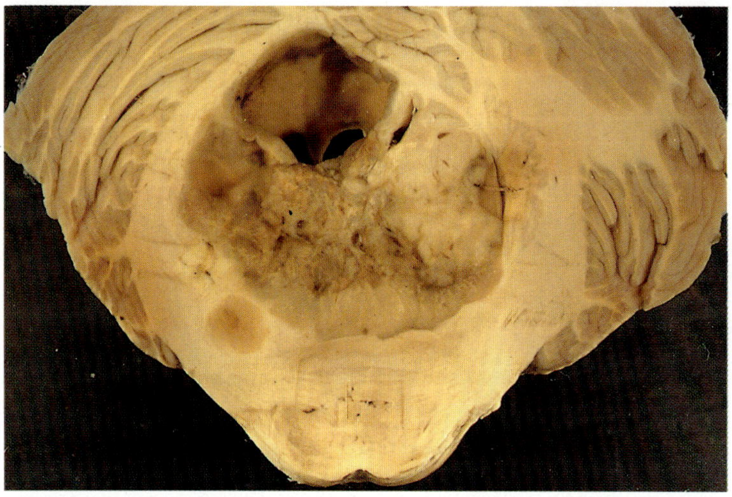

11.57 Cerebellar Medulloblastoma

This is a post-mortem specimen from a 12-year-old girl, who presented with increasingly severe headaches associated with vomiting. Examination revealed bilateral papilloedema, nystagmus and cerebellar signs in the limbs. A subtentorial decompression was performed leading to temporary improvement, but she died some weeks later.

In the centre of the cerebellum, apparently arising from the vermis, is a reasonably circumscribed pale tumour showing focal necrosis. The cavity of the 4th ventricle was completely obliterated in the fresh state.

Medulloblastoma is the commonest primary neuronal neoplasm to arise in the brain, but is nevertheless rare. This tumour, which most often arises in the cerebellum, typically presents in the 1st decade of life and affects males more than females. It is a rapidly growing, primitive neoplasm which, in the past, carried a very poor prognosis. However, modern radiotherapeutic techniques now achieve a significant cure rate. (Courtesy of St. Thomas's Hospital Medical School Museum)

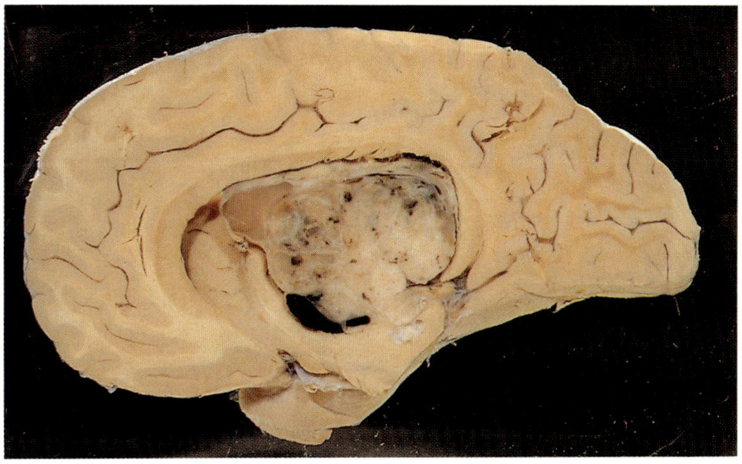

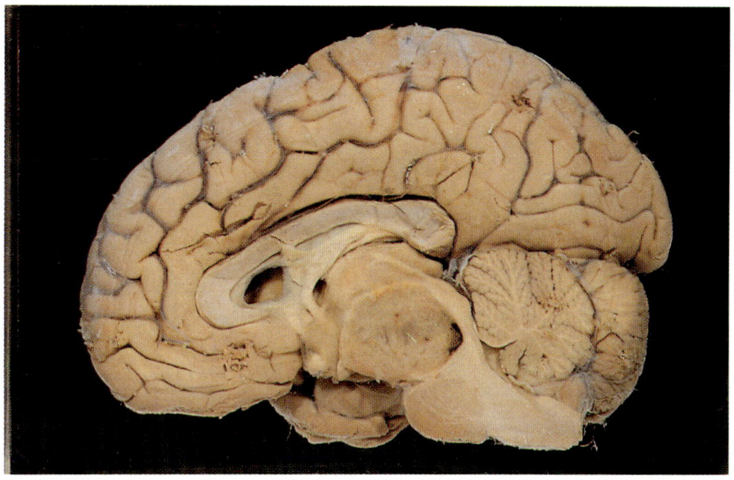

11.58 Teratoma of the Pineal Gland

This is a post-mortem specimen from a 26-year-old Italian man, who presented with a short history of frontal headache, vomiting, diplopia and dizziness. He developed weakness of the left-sided limbs, hemianopia and papilloedema. Ventriculography showed a tumour partly filling the right lateral ventricle and an exploratory craniotomy was performed. He died soon afterwards.

The right half of the brain, viewed from the medial aspect, shows a rounded tumour in the region of the mid-brain, measuring 6cm in maximum diameter. The neoplasm has extended forwards and superiorly to obliterate the 3rd ventricle and much of the right lateral ventricle. The cut surface has a variegated appearance, being focally solid, cystic and haemorrhagic.

Teratomas may arise from any mid-line body structure and the vast majority of such lesions, when located intracranially, develop in the region of the pineal gland. At this site adolescents and young adults, the vast majority of whom are male, are typically affected. This rare tumour often behaves in a very malignant fashion, showing extensive local invasion and often dissemination throughout the ventricular and meningeal systems.

11.59 Metastatic Breast Carcinoma

This is a post-mortem specimen from an adult woman, who had undergone a left mastectomy for adenocarcinoma of the breast 2 years previously. Five months before death, she developed intermittent diplopia and a tendency to fall towards her left side. Terminally she was unable to walk, through loss of balance, and suffered from persistent vomiting.

The right half of the brain, viewed from the medial aspect, shows a rounded, rather myxoid mass, measuring 3.5cm in diameter, situated in the mid-brain and interpeduncular fossa. This deposit of secondary tumour has displaced the thalamus upwards.

Metastatic deposits from malignant tumours elsewhere in the body are the commonest type of cerebral neoplasm, outnumbering primary intracranial lesions by about 100 to 1. The most frequent primary source is carcinoma of the bronchus but other tumours that show a particular tendency to spread to the brain are carcinomas of the breast, kidney, large bowel and cutaneous malignant melanoma.

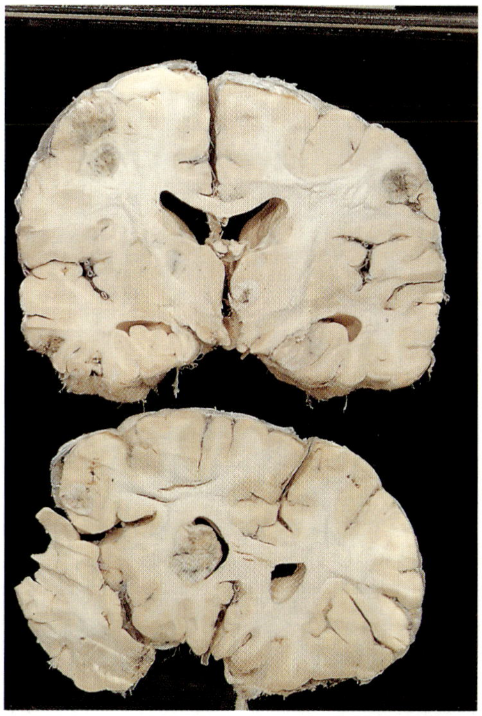

11.60 Metastatic Bronchial Carcinoma

This is a post-mortem specimen from a 64-year-old woman, who presented with symptoms of thyrotoxicosis, which was confirmed by thyroid function tests. Despite radioactive iodine and carbimazole treatment, her condition did not improve and she developed supraclavicular lymphadenopathy. Biopsy revealed metastatic carcinoma, compatible with a bronchial origin. She was admitted terminally with a right hemiparesis and died soon afterwards. At autopsy, there was an oat cell carcinoma of the right upper lobe bronchus which had metastasised to lymph nodes, the left adrenal gland, the pancreas and brain. The thyroid showed features compatible with radioactive iodine therapy with no histological evidence to explain the patient's thyrotoxicosis.

Two coronal sections through the cerebral hemispheres show multiple, discrete metastases, which are greyish in colour and measure up to 2cm in diameter.

This case shows the typical features of cerebral metastases. The lesions are most often multiple, are typically located at the junction of the white and grey matter, and tend to be sharply demarcated from the adjacent cerebral tissue (in contrast to gliomas). It would appear that this patient's bronchial carcinoma was ectopically secreting either thyroid stimulating hormone or thyroxine, a well-recognised paraneoplastic phenomenon (see Chapter 2).

SPINAL CORD

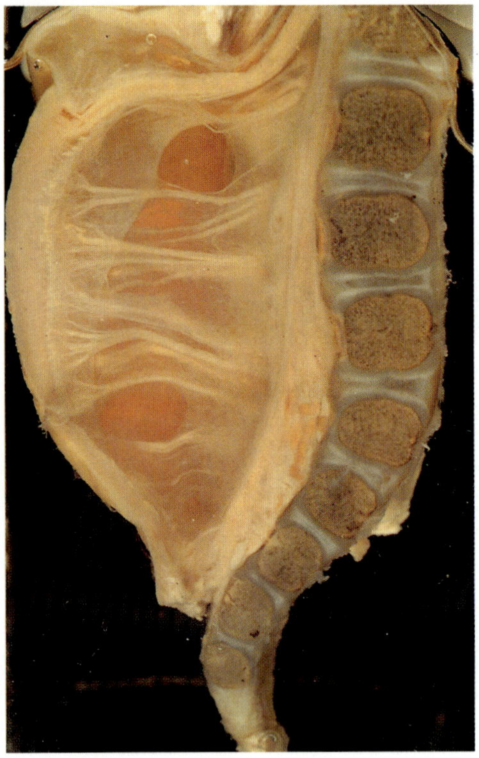

11.61 Meningomyelocele

No clinical details are available.

A sagittal section through the lumbar region of the vertebral column shows a large cystic structure posteriorly, composed of the cord and meninges which have herniated through the incomplete vertebral arches. Spinal nerves can be seen coursing over the surface.

Meningomyelocele represents the commonest form of spina bifida, a condition characterised by a variable degree of failed fusion between the neural tube and plate *in utero* which is then associated with an adjacent bony malformation. This variant often coexists with the Arnold-Chiari malformation (see Figure and Legend 11.18 et seq.). Social and dietary factors, in particular folate deficiency during pregnancy, are thought to be aetiologically important. The neurological consequences depend upon the level and extent of cord involvement and there is a significant risk of developing meningitis. (Courtesy of St. Thomas's Hospital Medical School Museum)

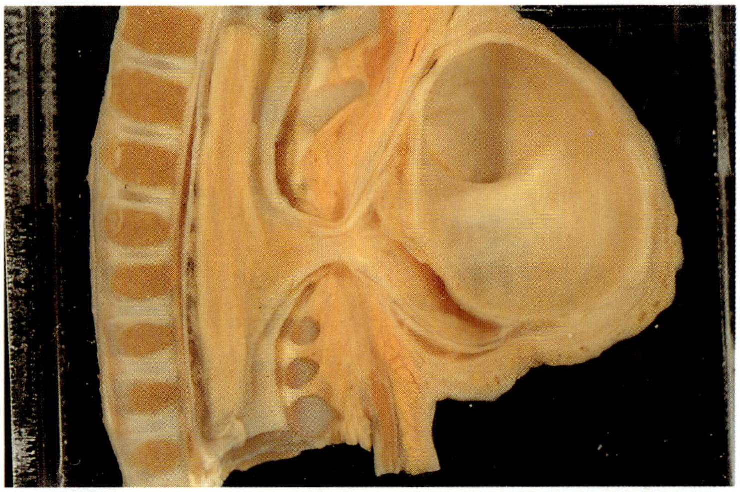

11.62 Meningocele

No clinical details are available.

A sagittal section through the lower thoracic and lumbar vertebral spine shows a well-formed spinal cord, over which a sac composed solely of meningeal tissue protrudes posteriorly through the incomplete vertebral arches.

A meningocele represents a less severe and clinically more treatable form of spina bifida than the preceding meningomyelocele. An even less serious form is spina bifida occulta, in which the cord and its meninges are normal but there is a defect in the vertebral arches, often associated with an overlying hairy or pigmented cutaneous naevus. (Courtesy of St. Thomas's Hospital Medical School Museum)

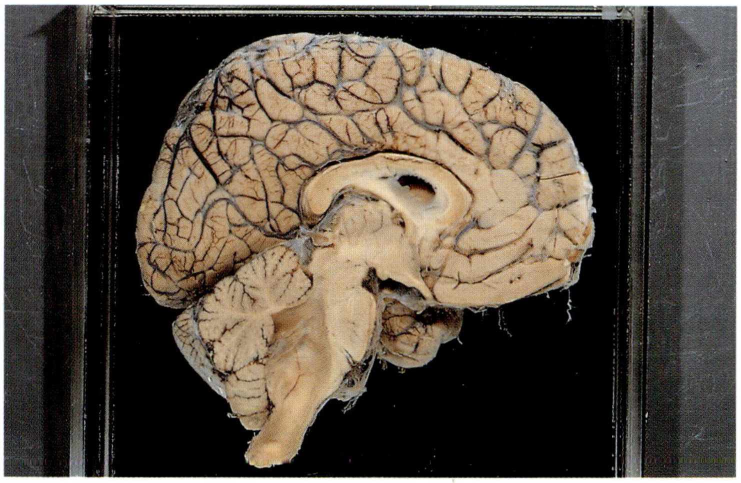

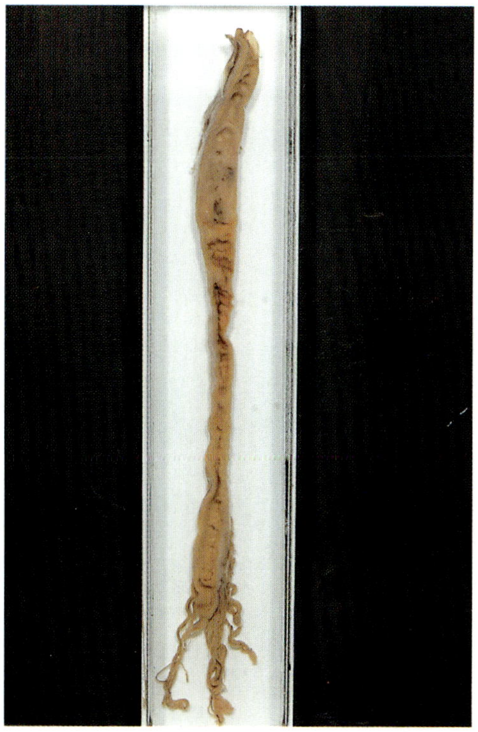

11.63 Brain and Spinal Cord: Hydromyelia with Astrocytoma

These are post-mortem specimens from a 7-year-old boy who had been noted to have a persistent stiff neck and who had developed a thoracic scoliosis at the age of 5. Four months before death, he developed weakness of the right arm which was followed by dysphagia and quadriplegia. An inoperable tumour of the spinal cord was detected and the patient died soon afterwards.

The left half of the brain (11.63a), viewed from the medial aspect, shows a central cavity in the brainstem separated from the 4th ventricle by a thin membrane. The medulla shows severe attenuation. A longitudinal section through the spinal cord (11.63b) shows dilatation of the central canal along its entire length, except in the mid-cervical segment where a pale tumour mass has obliterated the cavity and expanded the cord.

Hydromyelia, which is defined as dilatation of the central spinal canal, is an uncommon congenital malformation which may be seen in isolation or, more often, is associated with the Arnold-Chiari malformation (see Legend 11.18 et seq.). This anomaly, which is frequently most marked in the lumbar region, may give rise to surprisingly few symptoms. The coexistence of an astrocytoma, which was responsible for this patient's death, is not thought to be developmentally associated.

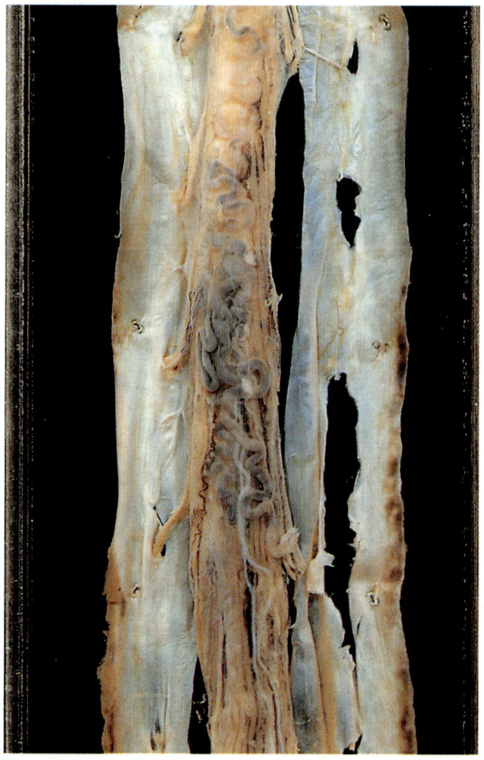

11.64 Plexiform Vascular Malformation

This is a post-mortem specimen from a 49-year-old man, who presented with a 9 month history of progressive weakness and numbness of the legs. Latterly he developed difficulty with micturition and the legs became paralysed. Myelography suggested a diffuse lesion extending from the 10th thoracic to the 1st lumbar segments which, at laminectomy, was found to be a diffuse vascular lesion. The patient died of a cerebral embolus on the 5th post-operative day.

A close-up view of the lower thoracic and upper lumbar portion of the cord, with the dura opened from behind, shows an extensive plexiform vascular abnormality, composed largely of tortuous vessels.

Vascular hamartomas (haemangiomas) of the cord are most often seen in the leptomeninges and may sometimes be associated with a cutaneous haemangioma in the corresponding dermatome (Cobb's syndrome). Occasionally such lesions may also coexist with underlying syringomyelia. The principal complications include thrombosis and intraspinal haemorrhage.

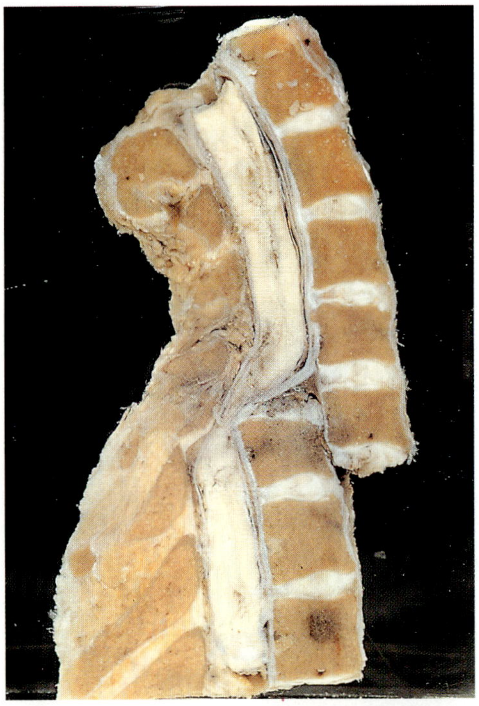

11.65 Transection due to Fracture Dislocation

This is a post-mortem specimen from a male adult who, following a fall from a hay cart, suffered complete paralysis of the trunk and legs. Breathing was purely diaphragmatic and he was unable to swallow. He gradually developed respiratory failure and died 16 days after the accident.

A sagittal section through the lower 6 cervical and upper 2 thoracic vertebrae shows an anterior fracture dislocation at the level of the disc between C6 and C7. The body of C7 has been forced upwards into the spinal canal and, at this point, the spinal cord is completely severed.

Fracture-dislocation of the vertebral column, leading to cord transection, most often follows a severe spinal flexion injury. Sudden or forcible flexion of the head gives rise to a similar injury in the upper cervical region (usually at the level of C2). Vertebral collapse, of whatever cause, may cause cord compression but very rarely leads to transection.

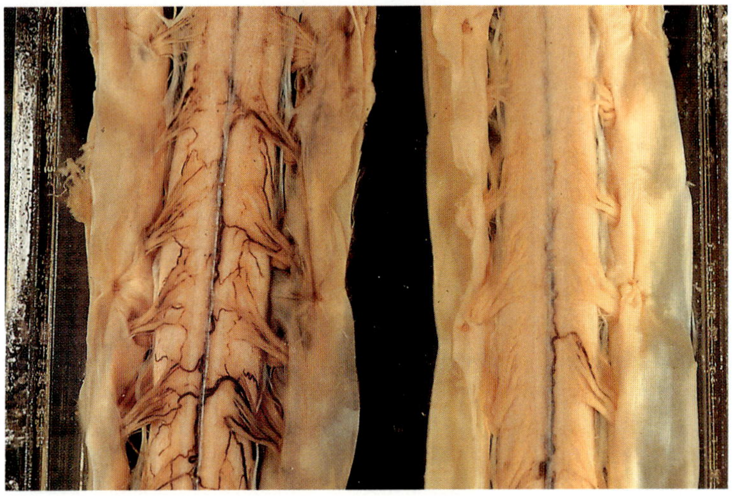

11.66 Motor Neuron Disease

This is a post-mortem specimen from a 53-year-old man known to suffer from motor neuron disease, who died of bronchial carcinomatosis.

The affected patient's cord is mounted on the left, and a normal control for comparison on the right. Note the relative wasting and atrophy of the anterior spinal roots on the left.

Motor neuron disease is a not uncommon degenerative disorder of both the upper and lower motor neurons which typically presents in late adulthood. It may take one of three forms; amyotrophic lateral sclerosis, progressive muscular atrophy and bulbar palsy. Clinical symptoms are dependent upon the type, but in general the prognosis is very poor. A very similar condition may be seen in association with a visceral carcinoma (particularly bronchial) and it is not certain if that was the cause in this case. (Courtesy of St. Thomas's Hospital Medical School Museum)

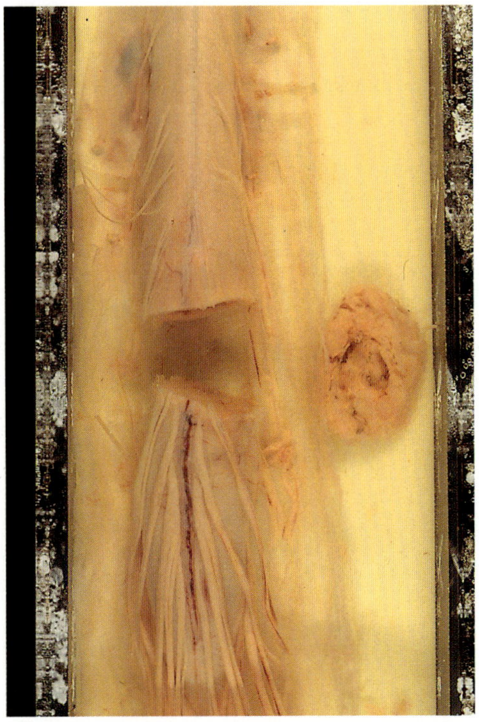

11.67 Ependymoma

This is a post-mortem specimen from a l-year-old boy, who had been noticed to have a lumbar scoliosis since the age of 8 months. He became constipated and developed a flaccid paresis of the lower limbs with complete loss of sensation below the 9th thoracic dermatome.

This lumbosacral segment of the spinal cord is markedly expanded and the segment seen in cross-section shows virtual replacement by brownish, necrotic tumour. The adjacent anterior spinal roots appear atrophic.

As already stated (see Legend 11.56), ependymomas are the commonest glioma to arise in the spinal cord, most often being located in the lumbosacral region or filum terminale. There is frequently an associated syringomyelia. (Courtesy of St. Thomas's Hospital Medical School Museum)

EYES AND EARS

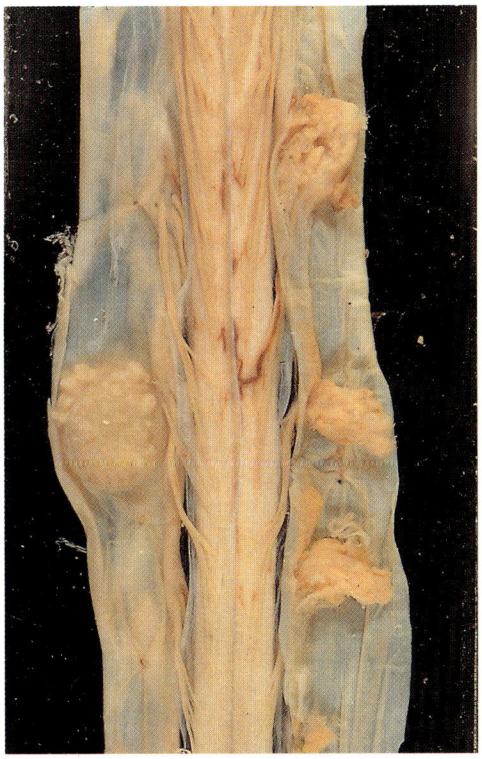

11.68 Meningioma

This is a post-mortem specimen from an adult male, who presented with a 4 month history of involuntary flexion spasm of the legs. He gradually developed a fixed flexion deformity of the lower limbs and examination revealed spastic rigidity and bilateral extensor plantar reflexes.

Adherent to the dura, adjacent to this segment of the lumbar cord, is a well circumscribed, lobulated and focally calcified tumour, measuring 1.5cm in maximum diameter.

Meningiomas arising from the spinal dura are much less common than their intracranial equivalent (see Legend 11.8 et seq.) but are seen most frequently in the thoracic region. (Courtesy of St. Thomas's Hospital Medical School Museum)

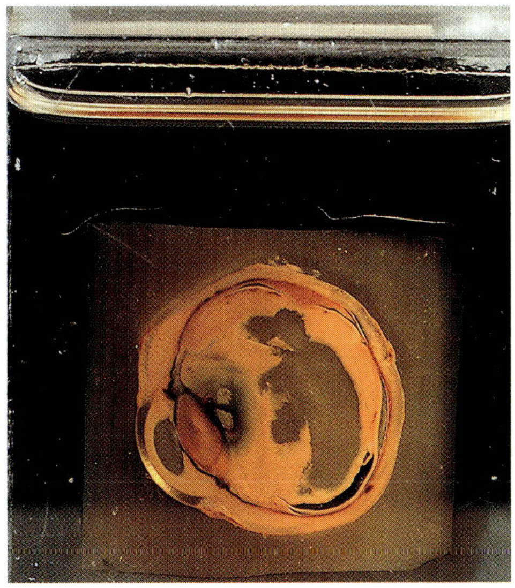

11.69 Eye: Siderosis Bulbi

This specimen was enucleated from a 9-year-old boy, whose eye became red and painful following a perforating corneal wound.

A coronal section through the whole eye shows inflammatory exudate filling the vitreous chamber, forming a layer beneath the retina and filling the angles of the anterior chamber. The lens is opaque and a fragment of steel (the source of the injury) was found in the space immediately behind it. The specimen has been stained for iron by the Prussian blue method and migration of iron particles from the site of injury into the surrounding tissues is clearly shown by the blue staining.

Siderosis bulbi is a well-recognised complication of penetrating eye injuries in which iron-containing foreign material is retained in the ocular tissues; such an event is usually an occupational hazard. The deposition of iron salts, derived from gradual dissolution of the embedded material, leads to extensive tissue damage and complications include lens opacity and atrophy of the retina, ciliary body or lens epithelium.

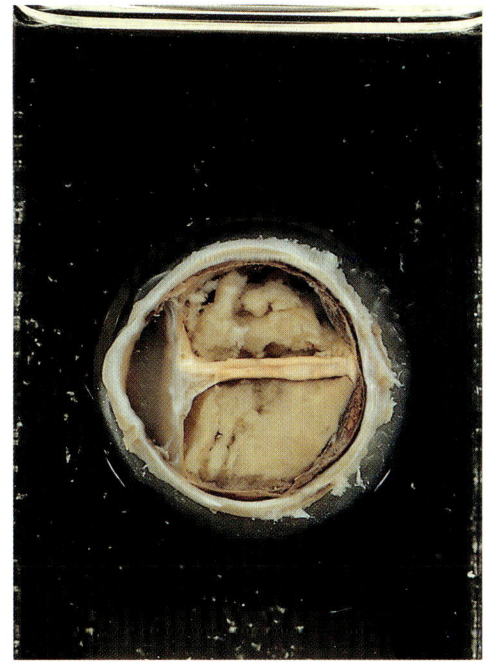

11.70 Eye: Ossification of the Choroid

This specimen was enucleated from a patient who had suffered from long-standing ophthalmitis due to diffuse corneal ulceration.

A section through the eye shows that the iris is adherent to the densely scarred cornea and the totally detached retina is similarly adherent to the lens, which has been replaced by inflammatory tissue. The post-retinal space is filled by a mass of purulent exudate and the posterior part of the choroid has undergone complete dystrophic ossification.

Panophthalmitis of this extent usually follows suppurative bacterial or viral infection of the uveal tract, often as a result of a penetrating injury. Infection may also be blood-borne from elsewhere. While perforation of the globe commonly results, dystrophic calcification and ossification of the inflamed, degenerate or necrotic tissues is a well-recognised phenomenon (as at other sites in the body).

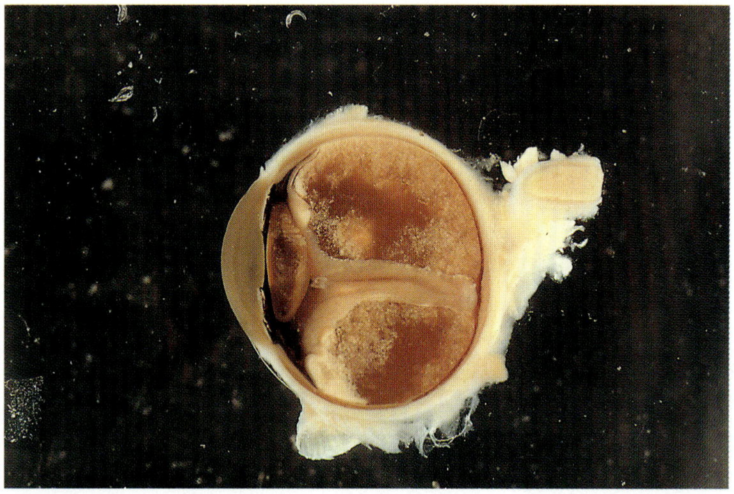

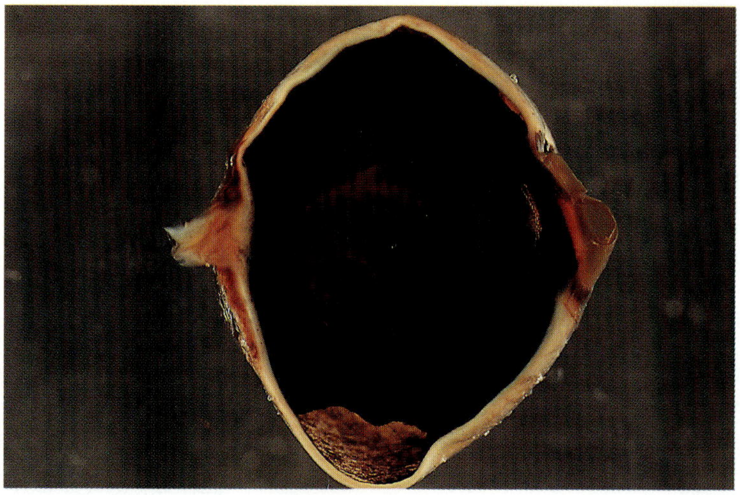

11.71 Eye: Retinal Detachment due to Coat's disease

This specimen was enucleated from a 5-year-old child, who was thought to have a retinoblastoma. No further clinical details are available.

The eye had been bisected to show complete detachment of the retina, except at the optic disc (centre right). Beneath the retina, there is a mass of loose organised exudate containing cholesterol crystals.

Retinal detachment which is not uncommon is, in fact, usually characterised by an *intraretinal* split between the pigment cell and neural layers. The commonest causes include subretinal haemorrhage, infection, a neoplasm, a traumatic tear leading to the passage of vitreous beneath the retina, or traction of vitreous fibrous scars that have resulted from previous infection or haemorrhage. If left untreated, the retina becomes ischaemic and undergoes atrophy. Coat's disease is an uncommon idiopathic condition typically seen in young people, which is characterised by a unilateral haemorrhagic exudate in the outer layers of the retina, which later becomes organised. Retinal detachment is almost invariable. (Courtesy of St. Thomas's Hospital Medical School Museum)

11.72 Eye: Subretinal Haemorrhage

No clinical details are available.

The retina of this eye is completely elevated by a mass of partially organised blood clot. The cornea has been removed for grafting purposes.

Subretinal haemorrhage (to be distinguished from the retinal haemorrhages of essential hypertension or diabetes mellitus) may be traumatic in origin, secondary to a coagulopathy, or a complication of retinal angiomatosis. (Courtesy of St. Thomas's Hospital Medical School Museum)

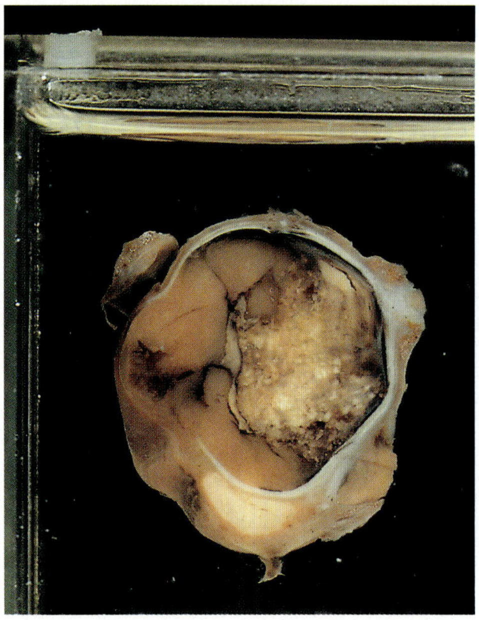

11.73 Eye: Retinoblastoma

This specimen was enucleated from a 7-year-old African boy from Malawi, who had presented with progressive proptosis of the left eye.

The eye has been bisected to show a greyish-white, irregularly calcified neoplasm which has distorted and replaced much of both the anterior and posterior segments.

Retinoblastoma is an uncommon embryonal tumour of the retina which typically arises in the first 2 years of life. While this neoplasm is usually sporadic, a proportion of cases show autosomal dominant inheritance. Multifocal origin is common and bilateral tumours develop in between 25-30 per cent of cases; extensive necrosis and calcification are common features. While in the past this lesion was regarded as highly aggressive, modern surgical and radiotherapeutic techniques now achieve up to a 90 per cent cure rate.

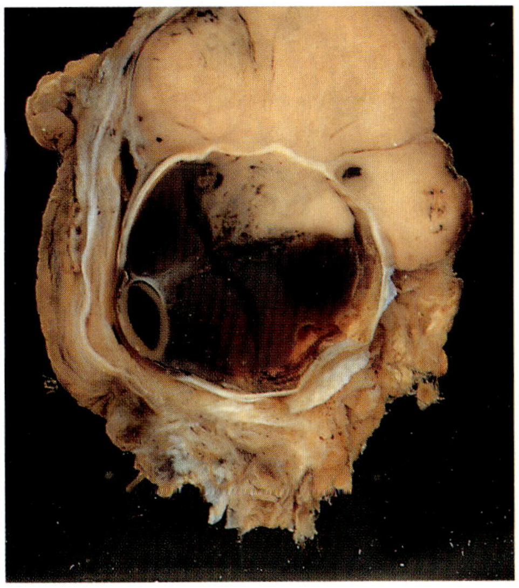

11.74 Eye: Malignant Melanoma of the Choroid

This specimen was enucleated from a 48-year-old man, who presented with gradual blurring of his vision and recent right-sided proptosis with a blood-stained discharge. Examination revealed anterior and infero-lateral displacement of the eye, which was fixed in the orbit, and there was secondary conjunctival inflammation. The contents of the orbit were radically excised.

A coronal section through the orbital contents shows a large primary choroidal tumour, situated postero-medially to the globe. Note that the neoplasm shows only focal pigmentation and that there has been extensive penetration of the sclera and extra-ocular spread.

Ocular malignant melanoma is an uncommon neoplasm which arises from the choroid in the majority of cases. Patients of either sex in late adulthood are typically affected. These lesions commonly show extensive local invasion, tending to spread in the subretinal region, within the globe and extra-ocularly. Metastatic dissemination to other parts of the body, particularly the liver, occurs by the bloodstream and is an extremely variable event in these tumours. It is a well-recognised, almost characteristic, feature that metastases may present up to 20 years after excision of the primary lesion. Note that penetration of Bruch's membrane (the choroidal basement membrane) by these lesions, which allows extension beneath the retina, often gives the neoplasm a 'collar-stud' appearance. Histologically, the spindle cell variant of ocular melanoma carries a better prognosis than the epitheloid type.

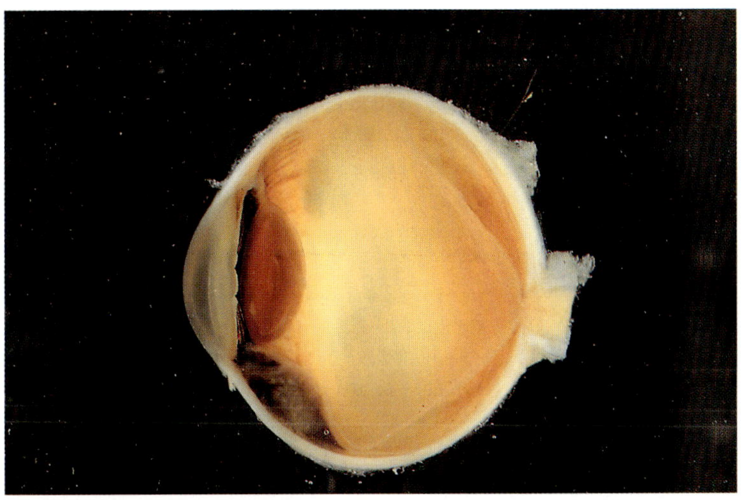

11.75 Eye: Malignant Melanoma of the Ciliary Body

No clinical details are available.

The eye has been bisected to show a small pigmented neoplasm arising in the region of the ciliary body and projecting into the posterior segment.

Up to 10 per cent of ocular malignant melanomas arise from the ciliary body. The prognosis is much the same as for choroidal tumours. (Courtesy of St. Thomas's Hospital Medical School Museum)

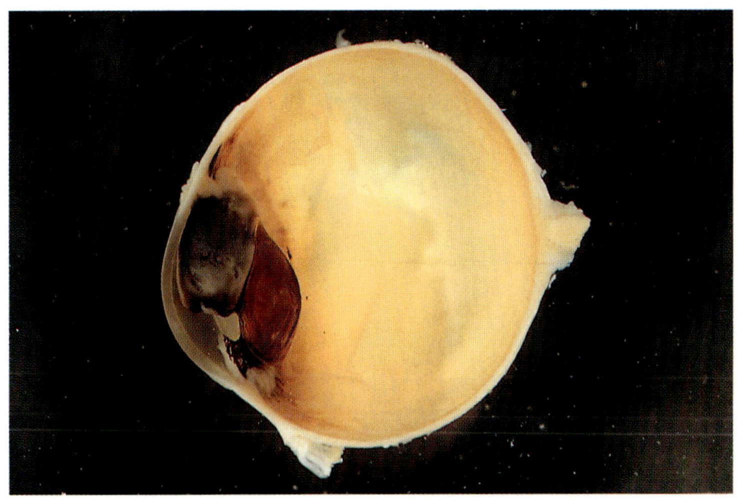

11.76 Eye: Malignant Melanoma of the Iris

No clinical details are available.

This eye has been bisected in the sagittal plane to show a rounded, pigmented tumour arising from the iris and projecting into the anterior chamber superiorly.

Approximately 5 per cent of ocular malignant melanomas arise from the iris. Typically they are seen on the anterior surface (as here) and in general the prognosis is extremely good. (Courtesy of St. Thomas's Hospital Medical School Museum)

INDEX

U

V

W

X

Z